THE WORDSWORTH DICTIONARY OF
PRESCRIPTION MEDICINES

THE WORDSWORTH DICTIONARY OF

PRESCRIPTION MEDICINES

*Compiled and edited by the Staff of
MedicaPress International, Inc. and MedicaPress,
AG., The National Encyclopedia, Inc.*

WORDSWORTH EDITIONS

First published in Great Britain 1999
by Wordsworth Editions Limited
Cumberland House, Crib Street, Ware, Herts SG12 9ET

Copyright this edition: © Wordsworth Editions 1999

Text copyright © MedicaPress Int., Inc.

This edition published 1999
by Wordsworth Editions Limited
Cumberland House, Crib Street, Ware,
Hertfordshire SG12 9ET

ISBN 1 84022 022 8

Wordsworth® is a registered trade mark of
Wordsworth Editions Limited

Printed and bound in Great Britain
by Mackays of Chatham plc, Chatham, Kent.

THE WORDSWORTH
DICTIONARY OF PRESCRIPTION MEDICINES

The *Dictionary of Prescription Medicines* gives you the information you need to take an active part in your own health care and help protect your family's health.

The Dictionary has been prepared by a committee of authors, consultants and editors and represents the committee's understanding of following important aspects of common medicines: chemical structure and function, indications, contra-indications, side effects, adverse reactions, use during pregnancy and lactation, etc.

The Dictionary has been reviewed by the committee at the latest possible date before publication to ensure that the information and advice given in the book is up to date.

The series of encyclopedias has been designed as a clear and comprehensive library for the lay public of information about medical, psychological and dental matters and also covers the field of healthy living with encyclopedias on Non-Prescription Medicines, Fitness Programmes, Healthy Food, Natural Medicine, Family First Aid, Women's Health and Children's Health etc.

COLLABORATING INSTITUTIONS

National Institutes of Health, USA
National Cancer Institute, USA
Department of Medicine, University of New York
Department of Pathology, University of San Francisco
Medical Library Foundation, Switzerland
Faculty of Medicine, Free University, Brussels
Faculty of Medicine, University of Utrecht

NOTE

In this *Wordsworth Dictionary of Prescription Medicines*, the authors and editors have done their best to outline the general characteristics of common prescription medicines. Also, recommendations are made regarding medications, and preparations; and descriptions of side effects and adverse reactions of medicines are offered.

Different people react to the same treatment, medication, preparation, test, or procedures in different ways. This dictionary does not attempt to answer all the questions about every situation that you may encounter in taking medicines.

Neither the editors of the *Wordsworth Dictionary of Prescription Medicines*, nor the consultants, authors, or publisher take responsibility for any possible consequences from any treatment, procedure, test, action, or application of medication or preparation by any person reading or following the information in this dictionary. The publication of this dictionary does not constitute the practice of medicine, and this book does not attempt to replace your physician. The authors, editors and publisher advise the reader to check with a physician before administering any medication or undertaking any course of teatment.

THE WORDSWORTH
DICTIONARY OF
PRESCRIPTION MEDICINES

I   General aspects

1. INTRODUCTION

A drug is a substance used as medicine in the treatment of disease, or a mood-altering substance, especially one that is addictive.

Drugs are chemical agents that affect the systems of the body. In general they are taken to treat or prevent disease, but certain drugs, such as the opium narcotics, amphetamines, barbiturates and hallucinogens, are taken for their psychological effects and are drugs of addiction or abuse.

Many drugs are the same as or similar to chemicals occurring naturally in the body and are used either to replace the natural substance (for instance, thyroid hormone) when deficient, or to induce effects that occur when these is an abnormal concentration of the substance, such as with steroids or oral contraceptives.

Other agents are known to interfere with a specific mechanism or to antagonize a normal process. Many other drugs are obtained from other biological systems; fungi, bacteria (antibiotics), plants (e.g. digitalis) and several others are chemical modifications of natural products.

In addition, there are a number of entirely synthetic drugs (e.g. barbiturates), some of which are based on active parts of naturally occurring drugs.

2. BASIC MECHANISMS

A medicine is any drug or other agent used to treat or prevent disease or to treat injury. The term medicine is generally used as a synonym for "drug."

In devising medicines for treating common conditions, an especially desirable factor is that the medicine should be capable of being taken by mouth - that is, that it should be able to pass into the body unchanged in spite of being exposed to stomach acidity and the enzymes of the digestive system.

In many cases, this is possible but there are some important exceptions, such as insulin that has to be given by injection.

This method may also be necessary if vomiting or a disease of the stomach or intestine prevent normal absorption. In most cases, the level of the drug in the blood or tissues determines its effectiveness.

Factors that can make a difference in the effectiveness of a drug include:
- the route of administration
- the rate of distribution in the body
- the degree of binding the proteins of the blood plasma
- the rate of breakdown
- the rate of excretion
- interactions with other drugs

In addition, there is an individual variation in drug responsiveness that is also apparent with undesired side-effects. These arise because drugs acting on one system commonly act on others.

Side effects

Side effects may be of various kinds, either non-specific, allergic or specific:
- non-specific side effects include nausea, vomiting, diarrhea, malaise or skin reactions;
- allergic side effects include urticaria (nettle rash), skin reactions and anaphylaxis (hypersensitivity leading to shock);
- specific side effects are related to the action of the medicine on the organ to be treated such as abnormal heart rhythm as a side effect of digitalis.

Mild side effects may be suppressed or simply accepted, but more serious ones must be watched for and the medicine stopped at the first sign of any adverse effect.

Drugs may cross the placenta to reach the fetus during pregnancy, interfering with its development and perhaps causing deformity, as happened with thalidomide.

Actions of medicines

Medicines may be used for relief of symptoms -for example, analgesics (painkillers) and anti-emetics (drugs to reduce nausea and vomiting) - or to control a disease.

This can be accomplished by various mechanisms, such as:

- killing the infecting agents;
- by preventing specific infections;
- by restoring normal control over muscle activity (e.g., drugs used in the treatment of Parkinson's disease);
- by restoring normal control over the mind (e.g., antidepressants);
- by replacing a lost nutrient or other vital substance (e.g., iron in anemia);
- by suppressing inflammatory responses (e.g., by giving steroids);
- by improving the functioning of an organ (e.g., digitalis in certain heart conditions);
- by protecting a diseased organ by altering the function of a normal one (e.g., diuretics to reduce fluid retention in heart failure);
- by toxic actions on cancer cells.

New medicines

The search for new medicines or drugs is mainly in the hands of a few giant firms whose products and markets span the world.

A large part of the industry is international in outlook, structure and organization, and its commitment to research is great: it has been estimated that the combined current expenditure is about $2,500 million yearly.

This high rate of investment reflects the continuing demand for drugs in world markets and the heavy costs of development.

For example, it has been calculated that, for every compound that is brought to therapeutic use, some 3000 or more substances have been made and tested; that the time of development is from five to ten years and the cost from $40 to $50 million.

Although one-third of this may be spent on tests of drug safety, risk and uncertainty still remain since it is not possible to specify all the actions that a drug might have.

Today the search for new therapeutic agents can be regarded as a collaborative exercise between the pharmaceutical industry, drug authorities, health services and academic institutions.

Thus private enterprise and government, representing the public interest, are joined in a system of complex activities involving many technical languages and skills. In this system the motives are humanitarian, scientific and commercial.

3. INTERACTIONS

Drug interactions are defined as the alteration of the effects of one drug by the prior or concurrent administration of another and the usual result is an increase or decrease of the effects of one of the drugs.

Desired interactions are usually considered in the context of "combination therapy" (for example, in the treatment of raised blood pressure, asthma, certain infections and malignant tumors), in which two or more drugs are used to increase the therapeutic effects and/or reduce the toxicity of drugs. Unwanted interactions can cause side effects or the ineffectiveness of the drugs.

Relatively few of the known or suggested drug interactions have been sufficiently analyzed to determine their clinical significance. If an interaction appears likely, a doctor will consider prescribing alternatives.

Drug interactions include the concurrent administration of drugs having the same (or opposing) pharmacological actions as well as alteration of the sensitivity or the responsiveness of the tissues to one drug or another. Many of these interactions can be predicted from a knowledge of the effects of each drug, and by monitoring patients, doctors will be able to detect deviations from expected effects and dosages can be adjusted accordingly.

Interactions that occur because of the way a drug passes through the body are more complicated and difficult to predict because the interacting drugs have unrelated actions. The interactions are mainly due to the processes of absorption, distribution, metabolism and excretion; the type of response expected from the drug is not changed, only the magnitude and duration.

The following general points concerning drug interactions warrant emphasis.
(1) The drugs for which interactions are

most significant are those with potent effect and low safety margins, such as
- anticoagulant drugs (used to reduce clotting of the blood);
- digitalis preparations (used in the treatment of heart failure);
- cytotoxic medicines (used to treat cancer);
- drugs for the treatment of hypertension (high blood pressure);
- drugs for the treatment of low blood sugar.

(2) It may be difficult to distinguish a drug interaction from symptoms of the illness or disease that can affect the body's response to a drug.

(3) Not all patients develop reactions, even when it is known that interactions may occur. Individual factors, such as dose and metabolism, determine whether the phenomenon occurs.

(4) When the effects of drugs are being closely monitored, an interaction usually requires a change of dosage or drug and does not result in significant problems for the patient.

Avoidance of drug interaction

To minimize the incidence and consequences of drug interactions, doctors should adhere to a number of general principles, and patients themselves should help doctors in detecting the symptoms of drug interaction.

(1) Doctors should know their patients' total drug intakes, including all agents prescribed by others and those that are purchased without a prescription. Patients should honestly tell their doctors about all chemicals and other agents they are using.

(2) Doctors should prescribe as few drugs in as low doses as possible for as short a time as needed to achieve a desired effect, and should avoid unnecessary combinations.

(3) Doctors should know the effects, both wanted and unwanted, of all the drugs used (since the spectrum of drug interactions is usually contained within these effects) and know which doses produce which responses.

(4) Doctors should observe and monitor their patients for the drugs' effects, particularly after any alteration in therapy.

(5) Doctors should, with the aid of accurate information from their patients, consider drug interactions as possible causes of any unanticipated trouble. If unexpected responses do occur, blood levels of drugs being taken should be measured, if possible. Most importantly, the doses of drugs should be altered until the desired effect is obtained. If this fails, the drugs should be changed to alternatives that will not interact with others being taken.

4. SIDE EFFECTS

The term side effects, or "adverse drug reactions" embodies a wide variety of toxic drug reactions that occur in numerous types of treatment. Assessing the incidence and consequences of side effects is extremely difficult, as cause-and-effect relationships are often difficult or impossible to prove.

The ultimate proof, which may be unobtainable in cases of severe reactions, depends on disappearance of the effect on withdrawal of the suspected drug (although some severe reactions are irreversible) and reappearance on the administration of the drug.

It is also difficult to select a control population in a clinical setting to differentiate drug-related symptoms and signs from those that are non-drug-related; thus, there is a wide variation in the methods used to collect data on side effects of drugs.

Some studies of side effects rely on reactions reported voluntarily by doctors; others involve selected patient groups; information from patients may also be collected by direct questioning or by patients volunteering information.

There is also a potential for both under- and overestimating the incidence of side effects of drugs. Perhaps 2 to 3 percent of admissions to hospital are due to drug reactions (excluding deliberate overdose or drug abuse), and among patients already in hospital, the incidence of mild to severe side effects may be as high as 8 to 10 percent.

These data are difficult to interpret in terms of cause-and-effect, mortality and physical damage. The incidence of drug-related deaths is unknown, but probably only a few deaths in medical units are drug-related, and these are often in patients with serious diseases that warrant such risks.

The most commonly reported causes of drug-related deaths are:
- Gastro-intestinal hemorrhage and peptic ulceration, caused by corticosteroids, aspirin and other anti-inflammatory drugs.
- Other hemorrhages, caused by anticoagulants (which reduce blood clotting) or cytostatic agents (anti-cancer drugs).
- Aplastic anemia, caused by chloramphenicol, phenylbutazone, gold salts or cytostatic agents.
- Damage to the liver, caused by paracetamol, chlorpromazine or isoniazid.
- Failure of the function of the kidney, caused by analgesics (painkillers).
- Infections, caused by corticosteroids or cytostatic drugs.
- Anaphylaxis, caused by penicillin or its derivatives or by antisera.

Although individuals vary considerably in their responsiveness to a particular drug effect, most toxic effects are related to the amount of drug taken. Previous contact with the drug is not necessary for the development of toxic reactions.

Side effects may be wanted under certain circumstances. For example, antihistamines given for hay fever may cause drowsiness as a side effect, but drowsiness may be a wanted effect when an antihistamine is given as a mild sleep remedy.

Management of minor side effects

Constipation
Increase the amount of fiber in your diet; drink plenty of fluids; exercise.

Decreased sweating
Avoid working or exercising in the sun or under warm conditions.

Diarrhea
Drink lots of water to replace lost fluids; if diarrhea lasts longer than three days, call your doctor.

Dizziness
Avoid operating machinery or driving a car.

Drowsiness
Avoid operating machinery or driving a car.

Dry mouth
Suck on candy or ice chips, or chew sugarless gum.

Fluid retention (mild)
Avoid adding salt to foods; keep legs raised, if possible.

Headache
Remain quiet; take aspirin or acetaminophen.

Insomnia
Take the last dose of the medicine earlier in the day (consult your doctor first); drink a glass of warm milk at bedtime; ask your doctor about an exercise program.

Itching
Take frequent baths or showers, or use wet soaks.

Palpitations (mild)
Rest often; avoid tension; do not drink coffee, tea, or cola; stop smoking.

Upset stomach
Take the medicine with milk or food (consult your doctor first).

Checklist

Checklist for safer medicine use

◆ Make sure you tell the doctor everything that is wrong with you. The more information he/she has, the more effective will be your treatment.

◆ Make sure each doctor you see knows all the medicines you use regularly - that is, all prescription and non-prescription drugs or medicines, including herbal and homeopathic remedies.

◆ Carry important medical facts about yourself in your handbag or wallet. Information about drug allergies, chronic diseases or special requirements can be very useful.

◆ Don't share your medicines with anyone. Your prescription was written for you and only you.

◆ Don't save unused medicine for future use unless you have consulted your doctor. Dispose of unused medicine by flushing it down the toilet.

◆ Tell your doctor about any medicine you take (even aspirin, allergy pills, cough and cold preparations, antacids, laxatives, vitamins, etc.) before you take any new medicine.

◆ Learn all you can about medicines you take before you take them. Information sources are your doctor, your nurse, your pharmacist, books in the public library, this computer database.

◆ Don't take medicines prescribed for someone else - even if your symptoms are the same.

◆ Keep your prescription drugs to yourself. Your drugs may be harmful to someone else.

◆ Tell your doctor about any symptoms you believe are caused by a medicine - prescription or non-prescription - that you take.

◆ Take only medicines that are necessary. Avoid taking non-prescription drugs while taking prescription drugs for a medical problem.

◆ Before your doctor prescribes for you, tell him about your previous experiences with any medicine -beneficial results, side effects, adverse reactions or allergies.

◆ Don't keep any medicines that change mood, alertness or judgment - such as sedatives, narcotics or tranquilizers -by your bedside. These cause many accidental deaths by overdose. You may unknowingly repeat a dose when you are half asleep or confused.

◆ Know the names of your medicines. These include the generic name, the brand name and the generic names of all ingredients in a medicine mixture. Your doctor, nurse or pharmacist can give you this information.

◆ Study the labels of all non-prescription medicines. If the information is incomplete or if you have questions, ask the pharmacist for more details.

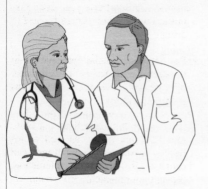

Checklist

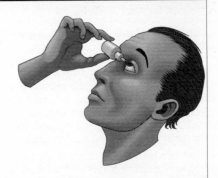

- If you must deviate from your prescribed dose schedule, tell your doctor.

- Shake liquid medicines before taking.

- Obtain a standard measuring spoon from your pharmacy for liquid medicines. Kitchen teaspoons and tablespoons are not accurate enough.

- Store all medicines away from moisture and heat. Bathroom medicine cabinets are usually unsuitable.

- If a medicine needs refrigeration, don't freeze.

- Follow diet instructions when you take medicines. Some work better on a full stomach, others on an empty stomach. Some drugs are more useful with special diets.

- Tell your doctor about any allergies you have. A previous allergy to a medicine may make it dangerous to prescribe again. People with other allergies, such as eczema, hay fever, asthma, bronchitis and food allergies, are more likely to be allergic to medicines.

- Prior to surgery, tell your doctor, anesthesiologist or dentist about any drugs you have taken in the past few weeks. Advise them of any cortisone drugs you have taken within two years.

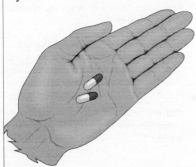

- If you become pregnant while taking any medicine, including birth control pills, tell your doctor immediately.

- Avoid all drugs while you are pregnant, if possible. If you must take medicines during pregnancy, record names, amounts, dates and reasons.

- If you see more than one doctor, tell each one about medicines others have prescribed.

- When you use non-prescription drugs, report it so the information is on your medical record.

- Store all drugs away from the reach of children.

- Note the expiration date on each drug label. Discard outdated ones safely. If no expiration date appears and it has been at least one year since taking the medication, it may be best to discard it.

- Pay attention to the information in the charts about safety while driving, piloting or working in dangerous places.

- Alcohol, cocaine, marijuana or other mood-altering drugs, as well as tobacco - mixed with some drugs - can cause a life-threatening interaction, prevent your medicine from being effective or delay your return to health.

Side effects may also be the result of allergic reactions. These depend on whether the person has become sensitive as a result of prior contact with a drug that functions as an antigen or allergen. Allergic reactions are not related to the level of the dose; the symptoms and signs that develop are determined by the interactions of antigens and antibodies and are largely independent of the specific properties of the drug molecule.

In a strict sense, allergic reactions are not completely unpredictable because a careful medical history and appropriate skin tests may make it possible to identify some of those at risk.

This is not possible with all drugs, however, and with penicillin in particular.

5. SKIN REACTIONS

The great number of reactions of the skin to the administration of drugs warrants a separate discussion.

The skin is the organ most commonly affected by severe, undesirable effects of drugs, and this can occur by a variety of different mechanisms: rashes and the like, which follow the taking of drugs, are often classed as allergic, but it must be said that the evidence for allergy is frequently scanty.

Allergic reactions

In order to be able, with absolute certainty, to classify such a drug reaction as "allergic" it is essential to demonstrate that antibodies or immune-competent cells directed against an antigen have been formed from the drug or one of its metabolites, and since drugs usually consist of fairly small molecules, the allergen that causes this reaction will as a rule be a compound formed by the drug and tissue protein.

In practice, the diagnosis of an allergic skin reaction to a drug is made only in those who have previously received the drug in question on one occasion and have tolerated it, but who, on renewed treatment, develop skin lesions with or without general symptoms such as high fever. Such people may develop an allergic reaction without having received exactly the same drug previously: for example, taking one sulphonamide drug can readily cause allergy to other sulphonamides in those sensitive to them.

Anaphylactic shock and nettle rash

These are caused by the formation of specific antibodies that become attached to tissue cells called mast cells.

When an individual is again exposed to the drug, the allergen reacts with the specific antibodies, and histamines and other active substances are released from the mast cells and cause urticaria and, in some cases, a fall in blood pressure, spasms of the muscles of the bronchi (airways), and edema (swelling) of the larynx.

In severe allergy, a person can die within minutes from allergic - or anaphylactic - shock. In moderate forms of allergy, urticaria alone may occur.

Penicillin, aspirin, heparin (a drug that reduces blood clotting) and X-ray contrast media are fairly common examples of drugs that can cause these reactions.

Cytotoxic allergy

This mechanism takes place when antibodies develop against drug-protein coupling with certain cells, and the immune reaction results in cell damage. Such allergic blood disorders (thrombocytopenias, leukopenias and hemolytic anemias) are well known in general medicine.

Toxic-complex syndrome

This syndrome, also called Arthus reaction, is the result of the formation of antibodies that, on reaction with a drug-protein coupling, produce damage to blood vessels via complement, a constituent of blood serum.

When antisera were in common use in the treatment of certain infections, they often produced these reactions.

At present, penicillin is the commonest cause.

The sufferers develop pain in the joints, fever and blood disorders, and their skin becomes tender and urticaria often occurs.

Delayed allergy

Allergic contact eczema due to drugs applied directly to the skin is a common reaction. The same type of allergic reaction may be caused by taking the same drugs by mouth, injected into a vein, as a pessary, etc. Sulphonamides, chlorothiazide and numerous other drugs may produce this effect.

6. ADDICTIVE AND ABUSED DRUGS

The drugs that are addictive and/or often abused include very valuable substances that, taken in moderate doses that have been properly prescribed, relieve pain and produce sleep, but in large doses cause various physical and psychological effects, including stupor, coma and, commonly, convulsions. Among the habit-forming drugs are opium and its derivatives, cocaine, amphetamines and barbiturates.

One of the major issues regarding drug dependence refers to the question of why young people take such drugs. There appear to be three major reasons for doing so:

(1) To obtain something valued. For instance, to be accepted among their circle of friends (one of the main reasons for the epidemic quality of drug-taking), or to be awake, alert and lively, throughout weekend parties that may in themselves be a means of filling in time away from an unacceptable or unaccepting home.

(2) To remove discomfort or anxiety. For example, a person who is shy and lonely finds that he can overcome his handicap with the help of alcohol or amphetamines.

Another who is despondent or who has accepted social failure (especially with the opposite sex) may find temporary relief, a new identity, and at the same time may express, against himself, the resentment and aggression that frustration always produces (hence the seemingly self-destructive element of much drug-taking).

(3) To dispel boredom. All humans, especially the vigorous and intelligent young, have exploratory drives towards mastering things and towards new and exciting, even dangerous, experiences; in their words they seek "kicks."

The problem is complicated by the varied effects of different drugs (not always the same in all people) and by the development of physical as well as psychological dependence. Thus, while drug-taking may be initiated in one way, it may be continued for quite different reasons.

One further general point concerns what is not known, and unfortunately the list is long. For example, we do not know the full extent of the problem - that is, how many are flirting with drugs, not just the factors that "hook" the few.

In particular, we do not know about treatment of severe cases; doctors are good at getting patients "off the hook" but very poor in keeping them off -all the more reason for trying to prevent addiction, and for the cooperation of lay people in the aftercare of former addicts.

Reflection on the above facts will suggest the principal ways of tackling the problem and where we, the general public, may help. Controlling sources of addictive drugs, law enforcement, the provision of treatment centers and research facilities are all of primary importance but are hardly our problems, except that, if responsible people repeatedly asked what was being done in these directions, there would be a powerful stimulus to getting something done, or getting something more done.

The most important thing for lay adults to be, if they are to help, is inquisitive, because if they are truly inquisitive either about the problem as a whole or about particular young persons, they will become concerned. They will not act on preconceived or emotional judgements but will try to find out, and that means that communication will be two-way and therefore potentially useful.

We know that it is no use talking at young people, or trying to scare them by depicting horrific consequences, but if there is a real exchange of facts, opinions and feelings between two parties, or within a group, understanding and perhaps trust will have been gained on both sides and something practical may develop. In this way, if young people admit to or are reported as misusing drugs, or if their erratic and variable behavior (their unhappiness and irritability, their exhaustion on Monday mornings, deterioration in their work, health and social relationships) suggests it, then we should begin thinking about the possible reasons as given here, and should make an opportunity to talk with them and to make plans with them. A high priority in the discussion will be whom to call in, and of course parents must first be considered, as well as school principals, priests, doctors or social workers. The majority of these cases, especially in the young, turn out to be based on familiar personal and family problems, directed into these new channels by unfortunate, but increasingly common, local conditions and opportunities. It is not quite such a new problem as may be supposed but it does need the active consideration and help of all responsible people, especially parents.

7. HOW TO USE MEDICINES

Important questions to ask your doctor or pharmacist.

(1) What is the name of this medicine or drug?

(2) What results can be expected from taking it?

(3) How long should I wait before reporting if this medicine does not help me?

(4) How does the substance work?

(5) What is the exact dose of the medicine or drug?

(6) What time(s) of the day should I take it?

(7) Can I drink alcoholic beverages while taking this medicine?

(8) Do I have to take special precautions with this medicine in combination with other prescription or non-prescription medicines I am taking?

(9) Do I have to take special precautions with this medicine if I am or want to become pregnant?

(10) Do I have to take special precautions about driving and/or operating machinery while taking this medicine?

(11) Can I take this medicine without regard to whether it is mealtime?

(12) Are there any special instructions I should have about how to use this medicine or drug?

(13) How long should I continue to take this medicine?

(14) Can I have a repeat prescription?

(15) Which side effects should I report?

(16) Do I have to take all this medicine, or can I stop when symptoms disappear?

(17) Can I save any unused portion of this medicine for future use?

(18) How long can I keep this medicine?

(19) What should I do if I forget to take a dose of this medicine?

(20) If this medicine is available without a prescription would it be cheaper than the prescription medicine?

II   Drugs

1.   *Introduction*

2.   *Alcohol*

3.   *Amphetamines*

4.   *Barbiturates*

5.   *Cannabis (Marijuana)*

6.   *Cocaine*

7.   *Hallucinogens*

8.   *Opiates (morphine)*

9.   *Volatile solvents ("glue sniffing")*

1. INTRODUCTION

The use or abuse of narcotic drugs is characterized by dependence phenomena. Drug dependence is a psychological and sometimes physical state resulting from the interaction between a living organism and a drug, characterized by behavioral and other responses that always include a compulsion to take the drug on a continuous or periodic basis in order to experience its psychological effects and sometimes to avoid the physical/mental discomfort of its absence.

This definition of drug dependence gives only a broad indication of the nature of the phenomena that are, in large measure, common to the various types or groups of drugs.

The characteristics of drug dependence show significant differences from one type of drug to another, a situation that makes it essential to establish clearly the dependence pattern for each type.

Even though some variations occur between individual drugs in each generic group, the consistency of the pattern of pharmacological actions and responses (human-drug interactions) is sufficiently uniform to permit a delineation of the principal types of dependence.

Before describing these types, it should be recalled that not all persons who take dependence-producing drugs become dependent on them. It is well-known, for example, that most users of alcoholic beverages and cannabis preparations do not become dependent on them.

It is, perhaps, not so widely appreciated that the non-medical use of opium and some drugs with similar effects is not always accompanied by the development of dependence.

The risk of such dependence is, however, much greater with drugs of the opiate (morphine) type than with alcoholic beverages and cannabis preparations.

The route of administration is also important; administration into a vein involves not only a greater risk of dependence but also of life-threatening complications.

The following factors are important in the development of drug dependency.
- The frequency and regularity of drug use.
- The characteristics and experience of the user.
- The social acceptability of the drug.
- Community attitudes towards intoxication.

2. ALCOHOL

The signs and symptoms of alcohol and of barbiturate intoxication are similar, as are the signs and symptoms of abstinence of these drugs.

In addition, barbiturates will suppress the effects of alcohol withdrawal, and alcohol will suppress, at least partially, the symptoms of barbiturate withdrawal.

Drug dependence of the alcohol-type may be said to exist when the consumption of alcohol by individuals exceeds the limits that are valid in their culture, if they consume alcohol at times that are deemed inappropriate within that culture, or if their intake of alcohol becomes so great as to injure their health or impair their social relationships.

Since the use of alcoholic beverages is a relatively normal part of the cultures of many countries, dependence on alcohol is usually apparent as an exaggeration of culturally accepted drinking patterns.

The manifestations of dependence vary accordingly, depending on how the particular society views the use of alcohol.

Psychological dependence on alcohol occurs in all degrees. In the mildest grade, alcohol is missed or desired if not available at meals or at social functions.

A moderate degree of psychological dependence exists when the individual feels compelled to drink in order to work or to participate socially and takes steps to ensure a supply of alcohol for these purposes.

Strong dependence is present when amounts are consumed that far exceed the cultural norm, drinking takes place in situations that culturally do not call for it and the person is obsessed with maintaining a supply of alcohol, even to the extent of drinking unusual or poisonous mixtures.

Tolerance to alcohol does develop. During continuous drinking, there is a slight but definite increase in the amount of ingested alcohol required to maintain a given blood level.

In addition, some physiological adaptation occurs so that the alcoholic appears less intoxicated and is less impaired in performance tests at a given concentration of blood alcohol than is a non-alcoholic.

Characteristics

The characteristics of drug dependence of the alcohol-type are:

◆ Psychological dependence, varying in degree from mild to intense.

◆ The development of a definite physical dependence that can, however, generally be detected only after the consumption of amounts considerably above the usual socially acceptable levels.

Following the reduction of intake below a critical level, characteristic withdrawal symptoms occur that can be largely suppressed by the administration of a barbiturate-like agent.

◆ The development of tolerance that is irregular and incomplete, so that there is a considerable persistence of disturbances in behavior dependent on the drug effects of the alcohol.

◆ A frequent consequence of alcoholism is physical illness, particularly of the liver.

3. AMPHETAMINES

The capacity of the amphetamines and drugs with similar properties to elevate the mood and induce a state of well-being is probably largely the basis for their previously widespread, but now decreasing, medial use as stimulants and slimming drugs.

Since such therapy commonly involves continuous and prolonged administration, those taking drugs of this kind, for health reasons or otherwise, may develop varying degrees of psychological dependence on them.

The stimulation and euphoria induced by drugs of this type lead to their non-medical use, and the user may increase both the size of the dose and the frequency of administration in order to attain a continuing stimulation and state of elation.

When this increasing use is carried to an extreme, the psychotoxic effects of large amounts of amphetamine-type drugs may lead to aggressive and dangerous anti-social behavior.

Qualitatively, the psychological effects are in many respects similar to those produced by cocaine.

It must be emphasized that the effects are dose-related. The occasional, or even the regular, consumption of relatively small doses taken by mouth produces primarily a sense of decreased fatigue, enhanced alertness and wakefulness.

A unique feature of the amphetamine-type drugs is their capacity to induce tolerance, a quality possessed by only a few central nervous system stimulants.

Although tolerance develops slowly when the amount taken is close to the usual therapeutic dosage, a progressive increase eventually permits the taking of amounts several hundred times as great as the original prescribed dose.

Although the amphetamines induce little, if any, physical dependence, as measured by the criterion of characteristic physical withdrawal symptoms, it would be inaccurate to state that withdrawal from very large dosages is symptomless.

The sudden stopping of a stimulant drug that has masked chronic fatigue, the need for sleep and, perhaps, depression permits these conditions to appear in an exaggerated fashion.

Thus, the withdrawal period is characteristically a state of depression, both psychological and physical, which probably reinforces the drive to resume using the drug.

Characteristics

♦ A variable, but sometimes intense, psychological dependence.

♦ Little, if any, physical dependence and, consequently, no characteristic physical withdrawal symptoms, although withdrawal is followed by a state of mental and physical depression.

♦ The development of a considerable degree of tolerance to many effects, which is not, however, shared equally by all; nervousness and sleeplessness therefore persist and psychotoxic effects, such as hallucinations and paranoid delusions, may occur.

4. BARBITURATES

Drugs producing dependence of the barbiturate-type include not only barbiturates but also some sedatives chemically related to them or to alcohol.

In addition, some (but not all) drugs commonly referred to as "tranquillizers" produce dependence of this kind; among those that produce barbiturate-type dependence are certain anti-anxiety agents, such as diazepam (Valium) and meprobamate (Equanil, Miltown).

Drug dependence of the barbiturate-type is a state arising from the repeated administration of drugs of this type on a continuous basis, generally in amounts that exceed the usual prescribed dosages.

There is a strong desire or need to continue the use of the drug, a need that can be satisfied by the drug used initially or by another with barbiturate-like properties.

There is a psychological dependence on the effects of the drug that is related to the way the individual appreciates those effects.

There is physical dependence requiring the presence of the drug for the maintenance of equilibrium and resulting in characteristic physical withdrawal symptoms when the drug is stopped.

Tolerance to barbiturate-type drugs does develop and, with relatively low doses, it will become evident within a few days.

However, there is - in contrast to the tolerance to morphine-like drugs - an upper limit to the size of dose to which a person may become tolerant.

During the chronic intoxication caused by the continual taking of the drug, there is some persistence of the sedative action, ataxia (unsteady gait), etc., on account of the incomplete development of tolerance; this makes the individual accident-prone.

There is also an impairment of mental ability, confusion, increased emotional instability and a risk of sudden over-dosage due to the delayed onset of activity, a distorted perception of time, and the relatively limited tolerance to the lethal dose.

The withdrawal symptoms are the most characteristic and destructive feature of drug dependence of the barbiturate-type.

They begin to appear within the first 24 hours after the cessation of drug-taking, reach a peak of intensity in two to three days, and subside slowly.

Abstinence syndrome

The complex of symptoms that constitutes what is called the "abstinence syndrome," in their approximate order of appearance, are:

- anxiety
- involuntary twitching of muscles
- tremor of the hand and fingers
- progressive weakness
- dizziness
- distortion in visual perception
- nausea and vomiting
- loss of weight
- precipitous drop in blood pressure
- not infrequently convulsions
- delirium resembling alcoholic delirium
- major psychotic episode.

Convulsions and delirium do not usually occur at the same time; generally, the person may have one or two convulsions during the first 48 hours of withdrawal and then become psychotic during the second or third night.

With respect to the psychotic episodes, paranoid reactions, reactions resembling schizophrenia with delusion and hallucinations, a withdrawn stuporous state and panic have all been observed.

In a person with a substantial physical dependence on a drug of the barbiturate-type, unsupported withdrawal of the drug is a life-threatening process. Carefully supervised gradual withdrawal is therefore essential.

Characteristics

◆ A variable, but often marked, psychological dependence related to the desired effects of the drug.

◆ A marked physical dependence when the dosage levels are substantially above prescribed levels; if the drug is stopped, the resulting withdrawal syndrome can be life-threatening, especially in the absence of appropriate medical treatment.

◆ The development of an incomplete and variable tolerance to the different pharmacological effects of the drug.

5. CANNABIS (MARIJUANA)

The hemp plant, Cannabis sativa, grows in most temperate to tropical parts of the world. It is used both for its fiber and its psychoactive properties.

Although it is still employed in some traditional systems of medicine, cannabis is of little importance in modern medical practice.

The amount of psychoactive material in a given cannabis preparation is influenced by a number of factors:
– the characteristic of the plant
– the place and circumstances of its growth
– the nature of the preparation

– the age of the harvested material
– the way in which it is stored.

The usual method of consuming cannabis is by smoking it, but it may be ingested as an ingredient of a food or beverage.

The effects of cannabis appear sooner when it is smoked, and greater amounts are required to produce comparable effects when cannabis is ingested.

Signs and symptoms

The usual immediate symptoms and signs resulting from low to moderate doses, in general order of appearance and increasing dose, may include:
– a mild to marked euphoria
– sensory and perceptual changes
– some decrease in the sense of identity and reality
– visual, but less often auditory, hallucinations.

Cannabis users often report a sense of increased auditory and visual sensitivity, with an enhanced appreciation of music and works of art. The perceptual changes involve mainly space and time.

At high dosage levels, a state of acute intoxication is usually observed, the major manifestations of which often include:
– paranoid ideas
– illusions and delusions
– depersonalization
– confusion and restlessness
– excitement
– hallucinations.

Inability to walk properly, however, does not normally occur, even after large doses of cannabis. It is possible that some long-term behavioral effects attributed to cannabis use are due largely, or in part, to the socio-cultural setting in which the drug is taken.

For example, in a society where the use of cannabis is illegal and generally disapproved of, the user is ipso facto engaged in non-conforming behavior.

Drug dependence of the cannabis-type is a state arising from the chronic, regular or periodic use of cannabis preparations.

Characteristics

♦ A moderate to strong psychological dependence related to the desired subjective effects.

♦ Little, if any, physical dependence (some possible withdrawal symptoms have been reported), but there is no evidence that the withdrawal of cannabis, even from an extremely "heavy" user, produces an abstinence syndrome that begins to approach in severity those produced by drugs of the alcohol, barbiturate, and opiate type.

♦ Perhaps some degree of tolerance associated with "heavy" use.

6. COCAINE

Cocaine is the prototype of stimulant drugs that are capable, in high dosages, of inducing euphoric excitement and hallucinatory experiences.

Because of these properties, cocaine ranks high in the esteem of experienced drug users, and it can lead to the highest degree of psychological dependence.

Cocaine induces feelings of muscular strength and mental alertness, leading individuals to overestimate their capabilities.

This, associated with paranoid delusions and auditory, visual and tactile hallucinations, often makes the user very dangerous and capable of serious anti-social acts.

Signs and symptoms

The use of cocaine in large amounts may lead to the following symptoms:
– digestive disorders
– nausea and vomiting
– loss of appetite
– loss of weight
– sleeplessness
– occasional convulsions.

No physical dependence on cocaine develops and, consequently, no characteristic withdrawal symptoms are noted when the drug is stopped abruptly, but

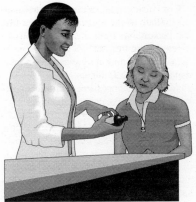

severe depression may persist for some time after withdrawal.

Characteristics

♦ A strong psychological dependence.

♦ The absence of physical dependence and, therefore, of characteristic withdrawal symptoms.

♦ The absence of tolerance; there is, rather, a sensitization to the drug's effects in some instances.

♦ A strong tendency to carry on taking the drug, as found in chewing coca leaves (from which cocaine is derived), or the rapid repetition of doses often observed when injecting the drug is involved.

7. HALLUCINOGENS

Drugs of this type include lysergic acid diethylamide (LSD, "acid"), psilocybin ("magic mushrooms") and mescaline (peyote). Drugs of the LSD-type induce a state of excitation of the brain that is manifested in a number of ways:
– changes in mood
– anxiety
– distortion in sensory perception
– visual hallucinations
– delusions
– depersonalization
– dilation of the pupils
– increase in body temperature
– rise in blood pressure.

Psychological dependence of drugs of the hallucinogen-type varies greatly, but it is usually not intense.

The users may enjoy the effects of these agents and may wish to repeat them, but if such agents are not readily available, these persons will either do without them or accept a substitute.

A minority of users may develop strong psychological dependence on these substances. No evidence of physical dependence has been detected when the drugs are withdrawn abruptly.

A high degree of tolerance to LSD and to psilocybin develops rapidly and disappears with equal rapidity. Tolerance to mescaline develops more slowly.

Persons who are tolerant to any one of these drugs will find they are tolerant to the other two.

The chief dangers to the individual arise from the psychological effects of hallucinogens. Serious impairment of judgement has led to dangerous decisions and accidents, while a "bad trip" with an associated panic reaction can be a most frightening experience.

8. OPIATES (MORPHINE)

The outstanding and distinctive characteristic of dependence on opium and morphine-like agents is that the major features - psychological and physical dependence, as well as tolerance - can be initiated by the repeated administration of small doses, and increase in intensity in direct relation to an increase in the dosage.

This characteristic implies that dependence on drugs of this generic type may be created within the dosage range generally used for medical purposes, and that the mechanism may be set in motion by the first dose administered.

The regular use of opiate-type drugs results in the development of strong physical dependence, and characteristic withdrawal symptoms occur when the narcotic is stopped.

With morphine, the abstinence syndrome appears within a few hours of the last dose, reaches a peak within 24 to 48 hours, and subsides spontaneously.

The most severe symptoms usually disappear within 10 days, although a few persist for a much longer period.

The time of onset, peak intensity and duration of adverse symptoms vary with the degree of dependence on the drug and with the characteristics of the specific agent involved.

The unique feature of the morphine abstinence syndrome is that it represents changes in all major areas of nervous activity, including alteration in behavior, excitation of the nervous system and depressive effects.

Signs and symptoms

The following general phenomena may occur:
- anxiety
- restlessness
- generalized body aches
- insomnia
- yawning
- watery eyes
- runny nose
- perspiration
- dilated pupils
- gooseflesh
- hot flushes
- nausea and vomiting
- diarrhea
- elevation of body temperature
- high respiratory rate
- raised blood pressure
- abdominal cramps
- dehydration and loss of appetite
- loss of body weight

A relationship between dose, pharmacological properties and intensity of physical dependence has been mentioned. Taking repeated doses of the drug while the previous doses are still being felt also hastens development of physical dependence.

The time from beginning to take the drug to the appearance of demonstrable physical dependence also varies with the agent.

With morphine, this interval (under clinical conditions of administration) is two or three weeks; it is shorter for ketobemidone, probably longer for phenazocine, and definitely longer for codeine, especially when this is administered by mouth.

Finally, with drug dependence of the morphine type, the harm to individuals is, in the main, indirect, arising from their preoccupation with drug-taking: personal neglect, malnutrition and infection. For society, too, the harm resulting from dependence is chiefly related to the preoccupation of the individual with drug-taking; disruption of personal relationships, economic loss and crimes against property are frequent consequences.

Characteristics

♦ A strong psychological dependence that manifests itself as an overpowering drive or compulsion to continue taking the drug for pleasure or to avoid physical/mental discomfort, and to obtain it by almost any means.

♦ An early development of physical dependence that increases in intensity, paralleling the increase in dosage; this requires continued administration of the same drug, or of an allied one, to maintain a semblance of equilibrium and to prevent the appearance of the symptoms and signs of withdrawal.

♦ Both the withdrawal of the drug and the administration of a specific antagonist precipitat definite, characteristic and self-limiting withdrawal symptoms.

♦ The development of tolerance that requires an increase in dosage to produce the effects obtained initially.

9. VOLATILE SOLVENTS ("GLUE SNIFFING")

Since anesthetics administered by inhalation became available, there have been instances of their self-administration, not to produce unconsciousness and anesthesia, but to induce a sense of giddiness, intoxication and sometimes euphoria.

Among the agents used in this way are ether, chloroform and nitrous oxide. More recently, certain volatile solvents - such as the acetone found in nail varnish remover, toluene found in the glue used to make models, and petrol - have been used for this purpose.

These substances are brain depressants and produce effects somewhat comparable to those produced by alcohol, although the symptoms vary from agent to agent. Initially, there may be mild euphoria and exhilaration, followed by confusion, disorientation and ataxia (disturbed gait), and the user may behave as though drunk.

Some of the substances, including petrol and toluene, may also produce symptoms rather like those sometimes induced by the hallucinogens, such as:
– a marked euphoria
– grandiose delusions
– recklessness
– other delusions and hallucinations
– substantial loss of self-control
– convulsions and coma

Certain of the substances, including petrol, benzene (used in solvents) and carbon tetrachloride (used in dry cleaning), are more likely to result in grave complications, such as liver or kidney damage.

Physical dependence, at least of the magnitude associated with the use of a drug of the alcohol, barbiturate or opium type, does not ordinarily occur. However, abrupt withdrawal after the person has been using substantial amounts may be associated with some degree of lethargy, depression and irritability.

In summary, a number of volatile solvents will produce psychological dependence of varying degrees because of a liking for the effects they produce. Some of these substances will also produce tolerance. The question of physical dependence remains open, but if it occurs, the syndrome is usually less intense than that associated with drugs such as alcohol, barbiturates and opiates.

Table of Drugs

AMPHETAMINES

To this category belong not only the original group of amphetamines but also a group of newly synthesized products (one well-known product is called "ice").

◆ Pharmacological category
Central nervous system stimulants.

◆ Mode of action
Amphetamines increase the release of norepinephrine from nerve endings and neurosynaptic junctions in the central nervous system and sympathetic part of the autonomic nervous system, yielding a generalized increase in nerve activity.

◆ Source
Synthesized primarily by the drug industry and illegal laboratories.

◆ Dosage forms abused
- capsules (time-released)
- tablets
- crystalline powder for injection in solution

◆ Routes of administration
- oral
- intravenous injection

◆ Slang terminology
- speed
- hearts
- bennys
- footballs
- crystal
- uppers
- meth
- copiots
- ice

◆ Medical uses
- for narcolepsy
- to reduce mental depression
- to control appetite and obesity
- for hyperkinetic or hyperactive children

◆ Short-term effects
- transient sense of alertness, wakefulness
- feeling of well-being and mental clarity
- hunger is diminished
- increased heart rate
- increased blood pressure
- dilation of pupils
- dryness in mouth and throat
- sweating

◆ Long-term effects
- damage to heart and brain
- general exhaustion
- nutritional deficiencies
- psychotic episodes
- infections due to unsanitary injections

◆ Unique problems
- Amphetamine abuse causes overexertion of normal body function, yielding such symptoms as nausea, exhaustion and cramps.
- Depressants (alcohol, heroin, tranquilizers and barbiturates) are often taken to relieve these symptoms.

◆ Tolerance potential
- Yes

◆ Psychological dependence
- Yes

◆ Physical dependence
- Questionable

BARBITURATES

◆ Pharmacological category
Central nervous system depressants which act as sedatives and hypnotics.

◆ Mode of action
The drugs interfere with the transmission of impulses to the cortex of the brain.

◆ Examples
(1) long-acting barbiturates
- phenobarbital.
(2) intermediate to short-acting barbiturates
- amobarbital (blue heavens, blue birds)

Table of Drugs

– pentobarbital (yellow jackets, membies)
– secobarbital (reds, pinks, red devils)
– amobarbital + secobarbital

♦ Source
Manufactured by the drug industry.

♦ Dosage form
– capsules
– tablets

♦ Route of administration
– oral
– parenteral

♦ Medical indications
– preoperative sedation
– insomnia
– epilepsy
– anxiety
– tension

♦ Short-term effects

LOW DOSAGE (30 mg)
– depression of sensory function
– sedation without analgesia
– drowsiness

HIGH DOSAGE (100 mg)
– depression of motor function
– depression of brain stem function
– depression of circulation
– sleep
– anesthesia

♦ Long-term effects with overdose
– mental confusion
– venous system damage
– dermatitis
– liver damage

♦ Unique problems
– Death due overdosage is common because the fatal dose for an individual does not increase with tolerance to the psychoactive effects of the drug. There is also a narrower range between toxic and therapeutic levels than with other depressants.
– Withdrawal effects from barbiturates are more severe than those from heroin.

♦ Tolerance potential
Yes

♦ Psychological dependence
Yes; with withdrawal symptoms such as
– weakness
– increased blood pressure
– anxiety
– motor incoordination
– behavior problems
– apprehension
– agitation
– dehydration
– weight loss
– psychosis (similar to delirium tremens)

COCAINE - CRACK - XTC

♦ Pharmacological category
Stimulant and local; anesthetic.

♦ Mode of action
Cocaine elevates the threshold of inhibitory nerve excitability and thus enhances normal stimulation of the central nervous system.

♦ Slang terminology
– coke
– snow
– stardust
– flade
– speedball (combination with heroin)
– crack (new synthetic preparation)

♦ Source
Cocaine is an odorless, white fluffy powder derived from the coca tree, grown in Bolivia, Colombia, Peru and Chili.

♦ Route of administration
– through nasal mucous membranes
– intravenous injection

♦ Medical use
None; has been used as local anesthetic.

♦ Short-term effects
– euphoria
– energetic sensations
– possible hallucinations

Table of Drugs

- possible delusions
- dilated pupils
- loss of appetite

◆ Long-term effects
- digestive disorders
- loss of weight
- insomnia
- occasional convulsions
- sometimes heart troubles
- memory disturbances
- social disorders
- possible perforation of the septum of the nose

◆ Tolerance potential
- None

◆ Psychological dependence
- Yes, very strong

◆ Physical dependence
- No

HALLUCINOGENS

To this category of drugs belong such substances as:
- STP, DOM
- Mescaline
- Phenyclydine
- DMT

These drugs have short-term activity comparable to that of LSD, but even less is known about their long term effects

◆ Characteristics of STP
- one-tenth as potent as LSD
- synthetic
- taken orally in tablet or capsule form

◆ Characteristics of mescaline
- 1/200 as potent as LSD
- active ingredient of the peyote cactus
- taken orally

◆ Characteristics of phenycyclidine
- taken by injection or orally
- sometimes smoked in tobacco
- once used as a general anesthetic
- used in counterfeit drugs

◆ Characteristics of DMT (dimethyltryptamine)
- short-acting
- taken by injection
- smoked in tobacco
- causes more pronounced rise in blood pressure

LSD

◆ Pharmacological category
LSD belongs to the group of hallucinogens. The hallucinogens represent a broad group of drugs, both natural and synthetic, which have the ability to induce hallucinations and illusions through alterations of sensory perception.

◆ Mode of action
LSD may alter the levels of certain natural chemicals in the brain, including serotonin, which could produce changes in the brain's electrical activity.

◆ Source
LSD is a modified form of lysergic acid, a chemical obtained from a fungus that grows on rye and wheat.

◆ Routes of administration
- oral
- injection

◆ Common dosage forms
LSD in pure form is a white powder that is easily dissolved and may be incorporated into numerous substances for oral administration:
- sugar cubes
- cookies
- tablets
- capsules
- beverages
- glycerin wafers

◆ Medical uses
LSD has no specific medical use. Sometimes LSD is being used in special cases such as:
- alcoholism
- emotional disorders
- terminal illnesses

Table of Drugs

– concentration camp syndrome

◆ Short-term physical effects (lasting 8-10 hours)
– slight increase in heart rate
– slight increase in blood pressure
– slight increase in temperature
– dilated pupils
– shaking of hands and feet
– cold, sweaty palms
– loss of appetite and nausea
– irregular breathing

◆ Short-term psychological effects
– sudden changes in sensory perception
– synesthesia (scrambling of sensory input)
– feeling of detachment from reality
– alteration of mood
– altered perception of time
– altered perception of space
– alteration of thinking and feelings
– depersonalization
– loss of identity

◆ Long-term effects
– severe mental illness is the only documented long-term effect of LSD.

◆ Unique problems
– severe panic may accompany LSD trips
– paranoia may persist up to 72 hours
– accidental deaths
– the drug state may recur days, or even months after using LSD.

◆ Tolerance potential
– Possible

◆ Psychological dependence
– Possible

◆ Physical dependence
– No

MARIJUANA AND ITS DERIVATIVES

◆ Pharmacological category
– marijuana: intoxicant

– hashish: intoxicant to hallucinogen
– THC: intoxicant to hallucinogen

◆ Mode of action
The active ingredient ion marijuana is 9-THC (tetrahydrocannabinol); and its mode of action is unknown. Research has shown that it affects the brain and nervous system.

◆ Slang terminology
– pot
– tea
– grass
– mary jane
– weed

◆ Abused dosage forms
– crude plant material
– hashish (resin)
– oil concentrates

◆ Routes of administration
– smoked
– added to food and taken orally

◆ Medical uses
– none

◆ Short-term physical effects (2-4 hours)
– enters blood stream quickly
– increased heart rate
– reddening of the eyes
– increased hunger
– irritation of mucous membranes of nose and bronchioles from smoke

◆ Short-term psychological effects
– alteration of moods
– alteration of thinking process
– tranquilizing effect
– alteration of spatial sense
– alteration of time perception
– uncontrollable hilarity
– illusions (in high doses)
– possible paranoia

◆ Long-term effects
– bronchitis
– alienation from society

◆ Tolerance potential
– mild to none

Table of Drugs

◆ Psychological dependence
– Yes

◆ Physical dependence
– No

MINOR TRANQUILIZERS

◆ Pharmacological category
Central nervous system depressants

◆ Mode of action
Tranquilizers generally act at a subcortical level by central nervous system depression.

◆ Examples
– meprobamate
– chlordiazepoxide
– diazepam (Valium)
– other benzodiazepines

◆ Sources
The drug industry manufactures tranquilizers from natural of synthetic products.

◆ Dosage forms abused
– capsules
– tablets

◆ Route of administration
– generally, oral

◆ Medical use
– muscle relaxants
– anticonvulsants
– relief of anxiety
– decrease of vomiting
– adjuvant in treatment of alcoholism

◆ Short-term effects
– reduction in motor activity
– mild drowsiness
– blockage of conditioned reflexes
– reduction of anxiety
– dermatitis
– disorientation
– blurred vision
– coordination problems

◆ Long-term effects
– obstructive hepatitis

– bone marrow depression
– induced nervous disorders

◆ Tolerance potential
– Yes

◆ Physical dependence
– Yes

◆ Psychological dependence
– Yes

OPIATES AND THEIR DERIVATIVES

◆ Pharmacological category
Central nervous system depressants which act as analgesics, sedatives, and cough depressants.

◆ Mode of action
Narcotics depress the following centers in the brain and spinal cord:
– pain perception center
– respiratory center
– smooth muscle stimulating center
– vasomotor center

◆ Examples

OPIUM DERIVATIVES
– morphine
– codeine
– paregoric
– heroin

SYNTHETIC FORMS
– hydromorphine
– meperidine
– oxymorphone
– methadone

◆ Sources
– Opium poppy
– Synthesized by drug industry

◆ Dosage forms abused
– capsules
– tablets
– powder for injections
– cough preparations

Table of Drugs

◆ Routes of administration
– oral
– nasal (sniffing)
– parental (intradermal or intravenous)

◆ Medical use
– morphine and morphine derivatives are used for the treatment of severe pain
– codeine is used to depress coughing and relieve pain
– paregoric is used to control diarrhea and to relieve pain of teething

◆ Short-term effects
– reduction in sensitivity to pain
– drowsiness
– induced sleep
– reduction in physical activity
– constipation
– constriction of pupils
– respiratory depression

◆ Long-term effects
– physical dependence
– tolerance
– psychological dependence

◆ Medical problems
– hepatitis due to septic administration
– death from overdosage
– skin infections due to septic administration
– AIDS due to use of dirty syringes

◆ Social problems
– Heroin eventually will most likely to be injected ("mainlined"), and the addict may resort to crude instruments for administration.
– The craving for heroin leads most addicts to commit crimes in order to obtain a substantial amount of money per day support the habit.

◆ Tolerance [potential
– Yes

VOLATILE SOLVENTS

◆ Pharmacological category
Central nervous system depressants.

◆ Mode of action
The solvents are extremely soluble in the mucous membranes of the respiratory tract and quickly depress the central nervous system and motor activity because they reach high concentrations in the blood shortly after inhalation.

◆ Examples
– glue
– fingernail polish and remover
– paint thinners
– freon and other aerosol propellants
– gasoline
– ether

◆ Source
Most of the solvents listed above may be found in the home.

◆ Route of administration
Inhalation, often with the aid of a paper or plastic bag, which concentrates the vapors of the solvent.

◆ Medicinal uses
None. It should be noted, however, that these solvents are similar in action to general anesthetics used during surgery.

◆ Short-term effects
– feeling of drunkenness
– slurring of speech
– dizziness
– impaired sensory perception
– disorganized behavior
– uncoordinated muscular activity
– unconsciousness, which can even lead to death

◆ Long-term effects
– damage to heart and lungs
– malfunctioning of kidneys and liver
– impaired perception
– impaired coordination and judgment

◆ Tolerance potential
– Unknown

◆ Psychological dependence
– Yes

◆ Physical dependence
– No

III Medicines A-Z

ACCURBRON

Properties
This medicine contains theophylline as active ingredient; it is used to treat or prevent breathing problems (wheezing and shortness of breath) caused by asthma, bronchitis, or emphysema. This medication belongs to a group known as xanthine-derivative bronchodilators. They work by opening up the bronchial tubes or air passages of the lungs and increasing the flow of air through them. These medicines are available only with your doctor's prescription.

Before using this medicine
Before you use this medicine check with your doctor, or pharmacist:
- if you ever had any unusual or allergic reaction to xanthine-derivative bronchodilators.
- if you are on a low-salt, low-sugar, or any other special diet, or if you are allergic to any substance, such as sulfites or other preservatives or dyes.
- if you are pregnant or intend to become pregnant while using this medicine.
- if you are breast-feeding an infant. Theophylline passes into the breast milk and may cause irritability, fretfulness, or trouble in sleeping in infants of mothers taking this medicine.
- if you have any of the following medical problems:
Diarrhea
Enlarged prostate
Fibrocystic breast disease
Heart disease
Stomach ulcer

Treatment
This medication is used to relieve or prevent the symptoms of your medical problem. Take them as directed. Do not take more of them and do not take them more often than recommended on the label, unless otherwise directed by your doctor. To do so may increase the chance of side effects. The medicine should be taking on an empty stomach 30 to 60 minutes before a meal or two hours after a meal. Try not to miss any doses of this medication. If you do miss a dose, take the missed dose as soon as possible, unless it is almost time for the next dose. Do not double the next dose. It works best when taken with a glass of water.

Side effects
The following minor side effects may occur:
    Dizziness or flushing
    Headache
    Diarrhea
    Heartburn
    Increased urination
    Nervousness or irritability
    Loss of appetite
    Nausea or stomach upset
    Stomach pain.
These side effects should disappear as your body adjusts to the medication. Tell your doctor about any side effects that are persistent or particularly bothersome. It is especially important to tell your doctor about black, tarry stools; confusion; convulsions; difficulty in breathing; fainting; muscle twitching; palpitations; rash; severe abdominal pain; or unusual weakness.

Interactions
This medicine interacts with several other drugs such as diuretics, reserpine, beta blockers, phenytoin, lithium, phenobarbital, birth control pills, and other medications.
- Be sure to tell your doctor about any medications you are currently taking.

Storage
Tablets, capsules, liquid and suspension should be stored at room temperature in tightly closed containers. Store away from heat and direct light. Keep out of reach of children, since overdose may be very dangerous in children. Discard any outdated medication.

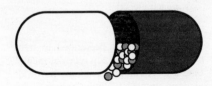

ACETAPHENAZINE

Properties
This medicine contains as active ingredient acetophenazine, a phenothiazine derivative. Phenothiazines are a family of medicines used to treat nervous, mental, and emotional conditions. Some are used to control anxiety, restlessness, nausea and vomiting, and severe hiccups. This medicine is available only with your doctor's prescription.

Before using this medicine
Before you use this medicine check with your doctor, or pharmacist:
- if you ever had any unusual or allergic reaction to phenothiazine medicines.
- if you are on a low-salt, low-sugar, or any other special diet, or if you are allergic to any substance, such as sulfites or other preservatives or dyes.
- if you are pregnant or intend to become pregnant while using this medicine. Although phenothiazines have not been shown to cause birth defects, some side effects such as jaundice and muscle tremors have occurred in a few newborns whose mothers received phenothiazines during pregnancy.
- if you are breast-feeding an infant. Although this medicine has not been shown to cause problems in humans the chance does exist since some phenothiazines are known to pass into the breast milk.
- if you have any of the following medical problems:
Alcoholism
Blood disease
Difficult urination
Enlarged prostate
Glaucoma
Heart or blood vessel disease
Liver or lung disease
Parkinson's disease
Stomach ulcers

Treatment
This medication is prescribed to treat the symptoms of certain types of mental illness or emotional problems. In order to avoid stomach irritation, you can take the tablet or capsule forms of this medication with a meal or with a glass of water or milk (unless your doctor or pharmacist directs you to do otherwise).

Side effects
Along with the needed effects, a medicine may cause some unwanted effects. Minor side effects are: blurred vision, constipation, decreased sweating, diarrhea, dizziness, drooling, drowsiness, dry mouth, fatigue, jitteriness, menstrual irregularities, nasal congestion, restlessness, tremors, vomiting, or weight gain.
- Tell your doctor about any side effects that are persistent or particularly bothersome. It is especially important to tell your doctor about:
Breast enlargement
Chest pain or convulsions
Darkened skin
Difficulty in swallowing
Fainting or fever
Involuntary movements
Palpitations or sleep disorders
Rash or sore throat
Uncoordinated movements
Unusual bleeding or bruising
Visual disturbances
Yellowing of the eyes or skin

Interactions
This medicine may interact with several other drugs such as barbiturates, sleeping pills, narcotics, other tranquilizers, or any other medication that may produce a sedative effect. Avoid alcohol.

Storage
Store this medication as directed on the label. Keep out of the reach of children.

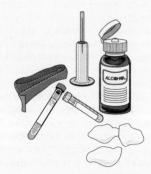

ACLOMETASONE DIPROPIONATE

Properties
This medicine contains aclometasone dipropionate, a corticosteroid, as active ingredient. Corticosteroids are used to help relieve redness, swelling, itching, inflammation, and discomfort of many skin problems. They exert this effect by interfering with natural body mechanisms that produce the rash, itching, or inflammation. They do not cure the underlying cause of the skin problem. This medication is applied to the skin.

Before using this medicine
Before you use this medicine check with your doctor, or pharmacist:
- if you ever had any unusual or allergic reaction to corticosteroids.
- if you are allergic to any substance, such as sulfites or other preservatives or dyes.
- if you are pregnant or intend to become pregnant while using this medicine. Studies have shown that corticosteroids applied to the skin in large amounts or over long periods of time can be the cause of birth defects.
- if you are breast-feeding an infant. Some corticosteroids pass into breast milk and may interfere with the infant's growth.

Treatment
Do not use this medicine more often or for a longer time than ordered. To do so may increase absorption through the skin and the chance of side effects. In addition, too much use, especially on areas with thinner skin (for example, face, armpits, groin), may result in thinning of the skin and stretch marks.

Before applying this medication, wash your hands. than, unless your doctor or pharmacist gives you different instructions, gently wash the area where the medication is to be applied. With a clean towel pat the area dry. Apply a small amount of the medication to the affected area in a thin layer. Do not bandage the area unless your doctor tells you to do so. If you miss a dose of this medication, apply the dose as soon as possible, unless it is almost time for the next application.
- ◆ Do not use this medicine for other skin problems without first checking with your doctor. You should not use a topical corticosteroid if you have a virus disease (such as herpes), fungal infection of the skin (such as athlete's foot), or tuberculosis of the skin.

Side effects
There are a number of side effects that usually do not require medical attention. Minor side effects are:
   Acne
   Burning sensations
   Itching
   Rash
   Skin dryness
These possible side effects may go away during treatment; however, if they continue or are bothersome, check with your doctor, nurse, or pharmacist. Tell your doctor about any side effects that are persistent or particularly bothersome, such as:
   Blistering
   Increased hair growth
   Irritation of the affected area
   Loss of skin
   Secondary infection in the area being treated
   Thinning of the skin with easy bruising

Interactions
None known as long as it is used according to the directions given to you by your doctor or pharmacist.

Storage
Cream, ointment, lotion, gel, spray, and aerosol should be stored at room temperature in tightly closed containers. This medication should never be frozen.

ACLOVATE

Properties

This medicine contains aclometasone dipropionate, a corticosteroid, as active ingredient. Corticosteroids are used to help relieve redness, swelling, itching, inflammation, and discomfort of many skin problems. They exert this effect by interfering with natural body mechanisms that produce the rash, itching, or inflammation. They do not cure the underlying cause of the skin problem. This medication is applied to the skin.

Before using this medicine

Before you use this medicine check with your doctor, or pharmacist:

- if you ever had any unusual or allergic reaction to corticosteroids.
- if you are allergic to any substance, such as sulfites or other preservatives or dyes.
- if you are pregnant or intend to become pregnant while using this medicine. Studies have shown that corticosteroids applied to the skin in large amounts or over long periods of time can be the cause of birth defects.
- if you are breast-feeding an infant. Some corticosteroids pass into breast milk and may interfere with the infant's growth.

Treatment

Do not use this medicine more often or for a longer time than ordered. To do so may increase absorption through the skin and the chance of side effects. In addition, too much use, especially on areas with thinner skin (for example, face, armpits, groin), may result in thinning of the skin and stretch marks.

Before applying this medication, wash your hands. than, unless your doctor or pharmacist gives you different instructions, gently wash the area where the medication is to be applied. With a clean towel pat the area dry. Apply a small amount of the medication to the affected area in a thin layer. Do not bandage the area unless your doctor tells you to do so.

If you miss a dose of this medication, apply the dose as soon as possible, unless it is almost time for the next application.

◆ Do not use this medicine for other skin problems without first checking with your doctor. You should not use a topical corticosteroid if you have a virus disease (such as herpes), fungal infection of the skin (such as athlete's foot), or tuberculosis of the skin.

Side effects

There are a number of side effects that usually do not require medical attention. Minor side effects are:

Acne

Burning sensations

Itching

Rash

Skin dryness

These possible side effects may go away during treatment; however, if they continue or are bothersome, check with your doctor, nurse, or pharmacist. Tell your doctor about any side effects that are persistent or particularly bothersome, such as:

- Blistering
- Increased hair growth
- Irritation of the affected area
- Loss of skin
- Secondary infection in the area being treated
- Thinning of the skin with easy bruising

Interactions

None known as long as it is used according to the directions given to you by your doctor or pharmacist.

Storage

Cream, ointment, lotion, gel, spray, and aerosol should be stored at room temperature in tightly closed containers. This medication should never be frozen.

ADALAT

Properties

This medicine contains nefedipine as active ingredient. It is a so-called calcium channel blocker, working by blocking the passage of calcium into heart and smooth muscle. Since calcium is an essential factor in muscle contraction, any medicine that affects calcium in this way will interfere with the contraction of these muscles.

The medicine works by:

◆ reducing the work that the heart must perform;

◆ reducing the normal arterial blood pressure;

◆ increasing oxygen to the heart muscle.

The medicine is prescribed for the treatment of attacks of angina pectoris, irregular heartbeat, and high blood pressure. In many cases it can be used for the treatment and prevention of migraine.

Before using this medicine

Before you use this medicine check with your doctor, or pharmacist:

– if you ever had any unusual or allergic reaction to this medicine or any calcium channel blocker;

– if you are pregnant or intend to become pregnant while using this medicine;

– if you have low blood pressure;

– if you have kidney or liver disease;

– if you are breast-feeding an infant;

– if you easily get a rash or intensity sunburn in areas exposed to sun or ultraviolet light.

Treatment

This medication is used for treatment of heart conditions (for instance, angina pectoris) and high blood pressure. Tablets, capsules or extended-release tablets should be taken with liquid. The usual dose amounts to 30 to 100 milligrams a day.

For safe and effective use of medicine:

◆ Follow your doctor's instructions if this medicine was prescribed.

◆ Follow the manufacturer's package directions if you are treating yourself.

Side effects

Along with the needed effects, a medicine may cause some unwanted effects. Possible side effects include:

Tiredness

Changes in heartbeat

Wheezing

Cough

Shortness of breath

Dizziness

Fainting

Numbness in hands and feet

Tingling in hands and feet

Difficult urination

Constipation

Overdose

The following symptoms may be a sign of overdose:

Unusually fast heartbeat

Unusually slow heartbeat

Loss of consciousness

Cardiac arrest

■ Call a doctor or hospital emergency room for instructions. If necessary start first aid immediately.

Interactions

The effect of this medicine may cause a blood pressure drop if taken together with antihypertensives. Cimetidine may increase the effect of the calcium blocker.

The simultaneous use of diuretics and calcium channel blockers may cause dangerous blood pressure drop.

◆ Be sure to tell your doctor about any medications you are currently taking.

Storage

Capsules, tablets, etc. should be stored at room temperature; store away from heat and direct light. Keep out of reach of children, since this medicine may be dangerous in children.

ADIPEX-P

Properties
This medicine contains phentermine as active ingredient; it is prescribed for appetite suppression.

Appetite suppressants are used in the short-term (a few weeks) treatment of obesity. In a few weeks (6 to 12), these medicines in combination with dieting, exercise, and changes in eating habits can help patients lose weight. However, since their appetite reducing effect is only temporary, they are useful only for the first weeks of dieting until new eating habits are established.

Before using this medicine
Before you use this medicine check with your doctor, or pharmacist:
- if you ever had any unusual or allergic reaction to any of the compounds of this medicine.
- if you are on a low-salt, low-sugar, or any other special diet, or if you are allergic to any substance, such as sulfites or other preservatives or dyes.
- if you are pregnant, intend to become pregnant or breast-feeding an infant while using this medicine.
- if you have any of the following medical problems:
Diabetes mellitus
Epilepsy
Glaucoma
Heart disease
High blood pressure
Mental illness (severe)

Treatment
This medication is used to relieve or prevent the symptoms of your medical problem.

Take them as directed. Do not take more of them and do not take them more often than recommended on the label. If too much of the drug is taken, it may become habit-forming.
- The medicine produces central nervous system stimulation, and it should not be taken by people with heart disease or high blood pressure.
- If you think this medicine is not working as well after you have taken it for a few weeks, do not increase the dose. Instead, check with your doctor.

Side effects
The following minor side effects may occur: irritability, nervousness, restlessness, trouble in sleeping.

These side effects should disappear as your body adjusts to the medication. Tell your doctor about any side effects that are persistent or particularly bothersome. It is especially important to tell your doctor about:
Mental depression
Nausea or vomiting
Stomach cramps or pain
Trembling
Unusual tiredness
- Discontinue use of the drug; call your doctor right away. Adverse reactions and side effects may be more frequent and severe in people over age 60 than in younger persons.

Interactions
This medicine interacts with several other drugs such as antihypertensives, other appetite suppressants, caffeine, central nervous system depressants, central nervous system stimulants, furazolidone, guanethidine, hydralazine, MAO inhibitors, methyldopa, molindone, phenothiazines, rauwolfia alkaloids, sodium bicarbonate.
- Be sure to tell your doctor about any medications you are currently taking.

Interaction with alcoholic beverages may produce drowsiness, sleepiness, and/or inability to concentrate.

Storage
This medicine should be stored at room temperature in tightly closed containers. Store away from heat and direct light. Keep out of reach of children, since overdose may be very dangerous in children. Do not store this medicine in the bathroom medicine cabinet because the heat and moisture cause the medicine to break down. Do not keep outdated medicine or medicine no longer needed. Flush the contents of the container down the toilet.

ADIPIN

Properties

This medicine contains doxepin as active ingredient. It belongs to the group of medicines known as tricyclic antidepressants or 'mood elevators.' It is used to relieve mental depression and depression that sometimes occurs with anxiety. The medication gradually relieves, but doesn't cure, symptoms of depression. The medication may also be used for the treatment of narcolepsy, bulimia, panic attacks, cocaine withdrawal, attention deficit disorder.

Before using this medicine

Before you use this medicine check with your doctor, or pharmacist:
- if you ever had any unusual or allergic reaction to any tricyclic antidepressant, maprotiline or trazodone.
- if you are on a low-salt, low-sugar, or any other special diet, or if you are allergic to any substance, such as sulfites or other preservatives or dyes.
- if you are pregnant or intend to become pregnant while using this medicine. There have been reports of newborns suffering from heart, breathing, and urinary problems when their mothers had taken tricyclic antidepressants before delivery.
- if you are breast-feeding an infant. Some tricyclic antidepressants pass into the breast milk.

Treatment

Take this medicine only as directed by your doctor, to benefit your condition as much as possible. Do not take more of it, do not take it more often, and do not take it for a longer period of time than your doctor ordered.

To lessen stomach upset, take this medicine with food, even for a daily bedtime dose, unless your doctor has told you to take it on an empty stomach. If you forget your once-a-day bedtime dose, don't take it more than 3 hours late. If more than 3 hours, wait for next scheduled dose.

Sometimes this medicine must be taken for several weeks before you begin to feel better.

Side effects

Along with the needed effects, a medicine may cause some unwanted effects. Side effects that usually do not require medical attention: difficult or frequent urination; decreased sex drive; muscle aches; abnormal dreams; nasal congestion; weakness and faintness when arising from bed or chair; back pain.
- Other side effects that should be reported to your doctor immediately are:
  Hallucinations
  Shakiness
  Dizziness or fainting
  Blurred vision, eye pain
  Irregular heartbeat or slow pulse
  Inflamed tongue
  Abdominal pain
  Jaundice
  Hair loss, rash
  Fever, chills
  Joint pain
  Palpitations

Interactions

This medicine may interact with several other drugs such as anticoagulants, anticholinergics, cold remedies, oral contraceptives, seizure medicines, sleeping medicines, thyroid medicines, etc.
- Be sure to tell your doctor about any medications you are currently taking.

Storage

Tablets, capsules, etc. should be stored at room temperature in tightly closed, light-resistant containers as directed by your pharmacist. Keep out of reach of children since overdose is especially dangerous in young children. Do not store in the bathroom medicine cabinet because the heart or moisture may cause the medicine to break down. Keep the liquid form of the medicine from freezing.

ADIPOST

Properties
This medicine contains phendimetrazine as active ingredient; it is prescribed for appetite suppression.

Appetite suppressants are used in the short-term (a few weeks) treatment of obesity. In a few weeks (6 to 12), these medicines in combination with dieting, exercise, and changes in eating habits can help patients lose weight. However, since their appetite reducing effect is only temporary, they are useful only for the first weeks of dieting until new eating habits are established.

Before using this medicine
Before you use this medicine check with your doctor, or pharmacist:
- if you ever had any unusual or allergic reaction to any of the compounds of this medicine.
- if you are on a low-salt, low-sugar, or any other special diet, or if you are allergic to any substance, such as sulfites or other preservatives or dyes.
- if you are pregnant, intend to become pregnant or breast-feeding an infant while using this medicine.
- if you have any of the following medical problems:
  Diabetes mellitus (sugar diabetes)
  Epilepsy
  Glaucoma
  Heart or blood vessel disease
  High blood pressure
  Mental illness (severe)

Treatment
This medication is used to relieve or prevent the symptoms of your medical problem. Take them as directed. Do not take more of them and do not take them more often than recommended on the label. If too much of the drug is taken, it may become habit-forming.

The medicine produces central nervous system stimulation, and it should not be taken by people with heart disease or high blood pressure.

If you think this medicine is not working as well after you have taken it for a few weeks, do not increase the dose. Instead, check with your doctor.

Side effects
The following minor side effects may occur: irritability, nervousness, restlessness, trouble in sleeping.

These side effects should disappear as your body adjusts to the medication. Tell your doctor about any side effects that are persistent or particularly bothersome. It is especially important to tell your doctor about:
  Mental depression
  Nausea or vomiting
  Stomach cramps or pain
  Trembling
  Unusual tiredness or weakness
- Discontinue use of the drug; call your doctor right away. Adverse reactions and side effects may be more frequent and severe in people over age 60 than in younger persons.

Interactions
This medicine interacts with several other drugs such as antihypertensives, other appetite suppressants, caffeine, central nervous system depressants, central nervous system stimulants, furazolidone, guanethidine, hydralazine, MAO inhibitors, methyldopa, molindone, phenothiazines, rauwolfia alkaloids, sodium bicarbonate.
- Be sure to tell your doctor about any medications you are currently taking.

Interaction with alcoholic beverages may produce drowsiness, sleepiness, and/or inability to concentrate.

Storage
This medicine should be stored at room temperature in tightly closed containers. Store away from heat and direct light. Keep out of reach of children, since overdose may be very dangerous in children. Do not store this medicine in the bathroom medicine cabinet because the heat and moisture cause the medicine to break down. Do not keep outdated medicine or medicine no longer needed. Flush the contents of the container down the toilet.

ADPHEN

Properties
This medicine contains phendimetrazine as active ingredient; it is prescribed for appetite suppression.

Appetite suppressants are used in the short-term (a few weeks) treatment of obesity. In a few weeks (6 to 12), these medicines in combination with dieting, exercise, and changes in eating habits can help patients lose weight. However, since their appetite reducing effect is only temporary, they are useful only for the first weeks of dieting until new eating habits are established.

Before using this medicine
Before you use this medicine check with your doctor, or pharmacist:
- if you ever had any unusual or allergic reaction to any of the compounds of this medicine.
- if you are on a low-salt, low-sugar, or any other special diet, or if you are allergic to any substance, such as sulfites or other preservatives or dyes.
- if you are pregnant, intend to become pregnant or breast-feeding an infant while using this medicine.
- if you have any of the following medical problems:
  Diabetes mellitus (sugar diabetes)
  Epilepsy
  Glaucoma
  Heart or blood vessel disease
  High blood pressure
  Mental illness (severe)

Treatment
This medication is used to relieve or prevent the symptoms of your medical problem. Take them as directed. Do not take more of them and do not take them more often than recommended on the label. If too much of the drug is taken, it may become habit-forming.

The medicine produces central nervous system stimulation, and it should not be taken by people with heart disease or high blood pressure.

If you think this medicine is not working as well after you have taken it for a few weeks, do not increase the dose. Instead, check with your doctor.

Side effects
The following minor side effects may occur: irritability, nervousness, restlessness, trouble in sleeping.

These side effects should disappear as your body adjusts to the medication. Tell your doctor about any side effects that are persistent or particularly bothersome. It is especially important to tell your doctor about:
  Mental depression
  Nausea or vomiting
  Stomach cramps or pain
  Trembling
  Unusual tiredness or weakness
- Discontinue use of the drug; call your doctor right away. Adverse reactions and side effects may be more frequent and severe in people over age 60 than in younger persons.

Interactions
This medicine interacts with several other drugs such as antihypertensives, other appetite suppressants, caffeine, central nervous system depressants, central nervous system stimulants, furazolidone, guanethidine, hydralazine, MAO inhibitors, methyldopa, molindone, phenothiazines, rauwolfia alkaloids, sodium bicarbonate.

Interaction with alcoholic beverages may produce drowsiness, sleepiness, and/or inability to concentrate.
- Be sure to tell your doctor about any medications you are currently taking.

Storage
This medicine should be stored at room temperature in tightly closed containers. Store away from heat and direct light. Keep out of reach of children, since overdose may be very dangerous in children.

Do not store this medicine in the bathroom medicine cabinet because the heat and moisture cause the medicine to break down. Do not keep outdated medicine or medicine no longer needed. Flush the contents of the container down the toilet.

AEROLATE

Properties
This medicine contains theophylline as active ingredient; it is used to treat or prevent breathing problems (wheezing and shortness of breath) caused by asthma, bronchitis, or emphysema. This medication belongs to a group known as xanthine-derivative bronchodilators. They work by opening up the bronchial tubes or air passages of the lungs and increasing the flow of air through them. These medicines are available only with your doctor's prescription.

Before using this medicine
Before you use this medicine check with your doctor, or pharmacist:
- if you ever had any unusual or allergic reaction to xanthine-derivative bronchodilators.
- if you are on a low-salt, low-sugar, or any other special diet, or if you are allergic to any substance, such as sulfites or other preservatives or dyes.
- if you are pregnant or intend to become pregnant while using this medicine.
- if you are breast-feeding an infant. Theophylline passes into the breast milk and may cause irritability, fretfulness, or trouble in sleeping in infants of mothers taking this medicine.
- if you have any of the following medical problems:
Diarrhea
Enlarged prostate
Fibrocystic breast disease
Heart disease
Stomach ulcer

Treatment
This medication is used to relieve or prevent the symptoms of your medical problem. Take them as directed. Do not take more of them and do not take them more often than recommended on the label, unless otherwise directed by your doctor. To do so may increase the chance of side effects. The medicine should be taken on an empty stomach 30 to 60 minutes before a meal or two hours after a meal. Try not to miss any doses of this medication. If you do miss a dose, take the missed dose as soon as possible, unless it is almost time for the next dose. Do not double the next dose. It works best when taken with a glass of water.

Side effects
The following minor side effects may occur:
Dizziness or flushing
Headache
Diarrhea
Heartburn
Increased urination
Insomnia
Nervousness or irritability
Loss of appetite
Nausea or stomach upset
Stomach pain.
These side effects should disappear as your body adjusts to the medication. Tell your doctor about any side effects that are persistent or particularly bothersome. It is especially important to tell your doctor about black, tarry stools; confusion; convulsions; difficulty in breathing; fainting; muscle twitching; palpitations; rash; severe abdominal pain; or unusual weakness.

Interactions
This medicine interacts with several other drugs such as diuretics, reserpine, beta blockers, phenytoin, lithium, phenobarbital, birth control pills, and other medications.
- Be sure to tell your doctor about any medications you are currently taking.

Storage
Tablets, capsules, liquid and suspension should be stored at room temperature in tightly closed containers. Store away from heat and direct light. Keep out of reach of children, since overdose may be very dangerous in children. Discard any outdated medication.

ALPHATREX

Properties
This medicine contains betamethasone, a corticosteroid, as active ingredient. Corticosteroids are used to help relieve redness, swelling, itching, inflammation, and discomfort of many skin problems. They exert this effect by interfering with natural body mechanisms that produce the rash, itching, or inflammation. They do not cure the underlying cause of the skin problem. This medication is applied to the skin.

Before using this medicine
Before you use this medicine check with your doctor, or pharmacist:
- if you ever had any unusual or allergic reaction to corticosteroids.
- if you are allergic to any substance, such as sulfites or other preservatives or dyes.
- if you are pregnant or intend to become pregnant while using this medicine. Studies have shown that corticosteroids applied to the skin in large amounts or over long periods of time can be the cause of birth defects.
- if you are breast-feeding an infant. Some corticosteroids pass into breast milk and may interfere with the infant's growth.

Treatment
Do not use this medicine more often or for a longer time than ordered. To do so may increase absorption through the skin and the chance of side effects. In addition, too much use, especially on areas with thinner skin (for example, face, armpits, groin), may result in thinning of the skin and stretch marks.

Before applying this medication, wash your hands. than, unless your doctor or pharmacist gives you different instructions, gently wash the area where the medication is to be applied. With a clean towel pat the area dry. Apply a small amount of the medication to the affected area in a thin layer. Do not bandage the area unless your doctor tells you to do so.

If you miss a dose of this medication, apply the dose as soon as possible, unless it is almost time for the next application.

- ◆ Do not use this medicine for other skin problems without first checking with your doctor. You should not use a topical corticosteroid if you have a virus disease (such as herpes), fungal infection of the skin (such as athlete's foot), or tuberculosis of the skin.

Side effects
There are a number of side effects that usually do not require medical attention. Minor side effects are:
  Acne
  Burning sensations
  Itching
  Rash
  Skin dryness

These possible side effects may go away during treatment; however, if they continue or are bothersome, check with your doctor, nurse, or pharmacist. Tell your doctor about any side effects that are persistent or particularly bothersome, such as:
  Blistering
  Increased hair growth
  Irritation of the affected area
  Loss of skin
  Secondary infection in the area being treated
  Thinning of the skin with easy bruising

Interactions
None known as long as it is used according to the directions given to you by your doctor or pharmacist.

Storage
Cream, ointment, lotion, gel, spray, and aerosol should be stored at room temperature in tightly closed containers. This medication should never be frozen.

ALURATE

Properties

This medicine contains as active ingredient the barbiturate aprobarbital. Barbiturates belong to the group of medicines called central nervous system depressants (medicines that slow down the nervous system).

Barbiturates may partially block nerve impulses at nerve-cell connections. They may be used to treat insomnia (sleeplessness) by helping patients fall asleep. Also, they may be used to relieve anxiety or tension. Some of the barbiturates are used as anticonvulsants to help control convulsions in certain disorders or diseases, such as epilepsy. If too much of the drug is used, it may become habit-forming (causing mental or physical dependence).

Before using this medicine

Before you use this medicine check with your doctor, or pharmacist:
- if you ever had any unusual or allergic reaction to this medicine or one of its components.
- if you are on a low-salt, low-sugar, or any other special diet, or if you are allergic to preservatives or dyes.
- if you are pregnant or intend to become pregnant while using this medicine, since barbiturates have been shown to increase the chance of birth defects in humans. Taking barbiturates regularly during the last 3 months of pregnancy may cause the baby to become dependent on the medicine. This may lead to withdrawal side effects in the baby after birth.
- if you have any of the following medical problems:
  Anemia (severe)
  Diabetes mellitus (sugar disease)
  Hyperactivity (in children)
  Kidney or liver disease
  Mental depression
  Overactive thyroid

Treatment

This medication is used to treat the symptoms of your medical condition. Barbiturates act in the central nervous system; some of their side effects are also caused by actions in the central nervous system. Use this medicine as directed by your doctor. Do not use more of it, do not use it more often, and do not use it for a longer period of time than your doctor ordered.

- If you are taking this medication on a regular schedule and you miss a dose, take the missed dose as soon as possible, unless it is almost time for your next dose. In that case do not take the missed dose at all.
- If a barbiturate is used for a long time, is may become habit-forming. Physical dependence may lead to withdrawal side effects when you stop taking this medicine.

Side effects

Along with the needed effects, a medicine may cause some unwanted effects. These side effects may go away during treatment as your body adjusts to the medicine. Such minor side effects are: depression, confusion, diarrhea, nausea, vomiting, joint or muscle pain, slurred speech, hallucinations, headache, decreased sex drive.

- Check with your doctor immediately if any of the following side effects occur:
  Rash or hives
  Face, lip or eyelid swelling
  Sore throat, fever
  Agitation
  Slow heartbeat
  Difficult breathing or chest pain

Interactions

This medicine may interact with several other drugs such as medicines acting on the central nervous system (e.g., antihistamines; beta-adrenergic blockers; MAO inhibitors; mind-altering drugs; nabilone; antidepressants; clozapine; anticonvulsants).

Storage

The medicine should be stored at room temperature in a tightly closed, light-resistant container. Keep out of reach of children since overdose is very dangerous in children.

ALZAPAM

Properties
This medicine contains as active ingredient lorazepam, a benzodiazepine preparation. Benzodiazepines belong to the group of psychoactive medicines that influence the activity of the brain. Some are used to relieve nervousness or tension. It is effective for this purpose for short periods. Others are used for sleeplessness or to relax muscles or relieve muscle spasm. The benzodiazepines may also be used for other conditions as determined by your doctor.

Before using this medicine
Before you use this medicine check with your doctor:
- if you ever had any unusual or allergic reaction to benzodiazepines.
- if you are on a low-salt, low-sugar, or any other special diet, or if you are allergic to any substance, such as sulfites or other preservatives or dyes.
- if you are pregnant or intend to become pregnant while using this medicine. Some benzodiazepines have been reported to increase the chance of birth defects when used during the first 3 months of pregnancy.
- if you are breast-feeding an infant. Benzodiazepines may pass into the breast milk and cause drowsiness, unusually slow heartbeat, shortness of breath, or troubled breathing in infants of mothers taking this medicine.
- if you have any of the following medical problems: asthma, bronchitis, emphysema, or other chronic lung disease; epilepsy or history of convulsions; hyperactivity (in children); kidney or liver disease; mental depression or illness; myasthania gravis, porphyria.

Treatment
This medication is used to relieve or prevent the symptoms of your medical problem. Benzodiazepines are mainly used as antianxiety agents, anticonvulsants, or sedatives. Take them as directed. Do not take more of them and do not take them more often than recommended on the label, unless otherwise directed by your doctor. Benzodiazepine tranquilizing drugs can be abused if taken for long periods of time and it is possible to develop withdrawal symptoms if you discontinue the therapy abruptly.

Side effects
Along with the needed effects, a medicine may cause some unwanted effects. Minor side effects are: bitter taste in the mouth, dizziness, drowsiness, depression, constipation, dry mouth, excessive salivation, fatigue, flushing, headache, heartburn, loss of appetite, nausea, nervousness, sweating or vomiting. As your body adjusts to the medicine, these side effects should disappear.
- Tell your doctor about any side effects that are persistent or particularly bothersome. It is especially important to tell your doctor about:
  Blurred or double vision
  Chest pain
  Difficulty in urinating
  Fainting or falling
  Fever or hallucinations
  Joint pain
  Mouth sores
  Nightmares
  Palpitations
  Severe depression
  Shortness of breath
  Slurred speech
  Uncoordinated movements
  Unusual tiredness
  Yellowing of the skin

Interactions
This medicine may interact with several other drugs. Be sure to tell your doctor about any medications you are currently taking. This medicine will add to the effects of alcohol, and CNS depressants.

Storage
Store at room temperature in tightly closed, light-resistant-resistant containers. Keep out of the reach of children since overdose may be especially dangerous in children.

AMITRIL

Properties
This medicine contains amitriptyline as active ingredient. It belongs to the group of medicines known as tricyclic antidepressants or 'mood elevators.' It is used to relieve mental depression and depression that sometimes occurs with anxiety. The medication gradually relieves, but doesn't cure, symptoms of depression. The medication may also be used for the treatment of narcolepsy, bulimia, panic attacks, cocaine withdrawal, attention deficit disorder.

Before using this medicine
Before you use this medicine check with your doctor, or pharmacist:
- if you ever had any unusual or allergic reaction to any tricyclic antidepressant, maprotiline or trazodone.
- if you are on a low-salt, low-sugar, or any other special diet, or if you are allergic to any substance, such as sulfites or other preservatives or dyes.
- if you are pregnant or intend to become pregnant while using this medicine. There have been reports of newborns suffering from heart, breathing, and urinary problems when their mothers had taken tricyclic antidepressants before delivery.
- if you are breast-feeding an infant. Some tricyclic antidepressants pass into the breast milk.

Treatment
Take this medicine only as directed by your doctor, to benefit your condition as much as possible.

Do not take more of it, do not take it more often, and do not take it for a longer period of time than your doctor ordered.

To lessen stomach upset, take this medicine with food, even for a daily bedtime dose, unless your doctor has told you to take it on an empty stomach.

If you forget your once-a-day bedtime dose, don't take it more than 3 hours late. If more than 3 hours, wait for next scheduled dose. Sometimes this medicine must be taken for several weeks before you begin to feel better.

Side effects
Along with the needed effects, a medicine may cause some unwanted effects. Side effects that usually do not require medical attention: difficult or frequent urination; decreased sex drive; muscle aches; abnormal dreams; nasal congestion; weakness and faintness when arising from bed or chair; back pain.
- Other side effects that should be reported to your doctor immediately are:
  Hallucinations
  Shakiness
  Dizziness or fainting
  Blurred vision, eye pain
  Irregular heartbeat or slow pulse
  Inflamed tongue
  Abdominal pain
  Jaundice
  Hair loss, rash
  Fever, chills
  Joint pain
  Palpitations

Interactions
This medicine may interact with several other drugs such as anticoagulants, anticholinergics, cold remedies, oral contraceptives, seizure medicines, sleeping medicines, thyroid medicines, etc.
- Be sure to tell your doctor about any medications you are currently taking.

Storage
Tablets, capsules, etc. should be stored at room temperature in tightly closed, light-resistant containers as directed by your pharmacist. Keep out of reach of children since overdose is especially dangerous in young children. Do not store in the bathroom medicine cabinet because the heat or moisture may cause the medicine to break down. Keep the liquid form of the medicine from freezing.

AMITRIPTYLINE

Properties

This medicine contains amitriptyline as active ingredient. It belongs to the group of medicines known as tricyclic antidepressants or 'mood elevators.' It is used to relieve mental depression and depression that sometimes occurs with anxiety. The medication gradually relieves, but doesn't cure, symptoms of depression. The medication may also be used for the treatment of narcolepsy, bulimia, panic attacks, cocaine withdrawal, attention deficit disorder.

Before using this medicine

Before you use this medicine check with your doctor, or pharmacist:
- if you ever had any unusual or allergic reaction to any tricyclic antidepressant, maprotiline or trazodone.
- if you are on a low-salt, low-sugar, or any other special diet, or if you are allergic to any substance, such as sulfites or other preservatives or dyes.
- if you are pregnant or intend to become pregnant while using this medicine. There have been reports of newborns suffering from heart, breathing, and urinary problems when their mothers had taken tricyclic antidepressants before delivery.
- if you are breast-feeding an infant. Some tricyclic antidepressants pass into the breast milk.

Treatment

Take this medicine only as directed by your doctor, to benefit your condition as much as possible. Do not take more of it, do not take it more often, and do not take it for a longer period of time than your doctor ordered.

To lessen stomach upset, take this medicine with food, even for a daily bedtime dose, unless your doctor has told you to take it on an empty stomach. If you forget your once-a-day bedtime dose, don't take it more than 3 hours late.

If more than 3 hours, wait for next scheduled dose. Sometimes this medicine must be taken for several weeks before you begin to feel better.

Side effects

Along with the needed effects, a medicine may cause some unwanted effects. Side effects that usually do not require medical attention: difficult or frequent urination; decreased sex drive; muscle aches; abnormal dreams; nasal congestion; weakness and faintness when arising from bed or chair; back pain.
- Other side effects that should be reported to your doctor immediately are:
  Hallucinations
  Shakiness
  Dizziness or fainting
  Blurred vision, eye pain
  Irregular heartbeat or slow pulse
  Inflamed tongue
  Abdominal pain
  Jaundice
  Hair loss, rash
  Fever, chills
  Joint pain
  Palpitations

Interactions

This medicine may interact with several other drugs such as anticoagulants, anticholinergics, cold remedies, oral contraceptives, seizure medicines, sleeping medicines, thyroid medicines, etc.
- Be sure to tell your doctor about any medications you are currently taking.

Storage

Tablets, capsules, etc. should be stored at room temperature in tightly closed, light-resistant containers as directed by your pharmacist. Keep out of reach of children since overdose is especially dangerous in young children. Do not store in the bathroom medicine cabinet because the heat or moisture may cause the medicine to break down. Keep the liquid form of the medicine from freezing.

AMLODIPINE

Properties
This medicine contains amlodipine as active ingredient. It is a so-called calcium channel blocker, working by blocking the passage of calcium into heart and smooth muscle. Since calcium is an essential factor in muscle contraction, any medicine that affects calcium in this way will interfere with the contraction of these muscles.

The medicine works by:
- reducing the work that the heart must perform;
- reducing the normal arterial blood pressure;
- increasing oxygen to the heart muscle.

The medicine is prescribed for the treatment of attacks of angina pectoris, irregular heartbeat, and high blood pressure. In many cases it can be used for the treatment and prevention of migraine.

Before using this medicine
Before you use this medicine check with your doctor, or pharmacist:
- if you ever had any unusual or allergic reaction to this medicine or any calcium channel blocker;
- if you are pregnant or intend to become pregnant while using this medicine;
- if you have low blood pressure;
- if you have kidney or liver disease;
- if you are breast-feeding an infant;
- if you easily get a rash or intensity sunburn in areas exposed to sun or ultraviolet light.

Treatment
This medication is used for treatment of heart conditions (for instance, angina pectoris) and high blood pressure. Tablets, capsules or extended-release tablets should be taken with liquid. The usual dose amounts to 30 to 100 milligrams a day.

For safe and effective use of medicine:
- Follow your doctor's instructions if this medicine was prescribed.
- Follow the manufacturer's package directions if you are treating yourself.

Side effects
Along with the needed effects, a medicine may cause some unwanted effects. Possible side effects include:
Tiredness
Changes in heartbeat
Wheezing
Cough
Shortness of breath
Dizziness
Fainting
Numbness in hands and feet
Tingling in hands and feet
Difficult urination
Constipation

Overdose
The following symptoms may be a sign of overdose:
Unusually fast heartbeat
Unusually slow heartbeat
Loss of consciousness
Cardiac arrest
- Call a doctor or hospital emergency room for instructions. If necessary start first aid immediately.

Interactions
The effect of this medicine may cause a blood pressure drop if taken together with antihypertensives. Cimetidine may increase the effect of the calcium blocker.

The simultaneous use of diuretics and calcium channel blockers may cause dangerous blood pressure drop.
- Be sure to tell your doctor about any medications you are currently taking.

Storage
Capsules, tablets, etc. should be stored at room temperature; store away from heat and direct light. Keep out of reach of children, since this medicine may be dangerous in children.

AMOBARBITAL

Properties
This medicine contains as active ingredient the barbiturate amobarbital. Barbiturates belong to the group of medicines called central nervous system depressants (medicines that slow down the nervous system).

Barbiturates may partially block nerve impulses at nerve-cell connections. They may be used to treat insomnia (sleeplessness) by helping patients fall asleep. Also, they may be used to relieve anxiety or tension. Some of the barbiturates are used as anticonvulsants to help control convulsions in certain disorders or diseases, such as epilepsy. If too much of the drug is used, it may become habit-forming (causing mental or physical dependence).

Before using this medicine
Before you use this medicine check with your doctor, or pharmacist:
- if you ever had any unusual or allergic reaction to this medicine or one of its components.
- if you are on a low-salt, low-sugar, or any other special diet, or if you are allergic to preservatives or dyes.
- if you are pregnant or intend to become pregnant while using this medicine, since barbiturates have been shown to increase the chance of birth defects in humans. Taking barbiturates regularly during the last 3 months of pregnancy may cause the baby to become dependent on the medicine. This may lead to withdrawal side effects in the baby after birth.
- if you have any of the following medical problems:
Anemia (severe)
Diabetes mellitus (sugar disease)
Hyperactivity (in children)
Kidney or liver disease
Mental depression
Overactive thyroid

Treatment
This medication is used to treat the symptoms of your medical condition. Barbiturates act in the central nervous system; some of their side effects are also caused by actions in the central nervous system. Use this medicine as directed by your doctor. Do not use more of it, do not use it more often, and do not use it for a longer period of time than your doctor ordered.
- If you are taking this medication on a regular schedule and you miss a dose, take the missed dose as soon as possible, unless it is almost time for your next dose. In that case do not take the missed dose at all.
- If a barbiturate is used for a long time, is may become habit-forming. Physical dependence may lead to withdrawal side effects when you stop taking this medicine.

Side effects
Along with the needed effects, a medicine may cause some unwanted effects. These side effects may go away during treatment as your body adjusts to the medicine. Such minor side effects are: depression, confusion, diarrhea, nausea, vomiting, joint or muscle pain, slurred speech, hallucinations, headache, decreased sex drive.
- Check with your doctor immediately if any of the following side effects occur:
Rash or hives
Face, lip or eyelid swelling
Sore throat, fever
Agitation
Slow heartbeat
Difficult breathing or chest pain

Interactions
This medicine may interact with several other drugs such as medicines acting on the central nervous system (e.g., antihistamines; beta-adrenergic blockers; MAO inhibitors; mind-altering drugs; nabilone; antidepressants; clozapine; anticonvulsants).

Storage
The medicine should be stored at room temperature in a tightly closed, light-resistant container. Keep out of reach of children since overdose is very dangerous in children.

AMOXAPINE

Properties

This medicine contains amoxapine as active ingredient. It belongs to the group of medicines known as tricyclic antidepressants or 'mood elevators.' It is used to relieve mental depression and depression that sometimes occurs with anxiety. The medication gradually relieves, but doesn't cure, symptoms of depression. The medication may also be used for the treatment of narcolepsy, bulimia, panic attacks, cocaine withdrawal, attention deficit disorder.

Before using this medicine

Before you use this medicine check with your doctor, or pharmacist:
- if you ever had any unusual or allergic reaction to any tricyclic antidepressant, maprotiline or trazodone.
- if you are on a low-salt, low-sugar, or any other special diet, or if you are allergic to any substance, such as sulfites or other preservatives or dyes.
- if you are pregnant or intend to become pregnant while using this medicine. There have been reports of newborns suffering from heart, breathing, and urinary problems when their mothers had taken tricyclic antidepressants before delivery.
- if you are breast-feeding an infant. Some tricyclic antidepressants pass into the breast milk.

Treatment

Take this medicine only as directed by your doctor, to benefit your condition as much as possible. Do not take more of it, do not take it more often, and do not take it for a longer period of time than your doctor ordered.

To lessen stomach upset, take this medicine with food, even for a daily bedtime dose, unless your doctor has told you to take it on an empty stomach. If you forget your once-a-day bedtime dose, don't take it more than 3 hours late. If more than 3 hours, wait for next scheduled dose.

Sometimes this medicine must be taken for several weeks before you begin to feel better.

Side effects

Along with the needed effects, a medicine may cause some unwanted effects. Side effects that usually do not require medical attention: difficult or frequent urination; decreased sex drive; muscle aches; abnormal dreams; nasal congestion; weakness and faintness when arising from bed or chair; back pain.
- Other side effects that should be reported to your doctor immediately are:
  Hallucinations
  Shakiness
  Dizziness or fainting
  Blurred vision, eye pain
  Irregular heartbeat or slow pulse
  Inflamed tongue
  Abdominal pain
  Jaundice
  Hair loss, rash
  Fever, chills
  Joint pain
  Palpitations

Interactions

This medicine may interact with several other drugs such as anticoagulants, anticholinergics, cold remedies, oral contraceptives, seizure medicines, sleeping medicines, thyroid medicines, etc.
- Be sure to tell your doctor about any medications you are currently taking.

Storage

Tablets, capsules, etc. should be stored at room temperature in tightly closed, light-resistant containers as directed by your pharmacist. Keep out of reach of children since overdose is especially dangerous in young children. Do not store in the bathroom medicine cabinet because the heat or moisture may cause the medicine to break down. Keep the liquid form of the medicine from freezing.

AMYTAL

Properties

This medicine contains as active ingredient the barbiturate amobarbital. Barbiturates belong to the group of medicines called central nervous system depressants (medicines that slow down the nervous system).

Barbiturates may partially block nerve impulses at nerve-cell connections. They may be used to treat insomnia (sleeplessness) by helping patients fall asleep. Also, they may be used to relieve anxiety or tension. Some of the barbiturates are used as anticonvulsants to help control convulsions in certain disorders or diseases, such as epilepsy. If too much of the drug is used, it may become habit-forming (causing mental or physical dependence).

Before using this medicine

Before you use this medicine check with your doctor, or pharmacist:
- if you ever had any unusual or allergic reaction to this medicine or one of its components.
- if you are on a low-salt, low-sugar, or any other special diet, or if you are allergic to preservatives or dyes.
- if you are pregnant or intend to become pregnant while using this medicine, since barbiturates have been shown to increase the chance of birth defects in humans. Taking barbiturates regularly during the last 3 months of pregnancy may cause the baby to become dependent on the medicine. This may lead to withdrawal side effects in the baby after birth.
- if you have any of the following medical problems:
Anemia (severe)
Diabetes mellitus (sugar disease)
Hyperactivity (in children)
Kidney or liver disease
Mental depression
Overactive thyroid

Treatment

This medication is used to treat the symptoms of your medical condition. Barbiturates act in the central nervous system; some of their side effects are also caused by actions in the central nervous system. Use this medicine as directed by your doctor. Do not use more of it, do not use it more often, and do not use it for a longer period of time than your doctor ordered.

- If you are taking this medication on a regular schedule and you miss a dose, take the missed dose as soon as possible, unless it is almost time for your next dose. In that case do not take the missed dose at all.
- If a barbiturate is used for a long time, is may become habit-forming. Physical dependence may lead to withdrawal side effects when you stop taking this medicine.

Side effects

Along with the needed effects, a medicine may cause some unwanted effects. These side effects may go away during treatment as your body adjusts to the medicine. Such minor side effects are: depression, confusion, diarrhea, nausea, vomiting, joint or muscle pain, slurred speech, hallucinations, headache, decreased sex drive.

- Check with your doctor immediately if any of the following side effects occur:
Rash or hives
Face, lip or eyelid swelling
Sore throat, fever
Agitation
Slow heartbeat
Difficult breathing or chest pain

Interactions

This medicine may interact with several other drugs such as medicines acting on the central nervous system (e.g., antihistamines; beta-adrenergic blockers; MAO inhibitors; mind-altering drugs; nabilone; antidepressants; clozapine; anticonvulsants).

Storage

The medicine should be stored at room temperature in a tightly closed, light-resistant container. Keep out of reach of children since overdose is very dangerous in children.

ANABOLIN

Properties

This medicine is a member of the androgenic, or male, hormone group, containing an androgenic preparation as active ingredient. It is used in diseases in which male hormone replacement or augmentation is needed and also in so-called male menopause. It is also used to decrease calcium loss in osteoporosis, to block growth of breast cancer cells in females and to reduce breast pain and fullness following childbirth.

Before using this medicine

Before you use this medicine check with your doctor, or pharmacist:
- if you ever had any unusual or allergic reaction to androgens or corticosteroids in general.
- if you are on a low-salt, low-sugar, or any other special diet, or if you are allergic to any substance, such as certain preservatives or dyes.
- if you have any of the following medical problems:
Cancer prostate
Heart disease or atherosclerosis
Kidney or liver disease
Breast cancer (males)
High blood pressure
High level of blood calcium
Epilepsy

Treatment

This medication is used to relieve or prevent the symptoms of your medical problem. Take them as directed. Do not take more of them and do not take them more often than recommended on the label. One should take the tablets or capsules with food to lessen stomach irritation. Take the medication at the same time each day. If you forget a dose take it as soon as you remember up to two hours late; wait for the next scheduled dose; don't double this dose. The risk to the unborn child outweighs the benefits of the drug.

Side effects

Females taking any androgenic drug should watch for deepening of the voice, oily skin, acne, hairiness, increased libido, and menstrual irregularities.

The following side effects may occur:
Acne or oily skin
Deep voice
Enlarged clitoris in females
Frequent erections in men
Sore mouth
Higher sex drive
Impotence in men
Yellow skin or eyes
These side effects should disappear as your body adjusts to the medication. Tell your doctor about any side effects that are persistent or particularly bothersome.
- Discontinue the use of the medication and seek
emergency treatment in the following situations:
Intense itching
Weakness
Loss of consciousness
Depression or confusion
Swollen feet or legs
Shortness of breath
Irregularities of heartbeat
Difficult urination
Vaginal bleeding in women
Scrotum pain in men

Interactions

This medicine interacts with several other drugs such as anticoagulants, oral antidiabetics, cyclosporine, hepatotoxic drugs, oxyphenbutazone, phenobarbital, and phenylbutazone.
- Be sure to tell your doctor about any medications you are currently taking.

Storage

This medicine should be stored at room temperature in closed containers. Store away from heat and direct light. Keep out of reach of children, since overdose may be dangerous in children.

ANADROL

Properties

This medicine is a member of the androgenic, or male, hormone group, containing an androgenic preparation as active ingredient. It is used in diseases in which male hormone replacement or augmentation is needed and also in so-called male menopause. It is also used to decrease calcium loss in osteoporosis, to block growth of breast cancer cells in females and to reduce breast pain and fullness following childbirth.

Before using this medicine

Before you use this medicine check with your doctor, or pharmacist:

- if you ever had any unusual or allergic reaction to androgens or corticosteroids in general.
- if you are on a low-salt, low-sugar, or any other special diet, or if you are allergic to any substance, such as certain preservatives or dyes.
- if you have any of the following medical problems:
  Cancer prostate
  Heart disease or atherosclerosis
  Kidney or liver disease
  Breast cancer (males)
  High blood pressure
  High level of blood calcium
  Epilepsy

Treatment

This medication is used to relieve or prevent the symptoms of your medical problem. Take them as directed. Do not take more of them and do not take them more often than recommended on the label. One should take the tablets or capsules with food to lessen stomach irritation. Take the medication at the same time each day. If you forget a dose take it as soon as you remember up to two hours late; wait for the next scheduled dose; don't double this dose. The risk to the unborn child outweighs the benefits of the drug.

Side effects

Females taking any androgenic drug should watch for deepening of the voice, oily skin, acne, hairiness, increased libido, and menstrual irregularities.

The following side effects may occur:
  Acne or oily skin
  Deep voice
  Enlarged clitoris in females
  Frequent erections in men
  Sore mouth
  Higher sex drive
  Impotence in men
  Yellow skin or eyes

These side effects should disappear as your body adjusts to the medication. Tell your doctor about any side effects that are persistent or particularly bothersome.

- Discontinue the use of the medication and seek emergency treatment in the following situations:
  Intense itching
  Weakness
  Loss of consciousness
  Depression or confusion
  Swollen feet or legs
  Shortness of breath
  Irregularities of heartbeat
  Difficult urination
  Vaginal bleeding in women
  Scrotum pain in men

Interactions

This medicine interacts with several other drugs such as anticoagulants, oral antidiabetics, cyclosporine, hepatotoxic drugs, oxyphenbutazone, phenobarbital, and phenylbutazone.

- Be sure to tell your doctor about any medications you are currently taking.

Storage

This medicine should be stored at room temperature in closed containers. Store away from heat and direct light. Keep out of reach of children, since overdose may be dangerous in children.

ANAFRANIL

Properties
This medicine contains clomipramine as active ingredient. It belongs to the group of medicines known as tricyclic antidepressants or 'mood elevators.' It is used to relieve mental depression and depression that sometimes occurs with anxiety. The medication gradually relieves, but doesn't cure, symptoms of depression. The medication may also be used for the treatment of narcolepsy, bulimia, panic attacks, cocaine withdrawal, attention deficit disorder.

Before using this medicine
Before you use this medicine check with your doctor, or pharmacist:
- if you ever had any unusual or allergic reaction to any tricyclic antidepressant, maprotiline or trazodone.
- if you are on a low-salt, low-sugar, or any other special diet, or if you are allergic to any substance, such as sulfites or other preservatives or dyes.
- if you are pregnant or intend to become pregnant while using this medicine. There have been reports of newborns suffering from heart, breathing, and urinary problems when their mothers had taken tricyclic antidepressants before delivery.
- if you are breast-feeding an infant. Some tricyclic antidepressants pass into the breast milk.

Treatment
Take this medicine only as directed by your doctor, to benefit your condition as much as possible. Do not take more of it, do not take it more often, and do not take it for a longer period of time than your doctor ordered.

To lessen stomach upset, take this medicine with food, even for a daily bedtime dose, unless your doctor has told you to take it on an empty stomach.

If you forget your once-a-day bedtime dose, don't take it more than 3 hours late.

If more than 3 hours, wait for next scheduled dose. Sometimes this medicine must be taken for several weeks before you begin to feel better.

Side effects
Along with the needed effects, a medicine may cause some unwanted effects. Side effects that usually do not require medical attention: difficult or frequent urination; decreased sex drive; muscle aches; abnormal dreams; nasal congestion; weakness and faintness when arising from bed or chair; back pain.
- Other side effects that should be reported to your doctor immediately are:
  Hallucinations
  Shakiness
  Dizziness or fainting
  Blurred vision, eye pain
  Irregular heartbeat or slow pulse
  Inflamed tongue
  Abdominal pain
  Jaundice
  Hair loss, rash
  Fever, chills
  Joint pain
  Palpitations

Interactions
This medicine may interact with several other drugs such as anticoagulants, anticholinergics, cold remedies, oral contraceptives, seizure medicines, sleeping medicines, thyroid medicines, etc.
- Be sure to tell your doctor about any medications you are currently taking.

Storage
Tablets, capsules, etc. should be stored at room temperature in tightly closed, light-resistant containers as directed by your pharmacist. Keep out of reach of children since overdose is especially dangerous in young children. Do not store in the bathroom medicine cabinet because the heart or moisture may cause the medicine to break down. Keep the liquid form of the medicine from freezing.

ANAPOLON 50

Properties
This medicine is a member of the androgenic, or male, hormone group, containing an androgenic preparation as active ingredient. It is used in diseases in which male hormone replacement or augmentation is needed and also in so-called male menopause. It is also used to decrease calcium loss in osteoporosis, to block growth of breast cancer cells in females and to reduce breast pain and fullness following childbirth.

Before using this medicine
Before you use this medicine check with your doctor, or pharmacist:
- if you ever had any unusual or allergic reaction to androgens or corticosteroids in general.
- if you are on a low-salt, low-sugar, or any other special diet, or if you are allergic to any substance, such as certain preservatives or dyes.
- if you have any of the following medical problems:
  Cancer prostate
  Heart disease or atherosclerosis
  Kidney or liver disease
  Breast cancer (males)
  High blood pressure
  High level of blood calcium
  Epilepsy

Treatment
This medication is used to relieve or prevent the symptoms of your medical problem. Take them as directed. Do not take more of them and do not take them more often than recommended on the label. One should take the tablets or capsules with food to lessen stomach irritation. Take the medication at the same time each day. If you forget a dose take it as soon as you remember up to two hours late; wait for the next scheduled dose don't double this dose. The risk to the unborn child outweighs the benefits of the drug.

Side effects
Females taking any androgenic drug should watch for deepening of the voice, oily skin, acne, hairiness, increased libido, and menstrual irregularities.

The following side effects may occur:
  Acne or oily skin
  Deep voice
  Enlarged clitoris in females
  Frequent erections in men
  Sore mouth
  Higher sex drive
  Impotence in men
  Yellow skin or eyes
These side effects should disappear as your body adjusts to the medication. Tell your doctor about any side effects that are persistent or particularly bothersome.
- Discontinue the use of the medication and seek emergency treatment in the following situations:
  Intense itching
  Weakness
  Loss of consciousness
  Depression or confusion
  Swollen feet or legs
  Shortness of breath
  Irregularities of heartbeat
  Difficult urination
  Vaginal bleeding in women
  Scrotum pain in men

Interactions
This medicine interacts with several other drugs such as anticoagulants, oral antidiabetics, cyclosporine, hepatotoxic drugs, oxyphenbutazone, phenobarbital, and phenylbutazone.
- Be sure to tell your doctor about any medications you are currently taking.

Storage
This medicine should be stored at room temperature in closed containers. Store away from heat and direct light. Keep out of reach of children, since overdose may be dangerous in children.

ANAVAR

Properties

This medicine is a member of the androgenic, or male, hormone group, containing an androgenic preparation as active ingredient. It is used in diseases in which male hormone replacement or augmentation is needed and also in so-called male menopause. It is also used to decrease calcium loss in osteoporosis, to block growth of breast cancer cells in females and to reduce breast pain and fullness following childbirth.

Before using this medicine

Before you use this medicine check with your doctor, or pharmacist:
- if you ever had any unusual or allergic reaction to androgens or corticosteroids in general.
- if you are on a low-salt, low-sugar, or any other special diet, or if you are allergic to any substance, such as certain preservatives or dyes.
- if you have any of the following medical problems:
  Cancer prostate
  Heart disease or atherosclerosis
  Kidney or liver disease
  Breast cancer (males)
  High blood pressure
  High level of blood calcium
  Epilepsy

Treatment

This medication is used to relieve or prevent the symptoms of your medical problem. Take them as directed. Do not take more of them and do not take them more often than recommended on the label. One should take the tablets or capsules with food to lessen stomach irritation. Take the medication at the same time each day. If you forget a dose take it as soon as you remember up to two hours late; wait for the next scheduled dos;e don't double this dose. The risk to the unborn child outweighs the benefits of the drug.

Side effects

Females taking any androgenic drug should watch for deepening of the voice, oily skin, acne, hairiness, increased libido, and menstrual irregularities.

The following side effects may occur:
  Acne or oily skin
  Deep voice
  Enlarged clitoris in females
  Frequent erections in men
  Sore mouth
  Higher sex drive
  Impotence in men
  Yellow skin or eyes

These side effects should disappear as your body adjusts to the medication. Tell your doctor about any side effects that are persistent or particularly bothersome.

- Discontinue the use of the medication and seek emergency treatment in the following situations:
  Intense itching
  Weakness
  Loss of consciousness
  Depression or confusion
  Swollen feet or legs
  Shortness of breath
  Irregularities of heartbeat
  Difficult urination
  Vaginal bleeding in women
  Scrotum pain in men

Interactions

This medicine interacts with several other drugs such as anticoagulants, oral antidiabetics, cyclosporine, hepatotoxic drugs, oxyphenbutazone, phenobarbital, and phenylbutazone.

- Be sure to tell your doctor about any medications you are currently taking.

Storage

This medicine should be stored at room temperature in closed containers. Store away from heat and direct light. Keep out of reach of children, since overdose may be dangerous in children.

ANCEF

Properties
This medicine contains cephalosporin as active ingredient. Cephalosporins belong to the general family of medicines called antibiotics, used in the treatment of infections caused by bacteria. They work by killing bacteria or preventing their growth. Cephalosporins will not work for colds, flu, or other viral infections.

Before using this medicine
Before you use this medicine check with your doctor:
- if you ever had any unusual or allergic reaction to any of the cephalosporins, penicillins, penicillin-like medicines, or penicillamine.
- if you are on a low-salt, low-sugar, or any other special diet, or if you are allergic to any substance, such as sulfites or other preservatives or dyes.
- if you are pregnant or intend to become pregnant while using this medicine. Although cephalosporins have not been shown to cause birth defects or other problems in humans, the chance always exists.
- if you are breast-feeding an infant. Most cephalosporins pass into the breast milk, usually in small amounts.
- if you have any of the following medical problems:
  Bleeding problem
  Kidney or liver disease

Treatment
This medication belongs to the general family of medicines called antibiotics. It is used to treat a wide variety of bacterial infections. It is also used to treat infections in persons who are allergic to penicillin.
- Keep taking this medicine for the full time of treatment even if you begin to feel better after a few days; do not miss any doses.
- If you do miss a dose of this medicine, take it as soon as possible. This will help to keep a constant amount of medicine in the blood. However, if it is almost time for your next dose, skip the missed dose and go back to your regular dosing schedule.
- This medication has been prescribed for your current infection only. Another infection later on, or one that someone else has, may require a different medicine. You should not give your medicine to other people or use it for other infections, unless your doctor specifically directs you to do so.
- Take the medicine at the same times each day, 1 hour before or 2 hours after eating.

Side effects
Along with the needed effects, a medicine may cause some unwanted effects. Side effects that usually do not require medical attention: rectal itching, oral or vaginal white spots, mild diarrhea. These side effects should disappear as your body adjusts to the medication.
- Other side effects that should be reported to your doctor immediately are:
  Hives, rash
  Intense itching
  Faintness soon after a dose
  Difficulty in breathing
  Nausea and vomiting
  Severe diarrhea
  Unusual weakness or tiredness
  Bleeding or bruising

Interactions
This medicine may interact with several other drugs such as anticoagulants, theophylline preparations, probenecid, tetracyclines, etc.
- Be sure to tell your doctor about any medications you are currently taking.

Storage
Tablets, capsules, etc. should be stored at room temperature. Store the liquid form in the refrigerator. Keep out of the reach of children. Do not keep outdated medicine or medicine no longer needed.

ANDRO 100

Properties
This medicine is a member of the androgenic, or male, hormone group, containing an androgenic preparation as active ingredient. It is used in diseases in which male hormone replacement or augmentation is needed and also in so-called male menopause. It is also used to decrease calcium loss in osteoporosis, to block growth of breast cancer cells in females and to reduce breast pain and fullness following childbirth.

Before using this medicine
Before you use this medicine check with your doctor, or pharmacist:
- if you ever had any unusual or allergic reaction to androgens or corticosteroids in general.
- if you are on a low-salt, low-sugar, or any other special diet, or if you are allergic to any substance, such as certain preservatives or dyes.
- if you have any of the following medical problems:
  Cancer prostate
  Heart disease or atherosclerosis
  Kidney or liver disease
  Breast cancer (males)
  High blood pressure
  High level of blood calcium
  Epilepsy

Treatment
This medication is used to relieve or prevent the symptoms of your medical problem. Take them as directed. Do not take more of them and do not take them more often than recommended on the label. One should take the tablets or capsules with food to lessen stomach irritation. Take the medication at the same time each day. If you forget a dose take it as soon as you remember up to two hours late; wait for the next scheduled dose; don't double this dose. The risk to the unborn child outweighs the benefits of the drug.

Side effects
Females taking any androgenic drug should watch for deepening of the voice, oily skin, acne, hairiness, increased libido, and menstrual irregularities.

The following side effects may occur:
  Acne or oily skin
  Deep voice
  Enlarged clitoris in females
  Frequent erections in men
  Sore mouth
  Higher sex drive
  Impotence in men
  Yellow skin or eyes
These side effects should disappear as your body adjusts to the medication. Tell your doctor about any side effects that are persistent or particularly bothersome.
- Discontinue the use of the medication and seek emergency treatment in the following situations:
  Intense itching
  Weakness
  Loss of consciousness
  Depression or confusion
  Swollen feet or legs
  Shortness of breath
  Irregularities of heartbeat
  Difficult urination
  Vaginal bleeding in women
  Scrotum pain in men

Interactions
This medicine interacts with several other drugs such as anticoagulants, oral antidiabetics, cyclosporine, hepatotoxic drugs, oxyphenbutazone, phenobarbital, and phenylbutazone.
- Be sure to tell your doctor about any medications you are currently taking.

Storage
This medicine should be stored at room temperature in closed containers. Store away from heat and direct light. Keep out of reach of children, since overdose may be dangerous in children.

ANDRO-CYP 100

Properties
This medicine is a member of the androgenic, or male, hormone group, containing an androgenic preparation as active ingredient. It is used in diseases in which male hormone replacement or augmentation is needed and also in so-called male menopause. It is also used to decrease calcium loss in osteoporosis, to block growth of breast cancer cells in females and to reduce breast pain and fullness following childbirth.

Before using this medicine
Before you use this medicine check with your doctor, or pharmacist:
- if you ever had any unusual or allergic reaction to androgens or corticosteroids in general.
- if you are on a low-salt, low-sugar, or any other special diet, or if you are allergic to any substance, such as certain preservatives or dyes.
- if you have any of the following medical problems:
Cancer prostate
Heart disease or atherosclerosis
Kidney or liver disease
Breast cancer (males)
High blood pressure
High level of blood calcium
Epilepsy

Treatment
This medication is used to relieve or prevent the symptoms of your medical problem. Take them as directed. Do not take more of them and do not take them more often than recommended on the label. One should take the tablets or capsules with food to lessen stomach irritation. Take the medication at the same time each day. If you forget a dose take it as soon as you remember up to two hours late; wait for the next scheduled dose; don't double this dose. The risk to the unborn child outweighs the benefits of the drug.

Side effects
Females taking any androgenic drug should watch for deepening of the voice, oily skin, acne, hairiness, increased libido, and menstrual irregularities.

The following side effects may occur:
Acne or oily skin
Deep voice
Enlarged clitoris in females
Frequent erections in men
Sore mouth
Higher sex drive
Impotence in men
Yellow skin or eyes
These side effects should disappear as your body adjusts to the medication. Tell your doctor about any side effects that are persistent or particularly bothersome.
- Discontinue the use of the medication and seek emergency treatment in the following situations:
Intense itching
Weakness
Loss of consciousness
Depression or confusion
Swollen feet or legs
Shortness of breath
Irregularities of heartbeat
Difficult urination
Vaginal bleeding in women
Scrotum pain in men

Interactions
This medicine interacts with several other drugs such as anticoagulants, oral antidiabetics, cyclosporine, hepatotoxic drugs, oxyphenbutazone, phenobarbital, and phenylbutazone.
- Be sure to tell your doctor about any medications you are currently taking.

Storage
This medicine should be stored at room temperature in closed containers. Store away from heat and direct light. Keep out of reach of children, since overdose may be dangerous in children.

ANDROID

Properties
This medicine is a member of the androgenic, or male, hormone group, containing an androgenic preparation as active ingredient. It is used in diseases in which male hormone replacement or augmentation is needed and also in so-called male menopause. It is also used to decrease calcium loss in osteoporosis, to block growth of breast cancer cells in females and to reduce breast pain and fullness following childbirth.

Before using this medicine
Before you use this medicine check with your doctor, or pharmacist:
- if you ever had any unusual or allergic reaction to androgens or corticosteroids in general.
- if you are on a low-salt, low-sugar, or any other special diet, or if you are allergic to any substance, such as certain preservatives or dyes.
- if you have any of the following medical problems:
  Cancer prostate
  Heart disease or atherosclerosis
  Kidney or liver disease
  Breast cancer (males)
  High blood pressure
  High level of blood calcium
  Epilepsy

Treatment
This medication is used to relieve or prevent the symptoms of your medical problem. Take them as directed. Do not take more of them and do not take them more often than recommended on the label. One should take the tablets or capsules with food to lessen stomach irritation. Take the medication at the same time each day. If you forget a dose take it as soon as you remember up to two hours late; wait for the next scheduled dose; don't double this dose. The risk to the unborn child outweighs the benefits of the drug.

Side effects
Females taking any androgenic drug should watch for deepening of the voice, oily skin, acne, hairiness, increased libido, and menstrual irregularities.

The following side effects may occur:
  Acne or oily skin
  Deep voice
  Enlarged clitoris in females
  Frequent erections in men
  Sore mouth
  Higher sex drive
  Impotence in men
  Yellow skin or eyes
These side effects should disappear as your body adjusts to the medication. Tell your doctor about any side effects that are persistent or particularly bothersome.
- Discontinue the use of the medication and seek emergency treatment in the following situations:
  Intense itching
  Weakness
  Loss of consciousness
  Depression or confusion
  Swollen feet or legs
  Shortness of breath
  Irregularities of heartbeat
  Difficult urination
  Vaginal bleeding in women
  Scrotum pain in men

Interactions
This medicine interacts with several other drugs such as anticoagulants, oral antidiabetics, cyclosporine, hepatotoxic drugs, oxyphenbutazone, phenobarbital, and phenylbutazone.
- Be sure to tell your doctor about any medications you are currently taking.

Storage
This medicine should be stored at room temperature in closed containers. Store away from heat and direct light. Keep out of reach of children, since overdose may be dangerous in children.

ANDROLONE

Properties

This medicine is a member of the androgenic, or male, hormone group, containing an androgenic preparation as active ingredient. It is used in diseases in which male hormone replacement or augmentation is needed and also in so-called male menopause. It is also used to decrease calcium loss in osteoporosis, to block growth of breast cancer cells in females and to reduce breast pain and fullness following childbirth.

Before using this medicine

Before you use this medicine check with your doctor, or pharmacist:
- if you ever had any unusual or allergic reaction to androgens or corticosteroids in general.
- if you are on a low-salt, low-sugar, or any other special diet, or if you are allergic to any substance, such as certain preservatives or dyes.
- if you have any of the following medical problems:
Cancer prostate
Heart disease or atherosclerosis
Kidney or liver disease
Breast cancer (males)
High blood pressure
High level of blood calcium
Epilepsy

Treatment

This medication is used to relieve or prevent the symptoms of your medical problem. Take them as directed. Do not take more of them and do not take them more often than recommended on the label. One should take the tablets or capsules with food to lessen stomach irritation. Take the medication at the same time each day. If you forget a dose take it as soon as you remember up to two hours late; wait for the next scheduled dose; don't double this dose. The risk to the unborn child outweighs the benefits of the drug.

Side effects

Females taking any androgenic drug should watch for deepening of the voice, oily skin, acne, hairiness, increased libido, and menstrual irregularities.

The following side effects may occur:
Acne or oily skin
Deep voice
Enlarged clitoris in females
Frequent erections in men
Sore mouth
Higher sex drive
Impotence in men
Yellow skin or eyes

These side effects should disappear as your body adjusts to the medication. Tell your doctor about any side effects that are persistent or particularly bothersome.

- Discontinue the use of the medication and seek emergency treatment in the following situations:
Intense itching
Weakness
Loss of consciousness
Depression or confusion
Swollen feet or legs
Shortness of breath
Irregularities of heartbeat
Difficult urination
Vaginal bleeding in women
Scrotum pain in men

Interactions

This medicine interacts with several other drugs such as anticoagulants, oral antidiabetics, cyclosporine, hepatotoxic drugs, oxyphenbutazone, phenobarbital, and phenylbutazone.

- Be sure to tell your doctor about any medications you are currently taking.

Storage

This medicine should be stored at room temperature in closed containers. Store away from heat and direct light. Keep out of reach of children, since overdose may be dangerous in children.

ANDRONAQ-50

Properties

This medicine is a member of the androgenic, or male, hormone group, containing an androgenic preparation as active ingredient. It is used in diseases in which male hormone replacement or augmentation is needed and also in so-called male menopause. It is also used to decrease calcium loss in osteoporosis, to block growth of breast cancer cells in females and to reduce breast pain and fullness following childbirth.

Before using this medicine

Before you use this medicine check with your doctor, or pharmacist:
- if you ever had any unusual or allergic reaction to androgens or corticosteroids in general.
- if you are on a low-salt, low-sugar, or any other special diet, or if you are allergic to any substance, such as certain preservatives or dyes.
- if you have any of the following medical problems:
Cancer prostate
Heart disease or atherosclerosis
Kidney or liver disease
Breast cancer (males)
High blood pressure
High level of blood calcium
Epilepsy

Treatment

This medication is used to relieve or prevent the symptoms of your medical problem. Take them as directed. Do not take more of them and do not take them more often than recommended on the label. One should take the tablets or capsules with food to lessen stomach irritation. Take the medication at the same time each day. If you forget a dose take it as soon as you remember up to two hours late; wait for the next scheduled dose; don't double this dose. The risk to the unborn child outweighs the benefits of the drug.

Side effects

Females taking any androgenic drug should watch for deepening of the voice, oily skin, acne, hairiness, increased libido, and menstrual irregularities.

The following side effects may occur:
Acne or oily skin
Deep voice
Enlarged clitoris in females
Frequent erections in men
Sore mouth
Higher sex drive
Impotence in men
Yellow skin or eyes

These side effects should disappear as your body adjusts to the medication. Tell your doctor about any side effects that are persistent or particularly bothersome.

- Discontinue the use of the medication and seek emergency treatment in the following situations:
Intense itching
Weakness
Loss of consciousness
Depression or confusion
Swollen feet or legs
Shortness of breath
Irregularities of heartbeat
Difficult urination
Vaginal bleeding in women
Scrotum pain in men

Interactions

This medicine interacts with several other drugs such as anticoagulants, oral antidiabetics, cyclosporine, hepatotoxic drugs, oxyphenbutazone, phenobarbital, and phenylbutazone.

- Be sure to tell your doctor about any medications you are currently taking.

Storage

This medicine should be stored at room temperature in closed containers. Store away from heat and direct light. Keep out of reach of children, since overdose may be dangerous in children.

ANDRONATE

Properties

This medicine is a member of the androgenic, or male, hormone group, containing an androgenic preparation as active ingredient. It is used in diseases in which male hormone replacement or augmentation is needed and also in so-called male menopause. It is also used to decrease calcium loss in osteoporosis, to block growth of breast cancer cells in females and to reduce breast pain and fullness following childbirth.

Before using this medicine

Before you use this medicine check with your doctor, or pharmacist:
- if you ever had any unusual or allergic reaction to androgens or corticosteroids in general.
- if you are on a low-salt, low-sugar, or any other special diet, or if you are allergic to any substance, such as certain preservatives or dyes.
- if you have any of the following medical problems:
Cancer prostate
Heart disease or atherosclerosis
Kidney or liver disease
Breast cancer (males)
High blood pressure
High level of blood calcium
Epilepsy

Treatment

This medication is used to relieve or prevent the symptoms of your medical problem. Take them as directed. Do not take more of them and do not take them more often than recommended on the label. One should take the tablets or capsules with food to lessen stomach irritation. Take the medication at the same time each day. If you forget a dose take it as soon as you remember up to two hours late; wait for the next scheduled dose; don't double this dose. The risk to the unborn child outweighs the benefits of the drug.

Side effects

Females taking any androgenic drug should watch for deepening of the voice, oily skin, acne, hairiness, increased libido, and menstrual irregularities.

The following side effects may occur:
Acne or oily skin
Deep voice
Enlarged clitoris in females
Frequent erections in men
Sore mouth
Higher sex drive
Impotence in men
Yellow skin or eyes
These side effects should disappear as your body adjusts to the medication. Tell your doctor about any side effects that are persistent or particularly bothersome.
- Discontinue the use of the medication and seek emergency treatment in the following situations:
Intense itching
Weakness
Loss of consciousness
Depression or confusion
Swollen feet or legs
Shortness of breath
Irregularities of heartbeat
Difficult urination
Vaginal bleeding in women
Scrotum pain in men

Interactions

This medicine interacts with several other drugs such as anticoagulants, oral antidiabetics, cyclosporine, hepatotoxic drugs, oxyphenbutazone, phenobarbital, and phenylbutazone.
- Be sure to tell your doctor about any medications you are currently taking.

Storage

This medicine should be stored at room temperature in closed containers. Store away from heat and direct light. Keep out of reach of children, since overdose may be dangerous in children.

ANDROPOSITORY 100

Properties
This medicine is a member of the androgenic, or male, hormone group, containing an androgenic preparation as active ingredient. It is used in diseases in which male hormone replacement or augmentation is needed and also in so-called male menopause. It is also used to decrease calcium loss in osteoporosis, to block growth of breast cancer cells in females and to reduce breast pain and fullness following childbirth.

Before using this medicine
Before you use this medicine check with your doctor, or pharmacist:
- if you ever had any unusual or allergic reaction to androgens or corticosteroids in general.
- if you are on a low-salt, low-sugar, or any other special diet, or if you are allergic to any substance, such as certain preservatives or dyes.
- if you have any of the following medical problems:
Cancer prostate
Heart disease or atherosclerosis
Kidney or liver disease
Breast cancer (males)
High blood pressure
High level of blood calcium
Epilepsy

Treatment
This medication is used to relieve or prevent the symptoms of your medical problem. Take them as directed. Do not take more of them and do not take them more often than recommended on the label. One should take the tablets or capsules with food to lessen stomach irritation. Take the medication at the same time each day. If you forget a dose take it as soon as you remember up to two hours late; wait for the next scheduled dose; don't double this dose. The risk to the unborn child outweighs the benefits of the drug.

Side effects
Females taking any androgenic drug should watch for deepening of the voice, oily skin, acne, hairiness, increased libido, and menstrual irregularities.

The following side effects may occur:
Acne or oily skin
Deep voice
Enlarged clitoris in females
Frequent erections in men
Sore mouth
Higher sex drive
Impotence in men
Yellow skin or eyes
These side effects should disappear as your body adjusts to the medication. Tell your doctor about any side effects that are persistent or particularly bothersome.
- Discontinue the use of the medication and seek emergency treatment in the following situations:
Intense itching
Weakness
Loss of consciousness
Depression or confusion
Swollen feet or legs
Shortness of breath
Difficult urination
Vaginal bleeding in women
Scrotum pain in men

Interactions
This medicine interacts with several other drugs such as anticoagulants, oral antidiabetics, cyclosporine, hepatotoxic drugs, oxyphenbutazone, phenobarbital, and phenylbutazone.
- Be sure to tell your doctor about any medications you are currently taking.

Storage
This medicine should be stored at room temperature in closed containers. Store away from heat and direct light. Keep out of reach of children, since overdose may be dangerous in children.

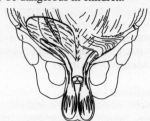

ANDRYL 200

Properties

This medicine is a member of the androgenic, or male, hormone group, containing an androgenic preparation as active ingredient. It is used in diseases in which male hormone replacement or augmentation is needed and also in so-called male menopause. It is also used to decrease calcium loss in osteoporosis, to block growth of breast cancer cells in females and to reduce breast pain and fullness following childbirth.

Before using this medicine

Before you use this medicine check with your doctor, or pharmacist:
- if you ever had any unusual or allergic reaction to androgens or corticosteroids in general.
- if you are on a low-salt, low-sugar, or any other special diet, or if you are allergic to any substance, such as certain preservatives or dyes.
- if you have any of the following medical problems:
  Cancer prostate
  Heart disease or atherosclerosis
  Kidney or liver disease
  Breast cancer (males)
  High blood pressure
  High level of blood calcium
  Epilepsy

Treatment

This medication is used to relieve or prevent the symptoms of your medical problem. Take them as directed. Do not take more of them and do not take them more often than recommended on the label. One should take the tablets or capsules with food to lessen stomach irritation. Take the medication at the same time each day. If you forget a dose take it as soon as you remember up to two hours late; wait for the next scheduled dose; don't double this dose. The risk to the unborn child outweighs the benefits of the drug.

Side effects

Females taking any androgenic drug should watch for deepening of the voice, oily skin, acne, hairiness, increased libido, and menstrual irregularities.

The following side effects may occur:
  Acne or oily skin
  Deep voice
  Enlarged clitoris in females
  Frequent erections in men
  Sore mouth
  Higher sex drive
  Impotence in men
  Yellow skin or eyes

These side effects should disappear as your body adjusts to the medication. Tell your doctor about any side effects that are persistent or particularly bothersome.

- Discontinue the use of the medication and seek emergency treatment in the following situations:
  Intense itching
  Weakness
  Loss of consciousness
  Depression or confusion
  Swollen feet or legs
  Shortness of breath
  Irregularities of heartbeat
  Difficult urination
  Vaginal bleeding in women
  Scrotum pain in men

Interactions

This medicine interacts with several other drugs such as anticoagulants, oral antidiabetics, cyclosporine, hepatotoxic drugs, oxyphenbutazone, phenobarbital, and phenylbutazone.

- Be sure to tell your doctor about any medications you are currently taking.

Storage

This medicine should be stored at room temperature in closed containers. Store away from heat and direct light. Keep out of reach of children, since overdose may be dangerous in children.

ANG-0-SPAN

Properties
This medicine contains nitroglycerin as active ingredient. Nitrates improve the supply of blood and oxygen to the heart. This medication is for oral use.

Before using this medicine
Before you use this medicine check with your doctor, or pharmacist:
- if you ever had any unusual or allergic reaction to nitrates or nitrites.
- if you are on a low-salt, low-sugar, or any other special diet, or if you are allergic to any substance, such as sulfites or other preservatives or dyes.
- if you are pregnant or intend to become pregnant while using this medicine. Although nitrates have not been shown to cause problems in humans, the chance always exists.
- if you are breast-feeding an infant.
- if you have recently had a heart attack or stroke.
- if you have any of the following medical problems:
  Anemia
  Glaucoma
  Intestinal problems
  Overactive thyroid
- if you are now taking any of the following medicines or types of medicines:
  Antihypertensives
  Asthma or hay fever medicine
  Cold medicine
  Decongestant
  Medicine for appetite control
  Narcotic
  Pain medicine
  Sinus congestion medicine

Treatment
This medication is used to treat and prevent angina (chest pain). Nitroglycerin is a vasodilator, which relaxes the muscles of the blood vessels, causing an increase in the oxygen supply to the heart. The oral tablets, capsules, ointment and patches do not act quickly; they are used to prevent chest pain. The sublingual tablets and oral spray act quickly and can be used to relieve chest pain after it has started.

- Take this medicine exactly as directed by your doctor or pharmacist. It will work only if taken correctly.
- If you are taking this medicine regularly and you miss a dose, take it as soon as possible. However, if your next scheduled dose is within 2 hours (or within 6 hours for extended-release capsules or tablets), skip the missed dose and go back to your regular dosing schedule.
- If you have been taking this medicine regularly for several weeks or more, do not suddenly stop using it. Stopping suddenly may bring on attacks of angina.

Side effects
There are a number of side effects that usually do not require medical attention. These possible side effects may go away during treatment; however, if they continue or are bothersome, check with your doctor, nurse, or pharmacist. More common are: dizziness, lightheadedness, or fainting when standing up; fast pulse; flushing of face and neck; headache; nausea or vomiting.
Side effects that should be reported to your doctor are: blurred vision; dry mouth; severe or prolonged headache; skin rash.

Interactions
This medicine may interact with several other drugs such as tricyclic antidepressants and cough medicines. Before starting to take or apply nitroglycerin, be sure to tell your doctor about any medications you are currently taking.

Storage
Tablets, capsules, and oral spray should be stored as in a tightly capped bottle in a cool, dry place. Ointment and patches should be stored at room temperature in their original containers. Keep out of reach of children. Do not keep outdated medicine or medicine no longer needed.

ANOREX

Properties

This medicine contains phendimetrazine as active ingredient; it is prescribed for appetite suppression.

Appetite suppressants are used in the short-term (a few weeks) treatment of obesity. In a few weeks (6 to 12), these medicines in combination with dieting, exercise, and changes in eating habits can help patients lose weight. However, since their appetite reducing effect is only temporary, they are useful only for the first weeks of dieting until new eating habits are established.

Before using this medicine

Before you use this medicine check with your doctor, or pharmacist:
– if you ever had any unusual or allergic reaction to any of the compounds of this medicine.
– if you are on a low-salt, low-sugar, or any other special diet, or if you are allergic to any substance, such as sulfites or other preservatives or dyes.
– if you are pregnant, intend to become pregnant or breast-feeding an infant while using this medicine.
– if you have any of the following medical problems:
Diabetes mellitus (sugar diabetes)
Epilepsy
Glaucoma
Heart or blood vessel disease
High blood pressure
Mental illness (severe)

Treatment

This medication is used to relieve or prevent the symptoms of your medical problem. Take them as directed. Do not take more of them and do not take them more often than recommended on the label. If too much of the drug is taken, it may become habit-forming.
The medicine produces central nervous system stimulation, and it should not be taken by people with heart disease or high blood pressure.

If you think this medicine is not working as well after you have taken it for a few weeks, do not increase the dose. Instead, check with your doctor.

Side effects

The following minor side effects may occur: irritability, nervousness, restlessness, trouble in sleeping.

These side effects should disappear as your body adjusts to the medication. Tell your doctor about any side effects that are persistent or particularly bothersome. It is especially important to tell your doctor about:
Mental depression
Nausea or vomiting
Stomach cramps or pain
Trembling
Unusual tiredness or weakness
■ Discontinue use of the drug; call your doctor right away. Adverse reactions and side effects may be more frequent and severe in people over age 60 than in younger persons.

Interactions

This medicine interacts with several other drugs such as antihypertensives, other appetite suppressants, caffeine, central nervous system depressants, central nervous system stimulants, furazolidone, guanethidine, hydralazine, MAO inhibitors, methyldopa, molindone, phenothiazines, rauwolfia alkaloids, sodium bicarbonate.

Interaction with alcoholic beverages may produce drowsiness, sleepiness, and/or inability to concentrate.
■ Be sure to tell your doctor about any medications you are currently taking.

Storage

This medicine should be stored at room temperature in tightly closed containers. Store away from heat and direct light. Keep out of reach of children, since overdose may be very dangerous in children.

Do not store this medicine in the bathroom medicine cabinet because the heat and moisture cause the medicine to break down. Do not keep outdated medicine or medicine no longer needed. Flush the contents of the container down the toilet.

ANTACEF

Properties
This medicine contains cephalosporin as active ingredient. Cephalosporins belong to the general family of medicines called antibiotics, used in the treatment of infections caused by bacteria. They work by killing bacteria or preventing their growth. Cephalosporins will not work for colds, flu, or other viral infections.

Before using this medicine
Before you use this medicine check with your doctor:
- if you ever had any unusual or allergic reaction to any of the cephalosporins, penicillins, penicillin-like medicines, or penicillamine.
- if you are on a low-salt, low-sugar, or any other special diet, or if you are allergic to any substance, such as sulfites or other preservatives or dyes.
- if you are pregnant or intend to become pregnant while using this medicine. Although cephalosporins have not been shown to cause birth defects or other problems in humans, the chance always exists.
- if you are breast-feeding an infant. Most cephalosporins pass into the breast milk, usually in small amounts.
- if you have any of the following medical problems:
  Bleeding problem
  Kidney or liver disease

Treatment
This medication belongs to the general family of medicines called antibiotics. It is used to treat a wide variety of bacterial infections. It is also used to treat infections in persons who are allergic to penicillin.
- Keep taking this medicine for the full time of treatment even if you begin to feel better after a few days; do not miss any doses.
- If you do miss a dose of this medicine, take it as soon as possible. This will help to keep a constant amount of medicine in the blood. However, if it is almost time for your next dose, skip the missed dose and go back to your regular dosing schedule.
- This medication has been prescribed for your current infection only. Another infection later on, or one that someone else has, may require a different medicine. You should not give your medicine to other people or use it for other infections, unless your doctor specifically directs you to do so.
- Take the medicine at the same times each day, 1 hour before or 2 hours after eating.

Side effects
Along with the needed effects, a medicine may cause some unwanted effects. Side effects that usually do not require medical attention: rectal itching, oral or vaginal white spots, mild diarrhea. These side effects should disappear as your body adjusts to the medication.
- Other side effects that should be reported to your doctor immediately are:
  Hives, rash
  Intense itching
  Faintness soon after a dose
  Difficulty in breathing
  Nausea and vomiting
  Severe diarrhea
  Unusual weakness or tiredness
  Bleeding or bruising

Interactions
This medicine may interact with several other drugs such as anticoagulants, theophylline preparations, probenecid, tetracyclines, etc.
- Be sure to tell your doctor about any medications you are currently taking.

Storage
Tablets, capsules, etc. should be stored at room temperature. Store the liquid form in the refrigerator. Keep out of the reach of children. Do not keep outdated medicine or medicine no longer needed.

AON-Cl

Properties
This medicine contains potassium chloride as active ingredient; it is used to treat or prevent potassium deficiency, especially potassium deficiency that is caused by the use of diuretics (water pills).

Potassium is needed to maintain good health. Potassium supplements may be needed by patients who do not have enough potassium in their regular diet and by those who have lost too much potassium because of illness or treatment with certain medicines.

Since too much potassium may also cause health problems, most potassium supplements are available only with your doctor's prescription.

Before using this medicine
Before you use this medicine check with your doctor, or pharmacist:
- if you ever had any unusual or allergic reaction to potassium preparations;
- if you are on a low-salt, low-sugar, or any other special diet, or if you are allergic to any substance, such as sulfites or other preservatives or dyes.
- if you are pregnant or intend to become pregnant while using this medicine. Although potassium supplements have not been shown to cause problems in humans, the chance always exists.
- if you are breast-feeding an infant. Although this medicine has not been shown to cause problems in humans, the chance always exists since small amounts of potassium pass into the breast milk.
- if you have any of the following medical problems:
Addison's disease
Heart disease
Diarrhea
Kidney disease
Stomach ulcer

Treatment
This medication is used to relieve or prevent the symptoms of your medical problem. Take them as directed. Do not take more of them and do not take them more often than recommended on the label, unless otherwise directed by your doctor. To do so may increase the chance of side effects.

In order to avoid stomach irritation, you should take potassium supplements with food or immediately after a meal. If you miss a dose of this medication, take the missed dose as soon as possible, unless it is within two hours of the next scheduled dose.

Side effects
The following minor side effects may occur:
Diarrhea
Nausea
Stomach pains
Vomiting.

These side effects should disappear as your body adjusts to the medication. Tell your doctor about any side effects that are persistent or particularly bothersome. It is especially important to tell your doctor about anxiety; bloody or black, tarry stools; confusion; difficulty in breathing; numbness or tingling in the arms, legs, or feet; palpitations; severe abdominal pain; or unusual weakness.

Interactions
This medicine interacts with several other drugs such as adrenocorticosteroids, antimuscarinics, calcium-containing medicines; heart medicines such as digitalis or digoxin; laxatives; other potassium-containing medicines.
- Be sure to tell your doctor about any medications you are currently taking.

Storage
Tablets, elixir, etc. should be stored at room temperature in tightly closed containers. Store away from heat and direct light. Keep out of reach of children, since overdose may be very dangerous in children. Do not keep outdated medicine or medicine no longer needed. Flush the contents of the container down the toilet, unless otherwise directed.

APO-AMITRIPTYLINE

Properties
This medicine contains amitriptyline as active ingredient. It belongs to the group of medicines known as tricyclic antidepressants or 'mood elevators.' It is used to relieve mental depression and depression that sometimes occurs with anxiety. The medication gradually relieves, but doesn't cure, symptoms of depression. The medication may also be used for the treatment of narcolepsy, bulimia, panic attacks, cocaine withdrawal, attention deficit disorder.

Before using this medicine
Before you use this medicine check with your doctor, or pharmacist:
- if you ever had any unusual or allergic reaction to any tricyclic antidepressant, maprotiline or trazodone.
- if you are on a low-salt, low-sugar, or any other special diet, or if you are allergic to any substance, such as sulfites or other preservatives or dyes.
- if you are pregnant or intend to become pregnant while using this medicine. There have been reports of newborns suffering from heart, breathing, and urinary problems when their mothers had taken tricyclic antidepressants before delivery.
- if you are breast-feeding an infant. Some tricyclic antidepressants pass into the breast milk.

Treatment
Take this medicine only as directed by your doctor, to benefit your condition as much as possible. Do not take more of it, do not take it more often, and do not take it for a longer period of time than your doctor ordered.

To lessen stomach upset, take this medicine with food, even for a daily bedtime dose, unless your doctor has told you to take it on an empty stomach. If you forget your once-a-day bedtime dose, don't take it more than 3 hours late. If more than 3 hours, wait for next scheduled dose.

Sometimes this medicine must be taken for several weeks before you begin to feel better.

Side effects
Along with the needed effects, a medicine may cause some unwanted effects. Side effects that usually do not require medical attention: difficult or frequent urination; decreased sex drive; muscle aches; abnormal dreams; nasal congestion; weakness and faintness when arising from bed or chair; back pain.
- Other side effects that should be reported to your doctor immediately are:
  Hallucinations
  Shakiness
  Dizziness or fainting
  Blurred vision, eye pain
  Irregular heartbeat or slow pulse
  Inflamed tongue
  Abdominal pain
  Jaundice
  Hair loss, rash
  Fever, chills
  Joint pain
  Palpitations

Interactions
This medicine may interact with several other drugs such as anticoagulants, anticholinergics, cold remedies, oral contraceptives, seizure medicines, sleeping medicines, thyroid medicines, etc.
- Be sure to tell your doctor about any medications you are currently taking.

Storage
Tablets, capsules, etc. should be stored at room temperature in tightly closed, light-resistant containers as directed by your pharmacist. Keep out of reach of children since overdose is especially dangerous in young children. Do not store in the bathroom medicine cabinet because the heat or moisture may cause the medicine to break down. Keep the liquid form of the medicine from freezing.

APO-CEPHALEX

Properties

This medicine contains cephalosporin as active ingredient. Cephalosporins belong to the general family of medicines called antibiotics, used in the treatment of infections caused by bacteria. They work by killing bacteria or preventing their growth. Cephalosporins will not work for colds, flu, or other viral infections.

Before using this medicine

Before you use this medicine check with your doctor:

- if you ever had any unusual or allergic reaction to any of the cephalosporins, penicillins, penicillin-like medicines, or penicillamine.
- if you are on a low-salt, low-sugar, or any other special diet, or if you are allergic to any substance, such as sulfites or other preservatives or dyes.
- if you are pregnant or intend to become pregnant while using this medicine. Although cephalosporins have not been shown to cause birth defects or other problems in humans, the chance always exists.
- if you are breast-feeding an infant. Most cephalosporins pass into the breast milk, usually in small amounts.
- if you have any of the following medical problems:
  Bleeding problem
  Kidney or liver disease

Treatment

This medication belongs to the general family of medicines called antibiotics. It is used to treat a wide variety of bacterial infections. It is also used to treat infections in persons who are allergic to penicillin.

- Keep taking this medicine for the full time of treatment even if you begin to feel better after a few days; do not miss any doses.
- If you do miss a dose of this medicine, take it as soon as possible. This will help to keep a constant amount of medicine in the blood. However, if it is almost time for your next dose, skip the missed dose and go back to your regular dosing schedule.
- This medication has been prescribed for your current infection only. Another infection later on, or one that someone else has, may require a different medicine. You should not give your medicine to other people or use it for other infections, unless your doctor specifically directs you to do so.
- Take the medicine at the same times each day, 1 hour before or 2 hours after eating.

Side effects

Along with the needed effects, a medicine may cause some unwanted effects. Side effects that usually do not require medical attention: rectal itching, oral or vaginal white spots, mild diarrhea. These side effects should disappear as your body adjusts to the medication.

- Other side effects that should be reported to your doctor immediately are:
  Hives, rash
  Intense itching
  Faintness soon after a dose
  Difficulty in breathing
  Nausea and vomiting
  Severe diarrhea
  Unusual weakness or tiredness
  Bleeding or bruising

Interactions

This medicine may interact with several other drugs such as anticoagulants, theophylline preparations, probenecid, tetracyclines, etc.

- Be sure to tell your doctor about any medications you are currently taking.

Storage

Tablets, capsules, etc. should be stored at room temperature. Store the liquid form in the refrigerator. Keep out of the reach of children. Do not keep outdated medicine or medicine no longer needed.

APO-FLURAZEPAM

Properties
This medicine contains as active ingredient flurazepam, a benzodiazepine preparation. Benzodiazepines belong to the group of psychoactive medicines that influence the activity of the brain. Some are used to relieve nervousness or tension. It is effective for this purpose for short periods. Others are used for sleeplessness or to relax muscles or relieve muscle spasm. The benzodiazepines may also be used for other conditions as determined by your doctor.

Before using this medicine
Before you use this medicine check with your doctor:
- if you ever had any unusual or allergic reaction to benzodiazepines.
- if you are on a low-salt, low-sugar, or any other special diet, or if you are allergic to any substance, such as sulfites or other preservatives or dyes.
- if you are pregnant or intend to become pregnant while using this medicine. Some benzodiazepines have been reported to increase the chance of birth defects when used during the first 3 months of pregnancy.
- if you are breast-feeding an infant. Benzodiazepines may pass into the breast milk and cause drowsiness, unusually slow heartbeat, shortness of breath, or troubled breathing in infants of mothers taking this medicine.
- if you have any of the following medical problems: asthma, bronchitis, emphysema, or other chronic lung disease; epilepsy or history of convulsions; hyperactivity (in children); kidney or liver disease; mental depression or illness; myasthania gravis, porphyria.

Treatment
This medication is used to relieve or prevent the symptoms of your medical problem. Benzodiazepines are mainly used as antianxiety agents, anticonvulsants, or sedatives. Take them as directed. Do not take more of them and do not take them more often than recommended on the label, unless otherwise directed by your doctor. Benzodiazepine tranquilizing drugs can be abused if taken for long periods of time and it is possible to develop withdrawal symptoms if you discontinue the therapy abruptly.

Side effects
Along with the needed effects, a medicine may cause some unwanted effects. Minor side effects are: bitter taste in the mouth, dizziness, drowsiness, depression, constipation, dry mouth, excessive salivation, fatigue, flushing, headache, heartburn, loss of appetite, nausea, nervousness, sweating or vomiting. As your body adjusts to the medicine, these side effects should disappear.
- Tell your doctor about any side effects that are persistent or particularly bothersome. It is especially important to tell your doctor about:
   Blurred or double vision
   Chest pain
   Difficulty in urinating
   Fainting or falling
   Fever or hallucinations
   Joint pain
   Mouth sores
   Nightmares
   Palpitations
   Severe depression
   Shortness of breath
   Slurred speech
   Uncoordinated movements
   Unusual tiredness
   Yellowing of the skin

Interactions
This medicine may interact with several other drugs. Be sure to tell your doctor about any medications you are currently taking. This medicine will add to the effects of alcohol, and CNS depressants.

Storage
Store at room temperature in tightly closed, light-resistant-resistant containers. Keep out of the reach of children since overdose may be especially dangerous in children.

APO-IMIPRAMINE

Properties
This medicine contains imipramine as active ingredient. It belongs to the group of medicines known as tricyclic antidepressants or 'mood elevators.' It is used to relieve mental depression and depression that sometimes occurs with anxiety. The medication gradually relieves, but doesn't cure, symptoms of depression. The medication may also be used for the treatment of narcolepsy, bulimia, panic attacks, cocaine withdrawal, attention deficit disorder.

Before using this medicine
Before you use this medicine check with your doctor, or pharmacist:
- if you ever had any unusual or allergic reaction to any tricyclic antidepressant, maprotiline or trazodone.
- if you are on a low-salt, low-sugar, or any other special diet, or if you are allergic to any substance, such as sulfites or other preservatives or dyes.
- if you are pregnant or intend to become pregnant while using this medicine. There have been reports of newborns suffering from heart, breathing, and urinary problems when their mothers had taken tricyclic antidepressants before delivery.
- if you are breast-feeding an infant. Some tricyclic antidepressants pass into the breast milk.

Treatment
Take this medicine only as directed by your doctor, to benefit your condition as much as possible. Do not take more of it, do not take it more often, and do not take it for a longer period of time than your doctor ordered.

To lessen stomach upset, take this medicine with food, even for a daily bedtime dose, unless your doctor has told you to take it on an empty stomach. If you forget your once-a-day bedtime dose, don't take it more than 3 hours late. If more than 3 hours, wait for next scheduled dose.

Sometimes this medicine must be taken for several weeks before you begin to feel better.

Side effects
Along with the needed effects, a medicine may cause some unwanted effects. Side effects that usually do not require medical attention: difficult or frequent urination; decreased sex drive; muscle aches; abnormal dreams; nasal congestion; weakness and faintness when arising from bed or chair; back pain.
- Other side effects that should be reported to your doctor immediately are:
Hallucinations
Shakiness
Dizziness or fainting
Blurred vision, eye pain
Irregular heartbeat or slow pulse
Inflamed tongue
Abdominal pain
Jaundice
Hair loss, rash
Fever, chills
Joint pain
Palpitations

Interactions
This medicine may interact with several other drugs such as anticoagulants, anticholinergics, cold remedies, oral contraceptives, seizure medicines, sleeping medicines, thyroid medicines, etc.
- Be sure to tell your doctor about any medications you are currently taking.

Storage
Tablets, capsules, etc. should be stored at room temperature in tightly closed, light-resistant containers as directed by your pharmacist. Keep out of reach of children since overdose is especially dangerous in young children. Do not store in the bathroom medicine cabinet because the heat or moisture may cause the medicine to break down. Keep the liquid form of the medicine from freezing.

APO-NIFED

Properties

This medicine contains nefedipine as active ingredient. It is a so-called calcium channel blocker, working by blocking the passage of calcium into heart and smooth muscle. Since calcium is an essential factor in muscle contraction, any medicine that affects calcium in this way will interfere with the contraction of these muscles.

The medicine works by:
◆ reducing the work that the heart must perform;
◆ reducing the normal arterial blood pressure;
◆ increasing oxygen to the heart muscle.

The medicine is prescribed for the treatment of attacks of angina pectoris, irregular heartbeat, and high blood pressure. In many cases it can be used for the treatment and prevention of migraine.

Before using this medicine

Before you use this medicine check with your doctor, or pharmacist:
– if you ever had any unusual or allergic reaction to this medicine or any calcium channel blocker;
– if you are pregnant or intend to become pregnant while using this medicine;
– if you have low blood pressure;
– if you have kidney or liver disease;
– if you are breast-feeding an infant;
– if you easily get a rash or intensity sunburn in areas exposed to sun or ultraviolet light.

Treatment

This medication is used for treatment of heart conditions (for instance, angina pectoris) and high blood pressure. Tablets, capsules or extended-release tablets should be taken with liquid. The usual dose amounts to 30 to 100 milligrams a day.

For safe and effective use of medicine:
◆ Follow your doctor's instructions if this medicine was prescribed.
◆ Follow the manufacturer's package directions if you are treating yourself.

Side effects

Along with the needed effects, a medicine may cause some unwanted effects. Possible side effects include:
   Tiredness
   Changes in heartbeat
   Wheezing
   Cough
   Shortness of breath
   Dizziness
   Fainting
   Numbness in hands and feet
   Tingling in hands and feet
   Difficult urination
   Constipation

Overdose

The following symptoms may be a sign of overdose:
   Unusually fast heartbeat
   Unusually slow heartbeat
   Loss of consciousness
   Cardiac arrest
▪ Call a doctor or hospital emergency room for instructions. If necessary start first aid immediately.

Interactions

The effect of this medicine may cause a blood pressure drop if taken together with antihypertensives. Cimetidine may increase the effect of the calcium blocker.

The simultaneous use of diuretics and calcium channel blockers may cause dangerous blood pressure drop.
▪ Be sure to tell your doctor about any medications you are currently taking.

Storage

Capsules, tablets, etc. should be stored at room temperature; store away from heat and direct light. Keep out of reach of children, since this medicine may be dangerous in children.

APO-OXAZEPAM

Properties
This medicine contains as active ingredient oxazepam, a benzodiazepine preparation. Benzodiazepines belong to the group of psychoactive medicines that influence the activity of the brain. Some are used to relieve nervousness or tension. It is effective for this purpose for short periods. Others are used for sleeplessness or to relax muscles or relieve muscle spasm. The benzodiazepines may also be used for other conditions as determined by your doctor.

Before using this medicine
Before you use this medicine check with your doctor:
- if you ever had any unusual or allergic reaction to benzodiazepines.
- if you are on a low-salt, low-sugar, or any other special diet, or if you are allergic to any substance, such as sulfites or other preservatives or dyes.
- if you are pregnant or intend to become pregnant while using this medicine. Some benzodiazepines have been reported to increase the chance of birth defects when used during the first 3 months of pregnancy.
- if you are breast-feeding an infant. Benzodiazepines may pass into the breast milk and cause drowsiness, unusually slow heartbeat, shortness of breath, or troubled breathing in infants of mothers taking this medicine.
- if you have any of the following medical problems: asthma, bronchitis, emphysema, or other chronic lung disease; epilepsy or history of convulsions; hyperactivity (in children); kidney or liver disease; mental depression or illness; myasthania gravis, porphyria.

Treatment
This medication is used to relieve or prevent the symptoms of your medical problem. Benzodiazepines are mainly used as antianxiety agents, anticonvulsants, or sedatives. Take them as directed. Do not take more of them and do not take them more often than recommended on the label, unless otherwise directed by your doctor. Benzodiazepine tranquilizing drugs can be abused if taken for long periods of time and it is possible to develop withdrawal symptoms if you discontinue the therapy abruptly.

Side effects
Along with the needed effects, a medicine may cause some unwanted effects. Minor side effects are: bitter taste in the mouth, dizziness, drowsiness, depression, constipation, dry mouth, excessive salivation, fatigue, flushing, headache, heartburn, loss of appetite, nausea, nervousness, sweating or vomiting. As your body adjusts to the medicine, these side effects should disappear.
- Tell your doctor about any side effects that are persistent or particularly bothersome. It is especially important to tell your doctor about:
  Blurred or double vision
  Chest pain
  Difficulty in urinating
  Fainting or falling
  Fever or hallucinations
  Joint pain
  Mouth sores
  Nightmares
  Palpitations
  Severe depression
  Shortness of breath
  Slurred speech
  Uncoordinated movements
  Unusual tiredness
  Yellowing of the skin

Interactions
- This medicine may interact with several other drugs. This medicine will add to the effects of alcohol, and CNS depressants.
- Be sure to tell your doctor about any medications you are currently taking.

Storage
Store at room temperature in tightly closed, light-resistant-resistant containers. Keep out of the reach of children since overdose may be especially dangerous in children.

APO-SULFATRIM

Properties
This medicine contains sulfamethoxazole, a sulfonamide, and trimethoprim as active ingredients. Sulfonamides are prescribed to treat infections caused by bacteria. They will not work for colds, flu, or other virus infections.

Before using this medicine
Before you use this medicine check with your doctor:
- if you ever had any unusual or allergic reaction to any of the compounds of the medicine.
- if you are on a low-salt, low-sugar, or any other special diet, or if you are allergic to any substance, such as sulfites or other preservatives or dyes.
- if you are pregnant or intend to become pregnant while using this medicine. Although sulfonamides have not been shown to cause defects in humans, the chance may exists.
- if you are breast-feeding an infant. Most sulfonamides pass into the breast milk in small amounts and may cause unwanted effects in infants with some specific conditions.
- if you have any of the following medical problems:
  Kidney disease
  Liver disease
  Porphyria
  Deficiency of enzymes such as
    G6PD

Treatment
This medication is used to treat an infection caused by bacteria. Most sulfonamides are best taken with a full glass (8 ounces) of water on an empty stomach, either one hour before or two hours after a meal. Follow your doctor's or pharmacist's directions on how to take your medicine.
- Keep taking this medicine for the full time of treatment even if you begin to feel better after a few days; do not miss any doses.
- If you do miss a dose of this medicine, take the missed dose immediately.
- This medication works best when the level of medicine in your bloodstream (and urine) is kept constant. It is best, therefore, to take the doses at evenly spaced intervals day and night. if you take two doses a day, the doses should be spaced 12 hours apart.

Side effects
Along with the needed effects, a medicine may cause some unwanted effects. Side effects that usually do not require medical attention: abdominal pain, diarrhea, dizziness, headache, loss of appetite, nausea, sore mouth, or vomiting. These side effects should disappear as your body adjusts to the medication.
Sulfonamides can increase sensitivity to sunlight. It is, therefore, important to avoid prolonged exposure to sunlight and sunlamps.
- Tell your doctor about any side effects that are persistent or particularly bothersome. It is especially important to tell your doctor about:
  Bloody urine
  Difficult urination
  Difficulty in breathing
  Difficulty in swallowing
  Fever or hallucinations
  Itching, rash, or pale skin
  Joint pain, lower back pain
  Ringing in the ears
  Sore throat
  Swollen or inflamed tongue
  Tingling in hands or feet
  Unusual bleeding
  Yellowing of the eyes or skin

Interactions
This medicine may interact with several other drugs such as anticoagulants, oral antidiabetic agents, aspirin, some antibiotics, or anticancer drugs.
- Be sure to tell your doctor about any medications you are currently taking.

Storage
Tablets, capsules, suspension, etc. should be stored at room temperature as directed by your pharmacist or according to instructions on the label.

APROBARBITAL

Properties
This medicine contains as active ingredient the barbiturate aprobarbital. Barbiturates belong to the group of medicines called central nervous system depressants (medicines that slow down the nervous system).

Barbiturates may partially block nerve impulses at nerve-cell connections. They may be used to treat insomnia (sleeplessness) by helping patients fall asleep. Also, they may be used to relieve anxiety or tension. Some of the barbiturates are used as anticonvulsants to help control convulsions in certain disorders or diseases, such as epilepsy. If too much of the drug is used, it may become habit-forming (causing mental or physical dependence).

Before using this medicine
Before you use this medicine check with your doctor, or pharmacist:
- if you ever had any unusual or allergic reaction to this medicine or one of its components.
- if you are on a low-salt, low-sugar, or any other special diet, or if you are allergic to preservatives or dyes.
- if you are pregnant or intend to become pregnant while using this medicine, since barbiturates have been shown to increase the chance of birth defects in humans. Taking barbiturates regularly during the last 3 months of pregnancy may cause the baby to become dependent on the medicine. This may lead to withdrawal side effects in the baby after birth.
- if you have any of the following medical problems:
  Anemia (severe)
  Diabetes mellitus (sugar disease)
  Hyperactivity (in children)
  Kidney or liver disease
  Mental depression
  Overactive thyroid

Treatment
This medication is used to treat the symptoms of your medical condition. Barbiturates act in the central nervous system; some of their side effects are also caused by actions in the central nervous system. Use this medicine as directed by your doctor. Do not use more of it, do not use it more often, and do not use it for a longer period of time than your doctor ordered.
- If you are taking this medication on a regular schedule and you miss a dose, take the missed dose as soon as possible, unless it is almost time for your next dose. In that case do not take the missed dose at all.
- If a barbiturate is used for a long time, is may become habit-forming. Physical dependence may lead to withdrawal side effects when you stop taking this medicine.

Side effects
Along with the needed effects, a medicine may cause some unwanted effects. These side effects may go away during treatment as your body adjusts to the medicine. Such minor side effects are: depression, confusion, diarrhea, nausea, vomiting, joint or muscle pain, slurred speech, hallucinations, headache, decreased sex drive.
- Check with your doctor immediately if any of the following side effects occur:
  Rash or hives
  Face, lip or eyelid swelling
  Sore throat, fever
  Agitation
  Slow heartbeat
  Difficult breathing or chest pain

Interactions
This medicine may interact with several other drugs such as medicines acting on the central nervous system (e.g., antihistamines; beta-adrenergic blockers; MAO inhibitors; mind-altering drugs; nabilone; antidepressants; clozapine; anticonvulsants).

Storage
The medicine should be stored at room temperature in a tightly closed, light-resistant container. Keep out of reach of children since overdose is very dangerous in children.

AQUAPHYLLIN

Properties
This medicine contains theophylline as active ingredient; it is used to treat or prevent breathing problems (wheezing and shortness of breath) caused by asthma, bronchitis, or emphysema. This medication belongs to a group known as xanthine-derivative bronchodilators. They work by opening up the bronchial tubes or air passages of the lungs and increasing the flow of air through them. These medicines are available only with your doctor's prescription.

Before using this medicine
Before you use this medicine check with your doctor, or pharmacist:
- if you ever had any unusual or allergic reaction to xanthine-derivative bronchodilators.
- if you are on a low-salt, low-sugar, or any other special diet, or if you are allergic to any substance, such as sulfites or other preservatives or dyes.
- if you are pregnant or intend to become pregnant while using this medicine.
- if you are breast-feeding an infant. Theophylline passes into the breast milk and may cause irritability, fretfulness, or trouble in sleeping in infants of mothers taking this medicine.
- if you have any of the following medical problems:
Diarrhea
Enlarged prostate
Fibrocystic breast disease
Heart disease
Stomach ulcer

Treatment
This medication is used to relieve or prevent the symptoms of your medical problem. Take them as directed. Do not take more of them and do not take them more often than recommended on the label, unless otherwise directed by your doctor. To do so may increase the chance of side effects. The medicine should be taken on an empty stomach 30 to 60 minutes before a meal or two hours after a meal. Try not to miss any doses of this medication. If you do miss a dose, take the missed dose as soon as possible, unless it is almost time for the next dose. Do not double the next dose. It works best when taken with a glass of water.

Side effects
The following minor side effects may occur:
Dizziness or flushing
Headache
Diarrhea
Heartburn
Increased urination
Insomnia
Nervousness or irritability
Loss of appetite
Nausea or stomach upset
Stomach pain.
These side effects should disappear as your body adjusts to the medication. Tell your doctor about any side effects that are persistent or particularly bothersome. It is especially important to tell your doctor about black, tarry stools; confusion; convulsions; difficulty in breathing; fainting; muscle twitching; palpitations; rash; severe abdominal pain; or unusual weakness.

Interactions
This medicine interacts with several other drugs such as diuretics, reserpine, beta blockers, phenytoin, lithium, phenobarbital, birth control pills, and other medications.
- Be sure to tell your doctor about any medications you are currently taking.

Storage
Tablets, capsules, liquid and suspension should be stored at room temperature in tightly closed containers. Store away from heat and direct light. Keep out of reach of children, since overdose may be very dangerous in children. Discard any outdated medication.

AQUATENSEN

Properties

This medicine contains as active ingredient methylclothiazide, a thiazide-like diuretic. Thiazide or thiazide-like diuretics are prescribed to treat high blood pressure (hypertension). They are also used to reduce fluid accumulation in the body caused by conditions such as heart failure, cirrhosis, kidney disease, and the long-term use of some medications. Thiazide diuretics may also be used for other conditions as determined by your doctor.

Before using this medicine

Before you use this medicine check with your doctor, or pharmacist:

- if you ever had any unusual or allergic reaction to sulfonamides (sulfa drugs) or any of the thiazide diuretics.
- if you are on a low-salt, low-sugar, or any other special diet, or if you are allergic to any substance, such as sulfites or other preservatives or dyes.
- if you are pregnant or intend to become pregnant while using this medicine. When this medicine is used during pregnancy, it may cause side effects including jaundice, blood problems, and low potassium in the newborn.
- if you are breast-feeding an infant. Although this medicine has not been shown to cause problems in humans, the chance always exists since thiazide diuretics pass into breast milk.
- if you have any of the following medical problems:
Diabetes
Gout
Kidney disease
Liver disease
Lupus erythematosus
Pancreas disease

Treatment

This medication is used to treat high blood pressure (hypertension) and also to help reduce the amount of water in the body by increasing the flow of urine. This medicine will not cure your high blood pressure but it does help control it. You must continue to take it - even if you feel well - if you expect to keep your blood pressure down. You may have to take high blood pressure medicine for the rest of your life.

Thiazide diuretics may cause an unusual feeling of tiredness when you begin to take them. You may also notice an increase in urine or in frequency of urination. To keep this from affecting sleep:
- if you are to take a single dose a day, take it in the morning after breakfast;
- if you are to take more than one dose, take the last one not later than 6 p.m.

Side effects

Along with the needed effects, a medicine may cause some unwanted effects. Side effects that usually do not require medical attention: decreased sexual ability; dizziness or lightheadedness when standing up; increased sensitivity of skin to sunlight; loss of appetite; upset stomach.
- Side effects that should be reported to your doctor: black, tarry stools; blood in urine or stools; cough or hoarseness; fever or chills; joint pain; lower back or side pains; painful or difficult urination; pinpoint red spots on skin; skin rash or hives; stomach pain (severe) with nausea; unusual bleeding or bruising; yellow eyes or skin. This medicine may cause a loss of potassium from your body. Signs of too much potassium loss are: dryness of mouth; increased thirst; mood changes; muscle cramps or pain; nausea or vomiting; unusual tiredness or weakness; weak or irregular heartbeat.

Interactions

This medicine may interact with several other drugs.
- Be sure to tell your doctor about any medications you are currently taking.

Storage

Store at room temperature in a tightly closed container.

AQUEST

Properties
This medicine contains estrone as active ingredient. The medicine is prescribed for treatment of estrogen deficiency; it restores normal estrogen levels in tissues. There is no evidence that this drug is effective for nervous symptoms or depression occurring during menopause. They should not be used to treat this condition; they should be used only to replace the estrogen that is naturally absent after menopause.

Before using this medicine
Before you use this medicine check with your doctor, or pharmacist:
- if you ever had any unusual or allergic reaction to estrogens;
- if you are pregnant or intend to become pregnant within three months;
- if you are breast-feeding an infant;
- if you have any of the following medical problems:
Diabetes
Breast cancer
Fibrocystic breast disease
Fibroid uterine tumors
Endometriosis
Migraine headaches
Epilepsy
Porphyria
High blood pressure
Asthma
Congestive heart failure
Kidney disease
Gallstones

Treatment
This medication is used to treat estrogen deficiency, specific symptoms of menopause, estrogen-deficiency osteoporosis, atrophic vaginitis, prostate cancer.
For safe and effective use of this medicine:
- ◆ Follow your doctor's instructions if this medicine was prescribed.
- ◆ Follow the manufacturer's package directions if you are treating yourself.
- ◆ Estrogens have been reported to increase the risk of endometrial carcinoma.

Side effects
Along with the needed effects, a medicine may cause some unwanted effects. Possible side effects include:
Stomach cramps
Profuse bleeding
Appetite loss
Nausea and vomiting
Swollen breasts
Change in menstruation
Rash, skin blisters
Depression
Dizziness

Overdose
The following symptoms may indicate an overdose:
Nausea and vomiting
Fluid retention
Breast enlargement
Abnormal vaginal bleeding
- ■ Call a doctor or hospital emergency room for instructions.

Interactions
This medicine may interact with several other drugs such as adrenocorticosteroids, antidepressants, oral antidiabetics, insulin, phenobarbital, primidone.
- ■ Be sure to tell your doctor about any medications you are currently taking.

Storage
Capsules, tablets, vaginal cream, transdermal patches, etc. should be stored at room temperature; store away from heat and direct light. Keep out of reach of children, since this medicine may be dangerous in children.

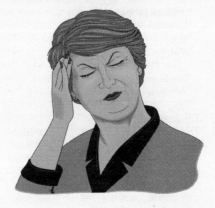

ASENDIN

Properties

This medicine contains amoxapine as active ingredient. It belongs to the group of medicines known as tricyclic antidepressants or 'mood elevators.' It is used to relieve mental depression and depression that sometimes occurs with anxiety. The medication gradually relieves, but doesn't cure, symptoms of depression. The medication may also be used for the treatment of narcolepsy, bulimia, panic attacks, cocaine withdrawal, attention deficit disorder.

Before using this medicine

Before you use this medicine check with your doctor, or pharmacist:

- if you ever had any unusual or allergic reaction to any tricyclic antidepressant, maprotiline or trazodone.
- if you are on a low-salt, low-sugar, or any other special diet, or if you are allergic to any substance, such as sulfites or other preservatives or dyes.
- if you are pregnant or intend to become pregnant while using this medicine. There have been reports of newborns suffering from heart, breathing, and urinary problems when their mothers had taken tricyclic antidepressants before delivery.
- if you are breast-feeding an infant. Some tricyclic antidepressants pass into the breast milk.

Treatment

Take this medicine only as directed by your doctor, to benefit your condition as much as possible. Do not take more of it, do not take it more often, and do not take it for a longer period of time than your doctor ordered.

To lessen stomach upset, take this medicine with food, even for a daily bedtime dose, unless your doctor has told you to take it on an empty stomach. If you forget your once-a-day bedtime dose, don't take it more than 3 hours late. If more than 3 hours, wait for next scheduled dose. Sometimes this medicine must be taken for several weeks before you begin to feel better.

Side effects

Along with the needed effects, a medicine may cause some unwanted effects. Side effects that usually do not require medical attention: difficult or frequent urination; decreased sex drive; muscle aches; abnormal dreams; nasal congestion; weakness and faintness when arising from bed or chair; back pain.

- Other side effects that should be reported to your doctor immediately are:
  Hallucinations
  Shakiness
  Dizziness or fainting
  Blurred vision, eye pain
  Irregular heartbeat or slow pulse
  Inflamed tongue
  Abdominal pain
  Jaundice
  Hair loss, rash
  Fever, chills
  Joint pain
  Palpitations

Interactions

This medicine may interact with several other drugs such as anticoagulants, anticholinergics, cold remedies, oral contraceptives, seizure medicines, sleeping medicines, thyroid medicines, etc.

- Be sure to tell your doctor about any medications you are currently taking.

Storage

Tablets, capsules, etc. should be stored at room temperature in tightly closed, light-resistant containers as directed by your pharmacist. Keep out of reach of children since overdose is especially dangerous in young children. Do not store in the bathroom medicine cabinet because the heat or moisture may cause the medicine to break down. Keep the liquid form of the medicine from freezing.

ASMALIX

Properties

This medicine contains theophylline as active ingredient; it is used to treat or prevent breathing problems (wheezing and shortness of breath) caused by asthma, bronchitis, or emphysema. This medication belongs to a group known as xanthine-derivative bronchodilators. They work by opening up the bronchial tubes or air passages of the lungs and increasing the flow of air through them. These medicines are available only with your doctor's prescription.

Before using this medicine

Before you use this medicine check with your doctor, or pharmacist:

- if you ever had any unusual or allergic reaction to xanthine-derivative bronchodilators.
- if you are on a low-salt, low-sugar, or any other special diet, or if you are allergic to any substance, such as sulfites or other preservatives or dyes.
- if you are pregnant or intend to become pregnant while using this medicine.
- if you are breast-feeding an infant. Theophylline passes into the breast milk and may cause irritability, fretfulness, or trouble in sleeping in infants of mothers taking this medicine.
- if you have any of the following medical problems:
Diarrhea
Enlarged prostate
Fibrocystic breast disease
Heart disease
Stomach ulcer

Treatment

This medication is used to relieve or prevent the symptoms of your medical problem. Take them as directed. Do not take more of them and do not take them more often than recommended on the label, unless otherwise directed by your doctor. To do so may increase the chance of side effects. The medicine should be taken on an empty stomach 30 to 60 minutes before a meal or two hours after a meal. Try not to miss any doses of this medication. If you do miss a dose, take the missed dose as soon as possible, unless it is almost time for the next dose. Do not double the next dose. It works best when taken with a glass of water.

Side effects

The following minor side effects may occur:

Dizziness or flushing
Headache
Diarrhea
Heartburn
Increased urination
Insomnia
Nervousness or irritability
Loss of appetite
Nausea or stomach upset
Stomach pain.

These side effects should disappear as your body adjusts to the medication. Tell your doctor about any side effects that are persistent or particularly bothersome. It is especially important to tell your doctor about black, tarry stools; confusion; convulsions; difficulty in breathing; fainting; muscle twitching; palpitations; rash; severe abdominal pain; or unusual weakness.

Interactions

This medicine interacts with several other drugs such as diuretics, reserpine, beta blockers, phenytoin, lithium, phenobarbital, birth control pills, and other medications.

- Be sure to tell your doctor about any medications you are currently taking.

Storage

Tablets, capsules, liquid and suspension should be stored at room temperature in tightly closed containers. Store away from heat and direct light. Keep out of reach of children, since overdose may be very dangerous in children. Discard any outdated medication.

ATIVAN

Properties
This medicine contains as active ingredient lorazepam, a benzodiazepine preparation. Benzodiazepines belong to the group of psychoactive medicines that influence the activity of the brain. Some are used to relieve nervousness or tension. It is effective for this purpose for short periods. Others are used for sleeplessness or to relax muscles or relieve muscle spasm. The benzodiazepines may also be used for other conditions as determined by your doctor.

Before using this medicine
Before you use this medicine check with your doctor:
- if you ever had any unusual or allergic reaction to benzodiazepines.
- if you are on a low-salt, low-sugar, or any other special diet, or if you are allergic to any substance, such as sulfites or other preservatives or dyes.
- if you are pregnant or intend to become pregnant while using this medicine. Some benzodiazepines have been reported to increase the chance of birth defects when used during the first 3 months of pregnancy.
- if you are breast-feeding an infant. Benzodiazepines may pass into the breast milk and cause drowsiness, unusually slow heartbeat, shortness of breath, or troubled breathing in infants of mothers taking this medicine.
- if you have any of the following medical problems: asthma, bronchitis, emphysema, or other chronic lung disease; epilepsy or history of convulsions; hyperactivity (in children); kidney or liver disease; mental depression or illness; myasthania gravis, porphyria.

Treatment
This medication is used to relieve or prevent the symptoms of your medical problem. Benzodiazepines are mainly used as antianxiety agents, anticonvulsants, or sedatives. Take them as directed. Do not take more of them and do not take them more often than recommended on the label, unless otherwise directed by your doctor. Benzodiazepine tranquilizing drugs can be abused if taken for long periods of time and it is possible to develop withdrawal symptoms if you discontinue the therapy abruptly.

Side effects
Along with the needed effects, a medicine may cause some unwanted effects. Minor side effects are: bitter taste in the mouth, dizziness, drowsiness, depression, constipation, dry mouth, excessive salivation, fatigue, flushing, headache, heartburn, loss of appetite, nausea, nervousness, sweating or vomiting. As your body adjusts to the medicine, these side effects should disappear.
- Tell your doctor about any side effects that are persistent or particularly bothersome. It is especially important to tell your doctor about:
  Blurred or double vision
  Chest pain
  Difficulty in urinating
  Fainting or falling
  Fever or hallucinations
  Joint pain
  Mouth sores
  Nightmares
  Palpitations
  Severe depression
  Shortness of breath
  Slurred speech
  Uncoordinated movements
  Unusual tiredness
  Yellowing of the skin

Interactions
This medicine may interact with several other drugs.
- Be sure to tell your doctor about any medications you are currently taking. This medicine will add to the effects of alcohol, and CNS depressants.

Storage
Store at room temperature in tightly closed, light-resistant-resistant containers. Keep out of the reach of children since overdose may be especially dangerous in children.

AUGMENTIN

Properties
This medicine contains penicillin as active ingredient. It is an antibiotic drug, belonging to the class of penicillins, particularly prescribed for infections of the upper and lower respiratory tract, middle ear infections, sinusitis, skin infections, urinary tract infections.

The antibiotic prevents growth and reproduction of certain types of bacteria that are susceptible to this medicine. It actually destroys bacteria.

Before using this medicine
Before you use this medicine check with your doctor, or pharmacist:
- if you ever had any unusual or allergic reaction to antibiotics;
- if you are pregnant or intend to become pregnant while using this medicine. Animal studies have shown an adverse effect on the fetus, but there are no adequate studies in humans. The drug may be used by pregnant women because of its benefits and despite its potential risks;
- if you are breast-feeding an infant. The medicine passes into breast milk in small amounts;
- if you have a serious kidney disorder;
- if you have congestive heart failure;
- if you have high blood pressure.

Treatment
This medication is used to treat the following ailments or disorders:
- bronchitis;
- pharyngitis;
- pneumonia;
- sinusitis;
- skin infections
- middle ear infections;
- urinary tract infections.

The tablets should be swallowed with liquid. If you forget a dose, take the dose as soon as you remember, than continue regular schedule.
- Follow your doctor's instructions if this medicine was prescribed.
- Follow the manufacturer's package directions if you are treating yourself.

Side effects
Along with the needed effects, a medicine may cause some unwanted effects. Possible side effects include:
- Abdominal discomfort
- Hives, rash
- Shortness of breath
- Vomiting
- Sore mouth
- Vaginal itching
- Sore tongue
- Stomach discharge

Interactions
This medicine may interact with several other drugs such as chloramphenicol (decreased effect of both drugs), colestipol (decreased penicillin effect) methotrexate (increased risk of methotrexate toxicity), tetracyclines (decreased effect of both drugs)
- Be sure to tell your doctor about any medications you are currently taking.

Overdose
Important symptoms are:
- Nausea
- Vomiting
- Severe diarrhea
- Consult a doctor or hospital emergency room if these symptoms persist and become more severe than regularly occurring side effects.

Storage
Capsules, tablets, etc. should be stored at room temperature; store away from heat and direct light. Keep out of reach of children.

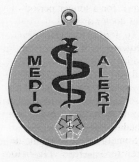

AVENTYL

Properties
This medicine contains nortriptyline as active ingredient. It belongs to the group of medicines known as tricyclic antidepressants or 'mood elevators.' It is used to relieve mental depression and depression that sometimes occurs with anxiety. The medication gradually relieves, but doesn't cure, symptoms of depression. The medication may also be used for the treatment of narcolepsy, bulimia, panic attacks, cocaine withdrawal, attention deficit disorder.

Before using this medicine
Before you use this medicine check with your doctor, or pharmacist:
- if you ever had any unusual or allergic reaction to any tricyclic antidepressant, maprotiline or trazodone.
- if you are on a low-salt, low-sugar, or any other special diet, or if you are allergic to any substance, such as sulfites or other preservatives or dyes.
- if you are pregnant or intend to become pregnant while using this medicine. There have been reports of newborns suffering from heart, breathing, and urinary problems when their mothers had taken tricyclic antidepressants before delivery.
- if you are breast-feeding an infant. Some tricyclic antidepressants pass into the breast milk.

Treatment
Take this medicine only as directed by your doctor, to benefit your condition as much as possible. Do not take more of it, do not take it more often, and do not take it for a longer period of time than your doctor ordered.

To lessen stomach upset, take this medicine with food, even for a daily bedtime dose, unless your doctor has told you to take it on an empty stomach. If you forget your once-a-day bedtime dose, don't take it more than 3 hours late. If more than 3 hours, wait for next scheduled dose.

Sometimes this medicine must be taken for several weeks before you begin to feel better.

Side effects
Along with the needed effects, a medicine may cause some unwanted effects. Side effects that usually do not require medical attention: difficult or frequent urination; decreased sex drive; muscle aches; abnormal dreams; nasal congestion; weakness and faintness when arising from bed or chair; back pain.
- Other side effects that should be reported to your doctor immediately are:
Hallucinations
Shakiness
Dizziness or fainting
Blurred vision, eye pain
Irregular heartbeat or slow pulse
Inflamed tongue
Abdominal pain
Jaundice
Hair loss, rash
Fever, chills
Joint pain
Palpitations

Interactions
This medicine may interact with several other drugs such as anticoagulants, anticholinergics, cold remedies, oral contraceptives, seizure medicines, sleeping medicines, thyroid medicines, etc.
- Be sure to tell your doctor about any medications you are currently taking.

Storage
Tablets, capsules, etc. should be stored at room temperature in tightly closed, light-resistant containers as directed by your pharmacist. Keep out of reach of children since overdose is especially dangerous in young children. Do not store in the bathroom medicine cabinet because the heat or moisture may cause the medicine to break down. Keep the liquid form of the medicine from freezing.

BACARATE

Properties
This medicine contains phendimetrazine as active ingredient; it is prescribed for appetite suppression.

Appetite suppressants are used in the short-term (a few weeks) treatment of obesity. In a few weeks (6 to 12), these medicines in combination with dieting, exercise, and changes in eating habits can help patients lose weight. However, since their appetite reducing effect is only temporary, they are useful only for the first weeks of dieting until new eating habits are established.

Before using this medicine
Before you use this medicine check with your doctor, or pharmacist:
- if you ever had any unusual or allergic reaction to any of the compounds of this medicine.
- if you are on a low-salt, low-sugar, or any other special diet, or if you are allergic to any substance, such as sulfites or other preservatives or dyes.
- if you are pregnant, intend to become pregnant or breast-feeding an infant while using this medicine.
- if you have any of the following medical problems:
Diabetes mellitus (sugar diabetes)
Epilepsy
Glaucoma
Heart or blood vessel disease
High blood pressure
Mental illness (severe)

Treatment
This medication is used to relieve or prevent the symptoms of your medical problem. Take them as directed. Do not take more of them and do not take them more often than recommended on the label. If too much of the drug is taken, it may become habit-forming.

The medicine produces central nervous system stimulation, and it should not be taken by people with heart disease or high blood pressure.

If you think this medicine is not working as well after you have taken it for a few weeks, do not increase the dose. Instead, check with your doctor.

Side effects
The following minor side effects may occur: irritability, nervousness, restlessness, trouble in sleeping.

These side effects should disappear as your body adjusts to the medication. Tell your doctor about any side effects that are persistent or particularly bothersome. It is especially important to tell your doctor about:
Mental depression
Nausea or vomiting
Stomach cramps or pain
Trembling
Unusual tiredness or weakness
- Discontinue use of the drug; call your doctor right away. Adverse reactions and side effects may be more frequent and severe in people over age 60 than in younger persons.

Interactions
This medicine interacts with several other drugs such as antihypertensives, other appetite suppressants, caffeine, central nervous system depressants, central nervous system stimulants, furazolidone, guanethidine, hydralazine, MAO inhibitors, methyldopa, molindone, phenothiazines, rauwolfia alkaloids, sodium bicarbonate.

Interaction with alcoholic beverages may produce drowsiness, sleepiness, and/or inability to concentrate.
- Be sure to tell your doctor about any medications you are currently taking.

Storage
This medicine should be stored at room temperature in tightly closed containers. Store away from heat and direct light. Keep out of reach of children, since overdose may be very dangerous in children.

Do not store this medicine in the bathroom medicine cabinet because the heat and moisture cause the medicine to break down. Do not keep outdated medicine or medicine no longer needed. Flush the contents of the container down the toilet.

BACTRIM

Properties
This medicine contains sulfamethoxazole, a sulfonamide, and trimethoprim as active ingredients. Sulfonamides are prescribed to treat infections caused by bacteria. They will not work for colds, flu, or other virus infections.

Before using this medicine
Before you use this medicine check with your doctor:
- if you ever had any unusual or allergic reaction to any of the compounds of the medicine.
- if you are on a low-salt, low-sugar, or any other special diet, or if you are allergic to any substance, such as sulfites or other preservatives or dyes.
- if you are pregnant or intend to become pregnant while using this medicine. Although sulfonamides have not been shown to cause defects in humans, the chance may exists.
- if you are breast-feeding an infant. Most sulfonamides pass into the breast milk in small amounts and may cause unwanted effects in infants with some specific conditions.
- if you have any of the following medical problems:
  Kidney disease
  Liver disease
  Porphyria
  Deficiency of enzymes such as G6PD

Treatment
This medication is used to treat an infection caused by bacteria. Most sulfonamides are best taken with a full glass (8 ounces) of water on an empty stomach, either one hour before or two hours after a meal. Follow your doctor's or pharmacist's directions on how to take your medicine.
- Keep taking this medicine for the full time of treatment even if you begin to feel better after a few days; do not miss any doses.
- If you do miss a dose of this medicine, take the missed dose immediately.
- This medication works best when the level of medicine in your bloodstream (and urine) is kept constant. It is best, therefore, to take the doses at evenly spaced intervals day and night. if you take two doses a day, the doses should be spaced 12 hours apart.

Side effects
Along with the needed effects, a medicine may cause some unwanted effects. Side effects that usually do not require medical attention: abdominal pain, diarrhea, dizziness, headache, loss of appetite, nausea, sore mouth, or vomiting. These side effects should disappear as your body adjusts to the medication.

Sulfonamides can increase sensitivity to sunlight. It is, therefore, important to avoid prolonged exposure to sunlight and sunlamps.
- Tell your doctor about any side effects that are persistent or particularly bothersome. It is especially important to tell your doctor about:
  Bloody urine
  Difficult urination
  Difficulty in breathing
  Difficulty in swallowing
  Fever or hallucinations
  Itching, rash, or pale skin
  Joint pain, lower back pain
  Ringing in the ears
  Sore throat
  Swollen or inflamed tongue
  Tingling in hands or feet
  Unusual bleeding
  Yellowing of the eyes or skin

Interactions
This medicine may interact with several other drugs such as anticoagulants, oral antidiabetic agents, aspirin, some antibiotics, or anticancer drugs.
- Be sure to tell your doctor about any medications you are currently taking.

Storage
Tablets, capsules, suspension, etc. should be stored at room temperature as directed by your pharmacist or according to instructions on the label.

BARBITA

Properties
This medicine contains as active ingredient the barbiturate phenobarbital. Barbiturates belong to the group of medicines called central nervous system depressants (medicines that slow down the nervous system).

Barbiturates may partially block nerve impulses at nerve-cell connections. They may be used to treat insomnia (sleeplessness) by helping patients fall asleep. Also, they may be used to relieve anxiety or tension. Some of the barbiturates are used as anticonvulsants to help control convulsions in certain disorders or diseases, such as epilepsy. If too much of the drug is used, it may become habit-forming (causing mental or physical dependence).

Before using this medicine
Before you use this medicine check with your doctor, or pharmacist:
- if you ever had any unusual or allergic reaction to this medicine or one of its components.
- if you are on a low-salt, low-sugar, or any other special diet, or if you are allergic to preservatives or dyes.
- if you are pregnant or intend to become pregnant while using this medicine, since barbiturates have been shown to increase the chance of birth defects in humans. Taking barbiturates regularly during the last 3 months of pregnancy may cause the baby to become dependent on the medicine. This may lead to withdrawal side effects in the baby after birth.
- if you have any of the following medical problems:
  Anemia (severe)
  Diabetes mellitus (sugar disease)
  Hyperactivity (in children)
  Kidney or liver disease
  Mental depression
  Overactive thyroid

Treatment
This medication is used to treat the symptoms of your medical condition. Barbiturates act in the central nervous system; some of their side effects are also caused by actions in the central nervous system. Use this medicine as directed by your doctor. Do not use more of it, do not use it more often, and do not use it for a longer period of time than your doctor ordered.
- If you are taking this medication on a regular schedule and you miss a dose, take the missed dose as soon as possible, unless it is almost time for your next dose. In that case do not take the missed dose at all.
- If a barbiturate is used for a long time, is may become habit-forming. Physical dependence may lead to withdrawal side effects when you stop taking this medicine.

Side effects
Along with the needed effects, a medicine may cause some unwanted effects. These side effects may go away during treatment as your body adjusts to the medicine. Such minor side effects are: depression, confusion, diarrhea, nausea, vomiting, joint or muscle pain, slurred speech, hallucinations, headache, decreased sex drive.
- Check with your doctor immediately if any of the following side effects occur:
  Rash or hives
  Face, lip or eyelid swelling
  Sore throat, fever
  Agitation
  Slow heartbeat
  Difficult breathing or chest pain

Interactions
This medicine may interact with several other drugs such as medicines acting on the central nervous system (e.g., antihistamines; beta-adrenergic blockers; MAO inhibitors; mind-altering drugs; nabilone; antidepressants; clozapine; anticonvulsants).

Storage
The medicine should be stored at room temperature in a tightly closed, light-resistant container. Keep out of reach of children since overdose is very dangerous in children.

BAYON

Properties
This medicine contains potassium gluconate as active ingredient; it is used to treat or prevent potassium deficiency, especially potassium deficiency that is caused by the use of diuretics (water pills).

Potassium is needed to maintain good health. Potassium supplements may be needed by patients who do not have enough potassium in their regular diet and by those who have lost too much potassium because of illness or treatment with certain medicines.

Since too much potassium may also cause health problems, most potassium supplements are available only with your doctor's prescription.

Before using this medicine
Before you use this medicine check with your doctor, or pharmacist:
- if you ever had any unusual or allergic reaction to potassium preparations;
- if you are on a low-salt, low-sugar, or any other special diet, or if you are allergic to any substance, such as sulfites or other preservatives or dyes.
- if you are pregnant or intend to become pregnant while using this medicine. Although potassium supplements have not been shown to cause problems in humans, the chance always exists.
- if you are breast-feeding an infant. Although this medicine has not been shown to cause problems in humans, the chance always exists since small amounts of potassium pass into the breast milk.
- if you have any of the following medical problems:
Addison's disease
Heart disease
Diarrhea
Kidney disease
Stomach ulcer

Treatment
This medication is used to relieve or prevent the symptoms of your medical problem. Take them as directed. Do not take more of them and do not take them more often than recommended on the label, unless otherwise directed by your doctor. To do so may increase the chance of side effects.

In order to avoid stomach irritation, you should take potassium supplements with food or immediately after a meal. If you miss a dose of this medication, take the missed dose as soon as possible, unless it is within two hours of the next scheduled dose.

Side effects
The following minor side effects may occur:
Diarrhea
Nausea
Stomach pains
Vomiting.
These side effects should disappear as your body adjusts to the medication. Tell your doctor about any side effects that are persistent or particularly bothersome. It is especially important to tell your doctor about anxiety; bloody or black, tarry stools; confusion; difficulty in breathing; numbness or tingling in the arms, legs, or feet; palpitations; severe abdominal pain; or unusual weakness.

Interactions
This medicine interacts with several other drugs such as adrenocorticosteroids, antimuscarinics, calcium-containing medicines; heart medicines such as digitalis or digoxin; laxatives; other potassium-containing medicines.
- Be sure to tell your doctor about any medications you are currently taking.

Storage
Tablets, elixir, etc. should be stored at room temperature in tightly closed containers. Store away from heat and direct light. Keep out of reach of children, since overdose may be very dangerous in children. Do not keep outdated medicine or medicine no longer needed. Flush the contents of the container down the toilet, unless otherwise directed.

BEBEN

Properties
This medicine contains betamethasone, a corticosteroid, as active ingredient. Corticosteroids are used to help relieve redness, swelling, itching, inflammation, and discomfort of many skin problems. They exert this effect by interfering with natural body mechanisms that produce the rash, itching, or inflammation. They do not cure the underlying cause of the skin problem. This medication is applied to the skin.

Before using this medicine
Before you use this medicine check with your doctor, or pharmacist:
- if you ever had any unusual or allergic reaction to corticosteroids.
- if you are allergic to any substance, such as sulfites or other preservatives or dyes.
- if you are pregnant or intend to become pregnant while using this medicine. Studies have shown that corticosteroids applied to the skin in large amounts or over long periods of time can be the cause of birth defects.
- if you are breast-feeding an infant. Some corticosteroids pass into breast milk and may interfere with the infant's growth.

Treatment
Do not use this medicine more often or for a longer time than ordered. To do so may increase absorption through the skin and the chance of side effects. In addition, too much use, especially on areas with thinner skin (for example, face, armpits, groin), may result in thinning of the skin and stretch marks.

Before applying this medication, wash your hands. than, unless your doctor or pharmacist gives you different instructions, gently wash the area where the medication is to be applied. With a clean towel pat the area dry. Apply a small amount of the medication to the affected area in a thin layer. Do not bandage the area unless your doctor tells you to do so.

If you miss a dose of this medication, apply the dose as soon as possible, unless it is almost time for the next application.
- ◆ Do not use this medicine for other skin problems without first checking with your doctor. You should not use a topical corticosteroid if you have a virus disease (such as herpes), fungal infection of the skin (such as athlete's foot), or tuberculosis of the skin.

Side effects
There are a number of side effects that usually do not require medical attention. Minor side effects are:
Acne
Burning sensations
Itching
Rash
Skin dryness
These possible side effects may go away during treatment; however, if they continue or are bothersome, check with your doctor, nurse, or pharmacist. Tell your doctor about any side effects that are persistent or particularly bothersome, such as:
Blistering
Increased hair growth
Irritation of the affected area
Loss of skin
Secondary infection in the area being treated
Thinning of the skin with easy bruising

Interactions
None known as long as it is used according to the directions given to you by your doctor or pharmacist.

Storage
Cream, ointment, lotion, gel, spray, and aerosol should be stored at room temperature in tightly closed containers. This medication should never be frozen.

BEEPEN-VK

Properties
This medicine contains penicillin V as active ingredient. Penicillins are prescribed to treat infections caused by bacteria. They will not work for colds, flu, or other virus infections. There are several different kinds of penicillins. Each is used to treat different kinds of infections.

Before using this medicine
Before you use this medicine check with your doctor, or pharmacist:
- if you ever had any unusual or allergic reaction to any of the penicillins, cefalosporins, griseofulvin, or penicillamine. Serious reactions may occur in patients who are allergic to penicillins.
- if you are on a low-salt, low-sugar, or any other special diet, or if you are allergic to any substance, such as sulfites or other preservatives or dyes.
- if you are pregnant or intend to become pregnant while using this medicine. Although penicillins have not been shown to cause problems in humans, the chance always exists.
- if you are breast-feeding an infant. Most penicillins (except amdinocillin) pass into the breast milk. Even though only small amounts may pass, allergic reaction, diarrhea, fungal infection, and skin rash may occur in the infant.
- if you have any of the following medical problems:
Allergy
Asthma
Bleeding problems
Eczema
Hay fever, hives
Kidney disease
Liver disease
Mononucleosis
Stomach or intestinal disease

Treatment
This medication is used to treat an infection caused by bacteria. Most penicillins are best taken with a full glass (8 ounces) of water on an empty stomach, some are best taken with a snack or meal. Follow your doctor's or pharmacist's directions on how to take your medicine.
- ◆ Keep taking this medicine for the full time of treatment even if you begin to feel better after a few days; do not miss any doses. This is especially important if you have a "strep" infection since serious heart problems could develop later if your infection is not cleared up completely.
- ◆ If you do miss a dose of this medicine, take it as soon as possible. However, if it is almost time for your next dose, skip the missed dose and go back to your regular dosing schedule.

Side effects
Along with the needed effects, a medicine may cause some unwanted effects. Side effects that usually do not require medical attention: diarrhea; nausea or vomiting; sore mouth or tongue.
- ◆ Stop taking this medicine and get emergency help immediately if you notice: difficulty in breathing; light-headedness; skin rash, hives, itching; wheezing.

Other side effects that should be reported to your doctor immediately are: abdominal bloating; blood in urine; convulsions (seizures); decreased amount of urine; diarrhea (watery and severe) which may also be bloody; fever; joint pain; sore throat and fever; stomach or abdominal cramps and pain; unusual bleeding or bruising.

Interactions
This medicine may interact with several other drugs such as anticoagulants, diarrhea medicines, heparin, ibuprofen, oral contraceptives, potassium-containing medicines, etc.
- ■ Be sure to tell your doctor about any medications you are currently taking.

Storage
Tablets, capsules, etc. should be stored as directed by your pharmacist or according to instructions on the label.

BENISONE

Properties

This medicine contains betamethasone, a corticosteroid, as active ingredient. Corticosteroids are used to help relieve redness, swelling, itching, inflammation, and discomfort of many skin problems. They exert this effect by interfering with natural body mechanisms that produce the rash, itching, or inflammation. They do not cure the underlying cause of the skin problem. This medication is applied to the skin.

Before using this medicine

Before you use this medicine check with your doctor, or pharmacist:
- if you ever had any unusual or allergic reaction to corticosteroids.
- if you are allergic to any substance, such as sulfites or other preservatives or dyes.
- if you are pregnant or intend to become pregnant while using this medicine. Studies have shown that corticosteroids applied to the skin in large amounts or over long periods of time can be the cause of birth defects.
- if you are breast-feeding an infant. Some corticosteroids pass into breast milk and may interfere with the infant's growth.

Treatment

Do not use this medicine more often or for a longer time than ordered. To do so may increase absorption through the skin and the chance of side effects. In addition, too much use, especially on areas with thinner skin (for example, face, armpits, groin), may result in thinning of the skin and stretch marks.

Before applying this medication, wash your hands. than, unless your doctor or pharmacist gives you different instructions, gently wash the area where the medication is to be applied. With a clean towel pat the area dry. Apply a small amount of the medication to the affected area in a thin layer. Do not bandage the area unless your doctor tells you to do so.

If you miss a dose of this medication, apply the dose as soon as possible, unless it is almost time for the next application.

♦ Do not use this medicine for other skin problems without first checking with your doctor. You should not use a topical corticosteroid if you have a virus disease (such as herpes), fungal infection of the skin (such as athlete's foot), or tuberculosis of the skin.

Side effects

There are a number of side effects that usually do not require medical attention. Minor side effects are:
Acne
Burning sensations
Itching
Rash
Skin dryness

These possible side effects may go away during treatment; however, if they continue or are bothersome, check with your doctor, nurse, or pharmacist. Tell your doctor about any side effects that are persistent or particularly bothersome, such as:
Blistering
Increased hair growth
Irritation of the affected area
Loss of skin
Secondary infection in the area being treated
Thinning of the skin with easy bruising

Interactions

None known as long as it is used according to the directions given to you by your doctor or pharmacist.

Storage

Cream, ointment, lotion, gel, spray, and aerosol should be stored at room temperature in tightly closed containers. This medication should never be frozen.

BENZPHETAMINE

Properties

This medicine contains benzphetamine as active ingredient; it is prescribed for appetite suppression.

Appetite suppressants are used in the short-term (a few weeks) treatment of obesity. In a few weeks (6 to 12), these medicines in combination with dieting, exercise, and changes in eating habits can help patients lose weight. However, since their appetite reducing effect is only temporary, they are useful only for the first weeks of dieting until new eating habits are established.

Before using this medicine

Before you use this medicine check with your doctor, or pharmacist:
- if you ever had any unusual or allergic reaction to any of the compounds of this medicine.
- if you are on a low-salt, low-sugar, or any other special diet, or if you are allergic to any substance, such as sulfites or other preservatives or dyes.
- if you are pregnant, intend to become pregnant or breast-feeding an infant while using this medicine.
- if you have any of the following medical problems:
Diabetes mellitus
Epilepsy
Glaucoma
Heart disease
High blood pressure
Mental illness (severe)

Treatment

This medication is used to relieve or prevent the symptoms of your medical problem. Take them as directed.

Do not take more of them and do not take them more often than recommended on the label. If too much of the drug is taken, it may become habit-forming.
- The medicine produces central nervous system stimulation, and it should not be taken by people with heart disease or high blood pressure.
- If you think this medicine is not working as well after you have taken it for a few weeks, do not increase the dose. Instead, check with your doctor.

Side effects

The following minor side effects may occur: irritability, nervousness, restlessness, trouble in sleeping.

These side effects should disappear as your body adjusts to the medication. Tell your doctor about any side effects that are persistent or particularly bothersome. It is especially important to tell your doctor about:
Mental depression
Nausea or vomiting
Stomach cramps or pain
Trembling
Unusual tiredness
- Discontinue use of the drug; call your doctor right away. Adverse reactions and side effects may be more frequent and severe in people over age 60 than in younger persons.

Interactions

This medicine interacts with several other drugs such as antihypertensives, other appetite suppressants, caffeine, central nervous system depressants, central nervous system stimulants, furazolidone, guanethidine, hydralazine, MAO inhibitors, methyldopa, molindone, phenothiazines, rauwolfia alkaloids, sodium bicarbonate.

Interaction with alcoholic beverages may produce drowsiness, sleepiness, and/or inability to concentrate.
- Be sure to tell your doctor about any medications you are currently taking.

Storage

This medicine should be stored at room temperature in tightly closed containers. Store away from heat and direct light. Keep out of reach of children, since overdose may be very dangerous in children.

Do not store this medicine in the bathroom medicine cabinet because the heat and moisture cause the medicine to break down. Do not keep outdated medicine or medicine no longer needed. Flush the contents of the container down the toilet.

BEPADIN

Properties
This medicine contains bepridil as active ingredient. It is a so-called calcium channel blocker, working by blocking the passage of calcium into heart and smooth muscle. Since calcium is an essential factor in muscle contraction, any medicine that affects calcium in this way will interfere with the contraction of these muscles.

The medicine works by:
♦ reducing the work that the heart must perform;
♦ reducing the normal arterial blood pressure;
♦ increasing oxygen to the heart muscle.

The medicine is prescribed for the treatment of attacks of angina pectoris, irregular heartbeat, and high blood pressure. In many cases it can be used for the treatment and prevention of migraine.

Before using this medicine
Before you use this medicine check with your doctor, or pharmacist:
- if you ever had any unusual or allergic reaction to this medicine or any calcium channel blocker;
- if you are pregnant or intend to become pregnant while using this medicine;
- if you have low blood pressure;
- if you have kidney or liver disease;
- if you are breast-feeding an infant;
- if you easily get a rash or intensity sunburn in areas exposed to sun or ultraviolet light.

Treatment
This medication is used for treatment of heart conditions (for instance, angina pectoris) and high blood pressure. Tablets, capsules or extended-release tablets should be taken with liquid. The usual dose amounts to 30 to 100 milligrams a day.

For safe and effective use of medicine:
♦ Follow your doctor's instructions if this medicine was prescribed.
♦ Follow the manufacturer's package directions if you are treating yourself.

Side effects
Along with the needed effects, a medicine may cause some unwanted effects. Possible side effects include:
Tiredness
Changes in heartbeat
Wheezing
Cough
Shortness of breath
Dizziness
Fainting
Numbness in hands and feet
Tingling in hands and feet
Difficult urination
Constipation

Overdose
The following symptoms may be a sign of overdose:
Unusually fast heartbeat
Unusually slow heartbeat
Loss of consciousness
Cardiac arrest
■ Call a doctor or hospital emergency room for instructions. If necessary start first aid immediately.

Interactions
The effect of this medicine may cause a blood pressure drop if taken together with antihypertensives. Cimetidine may increase the effect of the calcium blocker.
■ The simultaneous use of diuretics and calcium channel blockers may cause dangerous blood pressure drop. Be sure to tell your doctor about any medications you are currently taking.

Storage
Capsules, tablets, etc. should be stored at room temperature; store away from heat and direct light. Keep out of reach of children, since this medicine may be dangerous in children.

BEPRIDIL

Properties

This medicine contains bepridil as active ingredient. It is a so-called calcium channel blocker, working by blocking the passage of calcium into heart and smooth muscle. Since calcium is an essential factor in muscle contraction, any medicine that affects calcium in this way will interfere with the contraction of these muscles.

The medicine works by:

- reducing the work that the heart must perform;
- reducing the normal arterial blood pressure;
- increasing oxygen to the heart muscle.

The medicine is prescribed for the treatment of attacks of angina pectoris, irregular heartbeat, and high blood pressure. In many cases it can be used for the treatment and prevention of migraine.

Before using this medicine

Before you use this medicine check with your doctor, or pharmacist:

- if you ever had any unusual or allergic reaction to this medicine or any calcium channel blocker;
- if you are pregnant or intend to become pregnant while using this medicine;
- if you have low blood pressure;
- if you have kidney or liver disease;
- if you are breast-feeding an infant;
- if you easily get a rash or intensity sunburn in areas exposed to sun or ultraviolet light.

Treatment

This medication is used for treatment of heart conditions (for instance, angina pectoris) and high blood pressure. Tablets, capsules or extended-release tablets should be taken with liquid. The usual dose amounts to 30 to 100 milligrams a day.

For safe and effective use of medicine:

- Follow your doctor's instructions if this medicine was prescribed.
- Follow the manufacturer's package directions if you are treating yourself.

Side effects

Along with the needed effects, a medicine may cause some unwanted effects. Possible side effects include:

Tiredness
Changes in heartbeat
Wheezing
Cough
Shortness of breath
Dizziness
Fainting
Numbness in hands and feet
Tingling in hands and feet
Difficult urination
Constipation

Overdose

The following symptoms may be a sign of overdose:

Unusually fast heartbeat
Unusually slow heartbeat
Loss of consciousness
Cardiac arrest

- Call a doctor or hospital emergency room for instructions. If necessary start first aid immediately.

Interactions

The effect of this medicine may cause a blood pressure drop if taken together with antihypertensives. Cimetidine may increase the effect of the calcium blocker.

The simultaneous use of diuretics and calcium channel blockers may cause dangerous blood pressure drop.

- Be sure to tell your doctor about any medications you are currently taking.

Storage

Capsules, tablets, etc. should be stored at room temperature; store away from heat and direct light. Keep out of reach of children, since this medicine may be dangerous in children.

BETA-VAL

Properties

This medicine contains betamethasone, a corticosteroid, as active ingredient. Corticosteroids are used to help relieve redness, swelling, itching, inflammation, and discomfort of many skin problems. They exert this effect by interfering with natural body mechanisms that produce the rash, itching, or inflammation. They do not cure the underlying cause of the skin problem. This medication is applied to the skin.

Before using this medicine

Before you use this medicine check with your doctor, or pharmacist:
- if you ever had any unusual or allergic reaction to corticosteroids.
- if you are allergic to any substance, such as sulfites or other preservatives or dyes.
- if you are pregnant or intend to become pregnant while using this medicine. Studies have shown that corticosteroids applied to the skin in large amounts or over long periods of time can be the cause of birth defects.
- if you are breast-feeding an infant. Some corticosteroids pass into breast milk and may interfere with the infant's growth.

Treatment

Do not use this medicine more often or for a longer time than ordered. To do so may increase absorption through the skin and the chance of side effects. In addition, too much use, especially on areas with thinner skin (for example, face, armpits, groin), may result in thinning of the skin and stretch marks.

Before applying this medication, wash your hands. than, unless your doctor or pharmacist gives you different instructions, gently wash the area where the medication is to be applied. With a clean towel pat the area dry. Apply a small amount of the medication to the affected area in a thin layer. Do not bandage the area unless your doctor tells you to do so.

If you miss a dose of this medication, apply the dose as soon as possible, unless it is almost time for the next application.
- ◆ Do not use this medicine for other skin problems without first checking with your doctor. You should not use a topical corticosteroid if you have a virus disease (such as herpes), fungal infection of the skin (such as athlete's foot), or tuberculosis of the skin.

Side effects

There are a number of side effects that usually do not require medical attention. Minor side effects are:
Acne
Burning sensations
Itching
Rash
Skin dryness
These possible side effects may go away during treatment; however, if they continue or are bothersome, check with your doctor, nurse, or pharmacist. Tell your doctor about any side effects that are persistent or particularly bothersome, such as:
Blistering
Increased hair growth
Irritation of the affected area
Loss of skin
Secondary infection in the area being treated
Thinning of the skin with easy bruising

Interactions

None known as long as it is used according to the directions given to you by your doctor or pharmacist.

Storage

Cream, ointment, lotion, gel, spray, and aerosol should be stored at room temperature in tightly closed containers. This medication should never be frozen.

BETACORT SCALP LOTION

Properties

This medicine contains betamethasone, a corticosteroid, as active ingredient. Corticosteroids are used to help relieve redness, swelling, itching, inflammation, and discomfort of many skin problems. They exert this effect by interfering with natural body mechanisms that produce the rash, itching, or inflammation. They do not cure the underlying cause of the skin problem. This medication is applied to the skin.

Before using this medicine

Before you use this medicine check with your doctor, or pharmacist:
- if you ever had any unusual or allergic reaction to corticosteroids.
- if you are allergic to any substance, such as sulfites or other preservatives or dyes.
- if you are pregnant or intend to become pregnant while using this medicine. Studies have shown that corticosteroids applied to the skin in large amounts or over long periods of time can be the cause of birth defects.
- if you are breast-feeding an infant. Some corticosteroids pass into breast milk and may interfere with the infant's growth.

Treatment

Do not use this medicine more often or for a longer time than ordered. To do so may increase absorption through the skin and the chance of side effects. In addition, too much use, especially on areas with thinner skin (for example, face, armpits, groin), may result in thinning of the skin and stretch marks.

Before applying this medication, wash your hands. than, unless your doctor or pharmacist gives you different instructions, gently wash the area where the medication is to be applied. With a clean towel pat the area dry. Apply a small amount of the medication to the affected area in a thin layer. Do not bandage the area unless your doctor tells you to do so.

If you miss a dose of this medication, apply the dose as soon as possible, unless it is almost time for the next application.
- ◆ Do not use this medicine for other skin problems without first checking with your doctor. You should not use a topical corticosteroid if you have a virus disease (such as herpes), fungal infection of the skin (such as athlete's foot), or tuberculosis of the skin.

Side effects

There are a number of side effects that usually do not require medical attention. Minor side effects are:
Acne
Burning sensations
Itching
Rash
Skin dryness
These possible side effects may go away during treatment; however, if they continue or are bothersome, check with your doctor, nurse, or pharmacist. Tell your doctor about any side effects that are persistent or particularly bothersome, such as:
Blistering
Increased hair growth
Irritation of the affected area
Loss of skin
Secondary infection in the area being treated
Thinning of the skin with easy bruising

Interactions

None known as long as it is used according to the directions given to you by your doctor or pharmacist.

Storage

Cream, ointment, lotion, gel, spray, and aerosol should be stored at room temperature in tightly closed containers. This medication should never be frozen.

BETADERM

Properties
This medicine contains betamethasone, a corticosteroid, as active ingredient. Corticosteroids are used to help relieve redness, swelling, itching, inflammation, and discomfort of many skin problems. They exert this effect by interfering with natural body mechanisms that produce the rash, itching, or inflammation. They do not cure the underlying cause of the skin problem. This medication is applied to the skin.

Before using this medicine
Before you use this medicine check with your doctor, or pharmacist:
- if you ever had any unusual or allergic reaction to corticosteroids.
- if you are allergic to any substance, such as sulfites or other preservatives or dyes.
- if you are pregnant or intend to become pregnant while using this medicine. Studies have shown that corticosteroids applied to the skin in large amounts or over long periods of time can be the cause of birth defects.
- if you are breast-feeding an infant. Some corticosteroids pass into breast milk and may interfere with the infant's growth.

Treatment
Do not use this medicine more often or for a longer time than ordered. To do so may increase absorption through the skin and the chance of side effects. In addition, too much use, especially on areas with thinner skin (for example, face, armpits, groin), may result in thinning of the skin and stretch marks.

Before applying this medication, wash your hands. than, unless your doctor or pharmacist gives you different instructions, gently wash the area where the medication is to be applied. With a clean towel pat the area dry. Apply a small amount of the medication to the affected area in a thin layer. Do not bandage the area unless your doctor tells you to do so.

If you miss a dose of this medication, apply the dose as soon as possible, unless it is almost time for the next application.
- Do not use this medicine for other skin problems without first checking with your doctor. You should not use a topical corticosteroid if you have a virus disease (such as herpes), fungal infection of the skin (such as athlete's foot), or tuberculosis of the skin.

Side effects
There are a number of side effects that usually do not require medical attention. Minor side effects are:
Acne
Burning sensations
Itching
Rash
Skin dryness
These possible side effects may go away during treatment; however, if they continue or are bothersome, check with your doctor, nurse, or pharmacist. Tell your doctor about any side effects that are persistent or particularly bothersome, such as:
Blistering
Increased hair growth
Irritation of the affected area
Loss of skin
Secondary infection in the area being treated
Thinning of the skin with easy bruising

Interactions
None known as long as it is used according to the directions given to you by your doctor or pharmacist.

Storage
Cream, ointment, lotion, gel, spray, and aerosol should be stored at room temperature in tightly closed containers. This medication should never be frozen.

BETAMETHASONE

Properties

This medicine contains betamethasone, a corticosteroid, as active ingredient. Corticosteroids are used to help relieve redness, swelling, itching, inflammation, and discomfort of many skin problems. They exert this effect by interfering with natural body mechanisms that produce the rash, itching, or inflammation. They do not cure the underlying cause of the skin problem. This medication is applied to the skin.

Before using this medicine

Before you use this medicine check with your doctor, or pharmacist:
- if you ever had any unusual or allergic reaction to corticosteroids.
- if you are allergic to any substance, such as sulfites or other preservatives or dyes.
- if you are pregnant or intend to become pregnant while using this medicine. Studies have shown that corticosteroids applied to the skin in large amounts or over long periods of time can be the cause of birth defects.
- if you are breast-feeding an infant. Some corticosteroids pass into breast milk and may interfere with the infant's growth.

Treatment

Do not use this medicine more often or for a longer time than ordered. To do so may increase absorption through the skin and the chance of side effects. In addition, too much use, especially on areas with thinner skin (for example, face, armpits, groin), may result in thinning of the skin and stretch marks.

Before applying this medication, wash your hands. than, unless your doctor or pharmacist gives you different instructions, gently wash the area where the medication is to be applied. With a clean towel pat the area dry. Apply a small amount of the medication to the affected area in a thin layer. Do not bandage the area unless your doctor tells you to do so.

If you miss a dose of this medication, apply the dose as soon as possible, unless it is almost time for the next application.

◆ Do not use this medicine for other skin problems without first checking with your doctor. You should not use a topical corticosteroid if you have a virus disease (such as herpes), fungal infection of the skin (such as athlete's foot), or tuberculosis of the skin.

Side effects

There are a number of side effects that usually do not require medical attention. Minor side effects are:

Acne
Burning sensations
Itching
Rash
Skin dryness

These possible side effects may go away during treatment; however, if they continue or are bothersome, check with your doctor, nurse, or pharmacist. Tell your doctor about any side effects that are persistent or particularly bothersome, such as:

Blistering
Increased hair growth
Irritation of the affected area
Loss of skin
Secondary infection in the area being treated
Thinning of the skin with easy bruising

Interactions

None known as long as it is used according to the directions given to you by your doctor or pharmacist.

Storage

Cream, ointment, lotion, gel, spray, and aerosol should be stored at room temperature in tightly closed containers. This medication should never be frozen.

BETAPEN-VK

Properties
This medicine contains penicillin V as active ingredient. Penicillins are prescribed to treat infections caused by bacteria. They will not work for colds, flu, or other virus infections. There are several different kinds of penicillins. Each is used to treat different kinds of infections.

Before using this medicine
Before you use this medicine check with your doctor, or pharmacist:
− if you ever had any unusual or allergic reaction to any of the penicillins, cefalosporins, griseofulvin, or penicillamine. Serious reactions may occur in patients who are allergic to penicillins.
− if you are on a low-salt, low-sugar, or any other special diet, or if you are allergic to any substance, such as sulfites or other preservatives or dyes.
− if you are pregnant or intend to become pregnant while using this medicine. Although penicillins have not been shown to cause problems in humans, the chance always exists.
− if you are breast-feeding an infant. Most penicillins (except amdinocillin) pass into the breast milk. Even though only small amounts may pass, allergic reaction, diarrhea, fungal infection, and skin rash may occur in the infant.
− if you have any of the following medical problems:
Allergy
Asthma
Bleeding problems
Eczema
Hay fever, hives
Kidney disease
Liver disease
Mononucleosis
Stomach or intestinal disease

Treatment
This medication is used to treat an infection caused by bacteria. Most penicillins are best taken with a full glass (8 ounces) of water on an empty stomach, some are best taken with a snack or meal. Follow your doctor's or pharmacist's directions on how to take your medicine.
◆ Keep taking this medicine for the full time of treatment even if you begin to feel better after a few days; do not miss any doses. This is especially important if you have a "strep" infection since serious heart problems could develop later if your infection is not cleared up completely.
◆ If you do miss a dose of this medicine, take it as soon as possible. However, if it is almost time for your next dose, skip the missed dose and go back to your regular dosing schedule.

Side effects
Along with the needed effects, a medicine may cause some unwanted effects. Side effects that usually do not require medical attention: diarrhea; nausea or vomiting; sore mouth or tongue.
◆ Stop taking this medicine and get emergency help immediately if you notice: difficulty in breathing; lightheadedness; skin rash, hives, itching; wheezing.
Other side effects that should be reported to your doctor immediately are: abdominal bloating; blood in urine; convulsions (seizures); decreased amount of urine; diarrhea (watery and severe) which may also be bloody; fever; joint pain; sore throat and fever; stomach or abdominal cramps and pain; unusual bleeding or bruising.

Interactions
This medicine may interact with several other drugs such as anticoagulants, diarrhea medicines, heparin, ibuprofen, oral contraceptives, potassium-containing medicines, etc.
■ Be sure to tell your doctor about any medications you are currently taking.

Storage
Tablets, capsules, etc. should be stored as directed by your pharmacist or according to instructions on the label.

BETATREX

Properties

This medicine contains betamethasone, a corticosteroid, as active ingredient. Corticosteroids are used to help relieve redness, swelling, itching, inflammation, and discomfort of many skin problems. They exert this effect by interfering with natural body mechanisms that produce the rash, itching, or inflammation. They do not cure the underlying cause of the skin problem. This medication is applied to the skin.

Before using this medicine

Before you use this medicine check with your doctor, or pharmacist:
- if you ever had any unusual or allergic reaction to corticosteroids.
- if you are allergic to any substance, such as sulfites or other preservatives or dyes.
- if you are pregnant or intend to become pregnant while using this medicine. Studies have shown that corticosteroids applied to the skin in large amounts or over long periods of time can be the cause of birth defects.
- if you are breast-feeding an infant. Some corticosteroids pass into breast milk and may interfere with the infant's growth.

Treatment

Do not use this medicine more often or for a longer time than ordered. To do so may increase absorption through the skin and the chance of side effects. In addition, too much use, especially on areas with thinner skin (for example, face, armpits, groin), may result in thinning of the skin and stretch marks.

Before applying this medication, wash your hands. than, unless your doctor or pharmacist gives you different instructions, gently wash the area where the medication is to be applied. With a clean towel pat the area dry. Apply a small amount of the medication to the affected area in a thin layer. Do not bandage the area unless your doctor tells you to do so.

If you miss a dose of this medication, apply the dose as soon as possible, unless it is almost time for the next application.
- Do not use this medicine for other skin problems without first checking with your doctor. You should not use a topical corticosteroid if you have a virus disease (such as herpes), fungal infection of the skin (such as athlete's foot), or tuberculosis of the skin.

Side effects

There are a number of side effects that usually do not require medical attention. Minor side effects are:
  Acne
  Burning sensations
  Itching
  Rash
  Skin dryness
  These possible side effects may go away during treatment; however, if they continue or are bothersome, check with your doctor, nurse, or pharmacist. Tell your doctor about any side effects that are persistent or particularly bothersome, such as:
  Blistering
  Increased hair growth
  Irritation of the affected area
  Loss of skin
  Secondary infection in the area being treated
  Thinning of the skin with easy bruising

Interactions

None known as long as it is used according to the directions given to you by your doctor or pharmacist.

Storage

Cream, ointment, lotion, gel, spray, and aerosol should be stored at room temperature in tightly closed containers. This medication should never be frozen.

BETNOLATE

Properties
This medicine contains betamethasone, a corticosteroid, as active ingredient. Corticosteroids are used to help relieve redness, swelling, itching, inflammation, and discomfort of many skin problems. They exert this effect by interfering with natural body mechanisms that produce the rash, itching, or inflammation. They do not cure the underlying cause of the skin problem. This medication is applied to the skin.

Before using this medicine
Before you use this medicine check with your doctor, or pharmacist:
- if you ever had any unusual or allergic reaction to corticosteroids.
- if you are allergic to any substance, such as sulfites or other preservatives or dyes.
- if you are pregnant or intend to become pregnant while using this medicine. Studies have shown that corticosteroids applied to the skin in large amounts or over long periods of time can be the cause of birth defects.
- if you are breast-feeding an infant. Some corticosteroids pass into breast milk and may interfere with the infant's growth.

Treatment
Do not use this medicine more often or for a longer time than ordered. To do so may increase absorption through the skin and the chance of side effects. In addition, too much use, especially on areas with thinner skin (for example, face, armpits, groin), may result in thinning of the skin and stretch marks.

Before applying this medication, wash your hands. than, unless your doctor or pharmacist gives you different instructions, gently wash the area where the medication is to be applied. With a clean towel pat the area dry. Apply a small amount of the medication to the affected area in a thin layer. Do not bandage the area unless your doctor tells you to do so.

If you miss a dose of this medication, apply the dose as soon as possible, unless it is almost time for the next application.
- ◆ Do not use this medicine for other skin problems without first checking with your doctor. You should not use a topical corticosteroid if you have a virus disease (such as herpes), fungal infection of the skin (such as athlete's foot), or tuberculosis of the skin.

Side effects
There are a number of side effects that usually do not require medical attention. Minor side effects are:

Acne
Burning sensations
Itching
Rash
Skin dryness

These possible side effects may go away during treatment; however, if they continue or are bothersome, check with your doctor, nurse, or pharmacist. Tell your doctor about any side effects that are persistent or particularly bothersome, such as:

Blistering
Increased hair growth
Irritation of the affected area
Loss of skin
Secondary infection in the area being treated
Thinning of the skin with easy bruising

Interactions
None known as long as it is used according to the directions given to you by your doctor or pharmacist.

Storage
Cream, ointment, lotion, gel, spray, and aerosol should be stored at room temperature in tightly closed containers. This medication should never be frozen.

BIAXIN

Properties

This medicine contains clarithromycin as active ingredient. It is an antibiotic drug, belonging to the class of erythromycins, particularly prescribed for infections of the upper and lower respiratory tract such as bronchitis, pneumonia, and Legionnaire's disease. It may be used for other infections and inflammatory processes.

The antibiotic prevents growth and reproduction of certain types of bacteria that are susceptible to this medicine.

Before using this medicine

Before you use this medicine check with your doctor, or pharmacist:
- if you ever had any unusual or allergic reaction to antibiotics;
- if you are pregnant or intend to become pregnant while using this medicine. Animal studies have shown an adverse effect on the fetus, but there are no adequate studies in humans. The drug may be used by pregnant women because of its benefits and despite its potential risks;
- if you are breast-feeding an infant. The medicine passes into breast milk in small amounts. Avoid the medicine or discontinue nursing until you finish the medicine;
- if you have a serious kidney disorder.

Treatment

This medication is used to treat the following ailments or disorders:
- bronchitis;
- pharyngitis;
- pneumonia;
- Legionnaire's disease;
- sinusitis;
- skin infections;
- Heliobacter pylori infections of the stomach.
- Follow your doctor's instructions if this medicine was prescribed.
- Follow the manufacturer's package directions if you are treating yourself.

The tablets should be swallowed with liquid. If you forget a dose, take the dose as soon as you remember. Wait five to six hours for the next dose.

In patients over 60 years of age, adverse reactions and side effects may be more serious and frequent than in younger persons.

Side effects

Along with the needed effects, a medicine may cause some unwanted effects. Possible side effects include:
Abdominal discomfort
Diarrhea
Constipation or diarrhea
Change in taste
Unusual bleeding
Unusual bruising

Interactions

This medicine may interact with several other drugs such as antihistamines (heart rhythm problems), theophylline (increased concentration of theophylline), ziduvusine (decreased effect of this medicine).
- Be sure to tell your doctor about any medications you are currently taking.

Overdose

Important symptoms are:
Nausea
Vomiting
Abdominal discomfort
Diarrhea
- Consult a doctor or hospital emergency room if these symptoms persist and become more severe than regularly occurring side effects.

Storage

Capsules, tablets, etc. should be stored at room temperature; store away from heat and direct light. Keep out of reach of children.

BI-K

Properties

This medicine contains potassium citrate and potassium glucobate as active ingredients; it is used to treat or prevent potassium deficiency, especially potassium deficiency that is caused by the use of diuretics (water pills).

Potassium is needed to maintain good health. Potassium supplements may be needed by patients who do not have enough potassium in their regular diet and by those who have lost too much potassium because of illness or treatment with certain medicines.

Since too much potassium may also cause health problems, most potassium supplements are available only with your doctor's prescription.

Before using this medicine

Before you use this medicine check with your doctor, or pharmacist:
- if you ever had any unusual or allergic reaction to potassium preparations;
- if you are on a low-salt, low-sugar, or any other special diet, or if you are allergic to any substance, such as sulfites or other preservatives or dyes.
- if you are pregnant or intend to become pregnant while using this medicine. Although potassium supplements have not been shown to cause problems in humans, the chance always exists.
- if you are breast-feeding an infant. Although this medicine has not been shown to cause problems in humans, the chance always exists since small amounts of potassium pass into the breast milk.
- if you have any of the following medical problems:
Addison's disease
Heart disease
Diarrhea
Kidney disease
Stomach ulcer

Treatment

This medication is used to relieve or prevent the symptoms of your medical problem. Take them as directed. Do not take more of them and do not take them more often than recommended on the label, unless otherwise directed by your doctor. To do so may increase the chance of side effects.

In order to avoid stomach irritation, you should take potassium supplements with food or immediately after a meal. If you miss a dose of this medication, take the missed dose as soon as possible, unless it is within two hours of the next scheduled dose.

Side effects

The following minor side effects may occur:
Diarrhea
Nausea
Stomach pains
Vomiting.

These side effects should disappear as your body adjusts to the medication. Tell your doctor about any side effects that are persistent or particularly bothersome. It is especially important to tell your doctor about anxiety; bloody or black, tarry stools; confusion; difficulty in breathing; numbness or tingling in the arms, legs, or feet; palpitations; severe abdominal pain; or unusual weakness.

Interactions

This medicine interacts with several other drugs such as adrenocorticosteroids, antimuscarinics, calcium-containing medicines; heart medicines such as digitalis or digoxin; laxatives; other potassium-containing medicines.
- Be sure to tell your doctor about any medications you are currently taking.

Storage

Tablets, elixir, etc. should be stored at room temperature in tightly closed containers. Store away from heat and direct light. Keep out of reach of children, since overdose may be very dangerous in children. Do not keep outdated medicine or medicine no longer needed. Flush the contents of the container down the toilet, unless otherwise directed.

BONTRIL PDM

Properties
This medicine contains phendimetrazine as active ingredient; it is prescribed for appetite suppression.

Appetite suppressants are used in the short-term (a few weeks) treatment of obesity. In a few weeks (6 to 12), these medicines in combination with dieting, exercise, and changes in eating habits can help patients lose weight. However, since their appetite reducing effect is only temporary, they are useful only for the first weeks of dieting until new eating habits are established.

Before using this medicine
Before you use this medicine check with your doctor, or pharmacist:
- if you ever had any unusual or allergic reaction to any of the compounds of this medicine.
- if you are on a low-salt, low-sugar, or any other special diet, or if you are allergic to any substance, such as sulfites or other preservatives or dyes.
- if you are pregnant, intend to become pregnant or breast-feeding an infant while using this medicine.
- if you have any of the following medical problems:
  Diabetes mellitus (sugar diabetes)
  Epilepsy
  Glaucoma
  Heart or blood vessel disease
  High blood pressure
  Mental illness (severe)

Treatment
This medication is used to relieve or prevent the symptoms of your medical problem. Take them as directed. Do not take more of them and do not take them more often than recommended on the label. If too much of the drug is taken, it may become habit-forming.

The medicine produces central nervous system stimulation, and it should not be taken by people with heart disease or high blood pressure.

If you think this medicine is not working as well after you have taken it for a few weeks, do not increase the dose. Instead, check with your doctor.

Side effects
The following minor side effects may occur: irritability, nervousness, restlessness, trouble in sleeping.

These side effects should disappear as your body adjusts to the medication. Tell your doctor about any side effects that are persistent or particularly bothersome. It is especially important to tell your doctor about:
  Mental depression
  Nausea or vomiting
  Stomach cramps or pain
  Trembling
  Unusual tiredness or weakness
- Discontinue use of the drug; call your doctor right away. Adverse reactions and side effects may be more frequent and severe in people over age 60 than in younger persons.

Interactions
This medicine interacts with several other drugs such as antihypertensives, other appetite suppressants, caffeine, central nervous system depressants, central nervous system stimulants, furazolidone, guanethidine, hydralazine, MAO inhibitors, methyldopa, molindone, phenothiazines, rauwolfia alkaloids, sodium bicarbonate.

Interaction with alcoholic beverages may produce drowsiness, sleepiness, and/or inability to concentrate.
- Be sure to tell your doctor about any medications you are currently taking.

Storage
This medicine should be stored at room temperature in tightly closed containers. Store away from heat and direct light. Keep out of reach of children, since overdose may be very dangerous in children.

Do not store this medicine in the bathroom medicine cabinet because the heat and moisture cause the medicine to break down. Do not keep outdated medicine or medicine no longer needed. Flush the contents of the container down the toilet.

BREVICON

Properties
This medicine contains norethindrone and ethinyl estradiol as active ingredients. It is an oral contraceptive prescribed to prevent pregnancy and/or to regulate menstrual periods.

The drug works by altering the mucus at the cervix entrance to prevent the entry of sperm. It also alters the uterus lining to resist implantation of the fertilized egg. Oral contraceptives create the same chemical atmosphere in blood that exists during pregnancy.

Before using this medicine
Before you use this medicine check with your doctor, or pharmacist:
- if you ever had any unusual or allergic reaction to estrogens or progestogen;
- if you are pregnant or want to become pregnant within three months;
- if you are breast-feeding an infant;
- if you have any of the following medical problems:
  Diabetes
  Ailments of the breast
  Disorders of the uterus
  Migraine or epilepsy
  High blood pressure
  Asthma or heart conditions
  Kidney disease
  Gallstones

Treatment
This medication is used to prevent pregnancy or to regulate menstrual periods.

Adverse reactions
Along with the needed effects, a medicine may cause some unwanted effects or adverse reactions.
- *An increased risk of the following adverse reactions has been associated with the use of oral contraceptives:*
  Thrombophlebitis
  Venous thrombosis
  Arterial thromboembolism
  Pulmonary (lung) embolism
  Myocardial infarction
  Cerebral hemorrhage
  Cerebral thrombosis

Hypertension
Gallbladder disease
Hepatic (liver) hepatomas
Benign liver tumors
- *The following adverse reactions have been reported in patients receiving oral contraceptives and are believed to be drug-related:*
  Nausea and vomiting
  Abdominal cramps
  Breakthrough bleeding
  Spotting
  Change in menstrual flow
  Amenorrhea
  Temporary infertility
  Edema
  Breast changes
  Weight changes
  Cholestatic jaundice
  Migraine
  Rash (allergic)
  Mental depression
  Vaginal candidiasis

Interactions
This medicine may interact with several other drugs such as antibiotics, anticoagulants, anticonvulsants, antidepressants, oral antidiabetics, antihistamines, barbiturates, oral hypoglycemics, insulin, meperidine.
- Be sure to tell your doctor about any medications you are currently taking.

Storage
Tablets should be stored at room temperature; store away from heat and direct light. Keep out of reach of children, since this medicine may be dangerous in chidren.

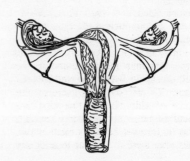

BRONKODYL

Properties
This medicine contains theophylline as active ingredient; it is used to treat or prevent breathing problems (wheezing and shortness of breath) caused by asthma, bronchitis, or emphysema. This medication belongs to a group known as xanthine-derivative bronchodilators. They work by opening up the bronchial tubes or air passages of the lungs and increasing the flow of air through them. These medicines are available only with your doctor's prescription.

Before using this medicine
Before you use this medicine check with your doctor, or pharmacist:
- if you ever had any unusual or allergic reaction to xanthine-derivative bronchodilators.
- if you are on a low-salt, low-sugar, or any other special diet, or if you are allergic to any substance, such as sulfites or other preservatives or dyes.
- if you are pregnant or intend to become pregnant while using this medicine.
- if you are breast-feeding an infant. Theophylline passes into the breast milk and may cause irritability, fretfulness, or trouble in sleeping in infants of mothers taking this medicine.
- if you have any of the following medical problems:
Diarrhea
Enlarged prostate
Fibrocystic breast disease
Heart disease
Stomach ulcer

Treatment
This medication is used to relieve or prevent the symptoms of your medical problem. Take them as directed. Do not take more of them and do not take them more often than recommended on the label, unless otherwise directed by your doctor. To do so may increase the chance of side effects. The medicine should be taken on an empty stomach 30 to 60 minutes before a meal or two hours after a meal. Try not to miss any doses of this medication. If you do miss a dose, take the missed dose as soon as possible, unless it is almost time for the next dose. Do not double the next dose. It works best when taken with a glass of water.

Side effects
The following minor side effects may occur:
Dizziness or flushing
Headache
Diarrhea
Heartburn
Increased urination
Insomnia
Nervousness or irritability
Loss of appetite
Nausea or stomach upset
Stomach pain.
These side effects should disappear as your body adjusts to the medication. Tell your doctor about any side effects that are persistent or particularly bothersome. It is especially important to tell your doctor about black, tarry stools; confusion; convulsions; difficulty in breathing; fainting; muscle twitching; palpitations; rash; severe abdominal pain; or unusual weakness.

Interactions
This medicine interacts with several other drugs such as diuretics, reserpine, beta blockers, phenytoin, lithium, phenobarbital, birth control pills, and other medications.
- Be sure to tell your doctor about any medications you are currently taking.

Storage
Tablets, capsules, liquid and suspension should be stored at room temperature in tightly closed containers. Store away from heat and direct light. Keep out of reach of children, since overdose may be very dangerous in children. Discard any outdated medication.

BRONKODYL S-R

Properties
This medicine contains theophylline as active ingredient; it is used to treat or prevent breathing problems (wheezing and shortness of breath) caused by asthma, bronchitis, or emphysema. This medication belongs to a group known as xanthine-derivative bronchodilators. They work by opening up the bronchial tubes or air passages of the lungs and increasing the flow of air through them. These medicines are available only with your doctor's prescription.

Before using this medicine
Before you use this medicine check with your doctor, or pharmacist:
- if you ever had any unusual or allergic reaction to xanthine-derivative bronchodilators.
- if you are on a low-salt, low-sugar, or any other special diet, or if you are allergic to any substance, such as sulfites or other preservatives or dyes.
- if you are pregnant or intend to become pregnant while using this medicine.
- if you are breast-feeding an infant. Theophylline passes into the breast milk and may cause irritability, fretfulness, or trouble in sleeping in infants of mothers taking this medicine.
- if you have any of the following medical problems:
Diarrhea
Enlarged prostate
Fibrocystic breast disease
Heart disease
Stomach ulcer

Treatment
This medication is used to relieve or prevent the symptoms of your medical problem. Take them as directed. Do not take more of them and do not take them more often than recommended on the label, unless otherwise directed by your doctor. To do so may increase the chance of side effects. The medicine should be taken on an empty stomach 30 to 60 minutes before a meal or two hours after a meal. Try not to miss any doses of this medication. If you do miss a dose, take the missed dose as soon as possible, unless it is almost time for the next dose. Do not double the next dose. It works best when taken with a glass of water.

Side effects
The following minor side effects may occur:
Dizziness or flushing
Headache
Diarrhea
Heartburn
Increased urination
Insomnia
Nervousness or irritability
Loss of appetite
Nausea or stomach upset
Stomach pain.
These side effects should disappear as your body adjusts to the medication. Tell your doctor about any side effects that are persistent or particularly bothersome. It is especially important to tell your doctor about black, tarry stools; confusion; convulsions; difficulty in breathing; fainting; muscle twitching; palpitations; rash; severe abdominal pain; or unusual weakness.

Interactions
This medicine interacts with several other drugs such as diuretics, reserpine, beta blockers, phenytoin, lithium, phenobarbital, birth control pills, and other medications.
- Be sure to tell your doctor about any medications you are currently taking.

Storage
Tablets, capsules, liquid and suspension should be stored at room temperature in tightly closed containers. Store away from heat and direct light. Keep out of reach of children, since overdose may be very dangerous in children. Discard any outdated medication.

BUTABARBITAL

Properties

This medicine contains as active ingredient the barbiturate butabarbital. Barbiturates belong to the group of medicines called central nervous system depressants (medicines that slow down the nervous system).

Barbiturates may partially block nerve impulses at nerve-cell connections. They may be used to treat insomnia (sleeplessness) by helping patients fall asleep. Also, they may be used to relieve anxiety or tension. Some of the barbiturates are used as anticonvulsants to help control convulsions in certain disorders or diseases, such as epilepsy. If too much of the drug is used, it may become habit-forming (causing mental or physical dependence).

Before using this medicine

Before you use this medicine check with your doctor, or pharmacist:

- if you ever had any unusual or allergic reaction to this medicine or one of its components.
- if you are on a low-salt, low-sugar, or any other special diet, or if you are allergic to preservatives or dyes.
- if you are pregnant or intend to become pregnant while using this medicine, since barbiturates have been shown to increase the chance of birth defects in humans. Taking barbiturates regularly during the last 3 months of pregnancy may cause the baby to become dependent on the medicine. This may lead to withdrawal side effects in the baby after birth.
- if you have any of the following medical problems:
  Anemia (severe)
  Diabetes mellitus (sugar disease)
  Hyperactivity (in children)
  Kidney or liver disease
  Mental depression
  Overactive thyroid

Treatment

This medication is used to treat the symptoms of your medical condition. Barbiturates act in the central nervous system; some of their side effects are also caused by actions in the central nervous system. Use this medicine as directed by your doctor. Do not use more of it, do not use it more often, and do not use it for a longer period of time than your doctor ordered.

- If you are taking this medication on a regular schedule and you miss a dose, take the missed dose as soon as possible, unless it is almost time for your next dose. In that case do not take the missed dose at all.
- If a barbiturate is used for a long time, is may become habit-forming. Physical dependence may lead to withdrawal side effects when you stop taking this medicine.

Side effects

Along with the needed effects, a medicine may cause some unwanted effects. These side effects may go away during treatment as your body adjusts to the medicine. Such minor side effects are: depression, confusion, diarrhea, nausea, vomiting, joint or muscle pain, slurred speech, hallucinations, headache, decreased sex drive.

- Check with your doctor immediately if any of the following side effects occur:
  Rash or hives
  Face, lip or eyelid swelling
  Sore throat, fever
  Agitation
  Slow heartbeat
  Difficult breathing or chest pain

Interactions

This medicine may interact with several other drugs such as medicines acting on the central nervous system (e.g., antihistamines; beta-adrenergic blockers; MAO inhibitors; mind-altering drugs; nabilone; antidepressants; clozapine; anticonvulsants).

Storage

The medicine should be stored at room temperature in a tightly closed, light-resistant container. Keep out of reach of children since overdose is very dangerous in children.

BUTACE

Properties

This medicine contains as active ingredient the barbiturate butabarbital. Barbiturates belong to the group of medicines called central nervous system depressants (medicines that slow down the nervous system).

Barbiturates may partially block nerve impulses at nerve-cell connections. They may be used to treat insomnia (sleeplessness) by helping patients fall asleep. Also, they may be used to relieve anxiety or tension. Some of the barbiturates are used as anticonvulsants to help control convulsions in certain disorders or diseases, such as epilepsy. If too much of the drug is used, it may become habit-forming (causing mental or physical dependence).

Before using this medicine

Before you use this medicine check with your doctor, or pharmacist:
- if you ever had any unusual or allergic reaction to this medicine or one of its components.
- if you are on a low-salt, low-sugar, or any other special diet, or if you are allergic to preservatives or dyes.
- if you are pregnant or intend to become pregnant while using this medicine, since barbiturates have been shown to increase the chance of birth defects in humans. Taking barbiturates regularly during the last 3 months of pregnancy may cause the baby to become dependent on the medicine. This may lead to withdrawal side effects in the baby after birth.
- if you have any of the following medical problems:
  Anemia (severe)
  Diabetes mellitus (sugar disease)
  Hyperactivity (in children)
  Kidney or liver disease
  Mental depression
  Overactive thyroid

Treatment

This medication is used to treat the symptoms of your medical condition. Barbiturates act in the central nervous system; some of their side effects are also caused by actions in the central nervous system. Use this medicine as directed by your doctor. Do not use more of it, do not use it more often, and do not use it for a longer period of time than your doctor ordered.
- If you are taking this medication on a regular schedule and you miss a dose, take the missed dose as soon as possible, unless it is almost time for your next dose. In that case do not take the missed dose at all.
- If a barbiturate it used for a long time, is may become habit-forming. Physical dependence may lead to withdrawal side effects when you stop taking this medicine.

Side effects

Along with the needed effects, a medicine may cause some unwanted effects. These side effects may go away during treatment as your body adjusts to the medicine. Such minor side effects are: depression, confusion, diarrhea, nausea, vomiting, joint or muscle pain, slurred speech, hallucinations, headache, decreased sex drive.
- Check with your doctor immediately if any of the following side effects occur:
  Rash or hives
  Face, lip or eyelid swelling
  Sore throat, fever
  Agitation
  Slow heartbeat
  Difficult breathing or chest pain

Interactions

This medicine may interact with several other drugs such as medicines acting on the central nervous system (e.g., antihistamines; beta-adrenergic blockers; MAO inhibitors; mind-altering drugs; nabilone; antidepressants; clozapine; anticonvulsants).

Storage

The medicine should be stored at room temperature in a tightly closed, light-resistant container. Keep out of reach of children since overdose is very dangerous in children.

BUTALAN

Properties

This medicine contains as active ingredient the barbiturate butabarbital. Barbiturates belong to the group of medicines called central nervous system depressants (medicines that slow down the nervous system).

Barbiturates may partially block nerve impulses at nerve-cell connections. They may be used to treat insomnia (sleeplessness) by helping patients fall asleep. Also, they may be used to relieve anxiety or tension. Some of the barbiturates are used as anticonvulsants to help control convulsions in certain disorders or diseases, such as epilepsy. If too much of the drug is used, it may become habit-forming (causing mental or physical dependence).

Before using this medicine

Before you use this medicine check with your doctor, or pharmacist:
- if you ever had any unusual or allergic reaction to this medicine or one of its components.
- if you are on a low-salt, low-sugar, or any other special diet, or if you are allergic to preservatives or dyes.
- if you are pregnant or intend to become pregnant while using this medicine, since barbiturates have been shown to increase the chance of birth defects in humans. Taking barbiturates regularly during the last 3 months of pregnancy may cause the baby to become dependent on the medicine. This may lead to withdrawal side effects in the baby after birth.
- if you have any of the following medical problems:
  Anemia (severe)
  Diabetes mellitus (sugar disease)
  Hyperactivity (in children)
  Kidney or liver disease
  Mental depression
  Overactive thyroid

Treatment

This medication is used to treat the symptoms of your medical condition. Barbiturates act in the central nervous system; some of their side effects are also caused by actions in the central nervous system. Use this medicine as directed by your doctor. Do not use more of it, do not use it more often, and do not use it for a longer period of time than your doctor ordered.

- If you are taking this medication on a regular schedule and you miss a dose, take the missed dose as soon as possible, unless it is almost time for your next dose. In that case do not take the missed dose at all.
- If a barbiturate is used for a long time, it may become habit-forming. Physical dependence may lead to withdrawal side effects when you stop taking this medicine.

Side effects

Along with the needed effects, a medicine may cause some unwanted effects. These side effects may go away during treatment as your body adjusts to the medicine. Such minor side effects are: depression, confusion, diarrhea, nausea, vomiting, joint or muscle pain, slurred speech, hallucinations, headache, decreased sex drive.

- Check with your doctor immediately if any of the following side effects occur:
  Rash or hives
  Face, lip or eyelid swelling
  Sore throat, fever
  Agitation
  Slow heartbeat
  Difficult breathing or chest pain

Interactions

This medicine may interact with several other drugs such as medicines acting on the central nervous system (e.g., antihistamines; beta-adrenergic blockers; MAO inhibitors; mind-altering drugs; nabilone; antidepressants; clozapine; anticonvulsants).

Storage

The medicine should be stored at room temperature in a tightly closed, light-resistant container. Keep out of reach of children since overdose is very dangerous in children.

BUTALBITAL

Properties
This medicine contains as active ingredient the barbiturate butabarbital. Barbiturates belong to the group of medicines called central nervous system depressants (medicines that slow down the nervous system).

Barbiturates may partially block nerve impulses at nerve-cell connections. They may be used to treat insomnia (sleeplessness) by helping patients fall asleep. Also, they may be used to relieve anxiety or tension. Some of the barbiturates are used as anticonvulsants to help control convulsions in certain disorders or diseases, such as epilepsy. If too much of the drug is used, it may become habit-forming (causing mental or physical dependence).

Before using this medicine
Before you use this medicine check with your doctor, or pharmacist:
- if you ever had any unusual or allergic reaction to this medicine or one of its components.
- if you are on a low-salt, low-sugar, or any other special diet, or if you are allergic to preservatives or dyes.
- if you are pregnant or intend to become pregnant while using this medicine, since barbiturates have been shown to increase the chance of birth defects in humans. Taking barbiturates regularly during the last 3 months of pregnancy may cause the baby to become dependent on the medicine. This may lead to withdrawal side effects in the baby after birth.
- if you have any of the following medical problems:
Anemia (severe)
Diabetes mellitus (sugar disease)
Hyperactivity (in children)
Kidney or liver disease
Mental depression
Overactive thyroid

Treatment
This medication is used to treat the symptoms of your medical condition. Barbiturates act in the central nervous system; some of their side effects are also caused by actions in the central nervous system. Use this medicine as directed by your doctor. Do not use more of it, do not use it more often, and do not use it for a longer period of time than your doctor ordered.
- If you are taking this medication on a regular schedule and you miss a dose, take the missed dose as soon as possible, unless it is almost time for your next dose. In that case do not take the missed dose at all.
- If a barbiturate is used for a long time, it may become habit-forming. Physical dependence may lead to withdrawal side effects when you stop taking this medicine.

Side effects
Along with the needed effects, a medicine may cause some unwanted effects. These side effects may go away during treatment as your body adjusts to the medicine. Such minor side effects are: depression, confusion, diarrhea, nausea, vomiting, joint or muscle pain, slurred speech, hallucinations, headache, decreased sex drive.
- Check with your doctor immediately if any of the following side effects occur:
Rash or hives
Face, lip or eyelid swelling
Sore throat, fever
Agitation
Slow heartbeat
Difficult breathing or chest pain

Interactions
This medicine may interact with several other drugs such as medicines acting on the central nervous system (e.g., antihistamines; beta-adrenergic blockers; MAO inhibitors; mind-altering drugs; nabilone; antidepressants; clozapine; anticonvulsants).

Storage
The medicine should be stored at room temperature in a tightly closed, light-resistant container. Keep out of reach of children since overdose is very dangerous in children.

BUTATRAN

Properties

This medicine contains as active ingredient the barbiturate butabarbital. Barbiturates belong to the group of medicines called central nervous system depressants (medicines that slow down the nervous system).

Barbiturates may partially block nerve impulses at nerve-cell connections. They may be used to treat insomnia (sleeplessness) by helping patients fall asleep. Also, they may be used to relieve anxiety or tension. Some of the barbiturates are used as anticonvulsants to help control convulsions in certain disorders or diseases, such as epilepsy. If too much of the drug is used, it may become habit-forming (causing mental or physical dependence).

Before using this medicine

Before you use this medicine check with your doctor, or pharmacist:
- if you ever had any unusual or allergic reaction to this medicine or one of its components.
- if you are on a low-salt, low-sugar, or any other special diet, or if you are allergic to preservatives or dyes.
- if you are pregnant or intend to become pregnant while using this medicine, since barbiturates have been shown to increase the chance of birth defects in humans. Taking barbiturates regularly during the last 3 months of pregnancy may cause the baby to become dependent on the medicine. This may lead to withdrawal side effects in the baby after birth.
- if you have any of the following medical problems:
  Anemia (severe)
  Diabetes mellitus (sugar disease)
  Hyperactivity (in children)
  Kidney or liver disease
  Mental depression
  Overactive thyroid

Treatment

This medication is used to treat the symptoms of your medical condition. Barbiturates act in the central nervous system; some of their side effects are also caused by actions in the central nervous system. Use this medicine as directed by your doctor. Do not use more of it, do not use it more often, and do not use it for a longer period of time than your doctor ordered.
- If you are taking this medication on a regular schedule and you miss a dose, take the missed dose as soon as possible, unless it is almost time for your next dose. In that case do not take the missed dose at all.
- If a barbiturate is used for a long time, it may become habit-forming. Physical dependence may lead to withdrawal side effects when you stop taking this medicine.

Side effects

Along with the needed effects, a medicine may cause some unwanted effects. These side effects may go away during treatment as your body adjusts to the medicine. Such minor side effects are: depression, confusion, diarrhea, nausea, vomiting, joint or muscle pain, slurred speech, hallucinations, headache, decreased sex drive.
- Check with your doctor immediately if any of the following side effects occur:
  Rash or hives
  Face, lip or eyelid swelling
  Sore throat, fever
  Agitation
  Slow heartbeat
  Difficult breathing or chest pain

Interactions

This medicine may interact with several other drugs such as medicines acting on the central nervous system (e.g., antihistamines; beta-adrenergic blockers; MAO inhibitors; mind-altering drugs; nabilone; antidepressants; clozapine; anticonvulsants).

Storage

The medicine should be stored at room temperature in a tightly closed, light-resistant container. Keep out of reach of children since overdose is very dangerous in children.

BUTICAPS

Properties

This medicine contains as active ingredient the barbiturate butabarbital. Barbiturates belong to the group of medicines called central nervous system depressants (medicines that slow down the nervous system).

Barbiturates may partially block nerve impulses at nerve-cell connections. They may be used to treat insomnia (sleeplessness) by helping patients fall asleep. Also, they may be used to relieve anxiety or tension. Some of the barbiturates are used as anticonvulsants to help control convulsions in certain disorders or diseases, such as epilepsy. If too much of the drug is used, it may become habit-forming (causing mental or physical dependence).

Before using this medicine

Before you use this medicine check with your doctor, or pharmacist:
- if you ever had any unusual or allergic reaction to this medicine or one of its components.
- if you are on a low-salt, low-sugar, or any other special diet, or if you are allergic to preservatives or dyes.
- if you are pregnant or intend to become pregnant while using this medicine, since barbiturates have been shown to increase the chance of birth defects in humans. Taking barbiturates regularly during the last 3 months of pregnancy may cause the baby to become dependent on the medicine. This may lead to withdrawal side effects in the baby after birth.
- if you have any of the following medical problems:
  Anemia (severe)
  Diabetes mellitus (sugar disease)
  Hyperactivity (in children)
  Kidney or liver disease
  Mental depression
  Overactive thyroid

Treatment

This medication is used to treat the symptoms of your medical condition. Barbiturates act in the central nervous system; some of their side effects are also caused by actions in the central nervous system. Use this medicine as directed by your doctor. Do not use more of it, do not use it more often, and do not use it for a longer period of time than your doctor ordered.

- If you are taking this medication on a regular schedule and you miss a dose, take the missed dose as soon as possible, unless it is almost time for your next dose. In that case do not take the missed dose at all.
- If a barbiturate is used for a long time, it may become habit-forming. Physical dependence may lead to withdrawal side effects when you stop taking this medicine.

Side effects

Along with the needed effects, a medicine may cause some unwanted effects. These side effects may go away during treatment as your body adjusts to the medicine. Such minor side effects are: depression, confusion, diarrhea, nausea, vomiting, joint or muscle pain, slurred speech, hallucinations, headache, decreased sex drive.

- Check with your doctor immediately if any of the following side effects occur:
  Rash or hives
  Face, lip or eyelid swelling
  Sore throat, fever
  Agitation
  Slow heartbeat
  Difficult breathing or chest pain

Interactions

This medicine may interact with several other drugs such as medicines acting on the central nervous system (e.g., antihistamines; beta-adrenergic blockers; MAO inhibitors; mind-altering drugs; nabilone; antidepressants; clozapine; anticonvulsants).

Storage

The medicine should be stored at room temperature in a tightly closed, light-resistant container. Keep out of reach of children since overdose is very dangerous in children.

BUTISOL

Properties

This medicine contains as active ingredient the barbiturate butabarbital. Barbiturates belong to the group of medicines called central nervous system depressants (medicines that slow down the nervous system).

Barbiturates may partially block nerve impulses at nerve-cell connections. They may be used to treat insomnia (sleeplessness) by helping patients fall asleep. Also, they may be used to relieve anxiety or tension. Some of the barbiturates are used as anticonvulsants to help control convulsions in certain disorders or diseases, such as epilepsy. If too much of the drug is used, it may become habit-forming (causing mental or physical dependence).

Before using this medicine

Before you use this medicine check with your doctor, or pharmacist:
- if you ever had any unusual or allergic reaction to this medicine or one of its components.
- if you are on a low-salt, low-sugar, or any other special diet, or if you are allergic to preservatives or dyes.
- if you are pregnant or intend to become pregnant while using this medicine, since barbiturates have been shown to increase the chance of birth defects in humans. Taking barbiturates regularly during the last 3 months of pregnancy may cause the baby to become dependent on the medicine. This may lead to withdrawal side effects in the baby after birth.
- if you have any of the following medical problems:
  Anemia (severe)
  Diabetes mellitus (sugar disease)
  Hyperactivity (in children)
  Kidney or liver disease
  Mental depression
  Overactive thyroid

Treatment

This medication is used to treat the symptoms of your medical condition. Barbiturates act in the central nervous system; some of their side effects are also caused by actions in the central nervous system. Use this medicine as directed by your doctor. Do not use more of it, do not use it more often, and do not use it for a longer period of time than your doctor ordered.

- If you are taking this medication on a regular schedule and you miss a dose, take the missed dose as soon as possible, unless it is almost time for your next dose. In that case do not take the missed dose at all.
- If a barbiturate is used for a long time, it may become habit-forming. Physical dependence may lead to withdrawal side effects when you stop taking this medicine.

Side effects

Along with the needed effects, a medicine may cause some unwanted effects. These side effects may go away during treatment as your body adjusts to the medicine. Such minor side effects are: depression, confusion, diarrhea, nausea, vomiting, joint or muscle pain, slurred speech, hallucinations, headache, decreased sex drive.

- Check with your doctor immediately if any of the following side effects occur:
  Rash or hives
  Face, lip or eyelid swelling
  Sore throat, fever
  Agitation
  Slow heartbeat
  Difficult breathing or chest pain

Interactions

This medicine may interact with several other drugs such as medicines acting on the central nervous system (e.g., antihistamines; beta-adrenergic blockers; MAO inhibitors; mind-altering drugs; nabilone; antidepressants; clozapine; anticonvulsants).

Storage

The medicine should be stored at room temperature in a tightly closed, light-resistant container. Keep out of reach of children since overdose is very dangerous in children.

BUTORPHANOL

Properties
This medicine contains as active ingredient buthorphanol.

It is a narcotic analgesic that acts directly on the central nervous system (brain and spinal cord). It is used to relieve pain or to suppress coughing.

Before using this medicine
Before you use this medicine check with your doctor, or pharmacist:
- if you ever had any unusual or allergic reaction to this medicine or one of its components.
- if you are on a low-salt, low-sugar, or any other special diet, or if you are allergic to any substance, such as sulfites or other preservatives or dyes.
- if you are pregnant or intend to become pregnant while using this medicine. Studies on birth defects have not been done in humans. Too much use of narcotics during pregnancy may cause the baby to become dependent on the medicine.
- if you are breast-feeding an infant. Although this medicine has not been shown to cause problems in humans, it passes into the breast milk in small amounts.
- if you have any of the following medical problems:
  Brain disease or head injury
  Colitis
  Convulsions
  Emphysema, asthma, or chronic lung disease
  Enlarged prostate
  Gallbladder disease or gallstones
  Heart disease
  Kidney or liver disease
  Underactive thyroid

Treatment
This medication is used to relieve pain or to suppress coughing. Narcotic analgesics act in the central nervous system; some of their side effects are also caused by actions in the central nervous system.
- If you are taking this medication on a regular schedule and you miss a dose, take the missed dose as soon as possible, unless it is almost time for your next dose. In that case do not take the missed dose at all.
- If a narcotic analgesic is used for a long time, is may become habit-forming (causing mental or physical dependence). Physical dependence may lead to withdrawal side effects when you stop taking this medicine.

Unless otherwise directed by your doctor or pharmacist take this as directed. Do not take more of them and do not take them more often than recommended on the label. Children up to 12 years of age should not take this medicine more than 3 times a day or for more than 5 days in a row.

Side effects
Along with the needed effects, a medicine may cause some unwanted effects. These side effects may go away during treatment as your body adjusts to the medicine. Such minor side effects are: constipation, dizziness, drowsiness, dry mouth, false sense of well-being, flushing, light-headedness, loss or appetite, nausea, painful or difficult urination, or sweating.
- Check with your doctor immediately if any of the following side effects occur:
  Anxiety or breathing difficulties
  Excitation or restlessness
  Fatigue, palpitations
  Rash, sore throat and fever
  Tremors or weakness

Interactions
This medicine may interact with several other drugs such as medicines acting on the central nervous system (e.g., antidepressants, tranquilizers), cimetidine, nitrates, quinidine, etc.
- Be sure to tell your doctor about any medications you are currently taking.

Storage
Tablets, elixir, suppository etc. should be stored at room temperature in a tightly closed, light-resistant container.

C.E.S.

Properties
This medicine contains conjugated estrogens as active ingredients. The medicine is prescribed for treatment of estrogen deficiency; it restores normal estrogen levels in tissues.

There is no evidence that this drug is effective for nervous symptoms or depression occurring during menopause. They should not be used to treat this condition; they should be used only to replace the estrogen that is naturally absent after menopause.

Before using this medicine
Before you use this medicine check with your doctor, or pharmacist:
- if you ever had any unusual or allergic reaction to estrogens;
- if you are pregnant or intend to become pregnant within three months;
- if you are breast-feeding an infant;
- if you have any of the following medical problems:
Diabetes
Breast cancer
Fibrocystic breast disease
Fibroid uterine tumors
Endometriosis
Migraine headaches
Epilepsy
Porphyria
High blood pressure
Asthma
Congestive heart failure
Kidney disease
Gallstones

Treatment
This medication is used to treat estrogen deficiency, specific symptoms of menopause, estrogen-deficiency osteoporosis, atrophic vaginitis, prostate cancer.

For safe and effective use of this medicine:
- ◆ Follow your doctor's instructions if this medicine was prescribed.
- ◆ Follow the manufacturer's package directions if you are treating yourself.
- ◆ Estrogens have been reported to increase the risk of endometrial carcinoma.

Side effects
Along with the needed effects, a medicine may cause some unwanted effects. Possible side effects include:
Stomach cramps
Profuse bleeding
Appetite loss
Nausea and vomiting
Swollen breasts
Change in menstruation
Rash, skin blisters
Depression
Dizziness

Overdose
The following symptoms may indicate an overdose:
Nausea and vomiting
Fluid retention
Breast enlargement
Abnormal vaginal bleeding
- ■ Call a doctor or hospital emergency room for instructions.

Interactions
This medicine may interact with several other drugs such as adrenocorticosteroids, antidepressants, oral antidiabetics, insulin, phenobarbital, primidone.
- ■ Be sure to tell your doctor about any medications you are currently taking.

Storage
Capsules, tablets, vaginal cream, transdermal patches, etc. should be stored at room temperature; store away from heat and direct light. Keep out of reach of children, since this medicine may be dangerous in children.

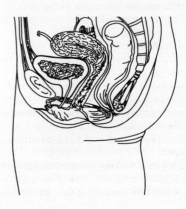

C-LEXIN

Properties

This medicine contains cephalosporin as active ingredient. Cephalosporins belong to the general family of medicines called antibiotics, used in the treatment of infections caused by bacteria. They work by killing bacteria or preventing their growth. Cephalosporins will not work for colds, flu, or other viral infections.

Before using this medicine

Before you use this medicine check with your doctor:
- if you ever had any unusual or allergic reaction to any of the cephalosporins, penicillins, penicillin-like medicines, or penicillamine.
- if you are on a low-salt, low-sugar, or any other special diet, or if you are allergic to any substance, such as sulfites or other preservatives or dyes.
- if you are pregnant or intend to become pregnant while using this medicine. Although cephalosporins have not been shown to cause birth defects or other problems in humans, the chance always exists.
- if you are breast-feeding an infant. Most cephalosporins pass into the breast milk, usually in small amounts.
- if you have any of the following medical problems:
  Bleeding problem
  Kidney or liver disease

Treatment

This medication belongs to the general family of medicines called antibiotics. It is used to treat a wide variety of bacterial infections. It is also used to treat infections in persons who are allergic to penicillin.
- Keep taking this medicine for the full time of treatment even if you begin to feel better after a few days; do not miss any doses.
- If you do miss a dose of this medicine, take it as soon as possible. This will help to keep a constant amount of medicine in the blood. However, if it is almost time for your next dose, skip the missed dose and go back to your regular dosing schedule.
- This medication has been prescribed for your current infection only. Another infection later on, or one that someone else has, may require a different medicine. You should not give your medicine to other people or use it for other infections, unless your doctor specifically directs you to do so.
- Take the medicine at the same times each day, 1 hour before or 2 hours after eating.

Side effects

Along with the needed effects, a medicine may cause some unwanted effects. Side effects that usually do not require medical attention: rectal itching, oral or vaginal white spots, mild diarrhea. These side effects should disappear as your body adjusts to the medication.
- Other side effects that should be reported to your doctor immediately are:
  Hives, rash
  Intense itching
  Faintness soon after a dose
  Difficulty in breathing
  Nausea and vomiting
  Severe diarrhea
  Unusual weakness or tiredness
  Bleeding or bruising

Interactions

This medicine may interact with several other drugs such as anticoagulants, theophylline preparations, probenecid, tetracyclines, etc.
- Be sure to tell your doctor about any medications you are currently taking.

Storage

Tablets, capsules, etc. should be stored at room temperature. Store the liquid form in the refrigerator. Keep out of the reach of children. Do not keep outdated medicine or medicine no longer needed.

CALAN

Properties

This medicine contains verapamil as active ingredient. It is a so-called calcium channel blocker, working by blocking the passage of calcium into heart and smooth muscle. Since calcium is an essential factor in muscle contraction, any medicine that affects calcium in this way will interfere with the contraction of these muscles.

The medicine works by:

♦ reducing the work that the heart must perform;
♦ reducing the normal arterial blood pressure;
♦ increasing oxygen to the heart muscle.

The medicine is prescribed for the treatment of attacks of angina pectoris, irregular heartbeat, and high blood pressure. In many cases it can be used for the treatment and prevention of migraine.

Before using this medicine

Before you use this medicine check with your doctor, or pharmacist:

– if you ever had any unusual or allergic reaction to this medicine or any calcium channel blocker;
– if you are pregnant or intend to become pregnant while using this medicine;
– if you have low blood pressure;
– if you have kidney or liver disease;
– if you are breast-feeding an infant;
– if you easily get a rash or intensity sunburn in areas exposed to sun or ultraviolet light.

Treatment

This medication is used for treatment of heart conditions (for instance, angina pectoris) and high blood pressure. Tablets, capsules or extended-release tablets should be taken with liquid. The usual dose amounts to 30 to 100 milligrams a day.

For safe and effective use of medicine:

♦ Follow your doctor's instructions if this medicine was prescribed.
♦ Follow the manufacturer's package directions if you are treating yourself.

Side effects

Along with the needed effects, a medicine may cause some unwanted effects. Possible side effects include:

Tiredness
Changes in heartbeat
Wheezing
Cough
Shortness of breath
Dizziness
Fainting
Numbness in hands and feet
Tingling in hands and feet
Difficult urination
Constipation

Overdose

The following symptoms may be a sign of overdose:

Unusually fast heartbeat
Unusually slow heartbeat
Loss of consciousness
Cardiac arrest

■ Call a doctor or hospital emergency room for instructions. If necessary start first aid immediately.

Interactions

The effect of this medicine may cause a blood pressure drop if taken together with antihypertensives. Cimetidine may increase the effect of the calcium blocker.

The simultaneous use of diuretics and calcium channel blockers may cause dangerous blood pressure drop.

■ Be sure to tell your doctor about any medications you are currently taking.

Storage

Capsules, tablets, etc. should be stored at room temperature; store away from heat and direct light. Keep out of reach of children, since this medicine may be dangerous in children.

CARDENE

Properties
This medicine contains nicardipine as active ingredient. It is a so-called calcium channel blocker, working by blocking the passage of calcium into heart and smooth muscle. Since calcium is an essential factor in muscle contraction, any medicine that affects calcium in this way will interfere with the contraction of these muscles.

The medicine works by:
♦ reducing the work that the heart must perform;
♦ reducing the normal arterial blood pressure;
♦ increasing oxygen to the heart muscle.

The medicine is prescribed for the treatment of attacks of angina pectoris, irregular heartbeat, and high blood pressure. In many cases it can be used for the treatment and prevention of migraine.

Before using this medicine
Before you use this medicine check with your doctor, or pharmacist:
– if you ever had any unusual or allergic reaction to this medicine or any calcium channel blocker;
– if you are pregnant or intend to become pregnant while using this medicine;
– if you have low blood pressure;
– if you have kidney or liver disease;
– if you are breast-feeding an infant;
– if you easily get a rash or intensity sunburn in areas exposed to sun or ultraviolet light.

Treatment
This medication is used for treatment of heart conditions (for instance, angina pectoris) and high blood pressure. Tablets, capsules or extended-release tablets should be taken with liquid. The usual dose amounts to 30 to 100 milligrams a day.

For safe and effective use of medicine:
♦ Follow your doctor's instructions if this medicine was prescribed.
♦ Follow the manufacturer's package

directions if you are treating yourself.

Side effects
Along with the needed effects, a medicine may cause some unwanted effects. Possible side effects include:
  Tiredness
  Changes in heartbeat
  Wheezing
  Cough
  Shortness of breath
  Dizziness
  Fainting
  Numbness in hands and feet
  Tingling in hands and feet
  Difficult urination
  Constipation

Overdose
The following symptoms may be a sign of overdose:
  Unusually fast heartbeat
  Unusually slow heartbeat
  Loss of consciousness
  Cardiac arrest
■ Call a doctor or hospital emergency room for instructions. If necessary start first aid immediately.

Interactions
The effect of this medicine may cause a blood pressure drop if taken together with antihypertensives. Cimetidine may increase the effect of the calcium blocker.

The simultaneous use of diuretics and calcium channel blockers may cause dangerous blood pressure drop.
■ Be sure to tell your doctor about any medications you are currently taking.

Storage
Capsules, tablets, etc. should be stored at room temperature; store away from heat and direct light. Keep out of reach of children, since this medicine may be dangerous in children.

CARDILATE

Properties
This medicine contains erythrityl tetranitrate as active ingredient. Nitrates improve the supply of blood and oxygen to the heart. This medication is for oral use.

Before using this medicine
Before you use this medicine check with your doctor, or pharmacist:
- if you ever had any unusual or allergic reaction to nitrates or nitrites.
- if you are on a low-salt, low-sugar, or any other special diet, or if you are allergic to any substance, such as sulfites or other preservatives or dyes.
- if you are pregnant or intend to become pregnant while using this medicine. Although nitrates have not been shown to cause problems in humans, the chance always exists.
- if you are breast-feeding an infant.
- if you have recently had a heart attack or stroke.
- if you have any of the following medical problems:
  Anemia
  Glaucoma
  Intestinal problems
  Overactive thyroid
- if you are now taking any of the following medicines or types of medicines:
  Antihypertensives
  Asthma or hay fever medicine
  Cold medicine
  Decongestant
  Medicine for appetite control
  Narcotic
  Pain medicine
  Sinus congestion medicine

Treatment
This medication is used to treat and prevent angina (chest pain). Nitroglycerin is a vasodilator, which relaxes the muscles of the blood vessels, causing an increase in the oxygen supply to the heart. The oral tablets, capsules, ointment and patches do not act quickly; they are used to prevent chest pain.

The sublingual tablets and oral spray act quickly and can be used to relieve chest pain after it has started.
- Take this medicine exactly as directed by your doctor or pharmacist. It will work only if taken correctly.
- If you are taking this medicine regularly and you miss a dose, take it as soon as possible. However, if your next scheduled dose is within 2 hours (or within 6 hours for extended-release capsules or tablets), skip the missed dose and go back to your regular dosing schedule.
- If you have been taking this medicine regularly for several weeks or more, do not suddenly stop using it. Stopping suddenly may bring on attacks of angina.

Side effects
There are a number of side effects that usually do not require medical attention. These possible side effects may go away during treatment; however, if they continue or are bothersome, check with your doctor, nurse, or pharmacist. More common are: dizziness, lightheadedness, or fainting when standing up; fast pulse; flushing of face and neck; headache; nausea or vomiting.

Side effects that should be reported to your doctor are: blurred vision; dry mouth; severe or prolonged headache; skin rash.

Interactions
This medicine may interact with several other drugs such as tricyclic antidepressants and cough medicines. Before starting to take or apply nitroglycerin, be sure to tell your doctor about any medications you are currently taking.

Storage
Tablets, capsules, and oral spray should be stored as in a tightly capped bottle in a cool, dry place. Ointment and patches should be stored at room temperature in their original containers. Keep out of reach of children. Do not keep outdated medicine or medicine no longer needed.

CARDIZEM

Properties

This medicine contains diltiazem as active ingredient. It is a so-called calcium channel blocker, working by blocking the passage of calcium into heart and smooth muscle. Since calcium is an essential factor in muscle contraction, any medicine that affects calcium in this way will interfere with the contraction of these muscles.

The medicine works by:
- reducing the work that the heart must perform;
- reducing the normal arterial blood pressure;
- increasing oxygen to the heart muscle.

The medicine is prescribed for the treatment of attacks of angina pectoris, irregular heartbeat, and high blood pressure. In many cases it can be used for the treatment and prevention of migraine.

Before using this medicine

Before you use this medicine check with your doctor, or pharmacist:
- if you ever had any unusual or allergic reaction to this medicine or any calcium channel blocker;
- if you are pregnant or intend to become pregnant while using this medicine;
- if you have low blood pressure;
- if you have kidney or liver disease;
- if you are breast-feeding an infant;
- if you easily get a rash or intensity sunburn in areas exposed to sun or ultraviolet light.

Treatment

This medication is used for treatment of heart conditions (for instance, angina pectoris) and high blood pressure. Tablets, capsules or extended-release tablets should be taken with liquid. The usual dose amounts to 30 to 100 milligrams a day.

For safe and effective use of medicine:
- Follow your doctor's instructions if this medicine was prescribed.
- Follow the manufacturer's package directions if you are treating yourself.

Side effects

Along with the needed effects, a medicine may cause some unwanted effects. Possible side effects include:
Tiredness
Changes in heartbeat
Wheezing
Cough
Shortness of breath
Dizziness
Fainting
Numbness in hands and feet
Tingling in hands and feet
Difficult urination
Constipation

Overdose

The following symptoms may be a sign of overdose:
Unusually fast heartbeat
Unusually slow heartbeat
Loss of consciousness
Cardiac arrest
- Call a doctor or hospital emergency room for instructions. If necessary start first aid immediately.

Interactions

The effect of this medicine may cause a blood pressure drop if taken together with antihypertensives. Cimetidine may increase the effect of the calcium blocker.

The simultaneous use of diuretics and calcium channel blockers may cause dangerous blood pressure drop.
- Be sure to tell your doctor about any medications you are currently taking.

Storage

Capsules, tablets, etc. should be stored at room temperature; store away from heat and direct light. Keep out of reach of children, since this medicine may be dangerous in children.

CECLOR

Properties

This medicine contains cephalosporin as active ingredient. Cephalosporins belong to the general family of medicines called antibiotics, used in the treatment of infections caused by bacteria. They work by killing bacteria or preventing their growth. Cephalosporins will not work for colds, flu, or other viral infections.

Before using this medicine

Before you use this medicine check with your doctor:

- if you ever had any unusual or allergic reaction to any of the cephalosporins, penicillins, penicillin-like medicines, or penicillamine.
- if you are on a low-salt, low-sugar, or any other special diet, or if you are allergic to any substance, such as sulfites or other preservatives or dyes.
- if you are pregnant or intend to become pregnant while using this medicine. Although cephalosporins have not been shown to cause birth defects or other problems in humans, the chance always exists.
- if you are breast-feeding an infant. Most cephalosporins pass into the breast milk, usually in small amounts.
- if you have any of the following medical problems:
Bleeding problem
Kidney or liver disease

Treatment

This medication belongs to the general family of medicines called antibiotics. It is used to treat a wide variety of bacterial infections. It is also used to treat infections in persons who are allergic to penicillin.

- Keep taking this medicine for the full time of treatment even if you begin to feel better after a few days; do not miss any doses.
- If you do miss a dose of this medicine, take it as soon as possible. This will help to keep a constant amount of medicine in the blood. However, if it is almost time for your next dose, skip the missed dose and go back to your regular dosing schedule.
- This medication has been prescribed for your current infection only. Another infection later on, or one that someone else has, may require a different medicine. You should not give your medicine to other people or use it for other infections, unless your doctor specifically directs you to do so.
- Take the medicine at the same times each day, 1 hour before or 2 hours after eating.

Side effects

Along with the needed effects, a medicine may cause some unwanted effects. Side effects that usually do not require medical attention: rectal itching, oral or vaginal white spots, mild diarrhea. These side effects should disappear as your body adjusts to the medication.

- Other side effects that should be reported to your doctor immediately are:
Hives, rash
Intense itching
Faintness soon after a dose
Difficulty in breathing
Nausea and vomiting
Severe diarrhea
Unusual weakness or tiredness
Bleeding or bruising

Interactions

This medicine may interact with several other drugs such as anticoagulants, theophylline preparations, probenecid, tetracyclines, etc.

- Be sure to tell your doctor about any medications you are currently taking.

Storage

Tablets, capsules, etc. should be stored at room temperature. Store the liquid form in the refrigerator. Keep out of the reach of children. Do not keep outdated medicine or medicine no longer needed.

CEFACLOR

Properties
This medicine contains cephalosporin as active ingredient. Cephalosporins belong to the general family of medicines called antibiotics, used in the treatment of infections caused by bacteria. They work by killing bacteria or preventing their growth. Cephalosporins will not work for colds, flu, or other viral infections.

Before using this medicine
Before you use this medicine check with your doctor:
– if you ever had any unusual or allergic reaction to any of the cephalosporins, penicillins, penicillin-like medicines, or penicillamine.
– if you are on a low-salt, low-sugar, or any other special diet, or if you are allergic to any substance, such as sulfites or other preservatives or dyes.
– if you are pregnant or intend to become pregnant while using this medicine. Although cephalosporins have not been shown to cause birth defects or other problems in humans, the chance always exists.
– if you are breast-feeding an infant. Most cephalosporins pass into the breast milk, usually in small amounts.
– if you have any of the following medical problems:
Bleeding problem
Kidney or liver disease

Treatment
This medication belongs to the general family of medicines called antibiotics. It is used to treat a wide variety of bacterial infections. It is also used to treat infections in persons who are allergic to penicillin.
■ Keep taking this medicine for the full time of treatment even if you begin to feel better after a few days; do not miss any doses.
■ If you do miss a dose of this medicine, take it as soon as possible. This will help to keep a constant amount of medicine in the blood. However, if it is almost time for your next dose,

skip the missed dose and go back to your regular dosing schedule.
■ This medication has been prescribed for your current infection only. Another infection later on, or one that someone else has, may require a different medicine. You should not give your medicine to other people or use it for other infections, unless your doctor specifically directs you to do so.
■ Take the medicine at the same times each day, 1 hour before or 2 hours after eating.

Side effects
Along with the needed effects, a medicine may cause some unwanted effects. Side effects that usually do not require medical attention: rectal itching, oral or vaginal white spots, mild diarrhea. These side effects should disappear as your body adjusts to the medication.
■ Other side effects that should be reported to your doctor immediately are:
Hives, rash
Intense itching
Faintness soon after a dose
Difficulty in breathing
Nausea and vomiting
Severe diarrhea
Unusual weakness or tiredness
Bleeding or bruising

Interactions
This medicine may interact with several other drugs such as anticoagulants, theophylline preparations, probenecid, tetracyclines, etc.
■ Be sure to tell your doctor about any medications you are currently taking.

Storage
Tablets, capsules, etc. should be stored at room temperature. Store the liquid form in the refrigerator. Keep out of the reach of children. Do not keep outdated medicine or medicine no longer needed.

CEFANEX

Properties

This medicine contains cephalosporin as active ingredient. Cephalosporins belong to the general family of medicines called antibiotics, used in the treatment of infections caused by bacteria. They work by killing bacteria or preventing their growth. Cephalosporins will not work for colds, flu, or other viral infections.

Before using this medicine

Before you use this medicine check with your doctor:
- if you ever had any unusual or allergic reaction to any of the cephalosporins, penicillins, penicillin-like medicines, or penicillamine.
- if you are on a low-salt, low-sugar, or any other special diet, or if you are allergic to any substance, such as sulfites or other preservatives or dyes.
- if you are pregnant or intend to become pregnant while using this medicine. Although cephalosporins have not been shown to cause birth defects or other problems in humans, the chance always exists.
- if you are breast-feeding an infant. Most cephalosporins pass into the breast milk, usually in small amounts.
- if you have any of the following medical problems:
Bleeding problem
Kidney or liver disease

Treatment

This medication belongs to the general family of medicines called antibiotics. It is used to treat a wide variety of bacterial infections. It is also used to treat infections in persons who are allergic to penicillin.

Keep taking this medicine for the full time of treatment even if you begin to feel better after a few days; do not miss any doses.
- If you do miss a dose of this medicine, take it as soon as possible. This will help to keep a constant amount of medicine in the blood. However, if it is almost time for your next dose, skip the missed dose and go back to your regular dosing schedule.
- This medication has been prescribed for your current infection only. Another infection later on, or one that someone else has, may require a different medicine. You should not give your medicine to other people or use it for other infections, unless your doctor specifically directs you to do so.
- Take the medicine at the same times each day, 1 hour before or 2 hours after eating.

Side effects

Along with the needed effects, a medicine may cause some unwanted effects. Side effects that usually do not require medical attention: rectal itching, oral or vaginal white spots, mild diarrhea. These side effects should disappear as your body adjusts to the medication.
- Other side effects that should be reported to your doctor immediately are:
Hives, rash
Intense itching
Faintness soon after a dose
Difficulty in breathing
Nausea and vomiting
Severe diarrhea
Unusual weakness or tiredness
Bleeding or bruising

Interactions

This medicine may interact with several other drugs such as anticoagulants, theophylline preparations, probenecid, tetracyclines, etc.
- Be sure to tell your doctor about any medications you are currently taking.

Storage

Tablets, capsules, etc. should be stored at room temperature. Store the liquid form in the refrigerator. Keep out of the reach of children. Do not keep outdated medicine or medicine no longer needed.

CEFIXIME

Properties

This medicine contains cephalosporin as active ingredient. Cephalosporins belong to the general family of medicines called antibiotics, used in the treatment of infections caused by bacteria. They work by killing bacteria or preventing their growth. Cephalosporins will not work for colds, flu, or other viral infections.

Before using this medicine

Before you use this medicine check with your doctor:
- if you ever had any unusual or allergic reaction to any of the cephalosporins, penicillins, penicillin-like medicines, or penicillamine.
- if you are on a low-salt, low-sugar, or any other special diet, or if you are allergic to any substance, such as sulfites or other preservatives or dyes.
- if you are pregnant or intend to become pregnant while using this medicine. Although cephalosporins have not been shown to cause birth defects or other problems in humans, the chance always exists.
- if you are breast-feeding an infant. Most cephalosporins pass into the breast milk, usually in small amounts.
- if you have any of the following medical problems:
  Bleeding problem
  Kidney or liver disease

Treatment

This medication belongs to the general family of medicines called antibiotics. It is used to treat a wide variety of bacterial infections. It is also used to treat infections in persons who are allergic to penicillin.
- Keep taking this medicine for the full time of treatment even if you begin to feel better after a few days; do not miss any doses.
- If you do miss a dose of this medicine, take it as soon as possible. This will help to keep a constant amount of medicine in the blood. However, if it is almost time for your next dose,

skip the missed dose and go back to your regular dosing schedule.
- This medication has been prescribed for your current infection only. Another infection later on, or one that someone else has, may require a different medicine. You should not give your medicine to other people or use it for other infections, unless your doctor specifically directs you to do so.
- Take the medicine at the same times each day, 1 hour before or 2 hours after eating.

Side effects

Along with the needed effects, a medicine may cause some unwanted effects. Side effects that usually do not require medical attention: rectal itching, oral or vaginal white spots, mild diarrhea. These side effects should disappear as your body adjusts to the medication.
- Other side effects that should be reported to your doctor immediately are:
  Hives, rash
  Intense itching
  Faintness soon after a dose
  Difficulty in breathing
  Nausea and vomiting
  Severe diarrhea
  Unusual weakness or tiredness
  Bleeding or bruising

Interactions

This medicine may interact with several other drugs such as anticoagulants, theophylline preparations, probenecid, tetracyclines, etc.
- Be sure to tell your doctor about any medications you are currently taking.

Storage

Tablets, capsules, etc. should be stored at room temperature. Store the liquid form in the refrigerator. Keep out of the reach of children. Do not keep outdated medicine or medicine no longer needed.

CEFIZOX

Properties
This medicine contains cephalosporin as active ingredient. Cephalosporins belong to the general family of medicines called antibiotics, used in the treatment of infections caused by bacteria. They work by killing bacteria or preventing their growth. Cephalosporins will not work for colds, flu, or other viral infections.

Before using this medicine
Before you use this medicine check with your doctor:
- if you ever had any unusual or allergic reaction to any of the cephalosporins, penicillins, penicillin-like medicines, or penicillamine.
- if you are on a low-salt, low-sugar, or any other special diet, or if you are allergic to any substance, such as sulfites or other preservatives or dyes.
- if you are pregnant or intend to become pregnant while using this medicine. Although cephalosporins have not been shown to cause birth defects or other problems in humans, the chance always exists.
- if you are breast-feeding an infant. Most cephalosporins pass into the breast milk, usually in small amounts.
- if you have any of the following medical problems:
  Bleeding problem
  Kidney or liver disease

Treatment
This medication belongs to the general family of medicines called antibiotics. It is used to treat a wide variety of bacterial infections. It is also used to treat infections in persons who are allergic to penicillin.
- Keep taking this medicine for the full time of treatment even if you begin to feel better after a few days; do not miss any doses.
- If you do miss a dose of this medicine, take it as soon as possible. This will help to keep a constant amount of medicine in the blood. However, if it is almost time for your next dose, skip the missed dose and go back to your regular dosing schedule.
- This medication has been prescribed for your current infection only. Another infection later on, or one that someone else has, may require a different medicine. You should not give your medicine to other people or use it for other infections, unless your doctor specifically directs you to do so.
- Take the medicine at the same times each day, 1 hour before or 2 hours after eating.

Side effects
Along with the needed effects, a medicine may cause some unwanted effects. Side effects that usually do not require medical attention: rectal itching, oral or vaginal white spots, mild diarrhea. These side effects should disappear as your body adjusts to the medication.
- Other side effects that should be reported to your doctor immediately are:
  Hives, rash
  Intense itching
  Faintness soon after a dose
  Difficulty in breathing
  Nausea and vomiting
  Severe diarrhea
  Unusual weakness or tiredness
  Bleeding or bruising

Interactions
This medicine may interact with several other drugs such as anticoagulants, theophylline preparations, probenecid, tetracyclines, etc.
- Be sure to tell your doctor about any medications you are currently taking.

Storage
Tablets, capsules, etc. should be stored at room temperature. Store the liquid form in the refrigerator. Keep out of the reach of children. Do not keep outdated medicine or medicine no longer needed.

CEFOBID

Properties
This medicine contains cephalosporin as active ingredient. Cephalosporins belong to the general family of medicines called antibiotics, used in the treatment of infections caused by bacteria. They work by killing bacteria or preventing their growth. Cephalosporins will not work for colds, flu, or other viral infections.

Before using this medicine
Before you use this medicine check with your doctor:
- if you ever had any unusual or allergic reaction to any of the cephalosporins, penicillins, penicillin-like medicines, or penicillamine.
- if you are on a low-salt, low-sugar, or any other special diet, or if you are allergic to any substance, such as sulfites or other preservatives or dyes.
- if you are pregnant or intend to become pregnant while using this medicine. Although cephalosporins have not been shown to cause birth defects or other problems in humans, the chance always exists.
- if you are breast-feeding an infant. Most cephalosporins pass into the breast milk, usually in small amounts.
- if you have any of the following medical problems:
  Bleeding problem
  Kidney or liver disease

Treatment
This medication belongs to the general family of medicines called antibiotics. It is used to treat a wide variety of bacterial infections. It is also used to treat infections in persons who are allergic to penicillin.
- Keep taking this medicine for the full time of treatment even if you begin to feel better after a few days; do not miss any doses.
- If you do miss a dose of this medicine, take it as soon as possible. This will help to keep a constant amount of medicine in the blood. However, if it is almost time for your next dose, skip the missed dose and go back to your regular dosing schedule.
- This medication has been prescribed for your current infection only. Another infection later on, or one that someone else has, may require a different medicine. You should not give your medicine to other people or use it for other infections, unless your doctor specifically directs you to do so.
- Take the medicine at the same times each day, 1 hour before or 2 hours after eating.

Side effects
Along with the needed effects, a medicine may cause some unwanted effects. Side effects that usually do not require medical attention: rectal itching, oral or vaginal white spots, mild diarrhea. These side effects should disappear as your body adjusts to the medication.
- Other side effects that should be reported to your doctor immediately are:
  Hives, rash
  Intense itching
  Faintness soon after a dose
  Difficulty in breathing
  Nausea and vomiting
  Severe diarrhea
  Unusual weakness or tiredness
  Bleeding or bruising

Interactions
This medicine may interact with several other drugs such as anticoagulants, theophylline preparations, probenecid, tetracyclines, etc.
- Be sure to tell your doctor about any medications you are currently taking.

Storage
Tablets, capsules, etc. should be stored at room temperature. Store the liquid form in the refrigerator. Keep out of the reach of children. Do not keep outdated medicine or medicine no longer needed.

CEFOBINE

Properties

This medicine contains cephalosporin as active ingredient. Cephalosporins belong to the general family of medicines called antibiotics, used in the treatment of infections caused by bacteria. They work by killing bacteria or preventing their growth. Cephalosporins will not work for colds, flu, or other viral infections.

Before using this medicine

Before you use this medicine check with your doctor:

– if you ever had any unusual or allergic reaction to any of the cephalosporins, penicillins, penicillin-like medicines, or penicillamine.

– if you are on a low-salt, low-sugar, or any other special diet, or if you are allergic to any substance, such as sulfites or other preservatives or dyes.

– if you are pregnant or intend to become pregnant while using this medicine. Although cephalosporins have not been shown to cause birth defects or other problems in humans, the chance always exists.

– if you are breast-feeding an infant. Most cephalosporins pass into the breast milk, usually in small amounts.

– if you have any of the following medical problems:
Bleeding problem
Kidney or liver disease

Treatment

This medication belongs to the general family of medicines called antibiotics. It is used to treat a wide variety of bacterial infections. It is also used to treat infections in persons who are allergic to penicillin.

■ Keep taking this medicine for the full time of treatment even if you begin to feel better after a few days; do not miss any doses.

■ If you do miss a dose of this medicine, take it as soon as possible. This will help to keep a constant amount of medicine in the blood. However, if it is almost time for your next dose, skip the missed dose and go back to your regular dosing schedule.

■ This medication has been prescribed for your current infection only. Another infection later on, or one that someone else has, may require a different medicine. You should not give your medicine to other people or use it for other infections, unless your doctor specifically directs you to do so.

■ Take the medicine at the same times each day, 1 hour before or 2 hours after eating.

Side effects

Along with the needed effects, a medicine may cause some unwanted effects. Side effects that usually do not require medical attention: rectal itching, oral or vaginal white spots, mild diarrhea. These side effects should disappear as your body adjusts to the medication.

■ Other side effects that should be reported to your doctor immediately are:
Hives, rash
Intense itching
Faintness soon after a dose
Difficulty in breathing
Nausea and vomiting
Severe diarrhea
Unusual weakness or tiredness
Bleeding or bruising

Interactions

This medicine may interact with several other drugs such as anticoagulants, theophylline preparations, probenecid, tetracyclines, etc.

■ Be sure to tell your doctor about any medications you are currently taking.

Storage

Tablets, capsules, etc. should be stored at room temperature. Store the liquid form in the refrigerator. Keep out of the reach of children. Do not keep outdated medicine or medicine no longer needed.

CEFOTAN

Properties

This medicine contains cephalosporin as active ingredient. Cephalosporins belong to the general family of medicines called antibiotics, used in the treatment of infections caused by bacteria. They work by killing bacteria or preventing their growth. Cephalosporins will not work for colds, flu, or other viral infections.

Before using this medicine

Before you use this medicine check with your doctor:

- if you ever had any unusual or allergic reaction to any of the cephalosporins, penicillins, penicillin-like medicines, or penicillamine.
- if you are on a low-salt, low-sugar, or any other special diet, or if you are allergic to any substance, such as sulfites or other preservatives or dyes.
- if you are pregnant or intend to become pregnant while using this medicine. Although cephalosporins have not been shown to cause birth defects or other problems in humans, the chance always exists.
- if you are breast-feeding an infant. Most cephalosporins pass into the breast milk, usually in small amounts.
- if you have any of the following medical problems:
  Bleeding problem
  Kidney or liver disease

Treatment

This medication belongs to the general family of medicines called antibiotics. It is used to treat a wide variety of bacterial infections. It is also used to treat infections in persons who are allergic to penicillin.

- Keep taking this medicine for the full time of treatment even if you begin to feel better after a few days; do not miss any doses.
- If you do miss a dose of this medicine, take it as soon as possible. This will help to keep a constant amount of medicine in the blood. However, if it is almost time for your next dose,

skip the missed dose and go back to your regular dosing schedule.
- This medication has been prescribed for your current infection only. Another infection later on, or one that someone else has, may require a different medicine. You should not give your medicine to other people or use it for other infections, unless your doctor specifically directs you to do so.
- Take the medicine at the same times each day, 1 hour before or 2 hours after eating.

Side effects

Along with the needed effects, a medicine may cause some unwanted effects. Side effects that usually do not require medical attention: rectal itching, oral or vaginal white spots, mild diarrhea. These side effects should disappear as your body adjusts to the medication.

- Other side effects that should be reported to your doctor immediately are:
  Hives, rash
  Intense itching
  Faintness soon after a dose
  Difficulty in breathing
  Nausea and vomiting
  Severe diarrhea
  Unusual weakness or tiredness
  Bleeding or bruising

Interactions

This medicine may interact with several other drugs such as anticoagulants, theophylline preparations, probenecid, tetracyclines, etc.

- Be sure to tell your doctor about any medications you are currently taking.

Storage

Tablets, capsules, etc. should be stored at room temperature. Store the liquid form in the refrigerator. Keep out of the reach of children. Do not keep outdated medicine or medicine no longer needed.

CEFOTETAN

Properties
This medicine contains cephalosporin as active ingredient. Cephalosporins belong to the general family of medicines called antibiotics, used in the treatment of infections caused by bacteria. They work by killing bacteria or preventing their growth. Cephalosporins will not work for colds, flu, or other viral infections.

Before using this medicine
Before you use this medicine check with your doctor:
- if you ever had any unusual or allergic reaction to any of the cephalosporins, penicillins, penicillin-like medicines, or penicillamine.
- if you are on a low-salt, low-sugar, or any other special diet, or if you are allergic to any substance, such as sulfites or other preservatives or dyes.
- if you are pregnant or intend to become pregnant while using this medicine. Although cephalosporins have not been shown to cause birth defects or other problems in humans, the chance always exists.
- if you are breast-feeding an infant. Most cephalosporins pass into the breast milk, usually in small amounts.
- if you have any of the following medical problems:
Bleeding problem
Kidney or liver disease

Treatment
This medication belongs to the general family of medicines called antibiotics. It is used to treat a wide variety of bacterial infections. It is also used to treat infections in persons who are allergic to penicillin.
- Keep taking this medicine for the full time of treatment even if you begin to feel better after a few days; do not miss any doses.
- If you do miss a dose of this medicine, take it as soon as possible. This will help to keep a constant amount of medicine in the blood. However, if it is almost time for your next dose, skip the missed dose and go back to your regular dosing schedule.
- This medication has been prescribed for your current infection only. Another infection later on, or one that someone else has, may require a different medicine. You should not give your medicine to other people or use it for other infections, unless your doctor specifically directs you to do so.
- Take the medicine at the same times each day, 1 hour before or 2 hours after eating.

Side effects
Along with the needed effects, a medicine may cause some unwanted effects. Side effects that usually do not require medical attention: rectal itching, oral or vaginal white spots, mild diarrhea. These side effects should disappear as your body adjusts to the medication.
- Other side effects that should be reported to your doctor immediately are:
Hives, rash
Intense itching
Faintness soon after a dose
Difficulty in breathing
Nausea and vomiting
Severe diarrhea
Unusual weakness or tiredness
Bleeding or bruising

Interactions
This medicine may interact with several other drugs such as anticoagulants, theophylline preparations, probenecid, tetracyclines, etc.
- Be sure to tell your doctor about any medications you are currently taking.

Storage
Tablets, capsules, etc. should be stored at room temperature. Store the liquid form in the refrigerator. Keep out of the reach of children. Do not keep outdated medicine or medicine no longer needed.

CEFROZIL

Properties

This medicine contains cephalosporin as active ingredient. Cephalosporins belong to the general family of medicines called antibiotics, used in the treatment of infections caused by bacteria. They work by killing bacteria or preventing their growth. Cephalosporins will not work for colds, flu, or other viral infections.

Before using this medicine

Before you use this medicine check with your doctor:

- if you ever had any unusual or allergic reaction to any of the cephalosporins, penicillins, penicillin-like medicines, or penicillamine.
- if you are on a low-salt, low-sugar, or any other special diet, or if you are allergic to any substance, such as sulfites or other preservatives or dyes.
- if you are pregnant or intend to become pregnant while using this medicine. Although cephalosporins have not been shown to cause birth defects or other problems in humans, the chance always exists.
- if you are breast-feeding an infant. Most cephalosporins pass into the breast milk, usually in small amounts.
- if you have any of the following medical problems:
  Bleeding problem
  Kidney or liver disease

Treatment

This medication belongs to the general family of medicines called antibiotics. It is used to treat a wide variety of bacterial infections. It is also used to treat infections in persons who are allergic to penicillin.

- Keep taking this medicine for the full time of treatment even if you begin to feel better after a few days; do not miss any doses.
- If you do miss a dose of this medicine, take it as soon as possible. This will help to keep a constant amount of medicine in the blood. However, if it is almost time for your next dose, skip the missed dose and go back to your regular dosing schedule.
- This medication has been prescribed for your current infection only. Another infection later on, or one that someone else has, may require a different medicine. You should not give your medicine to other people or use it for other infections, unless your doctor specifically directs you to do so.
- Take the medicine at the same times each day, 1 hour before or 2 hours after eating.

Side effects

Along with the needed effects, a medicine may cause some unwanted effects. Side effects that usually do not require medical attention: rectal itching, oral or vaginal white spots, mild diarrhea. These side effects should disappear as your body adjusts to the medication.

- Other side effects that should be reported to your doctor immediately are:
  Hives, rash
  Intense itching
  Faintness soon after a dose
  Difficulty in breathing
  Nausea and vomiting
  Severe diarrhea
  Unusual weakness or tiredness
  Bleeding or bruising

Interactions

This medicine may interact with several other drugs such as anticoagulants, theophylline preparations, probenecid, tetracyclines, etc.

- Be sure to tell your doctor about any medications you are currently taking.

Storage

Tablets, capsules, etc. should be stored at room temperature. Store the liquid form in the refrigerator. Keep out of the reach of children. Do not keep outdated medicine or medicine no longer needed.

CEFTIN

Properties
This medicine contains cephalosporin as active ingredient. Cephalosporins belong to the general family of medicines called antibiotics, used in the treatment of infections caused by bacteria. They work by killing bacteria or preventing their growth. Cephalosporins will not work for colds, flu, or other viral infections.

Before using this medicine
Before you use this medicine check with your doctor:
- if you ever had any unusual or allergic reaction to any of the cephalosporins, penicillins, penicillin-like medicines, or penicillamine.
- if you are on a low-salt, low-sugar, or any other special diet, or if you are allergic to any substance, such as sulfites or other preservatives or dyes.
- if you are pregnant or intend to become pregnant while using this medicine. Although cephalosporins have not been shown to cause birth defects or other problems in humans, the chance always exists.
- if you are breast-feeding an infant. Most cephalosporins pass into the breast milk, usually in small amounts.
- if you have any of the following medical problems:
  Bleeding problem
  Kidney or liver disease

Treatment
This medication belongs to the general family of medicines called antibiotics. It is used to treat a wide variety of bacterial infections. It is also used to treat infections in persons who are allergic to penicillin.
- Keep taking this medicine for the full time of treatment even if you begin to feel better after a few days; do not miss any doses.
- If you do miss a dose of this medicine, take it as soon as possible. This will help to keep a constant amount of medicine in the blood. However, if it is almost time for your next dose, skip the missed dose and go back to your regular dosing schedule.
- This medication has been prescribed for your current infection only. Another infection later on, or one that someone else has, may require a different medicine. You should not give your medicine to other people or use it for other infections, unless your doctor specifically directs you to do so.
- Take the medicine at the same times each day, 1 hour before or 2 hours after eating.

Side effects
Along with the needed effects, a medicine may cause some unwanted effects. Side effects that usually do not require medical attention: rectal itching, oral or vaginal white spots, mild diarrhea. These side effects should disappear as your body adjusts to the medication.
- Other side effects that should be reported to your doctor immediately are:
  Hives, rash
  Intense itching
  Faintness soon after a dose
  Difficulty in breathing
  Nausea and vomiting
  Severe diarrhea
  Unusual weakness or tiredness
  Bleeding or bruising

Interactions
This medicine may interact with several other drugs such as anticoagulants, theophylline preparations, probenecid, tetracyclines, etc.
- Be sure to tell your doctor about any medications you are currently taking.

Storage
Tablets, capsules, etc. should be stored at room temperature. Store the liquid form in the refrigerator. Keep out of the reach of children. Do not keep outdated medicine or medicine no longer needed.

CEFZIL

Properties

This medicine contains cephalosporin as active ingredient. Cephalosporins belong to the general family of medicines called antibiotics, used in the treatment of infections caused by bacteria. They work by killing bacteria or preventing their growth. Cephalosporins will not work for colds, flu, or other viral infections.

Before using this medicine

Before you use this medicine check with your doctor:
- if you ever had any unusual or allergic reaction to any of the cephalosporins, penicillins, penicillin-like medicines, or penicillamine.
- if you are on a low-salt, low-sugar, or any other special diet, or if you are allergic to any substance, such as sulfites or other preservatives or dyes.
- if you are pregnant or intend to become pregnant while using this medicine. Although cephalosporins have not been shown to cause birth defects or other problems in humans, the chance always exists.
- if you are breast-feeding an infant. Most cephalosporins pass into the breast milk, usually in small amounts.
- if you have any of the following medical problems:
  Bleeding problem
  Kidney or liver disease

Treatment

This medication belongs to the general family of medicines called antibiotics. It is used to treat a wide variety of bacterial infections. It is also used to treat infections in persons who are allergic to penicillin.
- Keep taking this medicine for the full time of treatment even if you begin to feel better after a few days; do not miss any doses.
- If you do miss a dose of this medicine, take it as soon as possible. This will help to keep a constant amount of medicine in the blood. However, if it is almost time for your next dose, skip the missed dose and go back to your regular dosing schedule.
- This medication has been prescribed for your current infection only. Another infection later on, or one that someone else has, may require a different medicine. You should not give your medicine to other people or use it for other infections, unless your doctor specifically directs you to do so.
- Take the medicine at the same times each day, 1 hour before or 2 hours after eating.

Side effects

Along with the needed effects, a medicine may cause some unwanted effects. Side effects that usually do not require medical attention: rectal itching, oral or vaginal white spots, mild diarrhea. These side effects should disappear as your body adjusts to the medication.
- Other side effects that should be reported to your doctor immediately are:
  Hives, rash
  Intense itching
  Faintness soon after a dose
  Difficulty in breathing
  Nausea and vomiting
  Severe diarrhea
  Unusual weakness or tiredness
  Bleeding or bruising

Interactions

This medicine may interact with several other drugs such as anticoagulants, theophylline preparations, probenecid, tetracyclines, etc.
- Be sure to tell your doctor about any medications you are currently taking.

Storage

Tablets, capsules, etc. should be stored at room temperature. Store the liquid form in the refrigerator. Keep out of the reach of children. Do not keep outdated medicine or medicine no longer needed.

CELESTODERM-V

Properties
This medicine contains betamethasone, a corticosteroid, as active ingredient. Corticosteroids are used to help relieve redness, swelling, itching, inflammation, and discomfort of many skin problems. They exert this effect by interfering with natural body mechanisms that produce the rash, itching, or inflammation. They do not cure the underlying cause of the skin problem. This medication is applied to the skin.

Before using this medicine
Before you use this medicine check with your doctor, or pharmacist:
- if you ever had any unusual or allergic reaction to corticosteroids.
- if you are allergic to any substance, such as sulfites or other preservatives or dyes.
- if you are pregnant or intend to become pregnant while using this medicine. Studies have shown that corticosteroids applied to the skin in large amounts or over long periods of time can be the cause of birth defects.
- if you are breast-feeding an infant. Some corticosteroids pass into breast milk and may interfere with the infant's growth.

Treatment
Do not use this medicine more often or for a longer time than ordered. To do so may increase absorption through the skin and the chance of side effects. In addition, too much use, especially on areas with thinner skin (for example, face, armpits, groin), may result in thinning of the skin and stretch marks.

Before applying this medication, wash your hands. than, unless your doctor or pharmacist gives you different instructions, gently wash the area where the medication is to be applied. With a clean towel pat the area dry. Apply a small amount of the medication to the affected area in a thin layer. Do not bandage the area unless your doctor tells you to do so.

If you miss a dose of this medication, apply the dose as soon as possible, unless it is almost time for the next application.
- ◆ Do not use this medicine for other skin problems without first checking with your doctor. You should not use a topical corticosteroid if you have a virus disease (such as herpes), fungal infection of the skin (such as athlete's foot), or tuberculosis of the skin.

Side effects
There are a number of side effects that usually do not require medical attention. Minor side effects are:

Acne
Burning sensations
Itching
Rash
Skin dryness

These possible side effects may go away during treatment; however, if they continue or are bothersome, check with your doctor, nurse, or pharmacist. Tell your doctor about any side effects that are persistent or particularly bothersome, such as:

Blistering
Increased hair growth
Irritation of the affected area
Loss of skin
Secondary infection in the area being treated
Thinning of the skin with easy bruising

Interactions
None known as long as it is used according to the directions given to you by your doctor or pharmacist.

Storage
Cream, ointment, lotion, gel, spray, and aerosol should be stored at room temperature in tightly closed containers. This medication should never be frozen.

CENA-K

Properties

This medicine contains potassium chloride as active ingredient; it is used to treat or prevent potassium deficiency, especially potassium deficiency that is caused by the use of diuretics (water pills).

Potassium is needed to maintain good health. Potassium supplements may be needed by patients who do not have enough potassium in their regular diet and by those who have lost too much potassium because of illness or treatment with certain medicines.

Since too much potassium may also cause health problems, most potassium supplements are available only with your doctor's prescription.

Before using this medicine

Before you use this medicine check with your doctor, or pharmacist:
- if you ever had any unusual or allergic reaction to potassium preparations;
- if you are on a low-salt, low-sugar, or any other special diet, or if you are allergic to any substance, such as sulfites or other preservatives or dyes.
- if you are pregnant or intend to become pregnant while using this medicine. Although potassium supplements have not been shown to cause problems in humans, the chance always exists.
- if you are breast-feeding an infant. Although this medicine has not been shown to cause problems in humans, the chance always exists since small amounts of potassium pass into the breast milk.
- if you have any of the following medical problems:
  Addison's disease
  Heart disease
  Diarrhea
  Kidney disease
  Stomach ulcer

Treatment

This medication is used to relieve or prevent the symptoms of your medical problem. Take them as directed. Do not take more of them and do not take them more often than recommended on the label, unless otherwise directed by your doctor. To do so may increase the chance of side effects.

In order to avoid stomach irritation, you should take potassium supplements with food or immediately after a meal. If you miss a dose of this medication, take the missed dose as soon as possible, unless it is within two hours of the next scheduled dose.

Side effects

The following minor side effects may occur:
  Diarrhea
  Nausea
  Stomach pains
  Vomiting.

These side effects should disappear as your body adjusts to the medication. Tell your doctor about any side effects that are persistent or particularly bothersome. It is especially important to tell your doctor about anxiety; bloody or black, tarry stools; confusion; difficulty in breathing; numbness or tingling in the arms, legs, or feet; palpitations; severe abdominal pain; or unusual weakness.

Interactions

This medicine interacts with several other drugs such as adrenocorticosteroids, antimuscarinics, calcium-containing medicines; heart medicines such as digitalis or digoxin; laxatives; other potassium-containing medicines.
- Be sure to tell your doctor about any medications you are currently taking.

Storage

Tablets, elixir, etc. should be stored at room temperature in tightly closed containers. Store away from heat and direct light. Keep out of reach of children, since overdose may be very dangerous in children. Do not keep outdated medicine or medicine no longer needed. Flush the contents of the container down the toilet, unless otherwise directed.

CENTRAX

Properties

This medicine contains as active ingredient prazepam, a benzodiazepine preparation. Benzodiazepines belong to the group of psychoactive medicines that influence the activity of the brain. Some are used to relieve nervousness or tension. It is effective for this purpose for short periods. Others are used for sleeplessness or to relax muscles or relieve muscle spasm. The benzodiazepines may also be used for other conditions as determined by your doctor.

Before using this medicine

Before you use this medicine check with your doctor:
- if you ever had any unusual or allergic reaction to benzodiazepines.
- if you are on a low-salt, low-sugar, or any other special diet, or if you are allergic to any substance, such as sulfites or other preservatives or dyes.
- if you are pregnant or intend to become pregnant while using this medicine. Some benzodiazepines have been reported to increase the chance of birth defects when used during the first 3 months of pregnancy.
- if you are breast-feeding an infant. Benzodiazepines may pass into the breast milk and cause drowsiness, unusually slow heartbeat, shortness of breath, or troubled breathing in infants of mothers taking this medicine.
- if you have any of the following medical problems: asthma, bronchitis, emphysema, or other chronic lung disease; epilepsy or history of convulsions; hyperactivity (in children); kidney or liver disease; mental depression or illness; myasthania gravis, porphyria.

Treatment

This medication is used to relieve or prevent the symptoms of your medical problem. Benzodiazepines are mainly used antianxiety agents, anticonvulsants, or sedatives. Take them as directed. Do not take more of them and do not take them more often than recommended on the label, unless otherwise directed by your doctor. Benzodiazepine tranquilizing drugs can be abused if taken for long periods of time and it is possible to develop withdrawal symptoms if you discontinue the therapy abruptly.

Side effects

Along with the needed effects, a medicine may cause some unwanted effects. Minor side effects are: bitter taste in the mouth, dizziness, drowsiness, depression, constipation, dry mouth, excessive salivation, fatigue, flushing, headache, heartburn, loss of appetite, nausea, nervousness, sweating or vomiting. As your body adjusts to the medicine, these side effects should disappear.

- Tell your doctor about any side effects that are persistent or particularly bothersome. It is especially important to tell your doctor about:
Blurred or double vision
Chest pain
Difficulty in urinating
Fainting or falling
Fever or hallucinations
Joint pain
Mouth sores
Nightmares
Palpitations
Severe depression
Shortness of breath
Slurred speech
Uncoordinated movements
Unusual tiredness
Yellowing of the skin

Interactions

This medicine may interact with several other drugs. This medicine will add to the effects of alcohol, and CNS depressants.

- Be sure to tell your doctor about any medications you are currently taking.

Storage

Store at room temperature in tightly closed, light-resistant-resistant containers. Keep out of the reach of children since overdose may be especially dangerous in children.

CHLOROTRIANISENE

Properties
This medicine contains chlorotrianisene as active ingredient. The medicine is prescribed for treatment of estrogen deficiency; it restores normal estrogen levels in tissues. There is no evidence that this drug is effective for nervous symptoms or depression occurring during menopause. They should not be used to treat this condition; they should be used only to replace the estrogen that is naturally absent after menopause.

Before using this medicine
Before you use this medicine check with your doctor, or pharmacist:
- if you ever had any unusual or allergic reaction to estrogens;
- if you are pregnant or intend to become pregnant within three months;
- if you are breast-feeding an infant;
- if you have any of the following medical problems:
  Diabetes
  Breast cancer
  Fibrocystic breast disease
  Fibroid uterine tumors
  Endometriosis
  Migraine headaches
  Epilepsy
  Porphyria
  High blood pressure
  Asthma
  Congestive heart failure
  Kidney disease
  Gallstones

Treatment
This medication is used to treat estrogen deficiency, specific symptoms of menopause, estrogen-deficiency osteoporosis, atrophic vaginitis, prostate cancer.
For safe and effective use of this medicine:
◆ Follow your doctor's instructions if this medicine was prescribed.
◆ Follow the manufacturer's package directions if you are treating yourself.
◆ Estrogens have been reported to increase the risk of endometrial carcinoma.

Side effects
Along with the needed effects, a medicine may cause some unwanted effects. Possible side effects include:
  Stomach cramps
  Profuse bleeding
  Appetite loss
  Nausea and vomiting
  Swollen breasts
  Change in menstruation
  Rash, skin blisters
  Depression
  Dizziness

Overdose
The following symptoms may indicate an overdose:
  Nausea and vomiting
  Fluid retention
  Breast enlargement
  Abnormal vaginal bleeding
■ Call a doctor or hospital emergency room for instructions.

Interactions
This medicine may interact with several other drugs such as adrenocorticosteroids, antidepressants, oral antidiabetics, insulin, phenobarbital, primidone.
■ Be sure to tell your doctor about any medications you are currently taking.

Storage
Capsules, tablets, vaginal cream, transdermal patches, etc. should be stored at room temperature; store away from heat and direct light. Keep out of reach of children, since this medicine may be dangerous in children.

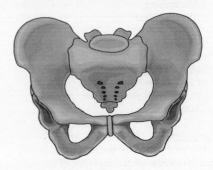

CHLORPROMAZINE

Properties

This medicine contains as active ingredient chlorpromazine, a phenothiazine derivative. Phenothiazines are a family of medicines used to treat nervous, mental, and emotional conditions. Some are used to control anxiety, restlessness, nausea and vomiting, and severe hiccups. This medicine is available only with your doctor's prescription.

Before using this medicine

Before you use this medicine check with your doctor, or pharmacist:
- if you ever had any unusual or allergic reaction to phenothiazine medicines.
- if you are on a low-salt, low-sugar, or any other special diet, or if you are allergic to any substance, such as sulfites or other preservatives or dyes.
- if you are pregnant or intend to become pregnant while using this medicine. Although phenothiazines have not been shown to cause birth defects, some side effects such as jaundice and muscle tremors have occurred in a few newborns whose mothers received phenothiazines during pregnancy.
- if you are breast-feeding an infant. Although this medicine has not been shown to cause problems in humans but the chance does exist since some phenothiazines are known to pass into the breast milk.
- if you have any of the following medical problems:
  Alcoholism
  Blood disease
  Difficult urination
  Enlarged prostate
  Glaucoma
  Heart or blood vessel disease
  Liver or lung disease
  Parkinson's disease
  Stomach ulcers

Treatment

This medication is prescribed to treat the symptoms of certain types of mental illness or emotional problems. In order to avoid stomach irritation, you can take the tablet or capsule forms of this medication with a meal or with a glass of water or milk (unless your doctor or pharmacist directs you to do otherwise).

Side effects

Along with the needed effects, a medicine may cause some unwanted effects.
Minor side effects are: blurred vision, constipation, decreased sweating, diarrhea, dizziness, drooling, drowsiness, dry mouth, fatigue, jitteriness, menstrual irregularities, nasal congestion, restlessness, tremors, vomiting, or weight gain.
- Tell your doctor about any side effects that are persistent or particularly bothersome. It is especially important to tell your doctor about:
  Breast enlargement
  Chest pain or convulsions
  Darkened skin
  Difficulty in swallowing
  Fainting or fever
  Involuntary movements
  Palpitations or sleep disorders
  Rash or sore throat
  Uncoordinated movements
  Unusual bleeding or bruising
  Visual disturbances
  Yellowing of the eyes

Interactions

This medicine may interact with several other drugs such as barbiturates, sleeping pills, narcotics, other tranquilizers, or any other medication that may produce a sedative effect. Avoid alcohol.

Storage

Store this medication as directed on the label. Keep out of the reach of children.

CIMETIDINE

Properties
This medicine contains cimetidine as active ingredient. It is a so-called H_2 receptor antagonist, a medicine prescribed for the short-term treatment of duodenal (intestinal) and gastric (stomach) ulcers. It is also prescribed for other gastrointestinal conditions characterized by the secretion of large amounts of gastric juice. In many cases it can be used for the treatment and prevention of heartburn. Good results have been obtained in maintenance of healing of erosive esophagitis (erosion of the mucosal membrane of the esophagus due to hydrochloric acid from the stomach.

Before using this medicine
Before you use this medicine check with your doctor, or pharmacist:
- if you ever had any unusual or allergic reaction to this medicine or any H_2 antagonist;
- if you are pregnant or intend to become pregnant while using this medicine;
- if you are breast-feeding an infant;
- if you take aspirin or an analogous medicine, since these preparations may irritate the mucosal lining (wall) of the stomach.

Treatment
This medication is used for treatment of peptic ulcers (duodenal or gastric ulcers), heartburn, and erosive esophagitis.

Tablets or capsules should be swallowed with liquid.

The usual dose amounts to 150 to 300 milligrams a day. If you forget to take a dose of this medicine, take it as soon as you remember.

Adverse reactions and side effects may be more frequent in elderly people.

For safe and effective use of medicine:
♦ Follow your doctor's instructions if this medicine was prescribed.
♦ Follow the manufacturer's package directions if you are treating yourself.

Side effects
Along with the needed effects, a medicine may cause some unwanted effects. Possible side effects include:
Dizziness
Headache
Diarrhea
Sore throat
Fever
Diminished sex drive
Hair loss
Confusion
Unusual bleeding
Unusual bruising
Irregular heartbeat
Fatigue or weakness
Constipation

Overdose
The following symptoms may be a sign of overdose:
Confusion
Slurred speech
Difficult breathing
Rapid heartbeat
Delirium
■ Call a doctor or hospital emergency room for instructions.

Interactions
The effect of this medicine may be reduced if it is taken together with antacids. It may decrease the effect of theophylline. Taken together with anticoagulants it may increase the effect of the latter.
■ Be sure to tell your doctor about any medications you are currently taking.

Storage
Capsules, tablets, elixir, etc. should be stored at room temperature; store away from heat and direct light. Keep out of reach of children, since overdose may be dangerous in children.

CLAFORAN

Properties
This medicine contains cephalosporin as active ingredient. Cephalosporins belong to the general family of medicines called antibiotics, used in the treatment of infections caused by bacteria. They work by killing bacteria or preventing their growth. Cephalosporins will not work for colds, flu, or other viral infections.

Before using this medicine
Before you use this medicine check with your doctor:
- if you ever had any unusual or allergic reaction to any of the cephalosporins, penicillins, penicillin-like medicines, or penicillamine.
- if you are on a low-salt, low-sugar, or any other special diet, or if you are allergic to any substance, such as sulfites or other preservatives or dyes.
- if you are pregnant or intend to become pregnant while using this medicine. Although cephalosporins have not been shown to cause birth defects or other problems in humans, the chance always exists.
- if you are breast-feeding an infant. Most cephalosporins pass into the breast milk, usually in small amounts.
- if you have any of the following medical problems:
  Bleeding problem
  Kidney or liver disease

Treatment
This medication belongs to the general family of medicines called antibiotics. It is used to treat a wide variety of bacterial infections. It is also used to treat infections in persons who are allergic to penicillin.
- Keep taking this medicine for the full time of treatment even if you begin to feel better after a few days; do not miss any doses.
- If you do miss a dose of this medicine, take it as soon as possible. This will help to keep a constant amount of medicine in the blood. However, if it is almost time for your next dose, skip the missed dose and go back to your regular dosing schedule.
- This medication has been prescribed for your current infection only. Another infection later on, or one that someone else has, may require a different medicine. You should not give your medicine to other people or use it for other infections, unless your doctor specifically directs you to do so.
- Take the medicine at the same times each day, 1 hour before or 2 hours after eating.

Side effects
Along with the needed effects, a medicine may cause some unwanted effects. Side effects that usually do not require medical attention: rectal itching, oral or vaginal white spots, mild diarrhea. These side effects should disappear as your body adjusts to the medication.
- Other side effects that should be reported to your doctor immediately are:
  Hives, rash
  Intense itching
  Faintness soon after a dose
  Difficulty in breathing
  Nausea and vomiting
  Severe diarrhea
  Unusual weakness or tiredness
  Bleeding or bruising

Interactions
This medicine may interact with several other drugs such as anticoagulants, theophylline preparations, probenecid, tetracyclines, etc.
- Be sure to tell your doctor about any medications you are currently taking.

Storage
Tablets, capsules, etc. should be stored at room temperature. Store the liquid form in the refrigerator. Keep out of the reach of children. Do not keep outdated medicine or medicine no longer needed.

CLARITIN

Properties
This medicine contains loratadine as active ingredient. It decreases blood volume in nasal tissues, shrinking tissues and enlarging airways. The medicine gives an effective seasonal allergy relief. Studies have shown that the incidence of drowsiness was similar to placebo at the recommended dose.

Before using this medicine
Before you use this medicine check with your doctor, or pharmacist:
- if you ever had any unusual or allergic reaction to iron medicine.
- if you are pregnant or intend to become pregnant while using this medicine. There is no proven harm to the unborn child. Avoid if possible;
- if you are breast-feeding an infant. The drug passes into the milk. Avoid the drug or discontinue nursing until you finish the medicine;
- if you have overactive thyroid;
- if you have diabetes;
- if you have high blood pressure or heart disease.

Treatment
This medication reduces congestion of nose, sinuses, eustachian tube and throat from allergies and infections.
  For safe and effective use of this iron supplement:
◆ Follow your doctor's instructions if this medicine was prescribed.
◆ Follow the manufacturer's package directions if you are treating yourself.

Side effects
Along with the needed effects, a medicine may cause some unwanted effects. Possible side effects include:
  Nervousness
  Wheezing
  Fatigue
  Hyperkinesia
  Abdominal pain
  Conjunctivitis
  Dysphonia
  Nausea
  Vomiting
  Slow heartbeat
  Difficult breathing
  Agitation
  Malaise
  Insomnia

Overdose
Important symptoms of overdose are:
  Restlessness
  Anxiety
  Vomiting
  Muscle tremors
  Rapid heartbeat
  Irregular heartbeat
  Confusion
  Delirium
  Convulsions
▪ Call a doctor or hospital emergency room.

Interactions
This medicine may interact with several other drugs such as tricyclic antidepressants (increased risk of heart toxicity), antihypertensives (decreased antihypertensive effect), epinephrine (increased epinephrine effect), guanethidine (decreased effect of both drugs), nitrates (possible decreased effect of both drugs).
▪ Be sure to tell your doctor about any medications you are currently taking.

Storage
Capsules, tablets, syrup, drops, oral solution should be stored at room temperature; store away from heat and direct light. Keep out of reach of children, since overdose may be very dangerous in children.

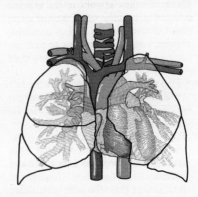

CLIMARA

Properties

This medicine contains estrogen as active ingredient. The medicine is prescribed for treatment of estrogen deficiency; it restores normal estrogen levels in tissues. There is no evidence that this drug is effective for nervous symptoms or depression occurring during menopause. They should not be used to treat this condition; they should be used only to replace the estrogen that is naturally absent after menopause.

Before using this medicine

Before you use this medicine check with your doctor, or pharmacist:
- if you ever had any unusual or allergic reaction to estrogens;
- if you are pregnant or intend to become pregnant within three months;
- if you are breast-feeding an infant;
- if you have any of the following medical problems:
  Diabetes
  Breast cancer
  Fibrocystic breast disease
  Fibroid uterine tumors
  Endometriosis
  Migraine headaches
  Epilepsy
  Porphyria
  High blood pressure
  Asthma
  Congestive heart failure
  Kidney disease
  Gallstones

Treatment

This medication is used to treat estrogen deficiency, specific symptoms of menopause, estrogen-deficiency osteoporosis, atrophic vaginitis, prostate cancer.
For safe and effective use of this medicine:
♦ Follow your doctor's instructions if this medicine was prescribed.
♦ Follow the manufacturer's package directions if you are treating yourself.
♦ Estrogens have been reported to increase the risk of endometrial carcinoma.

Side effects

Along with the needed effects, a medicine may cause some unwanted effects. Possible side effects include:
  Stomach cramps
  Profuse bleeding
  Appetite loss
  Nausea and vomiting
  Swollen breasts
  Change in menstruation
  Rash, skin blisters
  Depression
  Dizziness

Overdose

The following symptoms may indicate an overdose:
  Nausea and vomiting
  Fluid retention
  Breast enlargement
  Abnormal vaginal bleeding
■ Call a doctor or hospital emergency room for instructions.

Interactions

This medicine may interact with several other drugs such as adrenocorticosteroids, antidepressants, oral antidiabetics, insulin, phenobarbital, primidone.
■ Be sure to tell your doctor about any medications you are currently taking.

Storage

Capsules, tablets, vaginal cream, transdermal patches, etc. should be stored at room temperature; store away from heat and direct light. Keep out of reach of children, since this medicine may be dangerous in children.

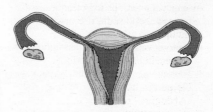

CLINAGEN LA 40

Properties
This medicine contains estrogen as active ingredient. The medicine is prescribed for treatment of estrogen deficiency; it restores normal estrogen levels in tissues. There is no evidence that this drug is effective for nervous symptoms or depression occurring during menopause. They should not be used to treat this condition; they should be used only to replace the estrogen that is naturally absent after menopause.

Before using this medicine
Before you use this medicine check with your doctor, or pharmacist:
- if you ever had any unusual or allergic reaction to estrogens;
- if you are pregnant or intend to become pregnant within three months;
- if you are breast-feeding an infant;
- if you have any of the following medical problems:
  Diabetes
  Breast cancer
  Fibrocystic breast disease
  Fibroid uterine tumors
  Endometriosis
  Migraine headaches
  Epilepsy
  Porphyria
  High blood pressure
  Asthma
  Congestive heart failure
  Kidney disease
  Gallstones

Treatment
This medication is used to treat estrogen deficiency, specific symptoms of menopause, estrogen-deficiency osteoporosis, atrophic vaginitis, prostate cancer.

For safe and effective use of this medicine:
- Follow your doctor's instructions if this medicine was prescribed.
- Follow the manufacturer's package directions if you are treating yourself.
- Estrogens have been reported to increase the risk of endometrial carcinoma.

Side effects
Along with the needed effects, a medicine may cause some unwanted effects. Possible side effects include:
  Stomach cramps
  Profuse bleeding
  Appetite loss
  Nausea and vomiting
  Swollen breasts
  Change in menstruation
  Rash, skin blisters
  Depression
  Dizziness

Overdose
The following symptoms may indicate an overdose:
  Nausea and vomiting
  Fluid retention
  Breast enlargement
  Abnormal vaginal bleeding
- Call a doctor or hospital emergency room for instructions.

Interactions
This medicine may interact with several other drugs such as adrenocorticosteroids, antidepressants, oral antidiabetics, insulin, phenobarbital, primidone.
- Be sure to tell your doctor about any medications you are currently taking.

Storage
Capsules, tablets, vaginal cream, transdermal patches, etc. should be stored at room temperature; store away from heat and direct light. Keep out of reach of children, since this medicine may be dangerous in children.

CLOBETASOL PROPIONATE

Properties

This medicine contains clobetasol propionate, a corticosteroid, as active ingredient. Corticosteroids are used to help relieve redness, swelling, itching, inflammation, and discomfort of many skin problems. They exert this effect by interfering with natural body mechanisms that produce the rash, itching, or inflammation. They do not cure the underlying cause of the skin problem. This medication is applied to the skin.

Before using this medicine

Before you use this medicine check with your doctor, or pharmacist:
- if you ever had any unusual or allergic reaction to corticosteroids.
- if you are allergic to any substance, such as sulfites or other preservatives or dyes.
- if you are pregnant or inintend to become pregnant while using this medicine. Studies have shown that corticosteroids applied to the skin in large amounts or over long periods of time can be the cause of birth defects.
- if you are breast-feeding an infant. Some corticosteroids pass into breast milk and may interfere with the infant's growth.

Treatment

Do not use this medicine more often or for a longer time than ordered. To do so may increase absorption through the skin and the chance of side effects. In addition, too much use, especially on areas with thinner skin (for example, face, armpits, groin), may result in thinning of the skin and stretch marks.

Before applying this medication, wash your hands. than, unless your doctor or pharmacist gives you different instructions, gently wash the area where the medication is to be applied. With a clean towel pat the area dry. Apply a small amount of the medication to the affected area in a thin layer. Do not bandage the area unless your doctor tells you to do so.

If you miss a dose of this medication, apply the dose as soon as possible, unless it is almost time for the next application.

- ◆ Do not use this medicine for other skin problems without first checking with your doctor. You should not use a topical corticosteroid if you have a virus disease (such as herpes), fungal infection of the skin (such as athlete's foot), or tuberculosis of the skin.

Side effects

There are a number of side effects that usually do not require medical attention. Minor side effects are:
Acne
Burning sensations
Itching
Rash
Skin dryness

These possible side effects may go away during treatment; however, if they continue or are bothersome, check with your doctor, nurse, or pharmacist. Tell your doctor about any side effects that are persistent or particularly bothersome, such as:
Blistering
Increased hair growth
Irritation of the affected area
Loss of skin
Secondary infection in the area being treated
Thinning of the skin with easy bruising

Interactions

None known as long as it is used according to the directions given to you by your doctor or pharmacist.

Storage

Cream, ointment, lotion, gel, spray, and aerosol should be stored at room temperature in tightly closed containers. This medication should never be frozen.

CLOCORTOLONE

Properties

This medicine contains clocortolone, a corticosteroid, as active ingredient. Corticosteroids are used to help relieve redness, swelling, itching, inflammation, and discomfort of many skin problems. They exert this effect by interfering with natural body mechanisms that produce the rash, itching, or inflammation. They do not cure the underlying cause of the skin problem. This medication is applied to the skin.

Before using this medicine

Before you use this medicine check with your doctor, or pharmacist:
- if you ever had any unusual or allergic reaction to corticosteroids.
- if you are allergic to any substance, such as sulfites or other preservatives or dyes.
- if you are pregnant or intend to become pregnant while using this medicine. Studies have shown that corticosteroids applied to the skin in large amounts or over long periods of time can be the cause of birth defects.
- if you are breast-feeding an infant. Some corticosteroids pass into breast milk and may interfere with the infant's growth.

Treatment

Do not use this medicine more often or for a longer time than ordered. To do so may increase absorption through the skin and the chance of side effects. In addition, too much use, especially on areas with thinner skin (for example, face, armpits, groin), may result in thinning of the skin and stretch marks.

Before applying this medication, wash your hands. than, unless your doctor or pharmacist gives you different instructions, gently wash the area where the medication is to be applied. With a clean towel pat the area dry. Apply a small amount of the medication to the affected area in a thin layer. Do not bandage the area unless your doctor tells you to do so.

If you miss a dose of this medication, apply the dose as soon as possible, unless it is almost time for the next application.
- ◆ Do not use this medicine for other skin problems without first checking with your doctor. You should not use a topical corticosteroid if you have a virus disease (such as herpes), fungal infection of the skin (such as athlete's foot), or tuberculosis of the skin.

Side effects

There are a number of side effects that usually do not require medical attention. Minor side effects are:

Acne
Burning sensations
Itching
Rash
Skin dryness

These possible side effects may go away during treatment; however, if they continue or are bothersome, check with your doctor, nurse, or pharmacist. Tell your doctor about any side effects that are persistent or particularly bothersome, such as:

Blistering
Increased hair growth
Irritation of the affected area
Loss of skin
Secondary infection in the area being treated
Thinning of the skin with easy bruising

Interactions

None known as long as it is used according to the directions given to you by your doctor or pharmacist.

Storage

Cream, ointment, lotion, gel, spray, and aerosol should be stored at room temperature in tightly closed containers. This medication should never be frozen.

CLODERM

Properties

This medicine contains clocortolone, a corticosteroid, as active ingredient. Corticosteroids are used to help relieve redness, swelling, itching, inflammation, and discomfort of many skin problems. They exert this effect by interfering with natural body mechanisms that produce the rash, itching, or inflammation. They do not cure the underlying cause of the skin problem. This medication is applied to the skin.

Before using this medicine

Before you use this medicine check with your doctor, or pharmacist:

- if you ever had any unusual or allergic reaction to corticosteroids.
- if you are allergic to any substance, such as sulfites or other preservatives or dyes.
- if you are pregnant or intend to become pregnant while using this medicine. Studies have shown that corticosteroids applied to the skin in large amounts or over long periods of time can be the cause of birth defects.
- if you are breast-feeding an infant. Some corticosteroids pass into breast milk and may interfere with the infant's growth.

Treatment

Do not use this medicine more often or for a longer time than ordered. To do so may increase absorption through the skin and the chance of side effects. In addition, too much use, especially on areas with thinner skin (for example, face, armpits, groin), may result in thinning of the skin and stretch marks.

Before applying this medication, wash your hands. than, unless your doctor or pharmacist gives you different instructions, gently wash the area where the medication is to be applied. With a clean towel pat the area dry. Apply a small amount of the medication to the affected area in a thin layer. Do not bandage the area unless your doctor tells you to do so.

If you miss a dose of this medication, apply the dose as soon as possible, unless it is almost time for the next application.

- ◆ Do not use this medicine for other skin problems without first checking with your doctor. You should not use a topical corticosteroid if you have a virus disease (such as herpes), fungal infection of the skin (such as athlete's foot), or tuberculosis of the skin.

Side effects

There are a number of side effects that usually do not require medical attention. Minor side effects are:

Acne

Burning sensations

Itching

Rash

Skin dryness

These possible side effects may go away during treatment; however, if they continue or are bothersome, check with your doctor, nurse, or pharmacist. Tell your doctor about any side effects that are persistent or particularly bothersome, such as:

Blistering

Increased hair growth

Irritation of the affected area

Loss of skin

Secondary infection in the area being treated

Thinning of the skin with easy bruising

Interactions

None known as long as it is used according to the directions given to you by your doctor or pharmacist.

Storage

Cream, ointment, lotion, gel, spray, and aerosol should be stored at room temperature in tightly closed containers. This medication should never be frozen.

CLOMIPRAMINE

Properties
This medicine contains clomipramine as active ingredient. It belongs to the group of medicines known as tricyclic antidepressants or 'mood elevators.' It is used to relieve mental depression and depression that sometimes occurs with anxiety. The medication gradually relieves, but doesn't cure, symptoms of depression. The medication may also be used for the treatment of narcolepsy, bulimia, panic attacks, cocaine withdrawal, attention deficit disorder.

Before using this medicine
Before you use this medicine check with your doctor, or pharmacist:
- if you ever had any unusual or allergic reaction to any tricyclic antidepressant, maprotiline or trazodone.
- if you are on a low-salt, low-sugar, or any other special diet, or if you are allergic to any substance, such as sulfites or other preservatives or dyes.
- if you are pregnant or intend to become pregnant while using this medicine. There have been reports of newborns suffering from heart, breathing, and urinary problems when their mothers had taken tricyclic antidepressants before delivery.
- if you are breast-feeding an infant. Some tricyclic antidepressants pass into the breast milk.

Treatment
Take this medicine only as directed by your doctor, to benefit your condition as much as possible. Do not take more of it, do not take it more often, and do not take it for a longer period of time than your doctor ordered.

To lessen stomach upset, take this medicine with food, even for a daily bedtime dose, unless your doctor has told you to take it on an empty stomach. If you forget your once-a-day bedtime dose, don't take it more than 3 hours late. If more than 3 hours, wait for next scheduled dose. Sometimes this medicine must be taken for several weeks before you begin to feel better.

Side effects
Along with the needed effects, a medicine may cause some unwanted effects. Side effects that usually do not require medical attention: difficult or frequent urination; decreased sex drive; muscle aches; abnormal dreams; nasal congestion; weakness and faintness when arising from bed or chair; back pain.
- Other side effects that should be reported to your doctor immediately are:
  Hallucinations
  Shakiness
  Dizziness or fainting
  Blurred vision, eye pain
  Irregular heartbeat or slow pulse
  Inflamed tongue
  Abdominal pain
  Jaundice
  Hair loss, rash
  Fever, chills
  Joint pain
  Palpitations

Interactions
This medicine may interact with several other drugs such as anticoagulants, anticholinergics, cold remedies, oral contraceptives, seizure medicines, sleeping medicines, thyroid medicines, etc.
- Be sure to tell your doctor about any medications you are currently taking.

Storage
Tablets, capsules, etc. should be stored at room temperature in tightly closed, light-resistant containers as directed by your pharmacist. Keep out of reach of children since overdose is especially dangerous in young children. Do not store in the bathroom medicine cabinet because the heat or moisture may cause the medicine to break down. Keep the liquid form of the medicine from freezing.

CLORAZINE

Properties
This medicine contains as active ingredient chlorpromazine, a phenothiazine derivative. Phenothiazines are a family of medicines used to treat nervous, mental, and emotional conditions. Some are used to control anxiety, restlessness, nausea and vomiting, and severe hiccups. This medicine is available only with your doctor's prescription.

Before using this medicine
Before you use this medicine check with your doctor, or pharmacist:
- if you ever had any unusual or allergic reaction to phenothiazine medicines.
- if you are on a low-salt, low-sugar, or any other special diet, or if you are allergic to any substance, such as sulfites or other preservatives or dyes.
- if you are pregnant or intend to become pregnant while using this medicine. Although phenothiazines have not been shown to cause birth defects, some side effects such as jaundice and muscle tremors have occurred in a few newborns whose mothers received phenothiazines during pregnancy.
- if you are breast-feeding an infant. Although this medicine has not been shown to cause problems in humans the chance does exist since some phenothiazines are known to pass into the breast milk.
- if you have any of the following medical problems:
  Alcoholism
  Blood disease
  Difficult urination
  Enlarged prostate
  Glaucoma
  Heart or blood vessel disease
  Liver or lung disease
  Parkinson's disease
  Stomach ulcers

Treatment
This medication is prescribed to treat the symptoms of certain types of mental illness or emotional problems. In order to avoid stomach irritation, you can take the tablet or capsule forms of this medication with a meal or with a glass of water or milk (unless your doctor or pharmacist directs you to do otherwise).

Side effects
Along with the needed effects, a medicine may cause some unwanted effects. Minor side effects are: blurred vision, constipation, decreased sweating, diarrhea, dizziness, drooling, drowsiness, dry mouth, fatigue, jitteriness, menstrual irregularities, nasal congestion, restlessness, tremors, vomiting, or weight gain.
- Tell your doctor about any side effects that are persistent or particularly bothersome. It is especially important to tell your doctor about:
  Breast enlargement
  Chest pain or convulsions
  Darkened skin
  Difficulty in swallowing
  Fainting or fever
  Involuntary movements
  Palpitations or sleep disorders
  Rash or sore throat
  Uncoordinated movements
  Unusual bleeding or bruising
  Visual disturbances
  Yellowing of the eyes

Interactions
This medicine may interact with several other drugs such as barbiturates, sleeping pills, narcotics, other tranquilizers, or any other medication that may produce a sedative effect. Avoid alcohol.

Storage
Store this medication as directed on the label. Keep out of the reach of children.

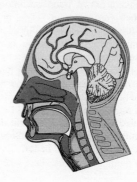

CO-TRIMOXAZOLE

Properties

This medicine contains sulfamethoxazole, a sulfonamide, and trimethoprim as active ingredients. Sulfonamides are prescribed to treat infections caused by bacteria. They will not work for colds, flu, or other virus infections.

Before using this medicine

Before you use this medicine check with your doctor:

- if you ever had any unusual or allergic reaction to any of the compounds of the medicine.
- if you are on a low-salt, low-sugar, or any other special diet, or if you are allergic to any substance, such as sulfites or other preservatives or dyes.
- if you are pregnant or intend to become pregnant while using this medicine. Although sulfonamides have not been shown to cause defects in humans, the chance may exists.
- if you are breast-feeding an infant. Most sulfonamides pass into the breast milk in small amounts and may cause unwanted effects in infants with some specific conditions.
- if you have any of the following medical problems:
  Kidney disease
  Liver disease
  Porphyria
  Deficiency of enzymes such as
   G6PD

Treatment

This medication is used to treat an infection caused by bacteria. Most sulfonamides are best taken with a full glass (8 ounces) of water on an empty stomach, either one hour before or two hours after a meal. Follow your doctor's or pharmacist's directions on how to take your medicine.

- Keep taking this medicine for the full time of treatment even if you begin to feel better after a few days; do not miss any doses.
- If you do miss a dose of this medicine, take the missed dose immediately.
- This medication works best when the level of medicine in your bloodstream (and urine) is kept constant. It is best, therefore, to take the doses at evenly spaced intervals day and night. if you take two doses a day, the doses should be spaced 12 hours apart.

Side effects

Along with the needed effects, a medicine may cause some unwanted effects. Side effects that usually do not require medical attention: abdominal pain, diarrhea, dizziness, headache, loss of appetite, nausea, sore mouth, or vomiting. These side effects should disappear as your body adjusts to the medication.

Sulfonamides can increase sensitivity to sunlight. It is, therefore, important to avoid prolonged exposure to sunlight and sunlamps.

Tell your doctor about any side effects that are persistent or particularly bothersome. It is especially important to tell your doctor about:

Bloody urine
Difficult urination
Difficulty in breathing
Difficulty in swallowing
Fever or hallucinations
Itching, rash, or pale skin
Joint pain, lower back pain
Ringing in the ears
Sore throat
Swollen or inflamed tongue
Tingling in hands or feet
Unusual bleeding
Yellowing of the eyes or skin

Interactions

This medicine may interact with several other drugs such as anticoagulants, oral antidiabetic agents, aspirin, some antibiotics, or anticancer drugs.

- Be sure to tell your doctor about any medications you are currently taking.

Storage

Tablets, capsules, suspension, etc. should be stored at room temperature as directed by your pharmacist or according to instructions on the label.

CODEINE

Properties

This medicine contains as active ingredient codeine.

It is a narcotic analgesic that acts directly on the central nervous system (brain and spinal cord). It is used to relieve pain or to suppress coughing.

Before using this medicine

Before you use this medicine check with your doctor, or pharmacist:

- if you ever had any unusual or allergic reaction to this medicine or one of its components.
- if you are on a low-salt, low-sugar, or any other special diet, or if you are allergic to any substance, such as sulfites or other preservatives or dyes.
- if you are pregnant or intend to become pregnant while using this medicine. Studies on birth defects have not been done in humans. Too much use of narcotics during pregnancy may cause the baby to become dependent on the medicine.
- if you are breast-feeding an infant. Although this medicine has not been shown to cause problems in humans, it passes into the breast milk in small amounts.
- if you have any of the following medical problems:
  Brain disease or head injury
  Colitis
  Convulsions
  Emphysema, asthma, or chronic lung disease
  Enlarged prostate
  Gallbladder disease or gallstones
  Heart disease
  Kidney or liver disease
  Underactive thyroid

Treatment

This medication is used to relieve pain or to suppress coughing. Narcotic analgesics act in the central nervous system; some of their side effects are also caused by actions in the central nervous system.

- If you are taking this medication on a regular schedule and you miss a dose, take the missed dose as soon as possible, unless it is almost time for your next dose. In that case do not take the missed dose at all.
- If a narcotic analgesic is used for a long time, is may become habit-forming (causing mental or physical dependence). Physical dependence may lead to withdrawal side effects when you stop taking this medicine.

Unless otherwise directed by your doctor or pharmacist take this as directed. Do not take more of them and do not take them more often than recommended on the label. Children up to 12 years of age should not take this medicine more than 3 times a day or for more than 5 days in a row.

Side effects

Along with the needed effects, a medicine may cause some unwanted effects. These side effects may go away during treatment as your body adjusts to the medicine. Such minor side effects are: constipation, dizziness, drowsiness, dry mouth, false sense of well-being, flushing, light-headedness, loss or appetite, nausea, painful or difficult urination, or sweating.

- Check with your doctor immediately if any of the following side effects occur:
  Anxiety or breathing difficulties
  Excitation or restlessness
  Fatigue, palpitations
  Rash, sore throat and fever
  Tremors or weakness

Interactions

This medicine may interact with several other drugs such as medicines acting on the central nervous system (e.g., antidepressants, tranquilizers), cimetidine, nitrates, quinidine, etc.

- Be sure to tell your doctor about any medications you are currently taking.

Storage

Tablets, elixir, suppository etc. should be stored at room temperature in a tightly closed, light-resistant container.

CONGEST

Properties
This medicine contains conjugated estrogens as active ingredients. The medicine is prescribed for treatment of estrogen deficiency; it restores normal estrogen levels in tissues. There is no evidence that this drug is effective for nervous symptoms or depression occurring during menopause. They should not be used to treat this condition; they should be used only to replace the estrogen that is naturally absent after menopause.

Before using this medicine
Before you use this medicine check with your doctor, or pharmacist:
- if you ever had any unusual or allergic reaction to estrogens;
- if you are pregnant or intend to become pregnant within three months;
- if you are breast-feeding an infant;
- if you have any of the following medical problems:
  Diabetes
  Breast cancer
  Fibrocystic breast disease
  Fibroid uterine tumors
  Endometriosis
  Migraine headaches
  Epilepsy
  Porphyria
  High blood pressure
  Asthma
  Congestive heart failure
  Kidney disease
  Gallstones

Treatment
This medication is used to treat estrogen deficiency, specific symptoms of menopause, estrogen-deficiency osteoporosis, atrophic vaginitis, prostate cancer.

For safe and effective use of this medicine:
- Follow your doctor's instructions if this medicine was prescribed.
- Follow the manufacturer's package directions if you are treating yourself.
- Estrogens have been reported to increase the risk of endometrial carcinoma.

Side effects
Along with the needed effects, a medicine may cause some unwanted effects. Possible side effects include:
  Stomach cramps
  Profuse bleeding
  Appetite loss
  Nausea and vomiting
  Swollen breasts
  Change in menstruation
  Rash, skin blisters
  Depression
  Dizziness

Overdose
The following symptoms may indicate an overdose:
  Nausea and vomiting
  Fluid retention
  Breast enlargement
  Abnormal vaginal bleeding
- Call a doctor or hospital emergency room for instructions.

Interactions
This medicine may interact with several other drugs such as adrenocorticosteroids, antidepressants, oral antidiabetics, insulin, phenobarbital, primidone.
- Be sure to tell your doctor about any medications you are currently taking.

Storage
Capsules, tablets, vaginal cream, transdermal patches, etc. should be stored at room temperature; store away from heat and direct light. Keep out of reach of children, since this medicine may be dangerous in children.

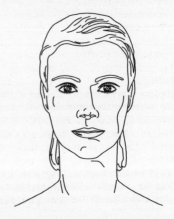

CONSTANT-T

Properties

This medicine contains theophylline as active ingredient; it is used to treat or prevent breathing problems (wheezing and shortness of breath) caused by asthma, bronchitis, or emphysema. This medication belongs to a group known as xanthine-derivative bronchodilators. They work by opening up the bronchial tubes or air passages of the lungs and increasing the flow of air through them. These medicines are available only with your doctor's prescription.

Before using this medicine

Before you use this medicine check with your doctor, or pharmacist:

- if you ever had any unusual or allergic reaction to xanthine-derivative bronchodilators.
- if you are on a low-salt, low-sugar, or any other special diet, or if you are allergic to any substance, such as sulfites or other preservatives or dyes.
- if you are pregnant or intend to become pregnant while using this medicine.
- if you are breast-feeding an infant. Theophylline passes into the breast milk and may cause irritability, fretfulness, or trouble in sleeping in infants of mothers taking this medicine.
- if you have any of the following medical problems:
Diarrhea
Enlarged prostate
Fibrocystic breast disease
Heart disease
Stomach ulcer

Treatment

This medication is used to relieve or prevent the symptoms of your medical problem. Take them as directed. Do not take more of them and do not take them more often than recommended on the label, unless otherwise directed by your doctor. To do so may increase the chance of side effects. The medicine should be taken on an empty stomach 30 to 60 minutes before a meal or two hours after a meal. Try not to miss any doses of this medication. If you do miss a dose, take the missed dose as soon as possible, unless it is almost time for the next dose. Do not double the next dose. It works best when taken with a glass of water.

Side effects

The following minor side effects may occur:

- Dizziness or flushing
- Headache
- Diarrhea
- Heartburn
- Increased urination
- Insomnia
- Nervousness or irritability
- Loss of appetite
- Nausea or stomach upset
- Stomach pain.

These side effects should disappear as your body adjusts to the medication. Tell your doctor about any side effects that are persistent or particularly bothersome. It is especially important to tell your doctor about black, tarry stools; confusion; convulsions; difficulty in breathing; fainting; muscle twitching; palpitations; rash; severe abdominal pain; or unusual weakness.

Interactions

This medicine interacts with several other drugs such as diuretics, reserpine, beta blockers, phenytoin, lithium, phenobarbital, birth control pills, and other medications.

- Be sure to tell your doctor about any medications you are currently taking.

Storage

Tablets, capsules, liquid and suspension should be stored at room temperature in tightly closed containers. Store away from heat and direct light. Keep out of reach of children, since overdose may be very dangerous in children. Discard any outdated medication.

CORONEX

Properties
This medicine contains isosorbide dinitrate as active ingredient. Nitrates improve the supply of blood and oxygen to the heart. This medication is for oral use.

Before using this medicine
Before you use this medicine check with your doctor, or pharmacist:
- if you ever had any unusual or allergic reaction to nitrates or nitrites.
- if you are on a low-salt, low-sugar, or any other special diet, or if you are allergic to any substance, such as sulfites or other preservatives or dyes.
- if you are pregnant or intend to become pregnant while using this medicine. Although nitrates have not been shown to cause problems in humans, the chance always exists.
- if you are breast-feeding an infant.
- if you have recently had a heart attack or stroke.
- if you have any of the following medical problems:
  Anemia
  Glaucoma
  Intestinal problems
  Overactive thyroid
- if you are now taking any of the following medicines or types of medicines:
  Antihypertensives
  Asthma or hay fever medicine
  Cold medicine
  Decongestant
  Medicine for appetite control
  Narcotic
  Pain medicine
  Sinus congestion medicine

Treatment
This medication is used to treat and prevent angina (chest pain). Nitroglycerin is a vasodilator, which relaxes the muscles of the blood vessels, causing an increase in the oxygen supply to the heart. The oral tablets, capsules, ointment and patches do not act quickly; they are used to prevent chest pain. The sublingual tablets and oral spray act quickly and can be used to relieve chest pain after it has started.

- Take this medicine exactly as directed by your doctor or pharmacist. It will work only if taken correctly.
- If you are taking this medicine regularly and you miss a dose, take it as soon as possible. However, if your next scheduled dose is within 2 hours (or within 6 hours for extended-release capsules or tablets), skip the missed dose and go back to your regular dosing schedule.
- If you have been taking this medicine regularly for several weeks or more, do not suddenly stop using it. Stopping suddenly may bring on attacks of angina.

Side effects
There are a number of side effects that usually do not require medical attention. These possible side effects may go away during treatment; however, if they continue or are bothersome, check with your doctor, nurse, or pharmacist. More common are: dizziness, lightheadedness, or fainting when standing up; fast pulse; flushing of face and neck; headache; nausea or vomiting.

Side effects that should be reported to your doctor are: blurred vision; dry mouth; severe or prolonged headache; skin rash.

Interactions
This medicine may interact with several other drugs such as tricyclic antidepressants and cough medicines. Before starting to take or apply nitroglycerin, be sure to tell your doctor about any medications you are currently taking.

Storage
Tablets, capsules, and oral spray should be stored as in a tightly capped bottle in a cool, dry place. Ointment and patches should be stored at room temperature in their original containers. Keep out of reach of children. Do not keep outdated medicine or medicine no longer needed.

COTRIM

Properties
This medicine contains sulfamethoxazole, a sulfonamide, and trimethoprim as active ingredients. Sulfonamides are prescribed to treat infections caused by bacteria. They will not work for colds, flu, or other virus infections.

Before using this medicine
Before you use this medicine check with your doctor:
- if you ever had any unusual or allergic reaction to any of the compounds of the medicine.
- if you are on a low-salt, low-sugar, or any other special diet, or if you are allergic to any substance, such as sulfites or other preservatives or dyes.
- if you are pregnant or intend to become pregnant while using this medicine. Although sulfonamides have not been shown to cause defects in humans, the chance may exists.
- if you are breast-feeding an infant. Most sulfonamides pass into the breast milk in small amounts and may cause unwanted effects in infants with some specific conditions.
- if you have any of the following medical problems:
Kidney disease
Liver disease
Porphyria
Deficiency of enzymes such as G6PD

Treatment
This medication is used to treat an infection caused by bacteria. Most sulfonamides are best taken with a full glass (8 ounces) of water on an empty stomach, either one hour before or two hours after a meal. Follow your doctor's or pharmacist's directions on how to take your medicine.
- Keep taking this medicine for the full time of treatment even if you begin to feel better after a few days; do not miss any doses.
- If you do miss a dose of this medicine, take the missed dose immediately.
- This medication works best when the level of medicine in your bloodstream (and urine) is kept constant. It is best, therefore, to take the doses at evenly spaced intervals day and night. if you take two doses a day, the doses should be spaced 12 hours apart.

Side effects
Along with the needed effects, a medicine may cause some unwanted effects. Side effects that usually do not require medical attention: abdominal pain, diarrhea, dizziness, headache, loss of appetite, nausea, sore mouth, or vomiting. These side effects should disappear as your body adjusts to the medication.

Sulfonamides can increase sensitivity to sunlight. It is, therefore, important to avoid prolonged exposure to sunlight and sunlamps.

Tell your doctor about any side effects that are persistent or particularly bothersome. It is especially important to tell your doctor about:
Bloody urine
Difficult urination
Difficulty in breathing
Difficulty in swallowing
Fever or hallucinations
Itching, rash, or pale skin
Joint pain, lower back pain
Ringing in the ears
Sore throat
Swollen or inflamed tongue
Tingling in hands or feet
Unusual bleeding
Yellowing of the eyes or skin

Interactions
This medicine may interact with several other drugs such as anticoagulants, oral antidiabetic agents, aspirin, some antibiotics, or anticancer drugs.
- Be sure to tell your doctor about any medications you are currently taking.

Storage
Tablets, capsules, suspension, etc. should be stored at room temperature as directed by your pharmacist or according to instructions on the label.

CYCLEN

Properties
This medicine contains norgestimate and ethinyl estradiol as active ingredients. It is an oral contraceptive prescribed to prevent pregnancy and/or to regulate menstrual periods.

The drug works by altering the mucus at the cervix entrance to prevent the entry of sperm. It also alters the uterus lining to resist implantation of the fertilized egg. Oral contraceptives create the same chemical atmosphere in blood that exists during pregnancy.

Before using this medicine
Before you use this medicine check with your doctor, or pharmacist:
- if you ever had any unusual or allergic reaction to estrogens or progestogen;
- if you are pregnant or want to become pregnant within three months;
- if you are breast-feeding an infant;
- if you have any of the following medical problems:
  Diabetes
  Ailments of the breast
  Disorders of the uterus
  Migraine or epilepsy
  High blood pressure
  Asthma or heart conditions
  Kidney disease
  Gallstones

Treatment
This medication is used to prevent pregnancy or to regulate menstrual periods.

Adverse reactions
Along with the needed effects, a medicine may cause some unwanted effects or adverse reactions.
- *An increased risk of the following adverse reactions has been associated with the use of oral contraceptives:*
  Thrombophlebitis
  Venous thrombosis
  Arterial thromboembolism
  Pulmonary (lung) embolism
  Myocardial infarction
  Cerebral hemorrhage
  Cerebral thrombosis
  Hypertension
  Gallbladder disease
  Hepatic (liver) hepatomas
  Benign liver tumors
- *The following adverse reactions have been reported in patients receiving oral contraceptives and are believed to be drug-related:*
  Nausea and vomiting
  Abdominal cramps
  Breakthrough bleeding
  Spotting
  Change in menstrual flow
  Amenorrhea
  Temporary infertility
  Edema
  Breast changes
  Weight changes
  Cholestatic jaundice
  Migraine
  Rash (allergic)
  Mental depression
  Vaginal candidiasis

Interactions
This medicine may interact with several other drugs such as antibiotics, anticoagulants, anticonvulsants, antidepressants, oral antidiabetics, antihistamines, barbiturates, oral hypoglycemics, insulin, meperidine.
- Be sure to tell your doctor about any medications you are currently taking.

Storage
Tablets should be stored at room temperature; store away from heat and direct light. Keep out of reach of children, since this medicine may be dangerous in children.

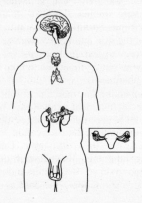

CYCLOCORT

Properties
This medicine contains amcinomide, a corticosteroid, as active ingredient. Corticosteroids are used to help relieve redness, swelling, itching, inflammation, and discomfort of many skin problems. They exert this effect by interfering with natural body mechanisms that produce the rash, itching, or inflammation. They do not cure the underlying cause of the skin problem. This medication is applied to the skin.

Before using this medicine
Before you use this medicine check with your doctor, or pharmacist:
- if you ever had any unusual or allergic reaction to corticosteroids.
- if you are allergic to any substance, such as sulfites or other preservatives or dyes.
- if you are pregnant or intend to become pregnant while using this medicine. Studies have shown that corticosteroids applied to the skin in large amounts or over long periods of time can be the cause of birth defects.
- if you are breast-feeding an infant. Some corticosteroids pass into breast milk and may interfere with the infant's growth.

Treatment
Do not use this medicine more often or for a longer time than ordered. To do so may increase absorption through the skin and the chance of side effects. In addition, too much use, especially on areas with thinner skin (for example, face, armpits, groin), may result in thinning of the skin and stretch marks.

Before applying this medication, wash your hands. than, unless your doctor or pharmacist gives you different instructions, gently wash the area where the medication is to be applied. With a clean towel pat the area dry. Apply a small amount of the medication to the affected area in a thin layer. Do not bandage the area unless your doctor tells you to do so. If you miss a dose of this medication, apply the dose as soon as possible, unless it is almost time for the next application.

◆ Do not use this medicine for other skin problems without first checking with your doctor. You should not use a topical corticosteroid if you have a virus disease (such as herpes), fungal infection of the skin (such as athlete's foot), or tuberculosis of the skin.

Side effects
There are a number of side effects that usually do not require medical attention. Minor side effects are:

Acne
Burning sensations
Itching
Rash
Skin dryness

These possible side effects may go away during treatment; however, if they continue or are bothersome, check with your doctor, nurse, or pharmacist. Tell your doctor about any side effects that are persistent or particularly bothersome, such as:

Blistering
Increased hair growth
Irritation of the affected area
Loss of skin
Secondary infection in the area being treated
Thinning of the skin with easy bruising

Interactions
None known as long as it is used according to the directions given to you by your doctor or pharmacist.

Storage
Cream, ointment, lotion, gel, spray, and aerosol should be stored at room temperature in tightly closed containers. This medication should never be frozen.

DAPEX-37.5

Properties

This medicine contains phentermine as active ingredient; it is prescribed for appetite suppression.

Appetite suppressants are used in the short-term (a few weeks) treatment of obesity. In a few weeks (6 to 12), these medicines in combination with dieting, exercise, and changes in eating habits can help patients lose weight. However, since their appetite reducing effect is only temporary, they are useful only for the first weeks of dieting until new eating habits are established.

Before using this medicine

Before you use this medicine check with your doctor, or pharmacist:
- if you ever had any unusual or allergic reaction to any of the compounds of this medicine.
- if you are on a low-salt, low-sugar, or any other special diet, or if you are allergic to any substance, such as sulfites or other preservatives or dyes.
- if you are pregnant, inintend to become pregnant or breast-feeding an infant while using this medicine.
- if you have any of the following medical problems:
  Diabetes mellitus
  Epilepsy
  Glaucoma
  Heart disease
  High blood pressure
  Mental illness (severe)

Treatment

This medication is used to relieve or prevent the symptoms of your medical problem.

Take them as directed. Do not take more of them and do not take them more often than recommended on the label. If too much of the drug is taken, it may become habit-forming.
- The medicine produces central nervous system stimulation, and it should not be taken by people with heart disease or high blood pressure.
- If you think this medicine is not working as well after you have taken it for a few weeks, do not increase the dose. Instead, check with your doctor.

Side effects

The following minor side effects may occur: irritability, nervousness, restlessness, trouble in sleeping.

These side effects should disappear as your body adjusts to the medication. Tell your doctor about any side effects that are persistent or particularly bothersome. It is especially important to tell your doctor about:
  Mental depression
  Nausea or vomiting
  Stomach cramps or pain
  Trembling
  Unusual tiredness
- Discontinue use of the drug; call your doctor right away. Adverse reactions and side effects may be more frequent and severe in people over age 60 than in younger persons.

Interactions

This medicine interacts with several other drugs such as antihypertensives, other appetite suppressants, caffeine, central nervous system depressants, central nervous system stimulants, furazolidone, guanethidine, hydralazine, MAO inhibitors, methyldopa, molindone, phenothiazines, rauwolfia alkaloids, sodium bicarbonate.

Interaction with alcoholic beverages may produce drowsiness, sleepiness, and/or inability to concentrate.
- Be sure to tell your doctor about any medications you are currently taking.

Storage

This medicine should be stored at room temperature in tightly closed containers. Store away from heat and direct light. Keep out of reach of children, since overdose may be very dangerous in children.

Do not store this medicine in the bathroom medicine cabinet because the heat and moisture cause the medicine to break down. Do not keep outdated medicine or medicine no longer needed. Flush the contents of the container down the toilet.

DAY-BARB

Properties

This medicine contains as active ingredient the barbiturate butabarbital. Barbiturates belong to the group of medicines called central nervous system depressants (medicines that slow down the nervous system).

Barbiturates may partially block nerve impulses at nerve-cell connections. They may be used to treat insomnia (sleeplessness) by helping patients fall asleep. Also, they may be used to relieve anxiety or tension. Some of the barbiturates are used as anticonvulsants to help control convulsions in certain disorders or diseases, such as epilepsy. If too much of the drug is used, it may become habit-forming (causing mental or physical dependence).

Before using this medicine

Before you use this medicine check with your doctor, or pharmacist:

- if you ever had any unusual or allergic reaction to this medicine or one of its components.
- if you are on a low-salt, low-sugar, or any other special diet, or if you are allergic to preservatives or dyes.
- if you are pregnant or inintend to become pregnant while using this medicine, since barbiturates have been shown to increase the chance of birth defects in humans. Taking barbiturates regularly during the last 3 months of pregnancy may cause the baby to become dependent on the medicine. This may lead to withdrawal side effects in the baby after birth.
- if you have any of the following medical problems:
Anemia (severe)
Diabetes mellitus (sugar disease)
Hyperactivity (in children)
Kidney or lifer disease
Mental depression
Overactive thyroid

Treatment

This medication is used to treat the symptoms of your medical condition. Barbiturates act in the central nervous system; some of their side effects are also caused by actions in the central nervous system. Use this medicine as directed by your doctor. Do not use more of it, do not use it more often, and do not use it for a longer period of time than your doctor ordered.

- If you are taking this medication on a regular schedule and you miss a dose, take the missed dose as soon as possible, unless it is almost time for your next dose. In that case do not take the missed dose at all.
- If a barbiturate is used for a long time, it may become habit-forming. Physical dependence may lead to withdrawal side effects when you stop taking this medicine.

Side effects

Along with the needed effects, a medicine may cause some unwanted effects. These side effects may go away during treatment as your body adjusts to the medicine. Such minor side effects are: depression, confusion, diarrhea, nausea, vomiting, joint or muscle pain, slurred speech, hallucinations, headache, decreased sex drive.

- Check with your doctor immediately if any of the following side effects occur:
Rash or hives
Face, lip or eyelid swelling
Sore throat, fever
Agitation
Slow heartbeat
Difficult breathing or chest pain

Interactions

This medicine may interact with several other drugs such as medicines acting on the central nervous system (e.g., antihistamines; beta-adrenergic blockers; MAO inhibitors; mind-altering drugs; nabilone; antidepressants; clozapine; anticonvulsants).

Storage

The medicine should be stored at room temperature in a tightly closed, light-resistant container. Keep out of reach of children since overdose is very dangerous in children.

DECA-DURABOLIN

Properties

This medicine is a member of the androgenic, or male, hormone group, containing an androgenic preparation as active ingredient. It is used in diseases in
which male hormone replacement or
augmentation is needed and also in so-
called male menopause. It is also used
to decrease calcium loss in
osteoporosis, to block growth of breast
cancer cells in females and to reduce
breast pain and fullness following childbirth.

Before using this medicine

Before you use this medicine check
with your doctor, or pharmacist:
- if you ever had any unusual or allergic reaction to androgens or corticosteroids in general.
- if you are on a low-salt, low-sugar,
  or any other special diet, or if you are
  allergic to any substance, such as
  certain preservatives or dyes.
- if you have any of the following
  medical problems:
  Cancer prostate
  Heart disease or atherosclerosis
  Kidney or lifer disease
  Breast cancer (males)
  High blood pressure
  High level of blood calcium
  Epilepsy

Treatment

This medication is used to relieve or
prevent the symptoms of your medical
problem. Take them as directed. Do not
take more of them and do not take them
more often than recommended on the
label. One should take the tablets or
capsules with food to lessen stomach irritation. Take the medication at the
same time each day. If you forget a
dose take it as soon as you remember up
to two hours late; wait for the next
scheduled dose;; don't double this dose.
The risk to the unborn child outweighs
the benefits of the drug.

Side effects

Females taking any androgenic drug
should watch for deepening of the
voice, oily skin, acne, hairiness, increased libido, and menstrual irregularities.

The following side effects may oc-
cur:
  Acne or oily skin
  Deep voice
  Enlarged clitoris in females
  Frequent erections in men
  Sore mouth
  Higher sex drive
  Impotence in men
  Yellow skin or eyes
These side effects should disappear
as your body adjusts to the medication.
Tell your doctor about any side effects
that are persistent or particularly bother-
some.
- Discontinue the use of the medica-
  tion and seek emergency treatment in
  the following situations:
  Intense itching
  Weakness
  Loss of consciousness
  Depression or confusion
  Swollen feet or legs
  Shortness of breath
  Irregularities of heartbeat
  Difficult urination
  Vaginal bleeding in women
  Scrotum pain in men

Interactions

This medicine interacts with several
other drugs such as anticoagulants, oral
antidiabetics, cyclosporine, hepatotoxic
drugs, oxyphenbutazone, phenobarbital,
and phenylbutazone.
- Be sure to tell your doctor about any
  medications you are currently taking.

Storage

This medicine should be stored at room
temperature in closed containers. Store
away from heat and direct light. Keep
out of reach of children, since overdose
may be dangerous in children.

DELADIOL-40

Properties

This medicine contains estrogen as active ingredient. The medicine is prescribed for treatment of estrogen deficiency; it restores normal estrogen levels in tissues. There is no evidence that this drug is effective for nervous symptoms or depression occurring during menopause. They should not be used to treat this condition; they should be used only to replace the estrogen that is naturally absent after menopause.

Before using this medicine

Before you use this medicine check with your doctor, or pharmacist:
- if you ever had any unusual or allergic reaction to estrogens;
- if you are pregnant or intend to become pregnant within three months;
- if you are breast-feeding an infant;
- if you have any of the following medical problems:
  Diabetes
  Breast cancer
  Fibrocystic breast disease
  Fibroid uterine tumors
  Endometriosis
  Migraine headaches
  Epilepsy
  Porphyria
  High blood pressure
  Asthma
  Congestive heart failure
  Kidney disease
  Gallstones

Treatment

This medication is used to treat estrogen deficiency, specific symptoms of menopause, estrogen-deficiency osteoporosis, atrophic vaginitis, prostate cancer.

For safe and effective use of this medicine:
- ◆ Follow your doctor's instructions if this medicine was prescribed.
- ◆ Follow the manufacturer's package directions if you are treating yourself.
- ◆ Estrogens have been reported to increase the risk of endometrial carcinoma.

Side effects

Along with the needed effects, a medicine may cause some unwanted effects. Possible side effects include:
  Stomach cramps
  Profuse bleeding
  Appetite loss
  Nausea and vomiting
  Swollen breasts
  Change in menstruation
  Rash, skin blisters
  Depression
  Dizziness

Overdose

The following symptoms may indicate an overdose:
  Nausea and vomiting
  Fluid retention
  Breast enlargement
  Abnormal vaginal bleeding
- ■ Call a doctor or hospital emergency room for instructions.

Interactions

This medicine may interact with several other drugs such as adrenocorticosteroids, antidepressants, oral antidiabetics, insulin, phenobarbital, primidone.
- ■ Be sure to tell your doctor about any medications you are currently taking.

Storage

Capsules, tablets, vaginal cream, transdermal patches, etc. should be stored at room temperature; store away from heat and direct light. Keep out of reach of children, since this medicine may be dangerous in children.

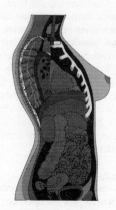

DELATEST

Properties
This medicine is a member of the androgenic, or male, hormone group, containing an androgenic preparation as active ingredient. It is used in diseases in which male hormone replacement or augmentation is needed and also in so-called male menopause. It is also used to decrease calcium loss in osteoporosis, to block growth of breast cancer cells in females and to reduce breast pain and fullness following childbirth.

Before using this medicine
Before you use this medicine check with your doctor, or pharmacist:
- if you ever had any unusual or allergic reaction to androgens or corticosteroids in general.
- if you are on a low-salt, low-sugar, or any other special diet, or if you are allergic to any substance, such as certain preservatives or dyes.
- if you have any of the following medical problems:
  Cancer prostate
  Heart disease or atherosclerosis
  Kidney or lifer disease
  Breast cancer (males)
  High blood pressure
  High level of blood calcium
  Epilepsy

Treatment
This medication is used to relieve or prevent the symptoms of your medical problem. Take them as directed. Do not take more of them and do not take them more often than recommended on the label. One should take the tablets or capsules with food to lessen stomach irritation. Take the medication at the same time each day. If you forget a dose take it as soon as you remember up to two hours late; wait for the next scheduled dose; don't double this dose. The risk to the unborn child outweighs the benefits of the drug.

Side effects
Females taking any androgenic drug should watch for deepening of the voice, oily skin, acne, hairiness, increased libido, and menstrual irregularities.

The following side effects may occur:
  Acne or oily skin
  Deep voice
  Enlarged clitoris in females
  Frequent erections in men
  Sore mouth
  Higher sex drive
  Impotence in men
  Yellow skin or eyes
These side effects should disappear as your body adjusts to the medication. Tell your doctor about any side effects that are persistent or particularly bothersome.
- Discontinue the use of the medication and seek emergency treatment in the following situations:
  Intense itching
  Weakness
  Loss of consciousness
  Depression or confusion
  Swollen feet or legs
  Shortness of breath
  Irregularities of heartbeat
  Difficult urination
  Vaginal bleeding in women
  Scrotum pain in men

Interactions
This medicine interacts with several other drugs such as anticoagulants, oral antidiabetics, cyclosporine, hepatotoxic drugs, oxyphenbutazone, phenobarbital, and phenylbutazone.
- Be sure to tell your doctor about any medications you are currently taking.

Storage
This medicine should be stored at room temperature in closed containers. Store away from heat and direct light. Keep out of reach of children, since overdose may be dangerous in children.

DELATESTRYL

Properties
This medicine is a member of the androgenic, or male, hormone group, containing an androgenic preparation as active ingredient. It is used in diseases in which male hormone replacement or augmentation is needed and also in so-called male menopause. It is also used to decrease calcium loss in osteoporosis, to block growth of breast cancer cells in females and to reduce breast pain and fullness following childbirth.

Before using this medicine
Before you use this medicine check with your doctor, or pharmacist:
- if you ever had any unusual or allergic reaction to androgens or corticosteroids in general.
- if you are on a low-salt, low-sugar, or any other special diet, or if you are allergic to any substance, such as certain preservatives or dyes.
- if you have any of the following medical problems:
  Cancer prostate
  Heart disease or atherosclerosis
  Kidney or lifer disease
  Breast cancer (males)
  High blood pressure
  High level of blood calcium
  Epilepsy

Treatment
This medication is used to relieve or prevent the symptoms of your medical problem. Take them as directed. Do not take more of them and do not take them more often than recommended on the label. One should take the tablets or capsules with food to lessen stomach irritation. Take the medication at the same time each day. If you forget a dose take it as soon as you remember up to two hours late; wait for the next scheduled dose; don't double this dose. The risk to the unborn child outweighs the benefits of the drug.

Side effects
Females taking any androgenic drug should watch for deepening of the voice, oily skin, acne, hairiness, increased libido, and menstrual irregularities.

The following side effects may occur:
  Acne or oily skin
  Deep voice
  Enlarged clitoris in females
  Frequent erections in men
  Sore mouth
  Higher sex drive
  Impotence in men
  Yellow skin or eyes
These side effects should disappear as your body adjusts to the medication. Tell your doctor about any side effects that are persistent or particularly bothersome.
- Discontinue the use of the medication and seek emergency treatment in the following situations:
  Intense itching
  Weakness
  Loss of consciousness
  Depression or confusion
  Swollen feet or legs
  Shortness of breath
  Irregularities of heartbeat
  Difficult urination
  Vaginal bleeding in women
  Scrotum pain in men

Interactions
This medicine interacts with several other drugs such as anticoagulants, oral antidiabetics, cyclosporine, hepatotoxic drugs, oxyphenbutazone, phenobarbital, and phenylbutazone.
- Be sure to tell your doctor about any medications you are currently taking.

Storage
This medicine should be stored at room temperature in closed containers. Store away from heat and direct light. Keep out of reach of children, since overdose may be dangerous in children.

DELESTROGEN

Properties
This medicine contains estrogen as active ingredient. The medicine is prescribed for treatment of estrogen deficiency; it restores normal estrogen levels in tissues. There is no evidence that this drug is effective for nervous symptoms or depression occurring during menopause. They should not be used to treat this condition; they should be used only to replace the estrogen that is naturally absent after menopause.

Before using this medicine
Before you use this medicine check with your doctor, or pharmacist:
- if you ever had any unusual or allergic reaction to estrogens;
- if you are pregnant or intend to become pregnant within three months;
- if you are breast-feeding an infant;
- if you have any of the following medical problems:
  Diabetes
  Breast cancer
  Fibrocystic breast disease
  Fibroid uterine tumors
  Endometriosis
  Migraine headaches
  Epilepsy
  Porphyria
  High blood pressure
  Asthma
  Congestive heart failure
  Kidney disease
  Gallstones

Treatment
This medication is used to treat estrogen deficiency, specific symptoms of menopause, estrogen-deficiency osteoporosis, atrophic vaginitis, prostate cancer.

For safe and effective use of this medicine:
- ◆ Follow your doctor's instructions if this medicine was prescribed.
- ◆ Follow the manufacturer's package directions if you are treating yourself.
- ◆ Estrogens have been reported to increase the risk of endometrial carcinoma.

Side effects
Along with the needed effects, a medicine may cause some unwanted effects. Possible side effects include:
  Stomach cramps
  Profuse bleeding
  Appetite loss
  Nausea and vomiting
  Swollen breasts
  Change in menstruation
  Rash, skin blisters
  Depression
  Dizziness

Overdose
The following symptoms may indicate an overdose:
  Nausea and vomiting
  Fluid retention
  Breast enlargement
  Abnormal vaginal bleeding
- ■ Call a doctor or hospital emergency room for instructions.

Interactions
This medicine may interact with several other drugs such as adrenocorticosteroids, antidepressants, oral antidiabetics, insulin, phenobarbital, primidone.
- ■ Be sure to tell your doctor about any medications you are currently taking.

Storage
Capsules, tablets, vaginal cream, transdermal patches, etc. should be stored at room temperature; store away from heat and direct light. Keep out of reach of children, since this medicine may be dangerous in children.

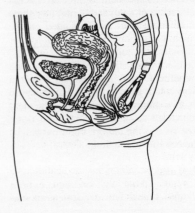

DEMER-IDINE

Properties
This medicine contains as active ingredient meperidine.

It is a narcotic analgesic that acts directly on the central nervous system (brain and spinal cord). It is used to relieve pain or to suppress coughing.

Before using this medicine
Before you use this medicine check with your doctor, or pharmacist:
- if you ever had any unusual or allergic reaction to this medicine or one of its components.
- if you are on a low-salt, low-sugar, or any other special diet, or if you are allergic to any substance, such as sulfites or other preservatives or dyes.
- if you are pregnant or inintend to become pregnant while using this medicine. Studies on birth defects have not been done in humans. Too much use of narcotics during pregnancy may cause the baby to become dependent on the medicine.
- if you are breast-feeding an infant. Although this medicine has not been shown to cause problems in humans, it passes into the breast milk in small amounts.
- if you have any of the following medical problems:
  Brain disease or head injury
  Colitis
  Convulsions
  Emphysema, asthma, or chronic lung disease
  Enlarged prostate
  Gallbladder disease or gallstones
  Heart disease
  Kidney or lifer disease
  Underactive thyroid

Treatment
This medication is used to relieve pain or to suppress coughing. Narcotic analgesics act in the central nervous system; some of their side effects are also caused by actions in the central nervous system.
- If you are taking this medication on a regular schedule and you miss a dose, take the missed dose as soon as possible, unless it is almost time for your next dose. In that case do not take the missed dose at all.
- If a narcotic analgesic is used for a long time, it may become habit-forming (causing mental or physical dependence). Physical dependence may lead to withdrawal side effects when you stop taking this medicine.

Unless otherwise directed by your doctor or pharmacist take this as directed. Do not take more of them and do not take them more often than recommended on the label. Children up to 12 years of age should not take this medicine more than 3 times a day or for more than 5 days in a row.

Side effects
Along with the needed effects, a medicine may cause some unwanted effects. These side effects may go away during treatment as your body adjusts to the medicine. Such minor side effects are: constipation, dizziness, drowsiness, dry mouth, false sense of well-being, flushing, light-headedness, loss of appetite, nausea, painful or difficult urination, or sweating.
- Check with your doctor immediately if any of the following side effects occur:
  Anxiety or breathing difficulties
  Excitation or restlessness
  Fatigue, palpitations
  Rash, sore throat and fever
  Tremors or weakness

Interactions
This medicine may interact with several other drugs such as medicines acting on the central nervous system (e.g., antidepressants, tranquilizers), cimetidine, nitrates, quinidine, etc.
- Be sure to tell your doctor about any medications you are currently taking.

Storage
Tablets, elixir, suppository etc. should be stored at room temperature in a tightly closed, light-resistant container.

DEMEROL

Properties
This medicine contains as active ingredient meperidine.

It is a narcotic analgesic that acts directly on the central nervous system (brain and spinal cord). It is used to relieve pain or to suppress coughing.

Before using this medicine
Before you use this medicine check with your doctor, or pharmacist:
- if you ever had any unusual or allergic reaction to this medicine or one of its components.
- if you are on a low-salt, low-sugar, or any other special diet, or if you are allergic to any substance, such as sulfites or other preservatives or dyes.
- if you are pregnant or inintend to become pregnant while using this medicine. Studies on birth defects have not been done in humans. Too much use of narcotics during pregnancy may cause the baby to become dependent on the medicine.
- if you are breast-feeding an infant. Although this medicine has not been shown to cause problems in humans, it passes into the breast milk in small amounts.
- if you have any of the following medical problems:
Brain disease or head injury
Colitis
Convulsions
Emphysema, asthma, or chronic lung disease
Enlarged prostate
Gallbladder disease or gallstones
Heart disease
Kidney or lifer disease
Underactive thyroid

Treatment
This medication is used to relieve pain or to suppress coughing. Narcotic analgesics act in the central nervous system; some of their side effects are also caused by actions in the central nervous system.
- If you are taking this medication on a regular schedule and you miss a dose, take the missed dose as soon as possible, unless it is almost time for your next dose. In that case do not take the missed dose at all.
- If a narcotic analgesic is used for a long time, it may become habit-forming (causing mental or physical dependence). Physical dependence may lead to withdrawal side effects when you stop taking this medicine.

Unless otherwise directed by your doctor or pharmacist take this as directed. Do not take more of them and do not take them more often than recommended on the label. Children up to 12 years of age should not take this medicine more than 3 times a day or for more than 5 days in a row.

Side effects
Along with the needed effects, a medicine may cause some unwanted effects. These side effects may go away during treatment as your body adjusts to the medicine. Such minor side effects are: constipation, dizziness, drowsiness, dry mouth, false sense of well-being, flushing, light-headedness, loss of appetite, nausea, painful or difficult urination, or sweating.
- Check with your doctor immediately if any of the following side effects occur:
Anxiety or breathing difficulties
Excitation or restlessness
Fatigue, palpitations
Rash, sore throat and fever
Tremors or weakness

Interactions
This medicine may interact with several other drugs such as medicines acting on the central nervous system (e.g., antidepressants, tranquilizers), cimetidine, nitrates, quinidine, etc.
- Be sure to tell your doctor about any medications you are currently taking.

Storage
Tablets, elixir, suppository etc. should be stored at room temperature in a tightly closed, light-resistant container.

DEMOVATE

Properties
This medicine contains clobetasol propionate, a corticosteroid, as active ingredient. Corticosteroids are used to help relieve redness, swelling, itching, inflammation, and discomfort of many skin problems. They exert this effect by interfering with natural body mechanisms that produce the rash, itching, or inflammation. They do not cure the underlying cause of the skin problem. This medication is applied to the skin.

Before using this medicine
Before you use this medicine check with your doctor, or pharmacist:
- if you ever had any unusual or allergic reaction to corticosteroids.
- if you are allergic to any substance, such as sulfites or other preservatives or dyes.
- if you are pregnant or inintend to become pregnant while using this medicine. Studies have shown that corticosteroids applied to the skin in large amounts or over long periods of time can be the cause of birth defects.
- if you are breast-feeding an infant. Some corticosteroids pass into breast milk and may interfere with the infant's growth.

Treatment
Do not use this medicine more often or for a longer time than ordered. To do so may increase absorption through the skin and the chance of side effects. In addition, too much use, especially on areas with thinner skin (for example, face, armpits, groin), may result in thinning of the skin and stretch marks.

Before applying this medication, wash your hands. than, unless your doctor or pharmacist gives you different instructions, gently wash the area where the medication is to be applied. With a clean towel pat the area dry. Apply a small amount of the medication to the affected area in a thin layer. Do not bandage the area unless your doctor tells you to do so.

If you miss a dose of this medication, apply the dose as soon as possible, unless it is almost time for the next application.
- ◆ Do not use this medicine for other skin problems without first checking with your doctor. You should not use a topical corticosteroid if you have a virus disease (such as herpes), fungal infection of the skin (such as athlete's foot), or tuberculosis of the skin.

Side effects
There are a number of side effects that usually do not require medical attention. Minor side effects are:
Acne
Burning sensations
Itching
Rash
Skin dryness
These possible side effects may go away during treatment; however, if they continue or are bothersome, check with your doctor, nurse, or pharmacist. Tell your doctor about any side effects that are persistent or particularly bothersome, such as:
Blistering
Increased hair growth
Irritation of the affected area
Loss of skin
Secondary infection in the area being treated
Thinning of the skin with easy bruising

Interactions
None known as long as it is used according to the directions given to you by your doctor or pharmacist.

Storage
Cream, ointment, lotion, gel, spray, and aerosol should be stored at room temperature in tightly closed containers. This medication should never be frozen.

DEMULEN

Properties
This medicine contains ethynodiol diacetate and ethinyl estradiol as active ingredients. It is an oral contraceptive prescribed to prevent pregnancy and/or to regulate menstrual periods.

The drug works by altering the mucus at the cervix entrance to prevent the entry of sperm. It also alters the uterus lining to resist implantation of the fertilized egg. Oral contraceptives create the same chemical atmosphere in blood that exists during pregnancy.

Before using this medicine
Before you use this medicine check with your doctor, or pharmacist:
- if you ever had any unusual or allergic reaction to estrogens or progestogen;
- if you are pregnant or want to become pregnant within three months;
- if you are breast-feeding an infant;
- if you have any of the following medical problems:
  Diabetes
  Ailments of the breast
  Disorders of the uterus
  Migraine or epilepsy
  High blood pressure
  Asthma or heart conditions
  Kidney disease
  Gallstones

Treatment
This medication is used to prevent pregnancy or to regulate menstrual periods.

Adverse reactions
Along with the needed effects, a medicine may cause some unwanted effects or adverse reactions.
- *An increased risk of the following adverse reactions has been associated with the use of oral contraceptives:*
  Thrombophlebitis
  Venous thrombosis
  Arterial thromboembolism
  Pulmonary (lung) embolism
  Myocardial infarction
  Cerebral hemorrhage
  Cerebral thrombosis
  Hypertension
  Gallbladder disease
  Hepatic (liver) hepatomas
  Benign lifer tumors
- *The following adverse reactions have been reported in patients receiving oral contraceptives and are believed to be drug-related:*
  Nausea and vomiting
  Abdominal cramps
  Breakthrough bleeding
  Spotting
  Change in menstrual flow
  Amenorrhea
  Temporary infertility
  Edema
  Breast changes
  Weight changes
  Cholestatic jaundice
  Migraine
  Rash (allergic)
  Mental depression
  Vaginal candidiasis

Interactions
This medicine may interact with several other drugs such as antibiotics, anticoagulants, anticonvulsants, antidepressants, oral antidiabetics, antihistamines, barbiturates, oral hypoglycemics, insulin, meperidine.
- Be sure to tell your doctor about any medications you are currently taking.

Storage
Tablets should be stored at room temperature; store away from heat and direct light. Keep out of reach of children, since this medicine may be dangerous in children.

DEP ANDRO

Properties
This medicine is a member of the androgenic, or male, hormone group, containing an androgenic preparation as active ingredient. It is used in diseases in which male hormone replacement or augmentation is needed and also in so-called male menopause. It is also used to decrease calcium loss in osteoporosis, to block growth of breast cancer cells in females and to reduce breast pain and fullness following childbirth.

Before using this medicine
Before you use this medicine check with your doctor, or pharmacist:
- if you ever had any unusual or allergic reaction to androgens or corticosteroids in general.
- if you are on a low-salt, low-sugar, or any other special diet, or if you are allergic to any substance, such as certain preservatives or dyes.
- if you have any of the following medical problems:
Cancer prostate
Heart disease or atherosclerosis
Kidney or lifer disease
Breast cancer (males)
High blood pressure
High level of blood calcium
Epilepsy

Treatment
This medication is used to relieve or prevent the symptoms of your medical problem. Take them as directed. Do not take more of them and do not take them more often than recommended on the label. One should take the tablets or capsules with food to lessen stomach irritation. Take the medication at the same time each day. If you forget a dose take it as soon as you remember up to two hours late; wait for the next scheduled dose; don't double this dose. The risk to the unborn child outweighs the benefits of the drug.

Side effects
Females taking any androgenic drug should watch for deepening of the voice, oily skin, acne, hairiness, increased libido, and menstrual irregularities.

The following side effects may occur:
Acne or oily skin
Deep voice
Enlarged clitoris in females
Frequent erections in men
Sore mouth
Higher sex drive
Impotence in men
Yellow skin or eyes

These side effects should disappear as your body adjusts to the medication. Tell your doctor about any side effects that are persistent or particularly bothersome.

- Discontinue the use of the medication and seek emergency treatment in the following situations:
Intense itching
Weakness
Loss of consciousness
Depression or confusion
Swollen feet or legs
Shortness of breath
Irregularities of heartbeat
Difficult urination
Vaginal bleeding in women
Scrotum pain in men

Interactions
This medicine interacts with several other drugs such as anticoagulants, oral antidiabetics, cyclosporine, hepatotoxic drugs, oxyphenbutazone, phenobarbital, and phenylbutazone.

- Be sure to tell your doctor about any medications you are currently taking.

Storage
This medicine should be stored at room temperature in closed containers. Store away from heat and direct light. Keep out of reach of children, since overdose may be dangerous in children.

DEPGYNOGEN

Properties

This medicine contains estradiol as active ingredient. The medicine is prescribed for treatment of estrogen deficiency; it restores normal estrogen levels in tissues. There is no evidence that this drug is effective for nervous symptoms or depression occurring during menopause. They should not be used to treat this condition; they should be used only to replace the estrogen that is naturally absent after menopause.

Before using this medicine

Before you use this medicine check with your doctor, or pharmacist:
- if you ever had any unusual or allergic reaction to estrogens;
- if you are pregnant or intend to become pregnant within three months;
- if you are breast-feeding an infant;
- if you have any of the following medical problems:
  Diabetes
  Breast cancer
  Fibrocystic breast disease
  Fibroid uterine tumors
  Endometriosis
  Migraine headaches
  Epilepsy
  Porphyria
  High blood pressure
  Asthma
  Congestive heart failure
  Kidney disease
  Gallstones

Treatment

This medication is used to treat estrogen deficiency, specific symptoms of menopause, estrogen-deficiency osteoporosis, atrophic vaginitis, prostate cancer.

For safe and effective use of this medicine:
- Follow your doctor's instructions if this medicine was prescribed.
- Follow the manufacturer's package directions if you are treating yourself.
- Estrogens have been reported to increase the risk of endometrial carcinoma.

Side effects

Along with the needed effects, a medicine may cause some unwanted effects. Possible side effects include:
  Stomach cramps
  Profuse bleeding
  Appetite loss
  Nausea and vomiting
  Swollen breasts
  Change in menstruation
  Rash, skin blisters
  Depression
  Dizziness

Overdose

The following symptoms may indicate an overdose:
  Nausea and vomiting
  Fluid retention
  Breast enlargement
  Abnormal vaginal bleeding
- Call a doctor or hospital emergency room for instructions.

Interactions

This medicine may interact with several other drugs such as adrenocorticosteroids, antidepressants, oral antidiabetics, insulin, phenobarbital, primidone.
- Be sure to tell your doctor about any medications you are currently taking.

Storage

Capsules, tablets, vaginal cream, transdermal patches, etc. should be stored at room temperature; store away from heat and direct light. Keep out of reach of children, since this medicine may be dangerous in children.

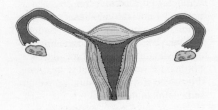

DEPO ESTRADIOL

Properties

This medicine contains estrogen as active ingredient. The medicine is prescribed for treatment of estrogen deficiency; it restores normal estrogen levels in tissues. There is no evidence that this drug is effective for nervous symptoms or depression occurring during menopause. They should not be used to treat this condition; they should be used only to replace the estrogen that is naturally absent after menopause.

Before using this medicine

Before you use this medicine check with your doctor, or pharmacist:
- if you ever had any unusual or allergic reaction to estrogens;
- if you are pregnant or intend to become pregnant within three months;
- if you are breast-feeding an infant;
- if you have any of the following medical problems:
  Diabetes
  Breast cancer
  Fibrocystic breast disease
  Fibroid uterine tumors
  Endometriosis
  Migraine headaches
  Epilepsy
  Porphyria
  High blood pressure
  Asthma
  Congestive heart failure
  Kidney disease
  Gallstones

Treatment

This medication is used to treat estrogen deficiency, specific symptoms of menopause, estrogen-deficiency osteoporosis, atrophic vaginitis, prostate cancer.

For safe and effective use of this medicine:
- ◆ Follow your doctor's instructions if this medicine was prescribed.
- ◆ Follow the manufacturer's package directions if you are treating yourself.
- ◆ Estrogens have been reported to increase the risk of endometrial carcinoma.

Side effects

Along with the needed effects, a medicine may cause some unwanted effects. Possible side effects include:
  Stomach cramps
  Profuse bleeding
  Appetite loss
  Nausea and vomiting
  Swollen breasts
  Change in menstruation
  Rash, skin blisters
  Depression
  Dizziness

Overdose

The following symptoms may indicate an overdose:
  Nausea and vomiting
  Fluid retention
  Breast enlargement
  Abnormal vaginal bleeding
- ▪ Call a doctor or hospital emergency room for instructions.

Interactions

This medicine may interact with several other drugs such as adrenocorticosteroids, antidepressants, oral antidiabetics, insulin, phenobarbital, primidone.
- ▪ Be sure to tell your doctor about any medications you are currently taking.

Storage

Capsules, tablets, vaginal cream, transdermal patches, etc. should be stored at room temperature; store away from heat and direct light. Keep out of reach of children, since this medicine may be dangerous in children.

DEPO-TESTOSTERONE

Properties
This medicine is a member of the androgenic, or male, hormone group, containing an androgenic preparation as active ingredient. It is used in diseases in which male hormone replacement or augmentation is needed and also in so-called male menopause. It is also used to decrease calcium loss in osteoporosis, to block growth of breast cancer cells in females and to reduce breast pain and fullness following childbirth.

Before using this medicine
Before you use this medicine check with your doctor, or pharmacist:
- if you ever had any unusual or allergic reaction to androgens or corticosteroids in general.
- if you are on a low-salt, low-sugar, or any other special diet, or if you are allergic to any substance, such as certain preservatives or dyes.
- if you have any of the following medical problems:
  Cancer prostate
  Heart disease or atherosclerosis
  Kidney or lifer disease
  Breast cancer (males)
  High blood pressure
  High level of blood calcium
  Epilepsy

Treatment
This medication is used to relieve or prevent the symptoms of your medical problem. Take them as directed. Do not take more of them and do not take them more often than recommended on the label. One should take the tablets or capsules with food to lessen stomach irritation. Take the medication at the same time each day. If you forget a dose take it as soon as you remember up to two hours late; wait for the next scheduled dose;; don't double this dose. The risk to the unborn child outweighs the benefits of the drug.

Side effects
Females taking any androgenic drug should watch for deepening of the voice, oily skin, acne, hairiness, increased libido, and menstrual irregularities.

The following side effects may occur:
  Acne or oily skin
  Deep voice
  Enlarged clitoris in females
  Frequent erections in men
  Sore mouth
  Higher sex drive
  Impotence in men
  Yellow skin or eyes
These side effects should disappear as your body adjusts to the medication. Tell your doctor about any side effects that are persistent or particularly bothersome.
- Discontinue the use of the medication and seek emergency treatment in the following situations:
  Intense itching
  Weakness
  Loss of consciousness
  Depression or confusion
  Swollen feet or legs
  Shortness of breath
  Irregularities of heartbeat
  Difficult urination
  Vaginal bleeding in women
  Scrotum pain in men

Interactions
This medicine interacts with several other drugs such as anticoagulants, oral antidiabetics, cyclosporine, hepatotoxic drugs, oxyphenbutazone, phenobarbital, and phenylbutazone.
- Be sure to tell your doctor about any medications you are currently taking.

Storage
This medicine should be stored at room temperature in closed containers. Store away from heat and direct light. Keep out of reach of children, since overdose may be dangerous in children.

DEPOGEN

Properties

This medicine contains estrogen as active ingredient. The medicine is prescribed for treatment of estrogen deficiency; it restores normal estrogen levels in tissues. There is no evidence that this drug is effective for nervous symptoms or depression occurring during menopause. They should not be used to treat this condition; they should be used only to replace the estrogen that is naturally absent after menopause.

Before using this medicine

Before you use this medicine check with your doctor, or pharmacist:
- if you ever had any unusual or allergic reaction to estrogens;
- if you are pregnant or intend to become pregnant within three months;
- if you are breast-feeding an infant;
- if you have any of the following medical problems:
  Diabetes
  Breast cancer
  Fibrocystic breast disease
  Fibroid uterine tumors
  Endometriosis
  Migraine headaches
  Epilepsy
  Porphyria
  High blood pressure
  Asthma
  Congestive heart failure
  Kidney disease
  Gallstones

Treatment

This medication is used to treat estrogen deficiency, specific symptoms of menopause, estrogen-deficiency osteoporosis, atrophic vaginitis, prostate cancer.

For safe and effective use of this medicine:
- ◆ Follow your doctor's instructions if this medicine was prescribed.
- ◆ Follow the manufacturer's package directions if you are treating yourself.
- ◆ Estrogens have been reported to increase the risk of endometrial carcinoma.

Side effects

Along with the needed effects, a medicine may cause some unwanted effects. Possible side effects include:
  Stomach cramps
  Profuse bleeding
  Appetite loss
  Nausea and vomiting
  Swollen breasts
  Change in menstruation
  Rash, skin blisters
  Depression
  Dizziness

Overdose

The following symptoms may indicate an overdose:
  Nausea and vomiting
  Fluid retention
  Breast enlargement
  Abnormal vaginal bleeding
- ■ Call a doctor or hospital emergency room for instructions.

Interactions

This medicine may interact with several other drugs such as adrenocorticosteroids, antidepressants, oral antidiabetics, insulin, phenobarbital, primidone.
- ■ Be sure to tell your doctor about any medications you are currently taking.

Storage

Capsules, tablets, vaginal cream, transdermal patches, etc. should be stored at room temperature; store away from heat and direct light. Keep out of reach of children, since this medicine may be dangerous in children.

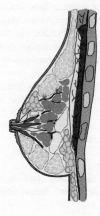

DEPOTEST

Properties
This medicine is a member of the androgenic, or male, hormone group, containing an androgenic preparation as active ingredient. It is used in diseases in which male hormone replacement or augmentation is needed and also in so-called male menopause. It is also used to decrease calcium loss in osteoporosis, to block growth of breast cancer cells in females and to reduce breast pain and fullness following childbirth.

Before using this medicine
Before you use this medicine check with your doctor, or pharmacist:
- if you ever had any unusual or allergic reaction to androgens or corticosteroids in general.
- if you are on a low-salt, low-sugar, or any other special diet, or if you are allergic to any substance, such as certain preservatives or dyes.
- if you have any of the following medical problems:
Cancer prostate
Heart disease or atherosclerosis
Kidney or lifer disease
Breast cancer (males)
High blood pressure
High level of blood calcium
Epilepsy

Treatment
This medication is used to relieve or prevent the symptoms of your medical problem. Take them as directed. Do not take more of them and do not take them more often than recommended on the label. One should take the tablets or capsules with food to lessen stomach irritation. Take the medication at the same time each day. If you forget a dose take it as soon as you remember up to two hours late; wait for the next scheduled dose; don't double this dose. The risk to the unborn child outweighs the benefits of the drug.

Side effects
Females taking any androgenic drug should watch for deepening of the voice, oily skin, acne, hairiness, increased libido, and menstrual irregularities.

The following side effects may occur:
Acne or oily skin
Deep voice
Enlarged clitoris in females
Frequent erections in men
Sore mouth
Higher sex drive
Impotence in men
Yellow skin or eyes
These side effects should disappear as your body adjusts to the medication. Tell your doctor about any side effects that are persistent or particularly bothersome.
- Discontinue the use of the medication and seek emergency treatment in the following situations:
Intense itching
Weakness
Loss of consciousness
Depression or confusion
Swollen feet or legs
Shortness of breath
Irregularities of heartbeat
Difficult urination
Vaginal bleeding in women
Scrotum pain in men

Interactions
This medicine interacts with several other drugs such as anticoagulants, oral antidiabetics, cyclosporine, hepatotoxic drugs, oxyphenbutazone, phenobarbital, and phenylbutazone.
- Be sure to tell your doctor about any medications you are currently taking.

Storage
This medicine should be stored at room temperature in closed containers. Store away from heat and direct light. Keep out of reach of children, since overdose may be dangerous in children.

DERMABET

Properties

This medicine contains betamethasone, a corticosteroid, as active ingredient. Corticosteroids are used to help relieve redness, swelling, itching, inflammation, and discomfort of many skin problems. They exert this effect by interfering with natural body mechanisms that produce the rash, itching, or inflammation. They do not cure the underlying cause of the skin problem. This medication is applied to the skin.

Before using this medicine

Before you use this medicine check with your doctor, or pharmacist:
- if you ever had any unusual or allergic reaction to corticosteroids.
- if you are allergic to any substance, such as sulfites or other preservatives or dyes.
- if you are pregnant or inintend to become pregnant while using this medicine. Studies have shown that corticosteroids applied to the skin in large amounts or over long periods of time can be the cause of birth defects.
- if you are breast-feeding an infant. Some corticosteroids pass into breast milk and may interfere with the infant's growth.

Treatment

Do not use this medicine more often or for a longer time than ordered. To do so may increase absorption through the skin and the chance of side effects. In addition, too much use, especially on areas with thinner skin (for example, face, armpits, groin), may result in thinning of the skin and stretch marks.

Before applying this medication, wash your hands. than, unless your doctor or pharmacist gives you different instructions, gently wash the area where the medication is to be applied. With a clean towel pat the area dry. Apply a small amount of the medication to the affected area in a thin layer. Do not bandage the area unless your doctor tells you to do so.

If you miss a dose of this medication, apply the dose as soon as possible, unless it is almost time for the next application.
- ◆ Do not use this medicine for other skin problems without first checking with your doctor. You should not use a topical corticosteroid if you have a virus disease (such as herpes), fungal infection of the skin (such as athlete's foot), or tuberculosis of the skin.

Side effects

There are a number of side effects that usually do not require medical attention. Minor side effects are:

Acne
Burning sensations
Itching
Rash
Skin dryness

These possible side effects may go away during treatment; however, if they continue or are bothersome, check with your doctor, nurse, or pharmacist. Tell your doctor about any side effects that are persistent or particularly bothersome, such as:

Blistering
Increased hair growth
Irritation of the affected area
Loss of skin
Secondary infection in the area being treated
Thinning of the skin with easy bruising

Interactions

None known as long as it is used according to the directions given to you by your doctor or pharmacist.

Storage

Cream, ointment, lotion, gel, spray, and aerosol should be stored at room temperature in tightly closed containers. This medication should never be frozen.

DES

Properties

This medicine contains diuethylstil-bestrol as active ingredient. The medicine is prescribed for treatment of estrogen deficiency; it restores normal estrogen levels in tissues. There is no evidence that this drug is effective for nervous symptoms or depression occurring during menopause. They should not be used to treat this condition; they should be used only to replace the estrogen that is naturally absent after menopause.

Before using this medicine

Before you use this medicine check with your doctor, or pharmacist:
- if you ever had any unusual or allergic reaction to estrogens;
- if you are pregnant or intend to become pregnant within three months;
- if you are breast-feeding an infant;
- if you have any of the following medical problems:
  Diabetes
  Breast cancer
  Fibrocystic breast disease
  Fibroid uterine tumors
  Endometriosis
  Migraine headaches
  Epilepsy
  Porphyria
  High blood pressure
  Asthma
  Congestive heart failure
  Kidney disease
  Gallstones

Treatment

This medication is used to treat estrogen deficiency, specific symptoms of menopause, estrogen-deficiency osteoporosis, atrophic vaginitis, prostate cancer.

For safe and effective use of this medicine:
- ◆ Follow your doctor's instructions if this medicine was prescribed.
- ◆ Follow the manufacturer's package directions if you are treating yourself.
- ◆ Estrogens have been reported to increase the risk of endometrial carcinoma.

Side effects

Along with the needed effects, a medicine may cause some unwanted effects. Possible side effects include:
  Stomach cramps
  Profuse bleeding
  Appetite loss
  Nausea and vomiting
  Swollen breasts
  Change in menstruation
  Rash, skin blisters
  Depression
  Dizziness

Overdose

The following symptoms may indicate an overdose:
  Nausea and vomiting
  Fluid retention
  Breast enlargement
  Abnormal vaginal bleeding
- ■ Call a doctor or hospital emergency room for instructions.

Interactions

This medicine may interact with several other drugs such as adrenocorticosteroids, antidepressants, oral antidiabetics, insulin, phenobarbital, primidone.
- ■ Be sure to tell your doctor about any medications you are currently taking.

Storage

Capsules, tablets, vaginal cream, transdermal patches, etc. should be stored at room temperature; store away from heat and direct light. Keep out of reach of children, since this medicine may be dangerous in children.

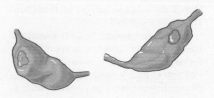

DERMABET

Properties

This medicine contains betamethasone, a corticosteroid, as active ingredient. Corticosteroids are used to help relieve redness, swelling, itching, inflammation, and discomfort of many skin problems. They exert this effect by interfering with natural body mechanisms that produce the rash, itching, or inflammation. They do not cure the underlying cause of the skin problem. This medication is applied to the skin.

Before using this medicine

Before you use this medicine check with your doctor, or pharmacist:

- if you ever had any unusual or allergic reaction to corticosteroids.
- if you are allergic to any substance, such as sulfites or other preservatives or dyes.
- if you are pregnant or inintend to become pregnant while using this medicine. Studies have shown that corticosteroids applied to the skin in large amounts or over long periods of time can be the cause of birth defects.
- if you are breast-feeding an infant. Some corticosteroids pass into breast milk and may interfere with the infant's growth.

Treatment

Do not use this medicine more often or for a longer time than ordered. To do so may increase absorption through the skin and the chance of side effects. In addition, too much use, especially on areas with thinner skin (for example, face, armpits, groin), may result in thinning of the skin and stretch marks.

Before applying this medication, wash your hands. than, unless your doctor or pharmacist gives you different instructions, gently wash the area where the medication is to be applied. With a clean towel pat the area dry. Apply a small amount of the medication to the affected area in a thin layer. Do not bandage the area unless your doctor tells you to do so.

If you miss a dose of this medication, apply the dose as soon as possible, unless it is almost time for the next application.

- ♦ Do not use this medicine for other skin problems without first checking with your doctor. You should not use a topical corticosteroid if you have a virus disease (such as herpes), fungal infection of the skin (such as athlete's foot), or tuberculosis of the skin.

Side effects

There are a number of side effects that usually do not require medical attention. Minor side effects are:

Acne
Burning sensations
Itching
Rash
Skin dryness

These possible side effects may go away during treatment; however, if they continue or are bothersome, check with your doctor, nurse, or pharmacist. Tell your doctor about any side effects that are persistent or particularly bothersome, such as:

Blistering
Increased hair growth
Irritation of the affected area
Loss of skin
Secondary infection in the area being treated
Thinning of the skin with easy bruising

Interactions

None known as long as it is used according to the directions given to you by your doctor or pharmacist.

Storage

Cream, ointment, lotion, gel, spray, and aerosol should be stored at room temperature in tightly closed containers. This medication should never be frozen.

DES

Properties

This medicine contains diuethylstilbestrol as active ingredient. The medicine is prescribed for treatment of estrogen deficiency; it restores normal estrogen levels in tissues. There is no evidence that this drug is effective for nervous symptoms or depression occurring during menopause. They should not be used to treat this condition; they should be used only to replace the estrogen that is naturally absent after menopause.

Before using this medicine

Before you use this medicine check with your doctor, or pharmacist:
- if you ever had any unusual or allergic reaction to estrogens;
- if you are pregnant or intend to become pregnant within three months;
- if you are breast-feeding an infant;
- if you have any of the following medical problems:
  Diabetes
  Breast cancer
  Fibrocystic breast disease
  Fibroid uterine tumors
  Endometriosis
  Migraine headaches
  Epilepsy
  Porphyria
  High blood pressure
  Asthma
  Congestive heart failure
  Kidney disease
  Gallstones

Treatment

This medication is used to treat estrogen deficiency, specific symptoms of menopause, estrogen-deficiency osteoporosis, atrophic vaginitis, prostate cancer.

For safe and effective use of this medicine:
- ◆ Follow your doctor's instructions if this medicine was prescribed.
- ◆ Follow the manufacturer's package directions if you are treating yourself.
- ◆ Estrogens have been reported to increase the risk of endometrial carcinoma.

Side effects

Along with the needed effects, a medicine may cause some unwanted effects. Possible side effects include:
  Stomach cramps
  Profuse bleeding
  Appetite loss
  Nausea and vomiting
  Swollen breasts
  Change in menstruation
  Rash, skin blisters
  Depression
  Dizziness

Overdose

The following symptoms may indicate an overdose:
  Nausea and vomiting
  Fluid retention
  Breast enlargement
  Abnormal vaginal bleeding
- ■ Call a doctor or hospital emergency room for instructions.

Interactions

This medicine may interact with several other drugs such as adrenocorticosteroids, antidepressants, oral antidiabetics, insulin, phenobarbital, primidone.
- ■ Be sure to tell your doctor about any medications you are currently taking.

Storage

Capsules, tablets, vaginal cream, transdermal patches, etc. should be stored at room temperature; store away from heat and direct light. Keep out of reach of children, since this medicine may be dangerous in children.

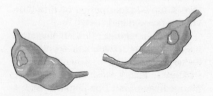

DESIPRAMINE

Properties
This medicine contains desipramine as active ingredient. It belongs to the group of medicines known as tricyclic antidepressants or 'mood elevators.' It is used to relieve mental depression and depression that sometimes occurs with anxiety. The medication gradually relieves, but doesn't cure, symptoms of depression. The medication may also be used for the treatment of narcolepsy, bulimia, panic attacks, cocaine withdrawal, attention deficit disorder.

Before using this medicine
Before you use this medicine check with your doctor, or pharmacist:
- if you ever had any unusual or allergic reaction to any tricyclic antidepressant, maprotiline or trazodone.
- if you are on a low-salt, low-sugar, or any other special diet, or if you are allergic to any substance, such as sulfites or other preservatives or dyes.
- if you are pregnant or inintend to become pregnant while using this medicine. There have been reports of newborns suffering from heart, breathing, and urinary problems when their mothers had taken tricyclic antidepressants before delivery.
- if you are breast-feeding an infant. Some tricyclic antidepressants pass into the breast milk.

Treatment
Take this medicine only as directed by your doctor, to benefit your condition as much as possible. Do not take more of it, do not take it more often, and do not take it for a longer period of time than your doctor ordered.

To lessen stomach upset, take this medicine with food, even for a daily bedtime dose, unless your doctor has told you to take it on an empty stomach. If you forget your once-a-day bedtime dose, don't take it more than 3 hours late. If more than 3 hours, wait for next scheduled dose;.

Sometimes this medicine must be taken for several weeks before you begin to feel better.

Side effects
Along with the needed effects, a medicine may cause some unwanted effects. Side effects that usually do not require medical attention: difficult or frequent urination; decreased sex drive; muscle aches; abnormal dreams; nasal congestion; weakness and faintness when arising from bed or chair; back pain.
- Other side effects that should be reported to your doctor immediately are:
Hallucinations
Shakiness
Dizziness or fainting
Blurred vision, eye pain
Irregular heartbeat or slow pulse
Inflamed tongue
Abdominal pain
Jaundice
Hair loss, rash
Fever, chills
Joint pain
Palpitations

Interactions
This medicine may interact with several other drugs such as anticoagulants, anticholinergics, cold remedies, oral contraceptives, seizure medicines, sleeping medicines, thyroid medicines, etc.
- Be sure to tell your doctor about any medications you are currently taking.

Storage
Tablets, capsules, etc. should be stored at room temperature in tightly closed, light-resistant containers as directed by your pharmacist. Keep out of reach of children since overdose is especially dangerous in young children. Do not store in the bathroom medicine cabinet because the heat or moisture may cause the medicine to break down. Keep the liquid form of the medicine from freezing.

DESOGEN

Properties
This medicine contains desogestrel and ethinyl estradiol as active ingredients. It is an oral contraceptive prescribed to prevent pregnancy and/or to regulate menstrual periods.

The drug works by altering the mucus at the cervix entrance to prevent the entry of sperm. It also alters the uterus lining to resist implantation of the fertilized egg. Oral contraceptives create the same chemical atmosphere in blood that exists during pregnancy.

Before using this medicine
Before you use this medicine check with your doctor, or pharmacist:
- if you ever had any unusual or allergic reaction to estrogens or progestogen;
- if you are pregnant or want to become pregnant within three months;
- if you are breast-feeding an infant;
- if you have any of the following medical problems:
Diabetes
Ailments of the breast
Disorders of the uterus
Migraine or epilepsy
High blood pressure
Asthma or heart conditions
Kidney disease
Gallstones

Treatment
This medication is used to prevent pregnancy or to regulate menstrual periods.

Adverse reactions
Along with the needed effects, a medicine may cause some unwanted effects or adverse reactions.
- *An increased risk of the following adverse reactions has been associated with the use of oral contraceptives:*
Thrombophlebitis
Venous thrombosis
Arterial thromboembolism
Pulmonary (lung) embolism
Myocardial infarction
Cerebral hemorrhage
Cerebral thrombosis

Hypertension
Gallbladder disease
Hepatic (liver) hepatomas
Benign lifer tumors
- *The following adverse reactions have been reported in patients receiving oral contraceptives and are believed to be drug-related:*
Nausea and vomiting
Abdominal cramps
Breakthrough bleeding
Spotting
Change in menstrual flow
Amenorrhea
Temporary infertility
Edema
Breast changes
Weight changes
Cholestatic jaundice
Migraine
Rash (allergic)
Mental depression
Vaginal candidiasis

Interactions
This medicine may interact with several other drugs such as antibiotics, anticoagulants, anticonvulsants, antidepressants, oral antidiabetics, antihistamines, barbiturates, oral hypoglycemics, insulin, meperidine.
- Be sure to tell your doctor about any medications you are currently taking.

Storage
Tablets should be stored at room temperature; store away from heat and direct light. Keep out of reach of children, since this medicine may be dangerous in children.

DESONIDE

Properties
This medicine contains desonide, a corticosteroid, as active ingredient. Corticosteroids are used to help relieve redness, swelling, itching, inflammation, and discomfort of many skin problems. They exert this effect by interfering with natural body mechanisms that produce the rash, itching, or inflammation. They do not cure the underlying cause of the skin problem. This medication is applied to the skin.

Before using this medicine
Before you use this medicine check with your doctor, or pharmacist:
- if you ever had any unusual or allergic reaction to corticosteroids.
- if you are allergic to any substance, such as sulfites or other preservatives or dyes.
- if you are pregnant or inintend to become pregnant while using this medicine. Studies have shown that corticosteroids applied to the skin in large amounts or over long periods of time can be the cause of birth defects.
- if you are breast-feeding an infant. Some corticosteroids pass into breast milk and may interfere with the infant's growth.

Treatment
Do not use this medicine more often or for a longer time than ordered. To do so may increase absorption through the skin and the chance of side effects. In addition, too much use, especially on areas with thinner skin (for example, face, armpits, groin), may result in thinning of the skin and stretch marks.

Before applying this medication, wash your hands. than, unless your doctor or pharmacist gives you different instructions, gently wash the area where the medication is to be applied. With a clean towel pat the area dry. Apply a small amount of the medication to the affected area in a thin layer. Do not bandage the area unless your doctor tells you to do so.

If you miss a dose of this medication, apply the dose as soon as possible, unless it is almost time for the next application.
- Do not use this medicine for other skin problems without first checking with your doctor. You should not use a topical corticosteroid if you have a virus disease (such as herpes), fungal infection of the skin (such as athlete's foot), or tuberculosis of the skin.

Side effects
There are a number of side effects that usually do not require medical attention. Minor side effects are:
  Acne
  Burning sensations
  Itching
  Rash
  Skin dryness
These possible side effects may go away during treatment; however, if they continue or are bothersome, check with your doctor, nurse, or pharmacist. Tell your doctor about any side effects that are persistent or particularly bothersome, such as:
  Blistering
  Increased hair growth
  Irritation of the affected area
  Loss of skin
  Secondary infection in the area being treated
  Thinning of the skin with easy bruising

Interactions
None known as long as it is used according to the directions given to you by your doctor or pharmacist.

Storage
Cream, ointment, lotion, gel, spray, and aerosol should be stored at room temperature in tightly closed containers. This medication should never be frozen.

DESOWEN

Properties
This medicine contains desonide, a corticosteroid, as active ingredient. Corticosteroids are used to help relieve redness, swelling, itching, inflammation, and discomfort of many skin problems. They exert this effect by interfering with natural body mechanisms that produce the rash, itching, or inflammation. They do not cure the underlying cause of the skin problem. This medication is applied to the skin.

Before using this medicine
Before you use this medicine check with your doctor, or pharmacist:
- if you ever had any unusual or allergic reaction to corticosteroids.
- if you are allergic to any substance, such as sulfites or other preservatives or dyes.
- if you are pregnant or inintend to become pregnant while using this medicine. Studies have shown that corticosteroids applied to the skin in large amounts or over long periods of time can be the cause of birth defects.
- if you are breast-feeding an infant. Some corticosteroids pass into breast milk and may interfere with the infant's growth.

Treatment
Do not use this medicine more often or for a longer time than ordered. To do so may increase absorption through the skin and the chance of side effects. In addition, too much use, especially on areas with thinner skin (for example, face, armpits, groin), may result in thinning of the skin and stretch marks.

Before applying this medication, wash your hands. than, unless your doctor or pharmacist gives you different instructions, gently wash the area where the medication is to be applied. With a clean towel pat the area dry. Apply a small amount of the medication to the affected area in a thin layer. Do not bandage the area unless your doctor tells you to do so.

If you miss a dose of this medication, apply the dose as soon as possible, unless it is almost time for the next application.
- ◆ Do not use this medicine for other skin problems without first checking with your doctor. You should not use a topical corticosteroid if you have a virus disease (such as herpes), fungal infection of the skin (such as athlete's foot), or tuberculosis of the skin.

Side effects
There are a number of side effects that usually do not require medical attention. Minor side effects are:
Acne
Burning sensations
Itching
Rash
Skin dryness
These possible side effects may go away during treatment; however, if they continue or are bothersome, check with your doctor, nurse, or pharmacist. Tell your doctor about any side effects that are persistent or particularly bothersome, such as:
Blistering
Increased hair growth
Irritation of the affected area
Loss of skin
Secondary infection in the area being treated
Thinning of the skin with easy bruising

Interactions
None known as long as it is used according to the directions given to you by your doctor or pharmacist.

Storage
Cream, ointment, lotion, gel, spray, and aerosol should be stored at room temperature in tightly closed containers. This medication should never be frozen.

DI-AP-TROL

Properties
This medicine contains phendimetrazine as active ingredient; it is prescribed for appetite suppression.

Appetite suppressants are used in the short-term (a few weeks) treatment of obesity. In a few weeks (6 to 12), these medicines in combination with dieting, exercise, and changes in eating habits can help patients lose weight. However, since their appetite reducing effect is only temporary, they are useful only for the first weeks of dieting until new eating habits are established.

Before using this medicine
Before you use this medicine check with your doctor, or pharmacist:
- if you ever had any unusual or allergic reaction to any of the compounds of this medicine.
- if you are on a low-salt, low-sugar, or any other special diet, or if you are allergic to any substance, such as sulfites or other preservatives or dyes.
- if you are pregnant, inintend to become pregnant or breast-feeding an infant while using this medicine.
- if you have any of the following medical problems:
Diabetes mellitus (sugar diabetes)
Epilepsy
Glaucoma
Heart or blood vessel disease
High blood pressure
Mental illness (severe)

Treatment
This medication is used to relieve or prevent the symptoms of your medical problem. Take them as directed. Do not take more of them and do not take them more often than recommended on the label. If too much of the drug is taken, it may become habit-forming.

The medicine produces central nervous system stimulation, and it should not be taken by people with heart disease or high blood pressure.

If you think this medicine is not working as well after you have taken it for a few weeks, do not increase the dose. Instead, check with your doctor.

Side effects
The following minor side effects may occur: irritability, nervousness, restlessness, trouble in sleeping.

These side effects should disappear as your body adjusts to the medication. Tell your doctor about any side effects that are persistent or particularly bothersome. It is especially important to tell your doctor about:
Mental depression
Nausea or vomiting
Stomach cramps or pain
Trembling
Unusual tiredness or weakness
- Discontinue use of the drug; call your doctor right away. Adverse reactions and side effects may be more frequent and severe in people over age 60 than in younger persons.

Interactions
This medicine interacts with several other drugs such as antihypertensives, other appetite suppressants, caffeine, central nervous system depressants, central nervous system stimulants, furazolidone, guanethidine, hydralazine, MAO inhibitors, methyldopa, molindone, phenothiazines, rauwolfia alkaloids, sodium bicarbonate.

Interaction with alcoholic beverages may produce drowsiness, sleepiness, and/or inability to concentrate.
- Be sure to tell your doctor about any medications you are currently taking.

Storage
This medicine should be stored at room temperature in tightly closed containers. Store away from heat and direct light. Keep out of reach of children, since overdose may be very dangerous in children.

Do not store this medicine in the bathroom medicine cabinet because the heat and moisture cause the medicine to break down. Do not keep outdated medicine or medicine no longer needed. Flush the contents of the container down the toilet.

DIAZEPAM INTENSOL

Properties

This medicine contains as active ingredient diazepam, a benzodiazepine preparation. Benzodiazepines belong to the group of psychoactive medicines that influence the activity of the brain. Some are used to relieve nervousness or tension. It is effective for this purpose for short periods. Others are used for sleeplessness or to relax muscles or relieve muscle spasm. The benzodiazepines may also be used for other conditions as determined by your doctor.

Before using this medicine

Before you use this medicine check with your doctor:

- if you ever had any unusual or allergic reaction to benzodiazepines.
- if you are on a low-salt, low-sugar, or any other special diet, or if you are allergic to any substance, such as sulfites or other preservatives or dyes.
- if you are pregnant or inintend to become pregnant while using this medicine. Some benzodiazepines have been reported to increase the chance of birth defects when used during the first 3 months of pregnancy.
- if you are breast-feeding an infant. Benzodiazepines may pass into the breast milk and cause drowsiness, unusually slow heartbeat, shortness of breath, or troubled breathing in infants of mothers taking this medicine.
- if you have any of the following medical problems: asthma, bronchitis, emphysema, or other chronic lung disease; epilepsy or history of convulsions; hyperactivity (in children); kidney or lifer disease; mental depression or illness; myasthania gravis, porphyria.

Treatment

This medication is used to relieve or prevent the symptoms of your medical problem. Benzodiazepines are mainly used as antianxiety agents, anticonvulsants, or sedatives. Take them as directed. Do not take more of them and do not take them more often than recommended on the label, unless otherwise directed by your doctor. Benzodiazepine tranquilizing drugs can be abused if taken for long periods of time and it is possible to develop withdrawal symptoms if you discontinue the therapy abruptly.

Side effects

Along with the needed effects, a medicine may cause some unwanted effects. Minor side effects are: bitter taste in the mouth, dizziness, drowsiness, depression, constipation, dry mouth, excessive salivation, fatigue, flushing, headache, heartburn, loss of appetite, nausea, nervousness, sweating or vomiting. As your body adjusts to the medicine, these side effects should disappear.

- Tell your doctor about any side effects that are persistent or particularly bothersome. It is especially important to tell your doctor about:
  Blurred or double vision
  Chest pain
  Difficulty in urinating
  Fainting or falling
  Fever or hallucinations
  Joint pain
  Mouth sores
  Nightmares
  Palpitations
  Severe depression
  Shortness of breath
  Slurred speech
  Uncoordinated movements
  Unusual tiredness
  Yellowing of the skin

Interactions

This medicine may interact with several other drugs. This medicine will add to the effects of alcohol, and CNS depressants.

- Be sure to tell your doctor about any medications you are currently taking.

Storage

Store at room temperature in tightly closed, light-resistant-resistant containers. Keep out of the reach of children since overdose may be especially dangerous in children.

DICODID

Properties
This medicine contains as active ingredient hydrocodone.

It is a narcotic analgesic that acts directly on the central nervous system (brain and spinal cord). It is used to relieve pain or to suppress coughing.

Before using this medicine
Before you use this medicine check with your doctor, or pharmacist:
- if you ever had any unusual or allergic reaction to this medicine or one of its components.
- if you are on a low-salt, low-sugar, or any other special diet, or if you are allergic to any substance, such as sulfites or other preservatives or dyes.
- if you are pregnant or inintend to become pregnant while using this medicine. Studies on birth defects have not been done in humans. Too much use of narcotics during pregnancy may cause the baby to become dependent on the medicine.
- if you are breast-feeding an infant. Although this medicine has not been shown to cause problems in humans, it passes into the breast milk in small amounts.
- if you have any of the following medical problems:
Brain disease or head injury
Colitis
Convulsions
Emphysema, asthma, or chronic lung disease
Enlarged prostate
Gallbladder disease or gallstones
Heart disease
Kidney or lifer disease
Underactive thyroid

Treatment
This medication is used to relieve pain or to suppress coughing. Narcotic analgesics act in the central nervous system; some of their side effects are also caused by actions in the central nervous system.
- If you are taking this medication on a regular schedule and you miss a dose, take the missed dose as soon as possible, unless it is almost time for your next dose. In that case do not take the missed dose at all.
- If a narcotic analgesic is used for a long time, it may become habit-forming (causing mental or physical dependence). Physical dependence may lead to withdrawal side effects when you stop taking this medicine.

Unless otherwise directed by your doctor or pharmacist take this as directed. Do not take more of them and do not take them more often than recommended on the label. Children up to 12 years of age should not take this medicine more than 3 times a day or for more than 5 days in a row.

Side effects
Along with the needed effects, a medicine may cause some unwanted effects. These side effects may go away during treatment as your body adjusts to the medicine. Such minor side effects are: constipation, dizziness, drowsiness, dry mouth, false sense of well-being, flushing, light-headedness, loss of appetite, nausea, painful or difficult urination, or sweating.
- Check with your doctor immediately if any of the following side effects occur:
Anxiety or breathing difficulties
Excitation or restlessness
Fatigue, palpitations
Rash, sore throat and fever
Tremors or weakness

Interactions
This medicine may interact with several other drugs such as medicines acting on the central nervous system (e.g., antidepressants, tranquilizers), cimetidine, nitrates, quinidine, etc.
- Be sure to tell your doctor about any medications you are currently taking.

Storage
Tablets, elixir, suppository etc. should be stored at room temperature in a tightly closed, light-resistant container.

DIDREX

Properties
This medicine contains benzphetamine as active ingredient; it is prescribed for appetite suppression.

Appetite suppressants are used in the short-term (a few weeks) treatment of obesity. In a few weeks (6 to 12), these medicines in combination with dieting, exercise, and changes in eating habits can help patients lose weight. However, since their appetite reducing effect is only temporary, they are useful only for the first weeks of dieting until new eating habits are established.

Before using this medicine
Before you use this medicine check with your doctor, or pharmacist:
- if you ever had any unusual or allergic reaction to any of the compounds of this medicine.
- if you are on a low-salt, low-sugar, or any other special diet, or if you are allergic to any substance, such as sulfites or other preservatives or dyes.
- if you are pregnant, inintend to become pregnant or breast-feeding an infant while using this medicine.
- if you have any of the following medical problems:
Diabetes mellitus
Epilepsy
Glaucoma
Heart disease
High blood pressure
Mental illness (severe)

Treatment
This medication is used to relieve or prevent the symptoms of your medical problem. Take them as directed.

Do not take more of them and do not take them more often than recommended on the label. If too much of the drug is taken, it may become habit-forming.
- The medicine produces central nervous system stimulation, and it should not be taken by people with heart disease or high blood pressure.
- If you think this medicine is not working as well after you have taken it for a few weeks, do not increase the dose. Instead, check with your doctor.

Side effects
The following minor side effects may occur: irritability, nervousness, restlessness, trouble in sleeping.

These side effects should disappear as your body adjusts to the medication. Tell your doctor about any side effects that are persistent or particularly bothersome. It is especially important to tell your doctor about:
Mental depression
Nausea or vomiting
Stomach cramps or pain
Trembling
Unusual tiredness
- Discontinue use of the drug; call your doctor right away. Adverse reactions and side effects may be more frequent and severe in people over age 60 than in younger persons.

Interactions
This medicine interacts with several other drugs such as antihypertensives, other appetite suppressants, caffeine, central nervous system depressants, central nervous system stimulants, furazolidone, guanethidine, hydralazine, MAO inhibitors, methyldopa, molindone, phenothiazines, rauwolfia alkaloids, sodium bicarbonate. Interaction with alcoholic beverages may produce drowsiness, sleepiness, and/or inability to concentrate.
- Be sure to tell your doctor about any medications you are currently taking.

Storage
This medicine should be stored at room temperature in tightly closed containers. Store away from heat and direct light. Keep out of reach of children, since overdose may be very dangerous in children.

Do not store this medicine in the bathroom medicine cabinet because the heat and moisture cause the medicine to break down. Do not keep outdated medicine or medicine no longer needed. Flush the contents of the container down the toilet.

DIETHYLPROPION

Properties
This medicine contains diethylpropion active ingredient; it is prescribed for appetite suppression.

Appetite suppressants are used in the short-term (a few weeks) treatment of obesity. In a few weeks (6 to 12), these medicines in combination with dieting, exercise, and changes in eating habits can help patients lose weight. However, since their appetite reducing effect is only temporary, they are useful only for the first weeks of dieting until new eating habits are established.

Before using this medicine
Before you use this medicine check with your doctor, or pharmacist:
- if you ever had any unusual or allergic reaction to any of the compounds of this medicine.
- if you are on a low-salt, low-sugar, or any other special diet, or if you are allergic to any substance, such as sulfites or other preservatives or dyes.
- if you are pregnant, inintend to become pregnant or breast-feeding an infant while using this medicine.
- if you have any of the following medical problems:
  Diabetes mellitus
  Epilepsy
  Glaucoma
  Heart disease
  High blood pressure
  Mental illness (severe)

Treatment
This medication is used to relieve or prevent the symptoms of your medical problem.

Take them as directed. Do not take more of them and do not take them more often than recommended on the label. If too much of the drug is taken, it may become habit-forming.
- The medicine produces central nervous system stimulation, and it should not be taken by people with heart disease or high blood pressure.
- If you think this medicine is not working as well after you have taken it for a few weeks, do not increase the dose. Instead, check with your doctor.

Side effects
The following minor side effects may occur: irritability, nervousness, restlessness, trouble in sleeping.

These side effects should disappear as your body adjusts to the medication. Tell your doctor about any side effects that are persistent or particularly bothersome. It is especially important to tell your doctor about:
  Mental depression
  Nausea or vomiting
  Stomach cramps or pain
  Trembling
  Unusual tiredness
- Discontinue use of the drug; call your doctor right away. Adverse reactions and side effects may be more frequent and severe in people over age 60 than in younger persons.

Interactions
This medicine interacts with several other drugs such as antihypertensives, other appetite suppressants, caffeine, central nervous system depressants, central nervous system stimulants, furazolidone, guanethidine, hydralazine, MAO inhibitors, methyldopa, molindone, phenothiazines, rauwolfia alkaloids, sodium bicarbonate. Interaction with alcoholic beverages may produce drowsiness, sleepiness, and/or inability to concentrate.
- Be sure to tell your doctor about any medications you are currently taking.

Storage
This medicine should be stored at room temperature in tightly closed containers. Store away from heat and direct light. Keep out of reach of children, since overdose may be very dangerous in children.

Do not store this medicine in the bathroom medicine cabinet because the heat and moisture cause the medicine to break down. Do not keep outdated medicine or medicine no longer needed. Flush the contents of the container down the toilet.

DIETHYLSTILBESTROL

Properties
This medicine contains diethylstilbestrol as active ingredient. The medicine is prescribed for treatment of estrogen deficiency; it restores normal estrogen levels in tissues. There is no evidence that this drug is effective for nervous symptoms or depression occurring during menopause. They should not be used to treat this condition; they should be used only to replace the estrogen that is naturally absent after menopause.

Before using this medicine
Before you use this medicine check with your doctor, or pharmacist:
- if you ever had any unusual or allergic reaction to estrogens;
- if you are pregnant or intend to become pregnant within three months;
- if you are breast-feeding an infant;
- if you have any of the following medical problems:
Diabetes
Breast cancer
Fibrocystic breast disease
Fibroid uterine tumors
Endometriosis
Migraine headaches
Epilepsy
Porphyria
High blood pressure
Asthma
Congestive heart failure
Kidney disease
Gallstones

Treatment
This medication is used to treat estrogen deficiency, specific symptoms of menopause, estrogen-deficiency osteoporosis, atrophic vaginitis, prostate cancer.

For safe and effective use of this medicine:
- ◆ Follow your doctor's instructions if this medicine was prescribed.
- ◆ Follow the manufacturer's package directions if you are treating yourself.
- ◆ Estrogens have been reported to increase the risk of endometrial carcinoma.

Side effects
Along with the needed effects, a medicine may cause some unwanted effects. Possible side effects include:
Stomach cramps
Profuse bleeding
Appetite loss
Nausea and vomiting
Swollen breasts
Change in menstruation
Rash, skin blisters
Depression
Dizziness

Overdose
The following symptoms may indicate an overdose:
Nausea and vomiting
Fluid retention
Breast enlargement
Abnormal vaginal bleeding
- ■ Call a doctor or hospital emergency room for instructions.

Interactions
This medicine may interact with several other drugs such as adrenocorticosteroids, antidepressants, oral antidiabetics, insulin, phenobarbital, primidone.
- ■ Be sure to tell your doctor about any medications you are currently taking.

Storage
Capsules, tablets, vaginal cream, transdermal patches, etc. should be stored at room temperature; store away from heat and direct light. Keep out of reach of children, since this medicine may be dangerous in children.

DIHYDROMORPHINONE

Properties
This medicine contains as active ingredient hydromorphone. It is a narcotic analgesic that acts directly on the central nervous system (brain and spinal cord). It is used to relieve pain or to suppress coughing.

Before using this medicine
Before you use this medicine check with your doctor, or pharmacist:
- if you ever had any unusual or allergic reaction to this medicine or one of its components.
- if you are on a low-salt, low-sugar, or any other special diet, or if you are allergic to any substance, such as sulfites or other preservatives or dyes.
- if you are pregnant or inintend to become pregnant while using this medicine. Studies on birth defects have not been done in humans. Too much use of narcotics during pregnancy may cause the baby to become dependent on the medicine.
- if you are breast-feeding an infant. Although this medicine has not been shown to cause problems in humans, it passes into the breast milk in small amounts.
- if you have any of the following medical problems:
  Brain disease or head injury
  Colitis
  Convulsions
  Emphysema, asthma, or chronic lung disease
  Enlarged prostate
  Gallbladder disease or gallstones
  Heart disease
  Kidney or lifer disease
  Underactive thyroid

Treatment
This medication is used to relieve pain or to suppress coughing. Narcotic analgesics act in the central nervous system; some of their side effects are also caused by actions in the central nervous system.
- If you are taking this medication on a regular schedule and you miss a dose, take the missed dose as soon as possible, unless it is almost time for your next dose. In that case do not take the missed dose at all.
- If a narcotic analgesic is used for a long time, it may become habit-forming (causing mental or physical dependence). Physical dependence may lead to withdrawal side effects when you stop taking this medicine.

Unless otherwise directed by your doctor or pharmacist take this as directed. Do not take more of them and do not take them more often than recommended on the label. Children up to 12 years of age should not take this medicine more than 3 times a day or for more than 5 days in a row.

Side effects
Along with the needed effects, a medicine may cause some unwanted effects. These side effects may go away during treatment as your body adjusts to the medicine. Such minor side effects are: constipation, dizziness, drowsiness, dry mouth, false sense of well-being, flushing, light-headedness, loss of appetite, nausea, painful or difficult urination, or sweating.
- Check with your doctor immediately if any of the following side effects occur:
  Anxiety or breathing difficulties
  Excitation or restlessness
  Fatigue, palpitations
  Rash, sore throat and fever
  Tremors or weakness

Interactions
This medicine may interact with several other drugs such as medicines acting on the central nervous system (e.g., antidepressants, tranquilizers), cimetidine, nitrates, quinidine, etc.
- Be sure to tell your doctor about any medications you are currently taking.

Storage
Tablets, elixir, suppository etc. should be stored at room temperature in a tightly closed, light-resistant container.

DILACOR-XR

Properties
This medicine contains diltiazem as active ingredient. It is a so-called calcium channel blocker, working by blocking the passage of calcium into heart and smooth muscle. Since calcium is an essential factor in muscle contraction, any medicine that affects calcium in this way will interfere with the contraction of these muscles.

The medicine works by:
- reducing the work that the heart must perform;
- reducing the normal arterial blood pressure;
- increasing oxygen to the heart muscle.

The medicine is prescribed for the treatment of attacks of angina pectoris, irregular heartbeat, and high blood pressure. In many cases it can be used for the treatment and prevention of migraine.

Before using this medicine
Before you use this medicine check with your doctor, or pharmacist:
- if you ever had any unusual or allergic reaction to this medicine or any calcium channel blocker;
- if you are pregnant or inintend to become pregnant while using this medicine;
- if you have low blood pressure;
- if you have kidney or lifer disease;
- if you are breast-feeding an infant;
- if you easily get a rash or intensity sunburn in areas exposed to sun or ultraviolet light.

Treatment
This medication is used for treatment of heart conditions (for instance, angina pectoris) and high blood pressure. Tablets, capsules or extended-release tablets should be taken with liquid. The usual dose amounts to 30 to 100 milligrams a day.

For safe and effective use of medicine:
- Follow your doctor's instructions if this medicine was prescribed.
- Follow the manufacturer's package directions if you are treating yourself.

Side effects
Along with the needed effects, a medicine may cause some unwanted effects. Possible side effects include:
Tiredness
Changes in heartbeat
Wheezing
Cough
Shortness of breath
Dizziness
Fainting
Numbness in hands and feet
Tingling in hands and feet
Difficult urination
Constipation

Overdose
The following symptoms may be a sign of overdose:
Unusually fast heartbeat
Unusually slow heartbeat
Loss of consciousness
Cardiac arrest
- Call a doctor or hospital emergency room for instructions. If necessary start first aid immediately.

Interactions
The effect of this medicine may cause a blood pressure drop if taken together with antihypertensives. Cimetidine may increase the effect of the calcium blocker.

The simultaneous use of diuretics and calcium channel blockers may cause dangerous blood pressure drop.
- Be sure to tell your doctor about any medications you are currently taking.

Storage
Capsules, tablets, etc. should be stored at room temperature; store away from heat and direct light. Keep out of reach of children, since this medicine may be dangerous in children.

DILATRATE SR

Properties
This medicine contains isosorbide dinitrate as active ingredient. Nitrates improve the supply of blood and oxygen to the heart. This medication is for oral use.

Before using this medicine
Before you use this medicine check with your doctor, or pharmacist:
- if you ever had any unusual or allergic reaction to nitrates or nitrites.
- if you are on a low-salt, low-sugar, or any other special diet, or if you are allergic to any substance, such as sulfites or other preservatives or dyes.
- if you are pregnant or inintend to become pregnant while using this medicine. Although nitrates have not been shown to cause problems in humans, the chance always exists.
- if you are breast-feeding an infant.
- if you have recently had a heart attack or stroke.
- if you have any of the following medical problems:
Anemia
Glaucoma
Intestinal problems
Overactive thyroid
- if you are now taking any of the following medicines or types of medicines:
Antihypertensives
Asthma or hay fever medicine
Cold medicine
Decongestant
Medicine for appetite control
Narcotic
Pain medicine
Sinus congestion medicine

Treatment
This medication is used to treat and prevent angina (chest pain). Nitroglycerin is a vasodilator, which relaxes the muscles of the blood vessels, causing an increase in the oxygen supply to the heart. The oral tablets, capsules, ointment and patches do not act quickly; they are used to prevent chest pain. The sublingual tablets and oral spray act quickly and can be used to relieve chest pain after it has started.

- Take this medicine exactly as directed by your doctor or pharmacist. It will work only if taken correctly.
- If you are taking this medicine regularly and you miss a dose, take it as soon as possible. However, if your next scheduled dose; is within 2 hours (or within 6 hours for extended-release capsules or tablets), skip the missed dose and go back to your regular dosing schedule.
- If you have been taking this medicine regularly for several weeks or more, do not suddenly stop using it. Stopping suddenly may bring on attacks of angina.

Side effects
There are a number of side effects that usually do not require medical attention. These possible side effects may go away during treatment; however, if they continue or are bothersome, check with your doctor, nurse, or pharmacist. More common are: dizziness, lightheadedness, or fainting when standing up; fast pulse; flushing of face and neck; headache; nausea or vomiting.

Side effects that should be reported to your doctor are: blurred vision; dry mouth; severe or prolonged headache; skin rash.

Interactions
This medicine may interact with several other drugs such as tricyclic antidepressants and cough medicines. Before starting to take or apply nitroglycerin, be sure to tell your doctor about any medications you are currently taking.

Storage
Tablets, capsules, and oral spray should be stored as in a tightly capped bottle in a cool, dry place. Ointment and patches should be stored at room temperature in their original containers. Keep out of reach of children. Do not keep outdated medicine or medicine no longer needed.

DILAUDID

Properties
This medicine contains as active ingredient hydromorphone. It is a narcotic analgesic that acts directly on the central nervous system (brain and spinal cord). It is used to relieve pain or to suppress coughing.

Before using this medicine
Before you use this medicine check with your doctor, or pharmacist:
- if you ever had any unusual or allergic reaction to this medicine or one of its components.
- if you are on a low-salt, low-sugar, or any other special diet, or if you are allergic to any substance, such as sulfites or other preservatives or dyes.
- if you are pregnant or inintend to become pregnant while using this medicine. Studies on birth defects have not been done in humans. Too much use of narcotics during pregnancy may cause the baby to become dependent on the medicine.
- if you are breast-feeding an infant. Although this medicine has not been shown to cause problems in humans, it passes into the breast milk in small amounts.
- if you have any of the following medical problems:
Brain disease or head injury
Colitis
Convulsions
Emphysema, asthma, or chronic lung disease
Enlarged prostate
Gallbladder disease or gallstones
Heart disease
Kidney or lifer disease
Underactive thyroid

Treatment
This medication is used to relieve pain or to suppress coughing. Narcotic analgesics act in the central nervous system; some of their side effects are also caused by actions in the central nervous system.
- If you are taking this medication on a regular schedule and you miss a dose, take the missed dose as soon as possible, unless it is almost time for your next dose. In that case do not take the missed dose at all.
- If a narcotic analgesic is used for a long time, it may become habit-forming (causing mental or physical dependence). Physical dependence may lead to withdrawal side effects when you stop taking this medicine.

Unless otherwise directed by your doctor or pharmacist take this as directed. Do not take more of them and do not take them more often than recommended on the label. Children up to 12 years of age should not take this medicine more than 3 times a day or for more than 5 days in a row.

Side effects
Along with the needed effects, a medicine may cause some unwanted effects. These side effects may go away during treatment as your body adjusts to the medicine. Such minor side effects are: constipation, dizziness, drowsiness, dry mouth, false sense of well-being, flushing, light-headedness, loss of appetite, nausea, painful or difficult urination, or sweating.
- Check with your doctor immediately if any of the following side effects occur:
Anxiety or breathing difficulties
Excitation or restlessness
Fatigue, palpitations
Rash, sore throat and fever
Tremors or weakness

Interactions
This medicine may interact with several other drugs such as medicines acting on the central nervous system (e.g., antidepressants, tranquilizers), cimetidine, nitrates, quinidine, etc.
- Be sure to tell your doctor about any medications you are currently taking.

Storage
Tablets, elixir, suppository etc. should be stored at room temperature in a tightly closed, light-resistant container.

DILTIAZEM

Properties

This medicine contains diltiazem as active ingredient. It is a so-called calcium channel blocker, working by blocking the passage of calcium into heart and smooth muscle. Since calcium is an essential factor in muscle contraction, any medicine that affects calcium in this way will interfere with the contraction of these muscles.

The medicine works by:

- reducing the work that the heart must perform;
- reducing the normal arterial blood pressure;
- increasing oxygen to the heart muscle.

The medicine is prescribed for the treatment of attacks of angina pectoris, irregular heartbeat, and high blood pressure. In many cases it can be used for the treatment and prevention of migraine.

Before using this medicine

Before you use this medicine check with your doctor, or pharmacist:

- if you ever had any unusual or allergic reaction to this medicine or any calcium channel blocker;
- if you are pregnant or inintend to become pregnant while using this medicine;
- if you have low blood pressure;
- if you have kidney or lifer disease;
- if you are breast-feeding an infant;
- if you easily get a rash or intensity sunburn in areas exposed to sun or ultraviolet light.

Treatment

This medication is used for treatment of heart conditions (for instance, angina pectoris) and high blood pressure. Tablets, capsules or extended-release tablets should be taken with liquid. The usual dose amounts to 30 to 100 milligrams a day.

For safe and effective use of medicine:

- Follow your doctor's instructions if this medicine was prescribed.
- Follow the manufacturer's package directions if you are treating yourself.

Side effects

Along with the needed effects, a medicine may cause some unwanted effects. Possible side effects include:

Tiredness
Changes in heartbeat
Wheezing
Cough
Shortness of breath
Dizziness
Fainting
Numbness in hands and feet
Tingling in hands and feet
Difficult urination
Constipation

Overdose

The following symptoms may be a sign of overdose:

Unusually fast heartbeat
Unusually slow heartbeat
Loss of consciousness
Cardiac arrest

- Call a doctor or hospital emergency room for instructions. If necessary start first aid immediately.

Interactions

The effect of this medicine may cause a blood pressure drop if taken together with antihypertensives. Cimetidine may increase the effect of the calcium blocker.

The simultaneous use of diuretics and calcium channel blockers may cause dangerous blood pressure drop.

- Be sure to tell your doctor about any medications you are currently taking.

Storage

Capsules, tablets, etc. should be stored at room temperature; store away from heat and direct light. Keep out of reach of children, since this medicine may be dangerous in children.

DIOVAL 40

Properties
This medicine contains estrogen as active ingredient. The medicine is prescribed for treatment of estrogen deficiency; it restores normal estrogen levels in tissues. There is no evidence that this drug is effective for nervous symptoms or depression occurring during menopause. They should not be used to treat this condition; they should be used only to replace the estrogen that is naturally absent after menopause.

Before using this medicine
Before you use this medicine check with your doctor, or pharmacist:
- if you ever had any unusual or allergic reaction to estrogens;
- if you are pregnant or intend to become pregnant within three months;
- if you are breast-feeding an infant;
- if you have any of the following medical problems:
  Diabetes
  Breast cancer
  Fibrocystic breast disease
  Fibroid uterine tumors
  Endometriosis
  Migraine headaches
  Epilepsy
  Porphyria
  High blood pressure
  Asthma
  Congestive heart failure
  Kidney disease
  Gallstones

Treatment
This medication is used to treat estrogen deficiency, specific symptoms of menopause, estrogen-deficiency osteoporosis, atrophic vaginitis, prostate cancer.

For safe and effective use of this medicine:
- Follow your doctor's instructions if this medicine was prescribed.
- Follow the manufacturer's package directions if you are treating yourself.
- Estrogens have been reported to increase the risk of endometrial carcinoma.

Side effects
Along with the needed effects, a medicine may cause some unwanted effects. Possible side effects include:
  Stomach cramps
  Profuse bleeding
  Appetite loss
  Nausea and vomiting
  Swollen breasts
  Change in menstruation
  Rash, skin blisters
  Depression
  Dizziness

Overdose
The following symptoms may indicate an overdose:
  Nausea and vomiting
  Fluid retention
  Breast enlargement
  Abnormal vaginal bleeding
- Call a doctor or hospital emergency room for instructions.

Interactions
This medicine may interact with several other drugs such as adrenocorticosteroids, antidepressants, oral antidiabetics, insulin, phenobarbital, primidone.
- Be sure to tell your doctor about any medications you are currently taking.

Storage
Capsules, tablets, vaginal cream, transdermal patches, etc. should be stored at room temperature; store away from heat and direct light. Keep out of reach of children, since this medicine may be dangerous in children.

DIPROLENE

Properties

This medicine contains betamethasone, a corticosteroid, as active ingredient. Corticosteroids are used to help relieve redness, swelling, itching, inflammation, and discomfort of many skin problems. They exert this effect by interfering with natural body mechanisms that produce the rash, itching, or inflammation. They do not cure the underlying cause of the skin problem. This medication is applied to the skin.

Before using this medicine

Before you use this medicine check with your doctor, or pharmacist:
- if you ever had any unusual or allergic reaction to corticosteroids.
- if you are allergic to any substance, such as sulfites or other preservatives or dyes.
- if you are pregnant or inintend to become pregnant while using this medicine. Studies have shown that corticosteroids applied to the skin in large amounts or over long periods of time can be the cause of birth defects.
- if you are breast-feeding an infant. Some corticosteroids pass into breast milk and may interfere with the infant's growth.

Treatment

Do not use this medicine more often or for a longer time than ordered. To do so may increase absorption through the skin and the chance of side effects. In addition, too much use, especially on areas with thinner skin (for example, face, armpits, groin), may result in thinning of the skin and stretch marks.

Before applying this medication, wash your hands. than, unless your doctor or pharmacist gives you different instructions, gently wash the area where the medication is to be applied. With a clean towel pat the area dry. Apply a small amount of the medication to the affected area in a thin layer. Do not bandage the area unless your doctor tells you to do so.

If you miss a dose of this medication, apply the dose as soon as possible, unless it is almost time for the next application.

- ◆ Do not use this medicine for other skin problems without first checking with your doctor. You should not use a topical corticosteroid if you have a virus disease (such as herpes), fungal infection of the skin (such as athlete's foot), or tuberculosis of the skin.

Side effects

There are a number of side effects that usually do not require medical attention. Minor side effects are:

Acne

Burning sensations

Itching

Rash

Skin dryness

These possible side effects may go away during treatment; however, if they continue or are bothersome, check with your doctor, nurse, or pharmacist. Tell your doctor about any side effects that are persistent or particularly bothersome, such as:

Blistering

Increased hair growth

Irritation of the affected area

Loss of skin

Secondary infection in the area being treated

Thinning of the skin with easy bruising

Interactions

None known as long as it is used according to the directions given to you by your doctor or pharmacist.

Storage

Cream, ointment, lotion, gel, spray, and aerosol should be stored at room temperature in tightly closed containers. This medication should never be frozen.

DIPROSONE

Properties
This medicine contains betamethasone, a corticosteroid, as active ingredient. Corticosteroids are used to help relieve redness, swelling, itching, inflammation, and discomfort of many skin problems. They exert this effect by interfering with natural body mechanisms that produce the rash, itching, or inflammation. They do not cure the underlying cause of the skin problem. This medication is applied to the skin.

Before using this medicine
Before you use this medicine check with your doctor, or pharmacist:
- if you ever had any unusual or allergic reaction to corticosteroids.
- if you are allergic to any substance, such as sulfites or other preservatives or dyes.
- if you are pregnant or inintend to become pregnant while using this medicine. Studies have shown that corticosteroids applied to the skin in large amounts or over long periods of time can be the cause of birth defects.
- if you are breast-feeding an infant. Some corticosteroids pass into breast milk and may interfere with the infant's growth.

Treatment
Do not use this medicine more often or for a longer time than ordered. To do so may increase absorption through the skin and the chance of side effects. In addition, too much use, especially on areas with thinner skin (for example, face, armpits, groin), may result in thinning of the skin and stretch marks.

Before applying this medication, wash your hands. than, unless your doctor or pharmacist gives you different instructions, gently wash the area where the medication is to be applied. With a clean towel pat the area dry. Apply a small amount of the medication to the affected area in a thin layer. Do not bandage the area unless your doctor tells you to do so.

If you miss a dose of this medication, apply the dose as soon as possible, unless it is almost time for the next application.
- ◆ Do not use this medicine for other skin problems without first checking with your doctor. You should not use a topical corticosteroid if you have a virus disease (such as herpes), fungal infection of the skin (such as athlete's foot), or tuberculosis of the skin.

Side effects
There are a number of side effects that usually do not require medical attention. Minor side effects are:
Acne
Burning sensations
Itching
Rash
Skin dryness

These possible side effects may go away during treatment; however, if they continue or are bothersome, check with your doctor, nurse, or pharmacist. Tell your doctor about any side effects that are persistent or particularly bothersome, such as:
Blistering
Increased hair growth
Irritation of the affected area
Loss of skin
Secondary infection in the area being treated
Thinning of the skin with easy bruising

Interactions
None known as long as it is used according to the directions given to you by your doctor or pharmacist.

Storage
Cream, ointment, lotion, gel, spray, and aerosol should be stored at room temperature in tightly closed containers. This medication should never be frozen.

DIULO

Properties

This medicine contains as active ingredient metolazone, a thiazide-like diuretic. Thiazide or thiazide-like diuretics are prescribed to treat high blood pressure (hypertension). They are also used to reduce fluid accumulation in the body caused by conditions such as heart failure, cirrhosis, kidney disease, and the long-term use of some medications. Thiazide diuretics may also be used for other conditions as determined by your doctor.

Before using this medicine

Before you use this medicine check with your doctor, or pharmacist:
- if you ever had any unusual or allergic reaction to sulfonamides (sulfa drugs) or any of the thiazide diuretics.
- if you are on a low-salt, low-sugar, or any other special diet, or if you are allergic to any substance, such as sulfites or other preservatives or dyes.
- if you are pregnant or inintend to become pregnant while using this medicine. When this medicine is used during pregnancy, it may cause side effects including jaundice, blood problems, and low potassium in the newborn.
- if you are breast-feeding an infant. Although this medicine has not been shown to cause problems in humans, the chance always exists since thiazide diuretics pass into breast milk.
- if you have any of the following medical problems:
Diabetes
Gout
Kidney disease
Liver disease
Lupus erythematosus
Pancreas disease

Treatment

This medication is used to treat high blood pressure (hypertension) and also to help reduce the amount of water in the body by increasing the flow of urine. This medicine will not cure your high blood pressure but it does help control it. You must continue to take it - even if you feel well - if you expect to keep your blood pressure down. You may have to take high blood pressure medicine for the rest of your life.

Thiazide diuretics may cause an unusual feeling of tiredness when you begin to take them. You may also notice an increase in urine or in frequency of urination. To keep this from affecting sleep:
- if you are to take a single dose a day, take it in the morning after breakfast;
- if you are to take more than one dose, take the last one not later than 6 p.m.

Side effects

Along with the needed effects, a medicine may cause some unwanted effects. Side effects that usually do not require medical attention: decreased sexual ability; dizziness or lightheadedness when standing up; increased sensitivity of skin to sunlight; loss of appetite; upset stomach.
- Side effects that should be reported to your doctor: black, tarry stools; blood in urine or stools; cough or hoarseness; fever or chills; joint pain; lower back or side pains; painful or difficult urination; pinpoint red spots on skin; skin rash or hives; stomach pain (severe) with nausea; unusual bleeding or bruising; yellow eyes or skin. This medicine may cause a loss of potassium from your body. Signs of too much potassium loss are: dryness of mouth; increased thirst; mood changes; muscle cramps or pain; nausea or vomiting; unusual tiredness or weakness; weak or irregular heartbeat.

Interactions

This medicine may interact with several other drugs.
- Be sure to tell your doctor about any medications you are currently taking.

Storage

Store at room temperature in a tightly closed container.

DIURESE

Properties
This medicine contains as active ingredient trichlormethiazide, a thiazide-like diuretic. Thiazide or thiazide-like diuretics are prescribed to treat high blood pressure (hypertension). They are also used to reduce fluid accumulation in the body caused by conditions such as heart failure, cirrhosis, kidney disease, and the long-term use of some medications. Thiazide diuretics may also be used for other conditions as determined by your doctor.

Before using this medicine
Before you use this medicine check with your doctor, or pharmacist:
- if you ever had any unusual or allergic reaction to sulfonamides (sulfa drugs) or any of the thiazide diuretics.
- if you are on a low-salt, low-sugar, or any other special diet, or if you are allergic to any substance, such as sulfites or other preservatives or dyes.
- if you are pregnant or inintend to become pregnant while using this medicine. When this medicine is used during pregnancy, it may cause side effects including jaundice, blood problems, and low potassium in the newborn.
- if you are breast-feeding an infant. Although this medicine has not been shown to cause problems in humans, the chance always exists since thiazide diuretics pass into breast milk.
- if you have any of the following medical problems:
Diabetes
Gout
Kidney disease
Liver disease
Lupus erythematosus
Pancreas disease

Treatment
This medication is used to treat high blood pressure (hypertension) and also to help reduce the amount of water in the body by increasing the flow of urine. This medicine will not cure your high blood pressure but it does help control it. You must continue to take it - even if you feel well - if you expect to keep your blood pressure down. You may have to take high blood pressure medicine for the rest of your life.

Thiazide diuretics may cause an unusual feeling of tiredness when you begin to take them. You may also notice an increase in urine or in frequency of urination. To keep this from affecting sleep:
- if you are to take a single dose a day, take it in the morning after breakfast;
- if you are to take more than one dose, take the last one not later than 6 p.m.

Side effects
Along with the needed effects, a medicine may cause some unwanted effects. Side effects that usually do not require medical attention: decreased sexual ability; dizziness or lightheadedness when standing up; increased sensitivity of skin to sunlight; loss of appetite; upset stomach.
- Side effects that should be reported to your doctor: black, tarry stools; blood in urine or stools; cough or hoarseness; fever or chills; joint pain; lower back or side pains; painful or difficult urination; pinpoint red spots on skin; skin rash or hives; stomach pain (severe) with nausea; unusual bleeding or bruising; yellow eyes or skin. This medicine may cause a loss of potassium from your body. Signs of too much potassium loss are: dryness of mouth; increased thirst; mood changes; muscle cramps or pain; nausea or vomiting; unusual tiredness or weakness; weak or irregular heartbeat.

Interactions
This medicine may interact with several other drugs.
- Be sure to tell your doctor about any medications you are currently taking.

Storage
Store at room temperature in a tightly closed container.

DOLOPHINE

Properties

This medicine contains as active ingredient methadone.

It is a narcotic analgesic that acts directly on the central nervous system (brain and spinal cord). It is used to relieve pain or to suppress coughing.

Before using this medicine

Before you use this medicine check with your doctor, or pharmacist:

- if you ever had any unusual or allergic reaction to this medicine or one of its components.
- if you are on a low-salt, low-sugar, or any other special diet, or if you are allergic to any substance, such as sulfites or other preservatives or dyes.
- if you are pregnant or inintend to become pregnant while using this medicine. Studies on birth defects have not been done in humans. Too much use of narcotics during pregnancy may cause the baby to become dependent on the medicine.
- if you are breast-feeding an infant. Although this medicine has not been shown to cause problems in humans, it passes into the breast milk in small amounts.
- if you have any of the following medical problems:
  Brain disease or head injury
  Colitis
  Convulsions
  Emphysema, asthma, or chronic lung disease
  Enlarged prostate
  Gallbladder disease or gallstones
  Heart disease
  Kidney or lifer disease
  Underactive thyroid

Treatment

This medication is used to relieve pain or to suppress coughing. Narcotic analgesics act in the central nervous system; some of their side effects are also caused by actions in the central nervous system.

- If you are taking this medication on a regular schedule and you miss a dose, take the missed dose as soon as possible, unless it is almost time for your next dose. In that case do not take the missed dose at all.
- If a narcotic analgesic is used for a long time, it may become habit-forming (causing mental or physical dependence). Physical dependence may lead to withdrawal side effects when you stop taking this medicine.

Unless otherwise directed by your doctor or pharmacist take this as directed. Do not take more of them and do not take them more often than recommended on the label. Children up to 12 years of age should not take this medicine more than 3 times a day or for more than 5 days in a row.

Side effects

Along with the needed effects, a medicine may cause some unwanted effects. These side effects may go away during treatment as your body adjusts to the medicine. Such minor side effects are: constipation, dizziness, drowsiness, dry mouth, false sense of well-being, flushing, light-headedness, loss of appetite, nausea, painful or difficult urination, or sweating.

- Check with your doctor immediately if any of the following side effects occur:
  Anxiety or breathing difficulties
  Excitation or restlessness
  Fatigue, palpitations
  Rash, sore throat and fever
  Tremors or weakness

Interactions

This medicine may interact with several other drugs such as medicines acting on the central nervous system (e.g., antidepressants, tranquilizers), cimetidine, nitrates, quinidine, etc.

- Be sure to tell your doctor about any medications you are currently taking.

Storage

Tablets, elixir, suppository etc. should be stored at room temperature in a tightly closed, light-resistant container.

DOXEPIN

Properties

This medicine contains doxepin as active ingredient. It belongs to the group of medicines known as tricyclic antidepressants or 'mood elevators.' It is used to relieve mental depression and depression that sometimes occurs with anxiety. The medication gradually relieves, but doesn't cure, symptoms of depression. The medication may also be used for the treatment of narcolepsy, bulimia, panic attacks, cocaine withdrawal, attention deficit disorder.

Before using this medicine

Before you use this medicine check with your doctor, or pharmacist:

- if you ever had any unusual or allergic reaction to any tricyclic antidepressant, maprotiline or trazodone.
- if you are on a low-salt, low-sugar, or any other special diet, or if you are allergic to any substance, such as sulfites or other preservatives or dyes.
- if you are pregnant or inintend to become pregnant while using this medicine. There have been reports of newborns suffering from heart, breathing, and urinary problems when their mothers had taken tricyclic antidepressants before delivery.
- if you are breast-feeding an infant. Some tricyclic antidepressants pass into the breast milk.

Treatment

Take this medicine only as directed by your doctor, to benefit your condition as much as possible. Do not take more of it, do not take it more often, and do not take it for a longer period of time than your doctor ordered.

To lessen stomach upset, take this medicine with food, even for a daily bedtime dose, unless your doctor has told you to take it on an empty stomach. If you forget your once-a-day bedtime dose, don't take it more than 3 hours late. If more than 3 hours, wait for next scheduled dose;.

Sometimes this medicine must be taken for several weeks before you begin to feel better.

Side effects

Along with the needed effects, a medicine may cause some unwanted effects. Side effects that usually do not require medical attention: difficult or frequent urination; decreased sex drive; muscle aches; abnormal dreams; nasal congestion; weakness and faintness when arising from bed or chair; back pain.

- Other side effects that should be reported to your doctor immediately are:
  Hallucinations
  Shakiness
  Dizziness or fainting
  Blurred vision, eye pain
  Irregular heartbeat or slow pulse
  Inflamed tongue
  Abdominal pain
  Jaundice
  Hair loss, rash
  Fever, chills
  Joint pain
  Palpitations

Interactions

This medicine may interact with several other drugs such as anticoagulants, anticholinergics, cold remedies, oral contraceptives, seizure medicines, sleeping medicines, thyroid medicines, etc. Be sure to tell your doctor about any medications you are currently taking.

Storage

Tablets, capsules, etc. should be stored at room temperature in tightly closed, light-resistant containers as directed by your pharmacist. Keep out of reach of children since overdose is especially dangerous in young children. Do not store in the bathroom medicine cabinet because the heat or moisture may cause the medicine to break down. Keep the liquid form of the medicine from freezing.

DURA-ESTRIN

Properties
This medicine contains estrogen as active ingredient. The medicine is prescribed for treatment of estrogen deficiency; it restores normal estrogen levels in tissues. There is no evidence that this drug is effective for nervous symptoms or depression occurring during menopause. They should not be used to treat this condition; they should be used only to replace the estrogen that is naturally absent after menopause.

Before using this medicine
Before you use this medicine check with your doctor, or pharmacist:
- if you ever had any unusual or allergic reaction to estrogens;
- if you are pregnant or intend to become pregnant within three months;
- if you are breast-feeding an infant;
- if you have any of the following medical problems:
  Diabetes
  Breast cancer
  Fibrocystic breast disease
  Fibroid uterine tumors
  Endometriosis
  Migraine headaches
  Epilepsy
  Porphyria
  High blood pressure
  Asthma
  Congestive heart failure
  Kidney disease
  Gallstones

Treatment
This medication is used to treat estrogen deficiency, specific symptoms of menopause, estrogen-deficiency osteoporosis, atrophic vaginitis, prostate cancer.
  For safe and effective use of this medicine:
- ◆ Follow your doctor's instructions if this medicine was prescribed.
- ◆ Follow the manufacturer's package directions if you are treating yourself.
- ◆ Estrogens have been reported to increase the risk of endometrial carcinoma.

Side effects
Along with the needed effects, a medicine may cause some unwanted effects. Possible side effects include:
  Stomach cramps
  Profuse bleeding
  Appetite loss
  Nausea and vomiting
  Swollen breasts
  Change in menstruation
  Rash, skin blisters
  Depression
  Dizziness

Overdose
The following symptoms may indicate an overdose:
  Nausea and vomiting
  Fluid retention
  Breast enlargement
  Abnormal vaginal bleeding
- ■ Call a doctor or hospital emergency room for instructions.

Interactions
This medicine may interact with several other drugs such as adrenocorticosteroids, antidepressants, oral antidiabetics, insulin, phenobarbital, primidone.
- ■ Be sure to tell your doctor about any medications you are currently taking.

Storage
Capsules, tablets, vaginal cream, transdermal patches, etc. should be stored at room temperature; store away from heat and direct light. Keep out of reach of children, since this medicine may be dangerous in children.

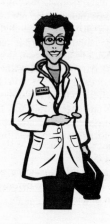

DURABOLIN

Properties
This medicine is a member of the androgenic, or male, hormone group, containing an androgenic preparation as active ingredient. It is used in diseases in which male hormone replacement or augmentation is needed and also in so-called male menopause. It is also used to decrease calcium loss in osteoporosis, to block growth of breast cancer cells in females and to reduce breast pain and fullness following childbirth.

Before using this medicine
Before you use this medicine check with your doctor, or pharmacist:
- if you ever had any unusual or allergic reaction to androgens or corticosteroids in general.
- if you are on a low-salt, low-sugar, or any other special diet, or if you are allergic to any substance, such as certain preservatives or dyes.
- if you have any of the following medical problems:
  Cancer prostate
  Heart disease or atherosclerosis
  Kidney or lifer disease
  Breast cancer (males)
  High blood pressure
  High level of blood calcium
  Epilepsy

Treatment
This medication is used to relieve or prevent the symptoms of your medical problem. Take them as directed. Do not take more of them and do not take them more often than recommended on the label. One should take the tablets or capsules with food to lessen stomach irritation. Take the medication at the same time each day. If you forget a dose take it as soon as you remember up to two hours late; wait for the next scheduled dose; don't double this dose. The risk to the unborn child outweighs the benefits of the drug.

Side effects
Females taking any androgenic drug should watch for deepening of the voice, oily skin, acne, hairiness, increased libido, and menstrual irregularities.

The following side effects may occur:
  Acne or oily skin
  Deep voice
  Enlarged clitoris in females
  Frequent erections in men
  Sore mouth
  Higher sex drive
  Impotence in men
  Yellow skin or eyes
These side effects should disappear as your body adjusts to the medication. Tell your doctor about any side effects that are persistent or particularly bothersome.
- Discontinue the use of the medication and seek emergency treatment in the following situations:
  Intense itching
  Weakness
  Loss of consciousness
  Depression or confusion
  Swollen feet or legs
  Shortness of breath
  Irregularities of heartbeat
  Difficult urination
  Vaginal bleeding in women
  Scrotum pain in men

Interactions
This medicine interacts with several other drugs such as anticoagulants, oral antidiabetics, cyclosporine, hepatotoxic drugs, oxyphenbutazone, phenobarbital, and phenylbutazone.
- Be sure to tell your doctor about any medications you are currently taking.

Storage
This medicine should be stored at room temperature in closed containers. Store away from heat and direct light. Keep out of reach of children, since overdose may be dangerous in children.

DURACILLIN A.S.

Properties

This medicine contains penicillin G as active ingredient. Penicillins are prescribed to treat infections caused by bacteria. They will not work for colds, flu, or other virus infections. There are several different kinds of penicillins. Each is used to treat different kinds of infections.

Before using this medicine

Before you use this medicine check with your doctor, or pharmacist:

- if you ever had any unusual or allergic reaction to any of the penicillins, cefalosporins, griseofulvin, or penicillamine. Serious reactions may occur in patients who are allergic to penicillins.
- if you are on a low-salt, low-sugar, or any other special diet, or if you are allergic to any substance, such as sulfites or other preservatives or dyes.
- if you are pregnant or inintend to become pregnant while using this medicine. Although penicillins have not been shown to cause problems in humans, the chance always exists.
- if you are breast-feeding an infant. Most penicillins (except amdinocillin) pass into the breast milk. Even though only small amounts may pass, allergic reaction, diarrhea, fungal infection, and skin rash may occur in the infant.
- if you have any of the following medical problems:
  Allergy
  Asthma
  Bleeding problems
  Eczema
  Hay fever, hives
  Kidney disease
  Liver disease
  Mononucleosis
  Stomach or intestinal disease

Treatment

This medication is used to treat an infection caused by bacteria. Most penicillins are best taken with a full glass (8 ounces) of water on an empty stomach, some are best taken with a snack or meal. Follow your doctor's or pharmacist's directions on how to take your medicine.

- ◆ Keep taking this medicine for the full time of treatment even if you begin to feel better after a few days; do not miss any doses. This is especially important if you have a "strep" infection since serious heart problems could develop later if your infection is not cleared up completely.
- ◆ If you do miss a dose of this medicine, take it as soon as possible. However, if it is almost time for your next dose, skip the missed dose and go back to your regular dosing schedule.

Side effects

Along with the needed effects, a medicine may cause some unwanted effects. Side effects that usually do not require medical attention: diarrhea; nausea or vomiting; sore mouth or tongue.

- ◆ Stop taking this medicine and get emergency help immediately if you notice: difficulty in breathing; lightheadedness; skin rash, hives, itching; wheezing.

Other side effects that should be reported to your doctor immediately are: abdominal bloating; blood in urine; convulsions (seizures); decreased amount of urine; diarrhea (watery and severe) which may also be bloody; fever; joint pain; sore throat and fever; stomach or abdominal cramps and pain; unusual bleeding or bruising.

Interactions

This medicine may interact with several other drugs such as anticoagulants, diarrhea medicines, heparin, ibuprofen, oral contraceptives, potassium-containing medicines, etc.

- ■ Be sure to tell your doctor about any medications you are currently taking.

Storage

Tablets, capsules, etc. should be stored as directed by your pharmacist or according to instructions on the label.

DURAGEN

Properties
This medicine contains estrogen as active ingredient. The medicine is prescribed for treatment of estrogen deficiency; it restores normal estrogen levels in tissues. There is no evidence that this drug is effective for nervous symptoms or depression occurring during menopause. They should not be used to treat this condition; they should be used only to replace the estrogen that is naturally absent after menopause.

Before using this medicine
Before you use this medicine check with your doctor, or pharmacist:
- if you ever had any unusual or allergic reaction to estrogens;
- if you are pregnant or intend to become pregnant within three months;
- if you are breast-feeding an infant;
- if you have any of the following medical problems:
  Diabetes
  Breast cancer
  Fibrocystic breast disease
  Fibroid uterine tumors
  Endometriosis
  Migraine headaches
  Epilepsy
  Porphyria
  High blood pressure
  Asthma
  Congestive heart failure
  Kidney disease
  Gallstones

Treatment
This medication is used to treat estrogen deficiency, specific symptoms of menopause, estrogen-deficiency osteoporosis, atrophic vaginitis, prostate cancer.

For safe and effective use of this medicine:
- ◆ Follow your doctor's instructions if this medicine was prescribed.
- ◆ Follow the manufacturer's package directions if you are treating yourself.
- ◆ Estrogens have been reported to increase the risk of endometrial carcinoma.

Side effects
Along with the needed effects, a medicine may cause some unwanted effects. Possible side effects include:
  Stomach cramps
  Profuse bleeding
  Appetite loss
  Nausea and vomiting
  Swollen breasts
  Change in menstruation
  Rash, skin blisters
  Depression
  Dizziness

Overdose
The following symptoms may indicate an overdose:
  Nausea and vomiting
  Fluid retention
  Breast enlargement
  Abnormal vaginal bleeding
- ■ Call a doctor or hospital emergency room for instructions.

Interactions
This medicine may interact with several other drugs such as adrenocorticosteroids, antidepressants, oral antidiabetics, insulin, phenobarbital, primidone.
- ■ Be sure to tell your doctor about any medications you are currently taking.

Storage
Capsules, tablets, vaginal cream, transdermal patches, etc. should be stored at room temperature; store away from heat and direct light. Keep out of reach of children, since this medicine may be dangerous in children.

DURAMORPH RF

Properties

This medicine contains as active ingredient morphine.

It is a narcotic analgesic that acts directly on the central nervous system (brain and spinal cord). It is used to relieve pain or to suppress coughing.

Before using this medicine

Before you use this medicine check with your doctor, or pharmacist:

- if you ever had any unusual or allergic reaction to this medicine or one of its components.
- if you are on a low-salt, low-sugar, or any other special diet, or if you are allergic to any substance, such as sulfites or other preservatives or dyes.
- if you are pregnant or inintend to become pregnant while using this medicine. Studies on birth defects have not been done in humans. Too much use of narcotics during pregnancy may cause the baby to become dependent on the medicine.
- if you are breast-feeding an infant. Although this medicine has not been shown to cause problems in humans, it passes into the breast milk in small amounts.
- if you have any of the following medical problems:
  Brain disease or head injury
  Colitis
  Convulsions
  Emphysema, asthma, or chronic lung disease
  Enlarged prostate
  Gallbladder disease or gallstones
  Heart disease
  Kidney or lifer disease
  Underactive thyroid

Treatment

This medication is used to relieve pain or to suppress coughing. Narcotic analgesics act in the central nervous system; some of their side effects are also caused by actions in the central nervous system.

- If you are taking this medication on a regular schedule and you miss a dose, take the missed dose as soon as possible, unless it is almost time for your next dose. In that case do not take the missed dose at all.
- If a narcotic analgesic is used for a long time, it may become habit-forming (causing mental or physical dependence). Physical dependence may lead to withdrawal side effects when you stop taking this medicine.

Unless otherwise directed by your doctor or pharmacist take this as directed. Do not take more of them and do not take them more often than recommended on the label. Children up to 12 years of age should not take this medicine more than 3 times a day or for more than 5 days in a row.

Side effects

Along with the needed effects, a medicine may cause some unwanted effects. These side effects may go away during treatment as your body adjusts to the medicine. Such minor side effects are: constipation, dizziness, drowsiness, dry mouth, false sense of well-being, flushing, light-headedness, loss of appetite, nausea, painful or difficult urination, or sweating.

- Check with your doctor immediately if any of the following side effects occur:
  Anxiety or breathing difficulties
  Excitation or restlessness
  Fatigue, palpitations
  Rash, sore throat and fever
  Tremors or weakness

Interactions

This medicine may interact with several other drugs such as medicines acting on the central nervous system (e.g., antidepressants, tranquilizers), cimetidine, nitrates, quinidine, etc.

- Be sure to tell your doctor about any medications you are currently taking.

Storage

Tablets, elixir, suppository etc. should be stored at room temperature in a tightly closed, light-resistant container.

DURAPHYL

Properties

This medicine contains theophylline as active ingredient; it is used to treat or prevent breathing problems (wheezing and shortness of breath) caused by asthma, bronchitis, or emphysema. This medication belongs to a group known as xanthine-derivative bronchodilators. They work by opening up the bronchial tubes or air passages of the lungs and increasing the flow of air through them. These medicines are available only with your doctor's prescription.

Before using this medicine

Before you use this medicine check with your doctor, or pharmacist:
- if you ever had any unusual or allergic reaction to xanthine-derivative bronchodilators.
- if you are on a low-salt, low-sugar, or any other special diet, or if you are allergic to any substance, such as sulfites or other preservatives or dyes.
- if you are pregnant or inintend to become pregnant while using this medicine.
- if you are breast-feeding an infant. Theophylline passes into the breast milk and may cause irritability, fretfulness, or trouble in sleeping in infants of mothers taking this medicine.
- if you have any of the following medical problems:
Diarrhea
Enlarged prostate
Fibrocystic breast disease
Heart disease
Stomach ulcer

Treatment

This medication is used to relieve or prevent the symptoms of your medical problem. Take them as directed. Do not take more of them and do not take them more often than recommended on the label, unless otherwise directed by your doctor. To do so may increase the chance of side effects. The medicine should be taken on an empty stomach 30 to 60 minutes before a meal or two hours after a meal. Try not to miss any doses of this medication. If you do miss a dose, take the missed dose as soon as possible, unless it is almost time for the next dose. Do not double the next dose. It works best when taken with a glass of water.

Side effects

The following minor side effects may occur:
Dizziness or flushing
Headache
Diarrhea
Heartburn
Increased urination
Insomnia
Nervousness or irritability
Loss of appetite
Nausea or stomach upset
Stomach pain.
These side effects should disappear as your body adjusts to the medication. Tell your doctor about any side effects that are persistent or particularly bothersome. It is especially important to tell your doctor about black, tarry stools; confusion; convulsions; difficulty in breathing; fainting; muscle twitching; palpitations; rash; severe abdominal pain; or unusual weakness.

Interactions

This medicine interacts with several other drugs such as diuretics, reserpine, beta blockers, phenytoin, lithium, phenobarbital, birth control pills, and other medications.
- Be sure to tell your doctor about any medications you are currently taking.

Storage

Tablets, capsules, liquid and suspension should be stored at room temperature in tightly closed containers. Store away from heat and direct light. Keep out of reach of children, since overdose may be very dangerous in children. Discard any outdated medication.

DURATEST

Properties

This medicine is a member of the androgenic, or male, hormone group, containing an androgenic preparation as active ingredient. It is used in diseases in which male hormone replacement or augmentation is needed and also in so-called male menopause. It is also used to decrease calcium loss in osteoporosis, to block growth of breast cancer cells in females and to reduce breast pain and fullness following childbirth.

Before using this medicine

Before you use this medicine check with your doctor, or pharmacist:
- if you ever had any unusual or allergic reaction to androgens or corticosteroids in general.
- if you are on a low-salt, low-sugar, or any other special diet, or if you are allergic to any substance, such as certain preservatives or dyes.
- if you have any of the following medical problems:
  Cancer prostate
  Heart disease or atherosclerosis
  Kidney or lifer disease
  Breast cancer (males)
  High blood pressure
  High level of blood calcium
  Epilepsy

Treatment

This medication is used to relieve or prevent the symptoms of your medical problem. Take them as directed. Do not take more of them and do not take them more often than recommended on the label. One should take the tablets or capsules with food to lessen stomach irritation. Take the medication at the same time each day. If you forget a dose take it as soon as you remember up to two hours late; wait for the next scheduled dose; don't double this dose. The risk to the unborn child outweighs the benefits of the drug.

Side effects

Females taking any androgenic drug should watch for deepening of the voice, oily skin, acne, hairiness, increased libido, and menstrual irregularities.

The following side effects may occur:
  Acne or oily skin
  Deep voice
  Enlarged clitoris in females
  Frequent erections in men
  Sore mouth
  Higher sex drive
  Impotence in men
  Yellow skin or eyes

These side effects should disappear as your body adjusts to the medication. Tell your doctor about any side effects that are persistent or particularly bothersome.

- Discontinue the use of the medication and seek emergency treatment in the following situations:
  Intense itching
  Weakness
  Loss of consciousness
  Depression or confusion
  Swollen feet or legs
  Shortness of breath
  Irregularities of heartbeat
  Difficult urination
  Vaginal bleeding in women
  Scrotum pain in men

Interactions

This medicine interacts with several other drugs such as anticoagulants, oral antidiabetics, cyclosporine, hepatotoxic drugs, oxyphenbutazone, phenobarbital, and phenylbutazone.

- Be sure to tell your doctor about any medications you are currently taking.

Storage

This medicine should be stored at room temperature in closed containers. Store away from heat and direct light. Keep out of reach of children, since overdose may be dangerous in children.

DURATHATE 200

Properties
This medicine is a member of the androgenic, or male, hormone group, containing an androgenic preparation as active ingredient. It is used in diseases in which male hormone replacement or augmentation is needed and also in so-called male menopause. It is also used to decrease calcium loss in osteoporosis, to block growth of breast cancer cells in females and to reduce breast pain and fullness following child-birth.

Before using this medicine
Before you use this medicine check with your doctor, or pharmacist:
- if you ever had any unusual or allergic reaction to androgens or corticosteroids in general.
- if you are on a low-salt, low-sugar, or any other special diet, or if you are allergic to any substance, such as certain preservatives or dyes.
- if you have any of the following medical problems:
  Cancer prostate
  Heart disease or atherosclerosis
  Kidney or lifer disease
  Breast cancer (males)
  High blood pressure
  High level of blood calcium
  Epilepsy

Treatment
This medication is used to relieve or prevent the symptoms of your medical problem. Take them as directed. Do not take more of them and do not take them more often than recommended on the label. One should take the tablets or capsules with food to lessen stomach irritation. Take the medication at the same time each day. If you forget a dose take it as soon as you remember up to two hours late; wait for the next scheduled dose; don't double this dose. The risk to the unborn child outweighs the benefits of the drug.

Side effects
Females taking any androgenic drug should watch for deepening of the voice, oily skin, acne, hairiness, increased libido, and menstrual irregularities.

The following side effects may occur:
  Acne or oily skin
  Deep voice
  Enlarged clitoris in females
  Frequent erections in men
  Sore mouth
  Higher sex drive
  Impotence in men
  Yellow skin or eyes
These side effects should disappear as your body adjusts to the medication. Tell your doctor about any side effects that are persistent or particularly bothersome.
- Discontinue the use of the medication and seek emergency treatment in the following situations:
  Intense itching
  Weakness
  Loss of consciousness
  Depression or confusion
  Swollen feet or legs
  Shortness of breath
  Irregularities of heartbeat
  Difficult urination
  Vaginal bleeding in women
  Scrotum pain in men

Interactions
This medicine interacts with several other drugs such as anticoagulants, oral antidiabetics, cyclosporine, hepatotoxic drugs, oxyphenbutazone, phenobarbital, and phenylbutazone.
- Be sure to tell your doctor about any medications you are currently taking.

Storage
This medicine should be stored at room temperature in closed containers. Store away from heat and direct light. Keep out of reach of children, since overdose may be dangerous in children.

DURETIC

Properties
This medicine contains as active ingredient methyclothiazide, a thiazide-like diuretic. Thiazide or thiazide-like diuretics are prescribed to treat high blood pressure (hypertension). They are also used to reduce fluid accumulation in the body caused by conditions such as heart failure, cirrhosis, kidney disease, and the long-term use of some medications. Thiazide diuretics may also be used for other conditions as determined by your doctor.

Before using this medicine
Before you use this medicine check with your doctor, or pharmacist:
- if you ever had any unusual or allergic reaction to sulfonamides (sulfa drugs) or any of the thiazide diuretics.
- if you are on a low-salt, low-sugar, or any other special diet, or if you are allergic to any substance, such as sulfites or other preservatives or dyes.
- if you are pregnant or inintend to become pregnant while using this medicine. When this medicine is used during pregnancy, it may cause side effects including jaundice, blood problems, and low potassium in the newborn.
- if you are breast-feeding an infant. Although this medicine has not been shown to cause problems in humans, the chance always exists since thiazide diuretics pass into breast milk.
- if you have any of the following medical problems:
  Diabetes
  Gout
  Kidney disease
  Liver disease
  Lupus erythematosus
  Pancreas disease

Treatment
This medication is used to treat high blood pressure (hypertension) and also to help reduce the amount of water in the body by increasing the flow of urine. This medicine will not cure your high blood pressure but it does help control it. You must continue to take it - even if you feel well - if you expect to keep your blood pressure down. You may have to take high blood pressure medicine for the rest of your life.

Thiazide diuretics may cause an unusual feeling of tiredness when you begin to take them. You may also notice an increase in urine or in frequency of urination. To keep this from affecting sleep:
- if you are to take a single dose a day, take it in the morning after breakfast;
- if you are to take more than one dose, take the last one not later than 6 p.m.

Side effects
Along with the needed effects, a medicine may cause some unwanted effects. Side effects that usually do not require medical attention: decreased sexual ability; dizziness or lightheadedness when standing up; increased sensitivity of skin to sunlight; loss of appetite; upset stomach.
- Side effects that should be reported to your doctor: black, tarry stools; blood in urine or stools; cough or hoarseness; fever or chills; joint pain; lower back or side pains; painful or difficult urination; pinpoint red spots on skin; skin rash or hives; stomach pain (severe) with nausea; unusual bleeding or bruising; yellow eyes or skin. This medicine may cause a loss of potassium from your body. Signs of too much potassium loss are: dryness of mouth; increased thirst; mood changes; muscle cramps or pain; nausea or vomiting; unusual tiredness or weakness; weak or irregular heartbeat.

Interactions
This medicine may interact with several other drugs.
- Be sure to tell your doctor about any medications you are currently taking.

Storage
Store at room temperature in a tightly closed container.

DURICEF

Properties

This medicine contains cephalosporin as active ingredient. Cephalosporins belong to the general family of medicines called antibiotics, used in the treatment of infections caused by bacteria. They work by killing bacteria or preventing their growth. Cephalosporins will not work for colds, fly, or other viral infections.

Before using this medicine

Before you use this medicine check with your doctor:
- if you ever had any unusual or allergic reaction to any of the cephalosporins, penicillins, penicillin-like medicines, or penicillamine.
- if you are on a low-salt, low-sugar, or any other special diet, or if you are allergic to any substance, such as sulfites or other preservatives or dyes.
- if you are pregnant or inintend to become pregnant while using this medicine. Although cephalosporins have not been shown to cause birth defects or other problems in humans, the chance always exists.
- if you are breast-feeding an infant. Most cephalosporins pass into the breast milk, usually in small amounts.
- if you have any of the following medical problems:
  Bleeding problem
  Kidney or lifer disease

Treatment

This medication belongs to the general family of medicines called antibiotics. It is used to treat a wide variety of bacterial infections. It is also used to treat infections in persons who are allergic to penicillin.
- Keep taking this medicine for the full time of treatment even if you begin to feel better after a few days; do not miss any doses.
- If you do miss a dose of this medicine, take it as soon as possible. This will help to keep a constant amount of medicine in the blood. However, if it is almost time for your next dose,

skip the missed dose and go back to your regular dosing schedule.
- This medication has been prescribed for your current infection only. Another infection later on, or one that someone else has, may require a different medicine. You should not give your medicine to other people or use it for other infections, unless your doctor specifically directs you to do so.
- Take the medicine at the same times each day, 1 hour before or 2 hours after eating.

Side effects

Along with the needed effects, a medicine may cause some unwanted effects. Side effects that usually do not require medical attention: rectal itching, oral or vaginal white spots, mild diarrhea. These side effects should disappear as your body adjusts to the medication.
- Other side effects that should be reported to your doctor immediately are:
  Hives, rash
  Intense itching
  Faintness soon after a dose
  Difficulty in breathing
  Nausea and vomiting
  Severe diarrhea
  Unusual weakness or tiredness
  Bleeding or bruising

Interactions

This medicine may interact with several other drugs such as anticoagulants, theophylline preparations, probenecid, tetracyclines, etc.
- Be sure to tell your doctor about any medications you are currently taking.

Storage

Tablets, capsules, etc. should be stored at room temperature. Store the liquid form in the refrigerator. Keep out of the reach of children. Do not keep outdated medicine or medicine no longer needed.

DYNA CIRC

Properties

This medicine contains isradipine as active ingredient. It is a so-called calcium channel blocker, working by blocking the passage of calcium into heart and smooth muscle. Since calcium is an essential factor in muscle contraction, any medicine that affects calcium in this way will interfere with the contraction of these muscles.

The medicine works by:

♦ reducing the work that the heart must perform;
♦ reducing the normal arterial blood pressure;
♦ increasing oxygen to the heart muscle.

The medicine is prescribed for the treatment of attacks of angina pectoris, irregular heartbeat, and high blood pressure. In many cases it can be used for the treatment and prevention of migraine.

Before using this medicine

Before you use this medicine check with your doctor, or pharmacist:

− if you ever had any unusual or allergic reaction to this medicine or any calcium channel blocker;
− if you are pregnant or inintend to become pregnant while using this medicine;
− if you have low blood pressure;
− if you have kidney or lifer disease;
− if you are breast-feeding an infant;
− if you easily get a rash or intensity sunburn in areas exposed to sun or ultraviolet light.

Treatment

This medication is used for treatment of heart conditions (for instance, angina pectoris) and high blood pressure. Tablets, capsules or extended-release tablets should be taken with liquid. The usual dose amounts to 30 to 100 milligrams a day.

For safe and effective use of medicine:

♦ Follow your doctor's instructions if this medicine was prescribed.
♦ Follow the manufacturer's package directions if you are treating yourself.

Side effects

Along with the needed effects, a medicine may cause some unwanted effects. Possible side effects include:

Tiredness
Changes in heartbeat
Wheezing
Cough
Shortness of breath
Dizziness
Fainting
Numbness in hands and feet
Tingling in hands and feet
Difficult urination
Constipation

Overdose

The following symptoms may be a sign of overdose:

Unusually fast heartbeat
Unusually slow heartbeat
Loss of consciousness
Cardiac arrest

▪ Call a doctor or hospital emergency room for instructions. If necessary start first aid immediately.

Interactions

The effect of this medicine may cause a blood pressure drop if taken together with antihypertensives. Cimetidine may increase the effect of the calcium blocker.

The simultaneous use of diuretics and calcium channel blockers may cause dangerous blood pressure drop.

▪ Be sure to tell your doctor about any medications you are currently taking.

Storage

Capsules, tablets, etc. should be stored at room temperature; store away from heat and direct light. Keep out of reach of children, since this medicine may be dangerous in children.

DYREXAN-OD

Properties
This medicine contains phendi-metrazine as active ingredient; it is prescribed for appetite suppression.

Appetite suppressants are used in the short-term (a few weeks) treatment of obesity. In a few weeks (6 to 12), these medicines in combination with dieting, exercise, and changes in eating habits can help patients lose weight. However, since their appetite reducing effect is only temporary, they are useful only for the first weeks of dieting until new eating habits are established.

Before using this medicine
Before you use this medicine check with your doctor, or pharmacist:
- if you ever had any unusual or allergic reaction to any of the compounds of this medicine.
- if you are on a low-salt, low-sugar, or any other special diet, or if you are allergic to any substance, such as sulfites or other preservatives or dyes.
- if you are pregnant, inintend to become pregnant or breast-feeding an infant while using this medicine.
- if you have any of the following medical problems:
  Diabetes mellitus (sugar diabetes)
  Epilepsy
  Glaucoma
  Heart or blood vessel disease
  High blood pressure
  Mental illness (severe)

Treatment
This medication is used to relieve or prevent the symptoms of your medical problem. Take them as directed. Do not take more of them and do not take them more often than recommended on the label. If too much of the drug is taken, it may become habit-forming.

The medicine produces central nervous system stimulation, and it should not be taken by people with heart disease or high blood pressure.

If you think this medicine is not working as well after you have taken it for a few weeks, do not increase the dose. Instead, check with your doctor.

Side effects
The following minor side effects may occur: irritability, nervousness, restlessness, trouble in sleeping.

These side effects should disappear as your body adjusts to the medication. Tell your doctor about any side effects that are persistent or particularly bothersome. It is especially important to tell your doctor about:
Mental depression
Nausea or vomiting
Stomach cramps or pain
Trembling
Unusual tiredness or weakness
- Discontinue use of the drug; call your doctor right away. Adverse reactions and side effects may be more frequent and severe in people over age 60 than in younger persons.

Interactions
This medicine interacts with several other drugs such as antihypertensives, other appetite suppressants, caffeine, central nervous system depressants, central nervous system stimulants, furazolidone, guanethidine, hydralazine, MAO inhibitors, methyldopa, molindone, phenothiazines, rauwolfia alkaloids, sodium bicarbonate. Interaction with alcoholic beverages may produce drowsiness, sleepiness, and/or inability to concentrate.
- Be sure to tell your doctor about any medications you are currently taking.

Storage
This medicine should be stored at room temperature in tightly closed containers. Store away from heat and direct light. Keep out of reach of children, since overdose may be very dangerous in children.

Do not store this medicine in the bathroom medicine cabinet because the heat and moisture cause the medicine to break down. Do not keep outdated medicine or medicine no longer needed. Flush the contents of the container down the toilet.

ECTOSONE

Properties

This medicine contains betamethasone, a corticosteroid, as active ingredient. Corticosteroids are used to help relieve redness, swelling, itching, inflammation, and discomfort of many skin problems. They exert this effect by interfering with natural body mechanisms that produce the rash, itching, or inflammation. They do not cure the underlying cause of the skin problem. This medication is applied to the skin.

Before using this medicine

Before you use this medicine check with your doctor, or pharmacist:
- if you ever had any unusual or allergic reaction to corticosteroids.
- if you are allergic to any substance, such as sulfites or other preservatives or dyes.
- if you are pregnant or inintend to become pregnant while using this medicine. Studies have shown that corticosteroids applied to the skin in large amounts or over long periods of time can be the cause of birth defects.
- if you are breast-feeding an infant. Some corticosteroids pass into breast milk and may interfere with the infant's growth.

Treatment

Do not use this medicine more often or for a longer time than ordered. To do so may increase absorption through the skin and the chance of side effects. In addition, too much use, especially on areas with thinner skin (for example, face, armpits, groin), may result in thinning of the skin and stretch marks.

Before applying this medication, wash your hands. than, unless your doctor or pharmacist gives you different instructions, gently wash the area where the medication is to be applied. With a clean towel pat the area dry. Apply a small amount of the medication to the affected area in a thin layer. Do not bandage the area unless your doctor tells you to do so.

If you miss a dose of this medication, apply the dose as soon as possible, unless it is almost time for the next application.
- ◆ Do not use this medicine for other skin problems without first checking with your doctor. You should not use a topical corticosteroid if you have a virus disease (such as herpes), fungal infection of the skin (such as athlete's foot), or tuberculosis of the skin.

Side effects

There are a number of side effects that usually do not require medical attention. Minor side effects are:
Acne
Burning sensations
Itching
Rash
Skin dryness

These possible side effects may go away during treatment; however, if they continue or are bothersome, check with your doctor, nurse, or pharmacist. Tell your doctor about any side effects that are persistent or particularly bothersome, such as:
Blistering
Increased hair growth
Irritation of the affected area
Loss of skin
Secondary infection in the area being treated
Thinning of the skin with easy bruising

Interactions

None known as long as it is used according to the directions given to you by your doctor or pharmacist.

Storage

Cream, ointment, lotion, gel, spray, and aerosol should be stored at room temperature in tightly closed containers. This medication should never be frozen.

E-CYPLONATE

Properties
This medicine contains estrogen as active ingredient. The medicine is prescribed for treatment of estrogen deficiency; it restores normal estrogen levels in tissues. There is no evidence that this drug is effective for nervous symptoms or depression occurring during menopause. They should not be used to treat this condition; they should be used only to replace the estrogen that is naturally absent after menopause.

Before using this medicine
Before you use this medicine check with your doctor, or pharmacist:
- if you ever had any unusual or allergic reaction to estrogens;
- if you are pregnant or intend to become pregnant within three months;
- if you are breast-feeding an infant;
- if you have any of the following medical problems:
  Diabetes
  Breast cancer
  Fibrocystic breast disease
  Fibroid uterine tumors
  Endometriosis
  Migraine headaches
  Epilepsy
  Porphyria
  High blood pressure
  Asthma
  Congestive heart failure
  Kidney disease
  Gallstones

Treatment
This medication is used to treat estrogen deficiency, specific symptoms of menopause, estrogen-deficiency osteoporosis, atrophic vaginitis, prostate cancer.
For safe and effective use of this medicine:
- ◆ Follow your doctor's instructions if this medicine was prescribed.
- ◆ Follow the manufacturer's package directions if you are treating yourself.
- ◆ Estrogens have been reported to increase the risk of endometrial carcinoma.

Side effects
Along with the needed effects, a medicine may cause some unwanted effects. Possible side effects include:
  Stomach cramps
  Profuse bleeding
  Appetite loss
  Nausea and vomiting
  Swollen breasts
  Change in menstruation
  Rash, skin blisters
  Depression
  Dizziness

Overdose
The following symptoms may indicate an overdose:
  Nausea and vomiting
  Fluid retention
  Breast enlargement
  Abnormal vaginal bleeding
- ■ Call a doctor or hospital emergency room for instructions.

Interactions
This medicine may interact with several other drugs such as adrenocorticosteroids, antidepressants, oral antidiabetics, insulin, phenobarbital, primidone.
- ■ Be sure to tell your doctor about any medications you are currently taking.

Storage
Capsules, tablets, vaginal cream, transdermal patches, etc. should be stored at room temperature; store away from heat and direct light. Keep out of reach of children, since this medicine may be dangerous in children.

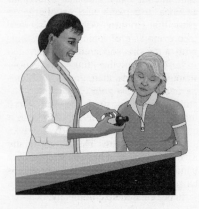

E.E.S.

Properties

This medicine contains erythromycin as active ingredient. This antibiotic is prescribed to treat infections caused by bacteria. They will not work for colds, flu, or other virus infections. Erythromycins are available only with your doctor's prescription.

Before using this medicine

Before you use this medicine check with your doctor, or pharmacist:

– if you ever had any unusual or allergic reaction to any of the erythromycins.
– if you are on a low-salt, low-sugar, or any other special diet, or if you are allergic to any substance, such as sulfites or other preservatives or dyes.
– if you are pregnant or inintend to become pregnant while using this medicine. Although erythromycins have not been shown to cause birth defects or other problems in humans, the chance always exists.
– if you are breast-feeding an infant. Most erythromycins pass into the breast milk. Although erythromycins have not been shown to cause problems in humans, the chance always exists.
– if you have lifer disease.

Treatment

This medication belongs to the general family of medicines called antibiotics. It is used to treat a wide variety of bacterial infections. It is also used to treat infections in persons who are allergic to penicillin. Erythromycins are also used to prevent "strep" infections in patients with a history of rheumatic heart disease. They may also be used in Legionnaires' disease and for other problems as determined by your doctor.

■ Keep taking this medicine for the full time of treatment even if you begin to feel better after a few days; do not miss any doses. This is especially important if you have a "strep" infection since serious heart problems could develop later if your infection is not cleared up completely.

■ If you do miss a dose of this medicine, take it as soon as possible. This will help to keep a constant amount of medicine in the blood. However, if it is almost time for your next dose, skip the missed dose and go back to your regular dosing schedule.

■ This medication has been prescribed for your current infection only. Another infection later on, or one that someone else has, may require a different medicine. You should not give your medicine to other people or use it for other infections, unless your doctor specifically directs you to do so.

Side effects

Along with the needed effects, a medicine may cause some unwanted effects. Side effects that usually do not require medical attention: abdominal cramps, black tongue, cough, diarrhea, fatigue, irritation of the mouth, loss of appetite, nausea, or vomiting. These side effects should disappear as your body adjusts to the medication.

■ Other side effects that should be reported to your doctor immediately are:
Fever
Hearing loss
Hives or rash
Rectal or vaginal itching
Yellowing of the eyes or skin

Interactions

This medicine may interact with several other drugs such as anticoagulants, theophylline preparations, carbamazepine, etc.

■ Be sure to tell your doctor about any medications you are currently taking.

Storage

Tablets, capsules, etc. should be stored at room temperature in tightly closed, light-resistant containers as directed by your pharmacist.

E-MYCIN E

Properties
This medicine contains erythromycin as active ingredient. This antibiotic is prescribed to treat infections caused by bacteria. They will not work for colds, flu, or other virus infections. Erythromycins are available only with your doctor's prescription.

Before using this medicine
Before you use this medicine check with your doctor, or pharmacist:
- if you ever had any unusual or allergic reaction to any of the erythromycins.
- if you are on a low-salt, low-sugar, or any other special diet, or if you are allergic to any substance, such as sulfites or other preservatives or dyes.
- if you are pregnant or inintend to become pregnant while using this medicine. Although erythromycins have not been shown to cause birth defects or other problems in humans, the chance always exists.
- if you are breast-feeding an infant. Most erythromycins pass into the breast milk. Although erythromycins have not been shown to cause problems in humans, the chance always exists.
- if you have lifer disease.

Treatment
This medication belongs to the general family of medicines called antibiotics. It is used to treat a wide variety of bacterial infections. It is also used to treat infections in persons who are allergic to penicillin. Erythromycins are also used to prevent "strep" infections in patients with a history of rheumatic heart disease. They may also be used in Legionnaires' disease and for other problems as determined by your doctor.
- Keep taking this medicine for the full time of treatment even if you begin to feel better after a few days; do not miss any doses. This is especially important if you have a "strep" infection since serious heart problems could develop later if your infection is not cleared up completely.
- If you do miss a dose of this medicine, take it as soon as possible. This will help to keep a constant amount of medicine in the blood. However, if it is almost time for your next dose, skip the missed dose and go back to your regular dosing schedule.
- This medication has been prescribed for your current infection only. Another infection later on, or one that someone else has, may require a different medicine. You should not give your medicine to other people or use it for other infections, unless your doctor specifically directs you to do so.

Side effects
Along with the needed effects, a medicine may cause some unwanted effects. Side effects that usually do not require medical attention: abdominal cramps, black tongue, cough, diarrhea, fatigue, irritation of the mouth, loss of appetite, nausea, or vomiting. These side effects should disappear as your body adjusts to the medication.
- Other side effects that should be reported to your doctor immediately are:
Fever
Hearing loss
Hives or rash
Rectal or vaginal itching
Yellowing of the eyes or skin

Interactions
This medicine may interact with several other drugs such as anticoagulants, theophylline preparations, carbamazepine, etc.
- Be sure to tell your doctor about any medications you are currently taking.

Storage
Tablets, capsules, etc. should be stored at room temperature in tightly closed, light-resistant containers as directed by your pharmacist.

E-MYCIN

Properties
This medicine contains erythromycin as active ingredient. This antibiotic is prescribed to treat infections caused by bacteria. They will not work for colds, flu, or other virus infections. Erythromycins are available only with your doctor's prescription.

Before using this medicine
Before you use this medicine check with your doctor, or pharmacist:
- if you ever had any unusual or allergic reaction to any of the erythromycins.
- if you are on a low-salt, low-sugar, or any other special diet, or if you are allergic to any substance, such as sulfites or other preservatives or dyes.
- if you are pregnant or inintend to become pregnant while using this medicine. Although erythromycins have not been shown to cause birth defects or other problems in humans, the chance always exists.
- if you are breast-feeding an infant. Most erythromycins pass into the breast milk. Although erythromycins have not been shown to cause problems in humans, the chance always exists.
- if you have lifer disease.

Treatment
This medication belongs to the general family of medicines called antibiotics. It is used to treat a wide variety of bacterial infections. It is also used to treat infections in persons who are allergic to penicillin. Erythromycins are also used to prevent "strep" infections in patients with a history of rheumatic heart disease. They may also be used in Legionnaires' disease and for other problems as determined by your doctor.
- Keep taking this medicine for the full time of treatment even if you begin to feel better after a few days; do not miss any doses. This is especially important if you have a "strep" infection since serious heart problems could develop later if your infection is not cleared up completely.
- If you do miss a dose of this medicine, take it as soon as possible. This will help to keep a constant amount of medicine in the blood. However, if it is almost time for your next dose, skip the missed dose and go back to your regular dosing schedule.
- This medication has been prescribed for your current infection only. Another infection later on, or one that someone else has, may require a different medicine. You should not give your medicine to other people or use it for other infections, unless your doctor specifically directs you to do so.

Side effects
Along with the needed effects, a medicine may cause some unwanted effects. Side effects that usually do not require medical attention: abdominal cramps, black tongue, cough, diarrhea, fatigue, irritation of the mouth, loss of appetite, nausea, or vomiting. These side effects should disappear as your body adjusts to the medication.
- Other side effects that should be reported to your doctor immediately are:
Fever
Hearing loss
Hives or rash
Rectal or vaginal itching
Yellowing of the eyes or skin

Interactions
This medicine may interact with several other drugs such as anticoagulants, theophylline preparations, carbamazepine, etc. Be sure to tell your doctor about any medications you are currently taking.

Storage
Tablets, capsules, etc. should be stored at room temperature in tightly closed, light-resistant containers as directed by your pharmacist.

E-MYCIN E

Properties
This medicine contains erythromycin as active ingredient. This antibiotic is prescribed to treat infections caused by bacteria. They will not work for colds, flu, or other virus infections. Erythromycins are available only with your doctor's prescription.

Before using this medicine
Before you use this medicine check with your doctor, or pharmacist:
- if you ever had any unusual or allergic reaction to any of the erythromycins.
- if you are on a low-salt, low-sugar, or any other special diet, or if you are allergic to any substance, such as sulfites or other preservatives or dyes.
- if you are pregnant or inintend to become pregnant while using this medicine. Although erythromycins have not been shown to cause birth defects or other problems in humans, the chance always exists.
- if you are breast-feeding an infant. Most erythromycins pass into the breast milk. Although erythromycins have not been shown to cause problems in humans, the chance always exists.
- if you have lifer disease.

Treatment
This medication belongs to the general family of medicines called antibiotics. It is used to treat a wide variety of bacterial infections. It is also used to treat infections in persons who are allergic to penicillin. Erythromycins are also used to prevent "strep" infections in patients with a history of rheumatic heart disease. They may also be used in Legionnaires' disease and for other problems as determined by your doctor.
- Keep taking this medicine for the full time of treatment even if you begin to feel better after a few days; do not miss any doses. This is especially important if you have a "strep" infection since serious heart problems could develop later if your infection is not cleared up completely.

- If you do miss a dose of this medicine, take it as soon as possible. This will help to keep a constant amount of medicine in the blood. However, if it is almost time for your next dose, skip the missed dose and go back to your regular dosing schedule.
- This medication has been prescribed for your current infection only. Another infection later on, or one that someone else has, may require a different medicine. You should not give your medicine to other people or use it for other infections, unless your doctor specifically directs you to do so.

Side effects
Along with the needed effects, a medicine may cause some unwanted effects. Side effects that usually do not require medical attention: abdominal cramps, black tongue, cough, diarrhea, fatigue, irritation of the mouth, loss of appetite, nausea, or vomiting. These side effects should disappear as your body adjusts to the medication.
- Other side effects that should be reported to your doctor immediately are:
Fever
Hearing loss
Hives or rash
Rectal or vaginal itching
Yellowing of the eyes or skin

Interactions
This medicine may interact with several other drugs such as anticoagulants, theophylline preparations, carbamazepine, etc.
- Be sure to tell your doctor about any medications you are currently taking.

Storage
Tablets, capsules, etc. should be stored at room temperature in tightly closed, light-resistant containers as directed by your pharmacist.

ELAVIL

Properties
This medicine contains amitriptyline as active ingredient. It belongs to the group of medicines known as tricyclic antidepressants or 'mood elevators.' It is used to relieve mental depression and depression that sometimes occurs with anxiety. The medication gradually relieves, but doesn't cure, symptoms of depression. The medication may also be used for the treatment of narcolepsy, bulimia, panic attacks, cocaine withdrawal, attention deficit disorder.

Before using this medicine
Before you use this medicine check with your doctor, or pharmacist:
- if you ever had any unusual or allergic reaction to any tricyclic antidepressant, maprotiline or trazodone.
- if you are on a low-salt, low-sugar, or any other special diet, or if you are allergic to any substance, such as sulfites or other preservatives or dyes.
- if you are pregnant or inintend to become pregnant while using this medicine. There have been reports of newborns suffering from heart, breathing, and urinary problems when their mothers had taken tricyclic antidepressants before delivery.
- if you are breast-feeding an infant. Some tricyclic antidepressants pass into the breast milk.

Treatment
Take this medicine only as directed by your doctor, to benefit your condition as much as possible. Do not take more of it, do not take it more often, and do not take it for a longer period of time than your doctor ordered.

To lessen stomach upset, take this medicine with food, even for a daily bedtime dose, unless your doctor has told you to take it on an empty stomach. If you forget your once-a-day bedtime dose, don't take it more than 3 hours late. If more than 3 hours, wait for next scheduled dose;.

Sometimes this medicine must be taken for several weeks before you begin to feel better.

Side effects
Along with the needed effects, a medicine may cause some unwanted effects. Side effects that usually do not require medical attention: difficult or frequent urination; decreased sex drive; muscle aches; abnormal dreams; nasal congestion; weakness and faintness when arising from bed or chair; back pain.
- Other side effects that should be reported to your doctor immediately are:
Hallucinations
Shakiness
Dizziness or fainting
Blurred vision, eye pain
Irregular heartbeat or slow pulse
Inflamed tongue
Abdominal pain
Jaundice
Hair loss, rash
Fever, chills
Joint pain
Palpitations

Interactions
This medicine may interact with several other drugs such as anticoagulants, anticholinergics, cold remedies, oral contraceptives, seizure medicines, sleeping medicines, thyroid medicines, etc.
- Be sure to tell your doctor about any medications you are currently taking.

Storage
Tablets, capsules, etc. should be stored at room temperature in tightly closed, light-resistant containers as directed by your pharmacist. Keep out of reach of children since overdose is especially dangerous in young children. Do not store in the bathroom medicine cabinet because the heat or moisture may cause the medicine to break down. Keep the liquid form of the medicine from freezing.

ELICOPHYLLIN

Properties

This medicine contains theophylline as active ingredient; it is used to treat or prevent breathing problems (wheezing and shortness of breath) caused by asthma, bronchitis, or emphysema. This medication belongs to a group known as xanthine-derivative bronchodilators. They work by opening up the bronchial tubes or air passages of the lungs and increasing the flow of air through them. These medicines are available only with your doctor's prescription.

Before using this medicine

Before you use this medicine check with your doctor, or pharmacist:

- if you ever had any unusual or allergic reaction to xanthine-derivative bronchodilators.
- if you are on a low-salt, low-sugar, or any other special diet, or if you are allergic to any substance, such as sulfites or other preservatives or dyes.
- if you are pregnant or inintend to become pregnant while using this medicine.
- if you are breast-feeding an infant. Theophylline passes into the breast milk and may cause irritability, fretfulness, or trouble in sleeping in infants of mothers taking this medicine.
- if you have any of the following medical problems:
Diarrhea
Enlarged prostate
Fibrocystic breast disease
Heart disease
Stomach ulcer

Treatment

This medication is used to relieve or prevent the symptoms of your medical problem. Take them as directed. Do not take more of them and do not take them more often than recommended on the label, unless otherwise directed by your doctor. To do so may increase the chance of side effects. The medicine should be taken on an empty stomach 30 to 60 minutes before a meal or two hours after a meal. Try not to miss any doses of this medication. If you do miss a dose, take the missed dose as soon as possible, unless it is almost time for the next dose. Do not double the next dose. It works best when taken with a glass of water.

Side effects

The following minor side effects may occur:

Dizziness or flushing
Headache
Diarrhea
Heartburn
Increased urination
Insomnia
Nervousness or irritability
Loss of appetite
Nausea or stomach upset
Stomach pain.

These side effects should disappear as your body adjusts to the medication. Tell your doctor about any side effects that are persistent or particularly bothersome. It is especially important to tell your doctor about black, tarry stools; confusion; convulsions; difficulty in breathing; fainting; muscle twitching; palpitations; rash; severe abdominal pain; or unusual weakness.

Interactions

This medicine interacts with several other drugs such as diuretics, reserpine, beta blockers, phenytoin, lithium, phenobarbital, birth control pills, and other medications.

- Be sure to tell your doctor about any medications you are currently taking.

Storage

Tablets, capsules, liquid and suspension should be stored at room temperature in tightly closed containers. Store away from heat and direct light. Keep out of reach of children, since overdose may be very dangerous in children. Discard any outdated medication.

ELIXICON

Properties

This medicine contains theophylline as active ingredient; it is used to treat or prevent breathing problems (wheezing and shortness of breath) caused by asthma, bronchitis, or emphysema. This medication belongs to a group known as xanthine-derivative bronchodilators. They work by opening up the bronchial tubes or air passages of the lungs and increasing the flow of air through them. These medicines are available only with your doctor's prescription.

Before using this medicine

Before you use this medicine check with your doctor, or pharmacist:
- if you ever had any unusual or allergic reaction to xanthine-derivative bronchodilators.
- if you are on a low-salt, low-sugar, or any other special diet, or if you are allergic to any substance, such as sulfites or other preservatives or dyes.
- if you are pregnant or inintend to become pregnant while using this medicine.
- if you are breast-feeding an infant. Theophylline passes into the breast milk and may cause irritability, fretfulness, or trouble in sleeping in infants of mothers taking this medicine.
- if you have any of the following medical problems:
  Diarrhea
  Enlarged prostate
  Fibrocystic breast disease
  Heart disease
  Stomach ulcer

Treatment

This medication is used to relieve or prevent the symptoms of your medical problem. Take them as directed. Do not take more of them and do not take them more often than recommended on the label, unless otherwise directed by your doctor. To do so may increase the chance of side effects. The medicine should be taken on an empty stomach 30 to 60 minutes before a meal or two hours after a meal. Try not to miss any doses of this medication. If you do miss a dose, take the missed dose as soon as possible, unless it is almost time for the next dose. Do not double the next dose. It works best when taken with a glass of water.

Side effects

The following minor side effects may occur:
  Dizziness or flushing
  Headache
  Diarrhea
  Heartburn
  Increased urination
  Insomnia
  Nervousness or irritability
  Loss of appetite
  Nausea or stomach upset
  Stomach pain.

These side effects should disappear as your body adjusts to the medication. Tell your doctor about any side effects that are persistent or particularly bothersome. It is especially important to tell your doctor about black, tarry stools; confusion; convulsions; difficulty in breathing; fainting; muscle twitching; palpitations; rash; severe abdominal pain; or unusual weakness.

Interactions

This medicine interacts with several other drugs such as diuretics, reserpine, beta blockers, phenytoin, lithium, phenobarbital, birth control pills, and other medications.
- Be sure to tell your doctor about any medications you are currently taking.

Storage

Tablets, capsules, liquid and suspension should be stored at room temperature in tightly closed containers. Store away from heat and direct light. Keep out of reach of children, since overdose may be very dangerous in children. Discard any outdated medication.

ELIXOMIN

Properties

This medicine contains theophylline as active ingredient; it is used to treat or prevent breathing problems (wheezing and shortness of breath) caused by asthma, bronchitis, or emphysema. This medication belongs to a group known as xanthine-derivative bronchodilators. They work by opening up the bronchial tubes or air passages of the lungs and increasing the flow of air through them. These medicines are available only with your doctor's prescription.

Before using this medicine

Before you use this medicine check with your doctor, or pharmacist:
- if you ever had any unusual or allergic reaction to xanthine-derivative bronchodilators.
- if you are on a low-salt, low-sugar, or any other special diet, or if you are allergic to any substance, such as sulfites or other preservatives or dyes.
- if you are pregnant or inintend to become pregnant while using this medicine.
- if you are breast-feeding an infant. Theophylline passes into the breast milk and may cause irritability, fretfulness, or trouble in sleeping in infants of mothers taking this medicine.
- if you have any of the following medical problems:
Diarrhea
Enlarged prostate
Fibrocystic breast disease
Heart disease
Stomach ulcer

Treatment

This medication is used to relieve or prevent the symptoms of your medical problem. Take them as directed. Do not take more of them and do not take them more often than recommended on the label, unless otherwise directed by your doctor. To do so may increase the chance of side effects. The medicine should be taken on an empty stomach 30 to 60 minutes before a meal or two hours after a meal. Try not to miss any doses of this medication. If you do miss a dose, take the missed dose as soon as possible, unless it is almost time for the next dose. Do not double the next dose. It works best when taken with a glass of water.

Side effects

The following minor side effects may occur:
Dizziness or flushing
Headache
Diarrhea
Heartburn
Increased urination
Insomnia
Nervousness or irritability
Loss of appetite
Nausea or stomach upset
Stomach pain.

These side effects should disappear as your body adjusts to the medication. Tell your doctor about any side effects that are persistent or particularly bothersome. It is especially important to tell your doctor about black, tarry stools; confusion; convulsions; difficulty in breathing; fainting; muscle twitching; palpitations; rash; severe abdominal pain; or unusual weakness.

Interactions

This medicine interacts with several other drugs such as diuretics, reserpine, beta blockers, phenytoin, lithium, phenobarbital, birth control pills, and other medications.
- Be sure to tell your doctor about any medications you are currently taking.

Storage

Tablets, capsules, liquid and suspension should be stored at room temperature in tightly closed containers. Store away from heat and direct light. Keep out of reach of children, since overdose may be very dangerous in children. Discard any outdated medication.

EM-K-10%

Properties

This medicine contains potassium chloride as active ingredient; it is used to treat or prevent potassium deficiency, especially potassium deficiency that is caused by the use of diuretics (water pills).

Potassium is needed to maintain good health. Potassium supplements may be needed by patients who do not have enough potassium in their regular diet and by those who have lost too much potassium because of illness or treatment with certain medicines.

Since too much potassium may also cause health problems, most potassium supplements are available only with your doctor's prescription.

Before using this medicine

Before you use this medicine check with your doctor, or pharmacist:

- if you ever had any unusual or allergic reaction to potassium preparations;
- if you are on a low-salt, low-sugar, or any other special diet, or if you are allergic to any substance, such as sulfites or other preservatives or dyes.
- if you are pregnant or inintend to become pregnant while using this medicine. Although potassium supplements have not been shown to cause problems in humans, the chance always exists.
- if you are breast-feeding an infant. Although this medicine has not been shown to cause problems in humans, the chance always exists since small amounts of potassium pass into the breast milk.
- if you have any of the following medical problems:
Addison's disease
Heart disease
Diarrhea
Kidney disease
Stomach ulcer

Treatment

This medication is used to relieve or prevent the symptoms of your medical problem. Take them as directed. Do not take more of them and do not take them more often than recommended on the label, unless otherwise directed by your doctor. To do so may increase the chance of side effects.

In order to avoid stomach irritation, you should take potassium supplements with food or immediately after a meal. If you miss a dose of this medication, take the missed dose as soon as possible, unless it is within two hours of the next scheduled dose;.

Side effects

The following minor side effects may occur:

Diarrhea
Nausea
Stomach Pains
Vomiting.

These side effects should disappear as your body adjusts to the medication. Tell your doctor about any side effects that are persistent or particularly bothersome. It is especially important to tell your doctor about anxiety; bloody or black, tarry stools; confusion; difficulty in breathing; numbness or tingling in the arms, legs, or feet; palpitations; severe abdominal pain; or unusual weakness.

Interactions

This medicine interacts with several other drugs such as adrenocorticosteroids, antimuscarinics, calcium-containing medicines; heart medicines such as digitalis or digoxin; laxatives; other potassium-containing medicines.

- Be sure to tell your doctor about any medications you are currently taking.

Storage

Tablets, elixir, etc. should be stored at room temperature in tightly closed containers. Store away from heat and direct light. Keep out of reach of children, since overdose may be very dangerous in children. Do not keep outdated medicine or medicine no longer needed. Flush the contents of the container down the toilet, unless otherwise directed.

EMITRIP

Properties
This medicine contains amitriptyline as active ingredient. It belongs to the group of medicines known as tricyclic antidepressants or 'mood elevators.' It is used to relieve mental depression and depression that sometimes occurs with anxiety. The medication gradually relieves, but doesn't cure, symptoms of depression. The medication may also be used for the treatment of narcolepsy, bulimia, panic attacks, cocaine withdrawal, attention deficit disorder.

Before using this medicine
Before you use this medicine check with your doctor, or pharmacist:
- if you ever had any unusual or allergic reaction to any tricyclic antidepressant, maprotiline or trazodone.
- if you are on a low-salt, low-sugar, or any other special diet, or if you are allergic to any substance, such as sulfites or other preservatives or dyes.
- if you are pregnant or inintend to become pregnant while using this medicine. There have been reports of newborns suffering from heart, breathing, and urinary problems when their mothers had taken tricyclic antidepressants before delivery.
- if you are breast-feeding an infant. Some tricyclic antidepressants pass into the breast milk.

Treatment
Take this medicine only as directed by your doctor, to benefit your condition as much as possible. Do not take more of it, do not take it more often, and do not take it for a longer period of time than your doctor ordered.

To lessen stomach upset, take this medicine with food, even for a daily bedtime dose, unless your doctor has told you to take it on an empty stomach. If you forget your once-a-day bedtime dose, don't take it more than 3 hours late. If more than 3 hours, wait for next scheduled dose;.

Sometimes this medicine must be taken for several weeks before you begin to feel better.

Side effects
Along with the needed effects, a medicine may cause some unwanted effects. Side effects that usually do not require medical attention: difficult or frequent urination; decreased sex drive; muscle aches; abnormal dreams; nasal congestion; weakness and faintness when arising from bed or chair; back pain.
- Other side effects that should be reported to your doctor immediately are:
  Hallucinations
  Shakiness
  Dizziness or fainting
  Blurred vision, eye pain
  Irregular heartbeat or slow pulse
  Inflamed tongue
  Abdominal pain
  Jaundice
  Hair loss, rash
  Fever, chills
  Joint pain
  Palpitations

Interactions
This medicine may interact with several other drugs such as anticoagulants, anticholinergics, cold remedies, oral contraceptives, seizure medicines, sleeping medicines, thyroid medicines, etc.
- Be sure to tell your doctor about any medications you are currently taking.

Storage
Tablets, capsules, etc. should be stored at room temperature in tightly closed, light-resistant containers as directed by your pharmacist. Keep out of reach of children since overdose is especially dangerous in young children. Do not store in the bathroom medicine cabinet because the heat or moisture may cause the medicine to break down. Keep the liquid form of the medicine from freezing.

ENDEP

Properties
This medicine contains amitriptyline as active ingredient. It belongs to the group of medicines known as tricyclic antidepressants or 'mood elevators.' It is used to relieve mental depression and depression that sometimes occurs with anxiety. The medication gradually relieves, but doesn't cure, symptoms of depression. The medication may also be used for the treatment of narcolepsy, bulimia, panic attacks, cocaine withdrawal, attention deficit disorder.

Before using this medicine
Before you use this medicine check with your doctor, or pharmacist:
- if you ever had any unusual or allergic reaction to any tricyclic antidepressant, maprotiline or trazodone.
- if you are on a low-salt, low-sugar, or any other special diet, or if you are allergic to any substance, such as sulfites or other preservatives or dyes.
- if you are pregnant or inintend to become pregnant while using this medicine. There have been reports of newborns suffering from heart, breathing, and urinary problems when their mothers had taken tricyclic antidepressants before delivery.
- if you are breast-feeding an infant. Some tricyclic antidepressants pass into the breast milk.

Treatment
Take this medicine only as directed by your doctor, to benefit your condition as much as possible. Do not take more of it, do not take it more often, and do not take it for a longer period of time than your doctor ordered.

To lessen stomach upset, take this medicine with food, even for a daily bedtime dose, unless your doctor has told you to take it on an empty stomach. If you forget your once-a-day bedtime dose, don't take it more than 3 hours late. If more than 3 hours, wait for next scheduled dose;.

Sometimes this medicine must be taken for several weeks before you begin to feel better.

Side effects
Along with the needed effects, a medicine may cause some unwanted effects. Side effects that usually do not require medical attention: difficult or frequent urination; decreased sex drive; muscle aches; abnormal dreams; nasal congestion; weakness and faintness when arising from bed or chair; back pain.
- Other side effects that should be reported to your doctor immediately are:
  Hallucinations
  Shakiness
  Dizziness or fainting
  Blurred vision, eye pain
  Irregular heartbeat or slow pulse
  Inflamed tongue
  Abdominal pain
  Jaundice
  Hair loss, rash
  Fever, chills
  Joint pain
  Palpitations

Interactions
This medicine may interact with several other drugs such as anticoagulants, anticholinergics, cold remedies, oral contraceptives, seizure medicines, sleeping medicines, thyroid medicines, etc.
- Be sure to tell your doctor about any medications you are currently taking.

Storage
Tablets, capsules, etc. should be stored at room temperature in tightly closed, light-resistant containers as directed by your pharmacist. Keep out of reach of children since overdose is especially dangerous in young children. Do not store in the bathroom medicine cabinet because the heat or moisture may cause the medicine to break down. Keep the liquid form of the medicine from freezing.

ENDURON

Properties

This medicine contains as active ingredient methyclothiazide, a thiazide-like diuretic. Thiazide or thiazide-like diuretics are prescribed to treat high blood pressure (hypertension). They are also used to reduce fluid accumulation in the body caused by conditions such as heart failure, cirrhosis, kidney disease, and the long-term use of some medications. Thiazide diuretics may also be used for other conditions as determined by your doctor.

Before using this medicine

Before you use this medicine check with your doctor, or pharmacist:

- if you ever had any unusual or allergic reaction to sulfonamides (sulfa drugs) or any of the thiazide diuretics.
- if you are on a low-salt, low-sugar, or any other special diet, or if you are allergic to any substance, such as sulfites or other preservatives or dyes.
- if you are pregnant or inintend to become pregnant while using this medicine. When this medicine is used during pregnancy, it may cause side effects including jaundice, blood problems, and low potassium in the newborn.
- if you are breast-feeding an infant. Although this medicine has not been shown to cause problems in humans, the chance always exists since thiazide diuretics pass into breast milk.
- if you have any of the following medical problems:
  Diabetes
  Gout
  Kidney disease
  Liver disease
  Lupus erythematosus
  Pancreas disease

Treatment

This medication is used to treat high blood pressure (hypertension) and also to help reduce the amount of water in the body by increasing the flow of urine. This medicine will not cure your high blood pressure but it does help control it. You must continue to take it - even if you feel well - if you expect to keep your blood pressure down. You may have to take high blood pressure medicine for the rest of your life.

Thiazide diuretics may cause an unusual feeling of tiredness when you begin to take them. You may also notice an increase in urine or in frequency of urination. To keep this from affecting sleep:

- if you are to take a single dose a day, take it in the morning after breakfast;
- if you are to take more than one dose, take the last one not later than 6 p.m.

Side effects

Along with the needed effects, a medicine may cause some unwanted effects. Side effects that usually do not require medical attention: decreased sexual ability; dizziness or lightheadedness when standing up; increased sensitivity of skin to sunlight; loss of appetite; upset stomach.

- Side effects that should be reported to your doctor: black, tarry stools; blood in urine or stools; cough or hoarseness; fever or chills; joint pain; lower back or side pains; painful or difficult urination; pinpoint red spots on skin; skin rash or hives; stomach pain (severe) with nausea; unusual bleeding or bruising; yellow eyes or skin. This medicine may cause a loss of potassium from your body. Signs of too much potassium loss are: dryness of mouth; increased thirst; mood changes; muscle cramps or pain; nausea or vomiting; unusual tiredness or weakness; weak or irregular heartbeat.

Interactions

This medicine may interact with several other drugs.

- Be sure to tell your doctor about any medications you are currently taking.

Storage

Store at room temperature in a tightly closed container.

ENOVIL

Properties

This medicine contains amitriptyline as active ingredient. It belongs to the group of medicines known as tricyclic antidepressants or 'mood elevators.' It is used to relieve mental depression and depression that sometimes occurs with anxiety. The medication gradually relieves, but doesn't cure, symptoms of depression. The medication may also be used for the treatment of narcolepsy, bulimia, panic attacks, cocaine withdrawal, attention deficit disorder.

Before using this medicine

Before you use this medicine check with your doctor, or pharmacist:
- if you ever had any unusual or allergic reaction to any tricyclic antidepressant, maprotiline or trazodone.
- if you are on a low-salt, low-sugar, or any other special diet, or if you are allergic to any substance, such as sulfites or other preservatives or dyes.
- if you are pregnant or inintend to become pregnant while using this medicine. There have been reports of newborns suffering from heart, breathing, and urinary problems when their mothers had taken tricyclic antidepressants before delivery.
- if you are breast-feeding an infant. Some tricyclic antidepressants pass into the breast milk.

Treatment

Take this medicine only as directed by your doctor, to benefit your condition as much as possible. Do not take more of it, do not take it more often, and do not take it for a longer period of time than your doctor ordered.

To lessen stomach upset, take this medicine with food, even for a daily bedtime dose, unless your doctor has told you to take it on an empty stomach. If you forget your once-a-day bedtime dose, don't take it more than 3 hours late. If more than 3 hours, wait for next scheduled dose;.

Sometimes this medicine must be taken for several weeks before you begin to feel better.

Side effects

Along with the needed effects, a medicine may cause some unwanted effects. Side effects that usually do not require medical attention: difficult or frequent urination; decreased sex drive; muscle aches; abnormal dreams; nasal congestion; weakness and faintness when arising from bed or chair; back pain.
- Other side effects that should be reported to your doctor immediately are:
  Hallucinations
  Shakiness
  Dizziness or fainting
  Blurred vision, eye pain
  Irregular heartbeat or slow pulse
  Inflamed tongue
  Abdominal pain
  Jaundice
  Hair loss, rash
  Fever, chills
  Joint pain
  Palpitations

Interactions

This medicine may interact with several other drugs such as anticoagulants, anticholinergics, cold remedies, oral contraceptives, seizure medicines, sleeping medicines, thyroid medicines, etc.
- Be sure to tell your doctor about any medications you are currently taking.

Storage

Tablets, capsules, etc. should be stored at room temperature in tightly closed, light-resistant containers as directed by your pharmacist. Keep out of reach of children since overdose is especially dangerous in young children. Do not store in the bathroom medicine cabinet because the heat or moisture may cause the medicine to break down. Keep the liquid form of the medicine from freezing.

EPIMORPH

Properties

This medicine contains as active ingredient morphine.

It is a narcotic analgesic that acts directly on the central nervous system (brain and spinal cord). It is used to relieve pain or to suppress coughing.

Before using this medicine

Before you use this medicine check with your doctor, or pharmacist:

- if you ever had any unusual or allergic reaction to this medicine or one of its components.
- if you are on a low-salt, low-sugar, or any other special diet, or if you are allergic to any substance, such as sulfites or other preservatives or dyes.
- if you are pregnant or inintend to become pregnant while using this medicine. Studies on birth defects have not been done in humans. Too much use of narcotics during pregnancy may cause the baby to become dependent on the medicine.
- if you are breast-feeding an infant. Although this medicine has not been shown to cause problems in humans, it passes into the breast milk in small amounts.
- if you have any of the following medical problems:
  Brain disease or head injury
  Colitis
  Convulsions
  Emphysema, asthma, or chronic lung disease
  Enlarged prostate
  Gallbladder disease or gallstones
  Heart disease
  Kidney or lifer disease
  Underactive thyroid

Treatment

This medication is used to relieve pain or to suppress coughing. Narcotic analgesics act in the central nervous system; some of their side effects are also caused by actions in the central nervous system.

- If you are taking this medication on a regular schedule and you miss a dose, take the missed dose as soon as possible, unless it is almost time for your next dose. In that case do not take the missed dose at all.
- If a narcotic analgesic is used for a long time, it may become habit-forming (causing mental or physical dependence). Physical dependence may lead to withdrawal side effects when you stop taking this medicine.

Unless otherwise directed by your doctor or pharmacist take this as directed. Do not take more of them and do not take them more often than recommended on the label. Children up to 12 years of age should not take this medicine more than 3 times a day or for more than 5 days in a row.

Side effects

Along with the needed effects, a medicine may cause some unwanted effects. These side effects may go away during treatment as your body adjusts to the medicine. Such minor side effects are: constipation, dizziness, drowsiness, dry mouth, false sense of well-being, flushing, light-headedness, loss of appetite, nausea, painful or difficult urination, or sweating.

- Check with your doctor immediately if any of the following side effects occur:
  Anxiety or breathing difficulties
  Excitation or restlessness
  Fatigue, palpitations
  Rash, sore throat and fever
  Tremors or weakness

Interactions

This medicine may interact with several other drugs such as medicines acting on the central nervous system (e.g., antidepressants, tranquilizers), cimetidine, nitrates, quinidine, etc.

- Be sure to tell your doctor about any medications you are currently taking.

Storage

Tablets, elixir, suppository etc. should be stored at room temperature in a tightly closed, light-resistant container.

ERAMYCIN

Properties
This medicine contains erythromycin as active ingredient. This antibiotic is prescribed to treat infections caused by bacteria. They will not work for colds, flu, or other virus infections. Erythromycins are available only with your doctor's prescription.

Before using this medicine
Before you use this medicine check with your doctor, or pharmacist:
- if you ever had any unusual or allergic reaction to any of the erythromycins.
- if you are on a low-salt, low-sugar, or any other special diet, or if you are allergic to any substance, such as sulfites or other preservatives or dyes.
- if you are pregnant or inintend to become pregnant while using this medicine. Although erythromycins have not been shown to cause birth defects or other problems in humans, the chance always exists.
- if you are breast-feeding an infant. Most erythromycins pass into the breast milk. Although erythromycins have not been shown to cause problems in humans, the chance always exists.
- if you have lifer disease.

Treatment
This medication belongs to the general family of medicines called antibiotics. It is used to treat a wide variety of bacterial infections. It is also used to treat infections in persons who are allergic to penicillin. Erythromycins are also used to prevent "strep" infections in patients with a history of rheumatic heart disease. They may also be used in Legionnaires' disease and for other problems as determined by your doctor.
- Keep taking this medicine for the full time of treatment even if you begin to feel better after a few days; do not miss any doses. This is especially important if you have a "strep" infection since serious heart problems could develop later if your infection is not cleared up completely.
- If you do miss a dose of this medicine, take it as soon as possible. This will help to keep a constant amount of medicine in the blood. However, if it is almost time for your next dose, skip the missed dose and go back to your regular dosing schedule.
- This medication has been prescribed for your current infection only. Another infection later on, or one that someone else has, may require a different medicine. You should not give your medicine to other people or use it for other infections, unless your doctor specifically directs you to do so.

Side effects
Along with the needed effects, a medicine may cause some unwanted effects. Side effects that usually do not require medical attention: abdominal cramps, black tongue, cough, diarrhea, fatigue, irritation of the mouth, loss of appetite, nausea, or vomiting. These side effects should disappear as your body adjusts to the medication.
- Other side effects that should be reported to your doctor immediately are:
Fever
Hearing loss
Hives or rash
Rectal or vaginal itching
Yellowing of the eyes or skin

Interactions
This medicine may interact with several other drugs such as anticoagulants, theophylline preparations, carbamazepine, etc.
- Be sure to tell your doctor about any medications you are currently taking.

Storage
Tablets, capsules, etc. should be stored at room temperature in tightly closed, light-resistant containers as directed by your pharmacist.

ERY-TAB

Properties
This medicine contains erythromycin as active ingredient. This antibiotic is prescribed to treat infections caused by bacteria. They will not work for colds, flu, or other virus infections. Erythromycins are available only with your doctor's prescription.

Before using this medicine
Before you use this medicine check with your doctor, or pharmacist:
- if you ever had any unusual or allergic reaction to any of the erythromycins.
- if you are on a low-salt, low-sugar, or any other special diet, or if you are allergic to any substance, such as sulfites or other preservatives or dyes.
- if you are pregnant or inintend to become pregnant while using this medicine. Although erythromycins have not been shown to cause birth defects or other problems in humans, the chance always exists.
- if you are breast-feeding an infant. Most erythromycins pass into the breast milk. Although erythromycins have not been shown to cause problems in humans, the chance always exists.
- if you have lifer disease.

Treatment
This medication belongs to the general family of medicines called antibiotics. It is used to treat a wide variety of bacterial infections. It is also used to treat infections in persons who are allergic to penicillin. Erythromycins are also used to prevent "strep" infections in patients with a history of rheumatic heart disease. They may also be used in Legionnaires' disease and for other problems as determined by your doctor.
- Keep taking this medicine for the full time of treatment even if you begin to feel better after a few days; do not miss any doses. This is especially important if you have a "strep" infection since serious heart problems could develop later if your infection is not cleared up completely.

- If you do miss a dose of this medicine, take it as soon as possible. This will help to keep a constant amount of medicine in the blood. However, if it is almost time for your next dose, skip the missed dose and go back to your regular dosing schedule.
- This medication has been prescribed for your current infection only. Another infection later on, or one that someone else has, may require a different medicine. You should not give your medicine to other people or use it for other infections, unless your doctor specifically directs you to do so.

Side effects
Along with the needed effects, a medicine may cause some unwanted effects. Side effects that usually do not require medical attention: abdominal cramps, black tongue, cough, diarrhea, fatigue, irritation of the mouth, loss of appetite, nausea, or vomiting. These side effects should disappear as your body adjusts to the medication.
- Other side effects that should be reported to your doctor immediately are:
Fever
Hearing loss
Hives or rash
Rectal or vaginal itching
Yellowing of the eyes or skin

Interactions
This medicine may interact with several other drugs such as anticoagulants, theophylline preparations, carbamazepine, etc.
- Be sure to tell your doctor about any medications you are currently taking.

Storage
Tablets, capsules, etc. should be stored at room temperature in tightly closed, light-resistant containers as directed by your pharmacist.

ERYC

Properties
This medicine contains erythromycin as active ingredient. This antibiotic is prescribed to treat infections caused by bacteria. They will not work for colds, flu, or other virus infections. Erythromycins are available only with your doctor's prescription.

Before using this medicine
Before you use this medicine check with your doctor, or pharmacist:
- if you ever had any unusual or allergic reaction to any of the erythromycins.
- if you are on a low-salt, low-sugar, or any other special diet, or if you are allergic to any substance, such as sulfites or other preservatives or dyes.
- if you are pregnant or inintend to become pregnant while using this medicine. Although erythromycins have not been shown to cause birth defects or other problems in humans, the chance always exists.
- if you are breast-feeding an infant. Most erythromycins pass into the breast milk. Although erythromycins have not been shown to cause problems in humans, the chance always exists.
- if you have lifer disease.

Treatment
This medication belongs to the general family of medicines called antibiotics. It is used to treat a wide variety of bacterial infections. It is also used to treat infections in persons who are allergic to penicillin. Erythromycins are also used to prevent "strep" infections in patients with a history of rheumatic heart disease. They may also be used in Legionnaires' disease and for other problems as determined by your doctor.
- Keep taking this medicine for the full time of treatment even if you begin to feel better after a few days; do not miss any doses. This is especially important if you have a "strep" infection since serious heart problems could develop later if your infection is not cleared up completely.
- If you do miss a dose of this medicine, take it as soon as possible. This will help to keep a constant amount of medicine in the blood. However, if it is almost time for your next dose, skip the missed dose and go back to your regular dosing schedule.
- This medication has been prescribed for your current infection only. Another infection later on, or one that someone else has, may require a different medicine. You should not give your medicine to other people or use it for other infections, unless your doctor specifically directs you to do so.

Side effects
Along with the needed effects, a medicine may cause some unwanted effects. Side effects that usually do not require medical attention: abdominal cramps, black tongue, cough, diarrhea, fatigue, irritation of the mouth, loss of appetite, nausea, or vomiting. These side effects should disappear as your body adjusts to the medication.
- Other side effects that should be reported to your doctor immediately are:
Fever
Hearing loss
Hives or rash
Rectal or vaginal itching
Yellowing of the eyes or skin

Interactions
This medicine may interact with several other drugs such as anticoagulants, theophylline preparations, carbamazepine, etc.
- Be sure to tell your doctor about any medications you are currently taking.

Storage
Tablets, capsules, etc. should be stored at room temperature in tightly closed, light-resistant containers as directed by your pharmacist.

ERYPAR

Properties
This medicine contains erythromycin as active ingredient. This antibiotic is prescribed to treat infections caused by bacteria. They will not work for colds, flu, or other virus infections. Erythromycins are available only with your doctor's prescription.

Before using this medicine
Before you use this medicine check with your doctor, or pharmacist:
- if you ever had any unusual or allergic reaction to any of the erythromycins.
- if you are on a low-salt, low-sugar, or any other special diet, or if you are allergic to any substance, such as sulfites or other preservatives or dyes.
- if you are pregnant or inintend to become pregnant while using this medicine. Although erythromycins have not been shown to cause birth defects or other problems in humans, the chance always exists.
- if you are breast-feeding an infant. Most erythromycins pass into the breast milk. Although erythromycins have not been shown to cause problems in humans, the chance always exists.
- if you have lifer disease.

Treatment
This medication belongs to the general family of medicines called antibiotics. It is used to treat a wide variety of bacterial infections. It is also used to treat infections in persons who are allergic to penicillin. Erythromycins are also used to prevent "strep" infections in patients with a history of rheumatic heart disease. They may also be used in Legionnaires' disease and for other problems as determined by your doctor.
- Keep taking this medicine for the full time of treatment even if you begin to feel better after a few days; do not miss any doses. This is especially important if you have a "strep" infection since serious heart problems could develop later if your infection is not cleared up completely.
- If you do miss a dose of this medicine, take it as soon as possible. This will help to keep a constant amount of medicine in the blood. However, if it is almost time for your next dose, skip the missed dose and go back to your regular dosing schedule.
- This medication has been prescribed for your current infection only. Another infection later on, or one that someone else has, may require a different medicine. You should not give your medicine to other people or use it for other infections, unless your doctor specifically directs you to do so.

Side effects
Along with the needed effects, a medicine may cause some unwanted effects. Side effects that usually do not require medical attention: abdominal cramps, black tongue, cough, diarrhea, fatigue, irritation of the mouth, loss of appetite, nausea, or vomiting. These side effects should disappear as your body adjusts to the medication.
- Other side effects that should be reported to your doctor immediately are:
Fever
Hearing loss
Hives or rash
Rectal or vaginal itching
Yellowing of the eyes or skin

Interactions
This medicine may interact with several other drugs such as anticoagulants, theophylline preparations, carbamazepine, etc.
- Be sure to tell your doctor about any medications you are currently taking.

Storage
Tablets, capsules, etc. should be stored at room temperature in tightly closed, light-resistant containers as directed by your pharmacist.

ERYPED

Properties
This medicine contains erythromycin as active ingredient. This antibiotic is prescribed to treat infections caused by bacteria. They will not work for colds, flu, or other virus infections. Erythromycins are available only with your doctor's prescription.

Before using this medicine
Before you use this medicine check with your doctor, or pharmacist:
- if you ever had any unusual or allergic reaction to any of the erythromycins.
- if you are on a low-salt, low-sugar, or any other special diet, or if you are allergic to any substance, such as sulfites or other preservatives or dyes.
- if you are pregnant or inintend to become pregnant while using this medicine. Although erythromycins have not been shown to cause birth defects or other problems in humans, the chance always exists.
- if you are breast-feeding an infant. Most erythromycins pass into the breast milk. Although erythromycins have not been shown to cause problems in humans, the chance always exists.
- if you have lifer disease.

Treatment
This medication belongs to the general family of medicines called antibiotics. It is used to treat a wide variety of bacterial infections. It is also used to treat infections in persons who are allergic to penicillin. Erythromycins are also used to prevent "strep" infections in patients with a history of rheumatic heart disease. They may also be used in Legionnaires' disease and for other problems as determined by your doctor.
■ Keep taking this medicine for the full time of treatment even if you begin to feel better after a few days; do not miss any doses. This is especially important if you have a "strep" infection since serious heart problems could develop later if your infection is not cleared up completely.

■ If you do miss a dose of this medicine, take it as soon as possible. This will help to keep a constant amount of medicine in the blood. However, if it is almost time for your next dose, skip the missed dose and go back to your regular dosing schedule.
■ This medication has been prescribed for your current infection only. Another infection later on, or one that someone else has, may require a different medicine. You should not give your medicine to other people or use it for other infections, unless your doctor specifically directs you to do so.

Side effects
Along with the needed effects, a medicine may cause some unwanted effects. Side effects that usually do not require medical attention: abdominal cramps, black tongue, cough, diarrhea, fatigue, irritation of the mouth, loss of appetite, nausea, or vomiting. These side effects should disappear as your body adjusts to the medication.
■ Other side effects that should be reported to your doctor immediately are:
Fever
Hearing loss
Hives or rash
Rectal or vaginal itching
Yellowing of the eyes or skin

Interactions
This medicine may interact with several other drugs such as anticoagulants, theophylline preparations, carbamazepine, etc.
■ Be sure to tell your doctor about any medications you are currently taking.

Storage
Tablets, capsules, etc. should be stored at room temperature in tightly closed, light-resistant containers as directed by your pharmacist.

ERYTHRITOL TETRANITRATE

Properties
This medicine contains erythritol tetranitrate as active ingredient. Nitrates improve the supply of blood and oxygen to the heart. This medication is for oral use.

Before using this medicine
Before you use this medicine check with your doctor, or pharmacist:
- if you ever had any unusual or allergic reaction to nitrates or nitrites.
- if you are on a low-salt, low-sugar, or any other special diet, or if you are allergic to any substance, such as sulfites or other preservatives or dyes.
- if you are pregnant or inintend to become pregnant while using this medicine. Although nitrates have not been shown to cause problems in humans, the chance always exists.
- if you are breast-feeding an infant.
- if you have recently had a heart attack or stroke.
- if you have any of the following medical problems:
  Anemia
  Glaucoma
  Intestinal problems
  Overactive thyroid
- if you are now taking any of the following medicines or types of medicines:
  Antihypertensives
  Asthma or hay fever medicine
  Cold medicine
  Decongestant
  Medicine for appetite control
  Narcotic
  Pain medicine
  Sinus congestion medicine

Treatment
This medication is used to treat and prevent angina (chest pain). Nitroglycerin is a vasodilator, which relaxes the muscles of the blood vessels, causing an increase in the oxygen supply to the heart. The oral tablets, capsules, ointment and patches do not act quickly; they are used to prevent chest pain. The sublingual tablets and oral spray act quickly and can be used to relieve chest pain after it has started.

- Take this medicine exactly as directed by your doctor or pharmacist. It will work only if taken correctly.
- If you are taking this medicine regularly and you miss a dose, take it as soon as possible. However, if your next scheduled dose; is within 2 hours (or within 6 hours for extended-release capsules or tablets), skip the missed dose and go back to your regular dosing schedule.
- If you have been taking this medicine regularly for several weeks or more, do not suddenly stop using it. Stopping suddenly may bring on attacks of angina.

Side effects
There are a number of side effects that usually do not require medical attention. These possible side effects may go away during treatment; however, if they continue or are bothersome, check with your doctor, nurse, or pharmacist. More common are: dizziness, lightheadedness, or fainting when standing up; fast pulse; flushing of face and neck; headache; nausea or vomiting.

Side effects that should be reported to your doctor are: blurred vision; dry mouth; severe or prolonged headache; skin rash.

Interactions
This medicine may interact with several other drugs such as tricyclic antidepressants and cough medicines. Before starting to take or apply nitroglycerin, be sure to tell your doctor about any medications you are currently taking.

Storage
Tablets, capsules, and oral spray should be stored as in a tightly capped bottle in a cool, dry place. Ointment and patches should be stored at room temperature in their original containers. Keep out of reach of children. Do not keep outdated medicine or medicine no longer needed.

ERYTHROCIN

Properties

This medicine contains erythromycin as active ingredient. This antibiotic is prescribed to treat infections caused by bacteria. They will not work for colds, flu, or other virus infections. Erythromycins are available only with your doctor's prescription.

Before using this medicine

Before you use this medicine check with your doctor, or pharmacist:
- if you ever had any unusual or allergic reaction to any of the erythromycins.
- if you are on a low-salt, low-sugar, or any other special diet, or if you are allergic to any substance, such as sulfites or other preservatives or dyes.
- if you are pregnant or inintend to become pregnant while using this medicine. Although erythromycins have not been shown to cause birth defects or other problems in humans, the chance always exists.
- if you are breast-feeding an infant. Most erythromycins pass into the breast milk. Although erythromycins have not been shown to cause problems in humans, the chance always exists.
- if you have lifer disease.

Treatment

This medication belongs to the general family of medicines called antibiotics. It is used to treat a wide variety of bacterial infections. It is also used to treat infections in persons who are allergic to penicillin. Erythromycins are also used to prevent "strep" infections in patients with a history of rheumatic heart disease. They may also be used in Legionnaires' disease and for other problems as determined by your doctor.
- Keep taking this medicine for the full time of treatment even if you begin to feel better after a few days; do not miss any doses. This is especially important if you have a "strep" infection since serious heart problems could develop later if your infection is not cleared up completely.
- If you do miss a dose of this medicine, take it as soon as possible. This will help to keep a constant amount of medicine in the blood. However, if it is almost time for your next dose, skip the missed dose and go back to your regular dosing schedule.
- This medication has been prescribed for your current infection only. Another infection later on, or one that someone else has, may require a different medicine. You should not give your medicine to other people or use it for other infections, unless your doctor specifically directs you to do so.

Side effects

Along with the needed effects, a medicine may cause some unwanted effects. Side effects that usually do not require medical attention: abdominal cramps, black tongue, cough, diarrhea, fatigue, irritation of the mouth, loss of appetite, nausea, or vomiting. These side effects should disappear as your body adjusts to the medication.
- Other side effects that should be reported to your doctor immediately are:
Fever
Hearing loss
Hives or rash
Rectal or vaginal itching
Yellowing of the eyes or skin

Interactions

This medicine may interact with several other drugs such as anticoagulants, theophylline preparations, carbamazepine, etc.
- Be sure to tell your doctor about any medications you are currently taking.

Storage

Tablets, capsules, etc. should be stored at room temperature in tightly closed, light-resistant containers as directed by your pharmacist.

ERYTHROMID

Properties

This medicine contains erythromycin as active ingredient. This antibiotic is prescribed to treat infections caused by bacteria. They will not work for colds, flu, or other virus infections. Erythromycins are available only with your doctor's prescription.

Before using this medicine

Before you use this medicine check with your doctor, or pharmacist:

- if you ever had any unusual or allergic reaction to any of the erythromycins.
- if you are on a low-salt, low-sugar, or any other special diet, or if you are allergic to any substance, such as sulfites or other preservatives or dyes.
- if you are pregnant or inintend to become pregnant while using this medicine. Although erythromycins have not been shown to cause birth defects or other problems in humans, the chance always exists.
- if you are breast-feeding an infant. Most erythromycins pass into the breast milk. Although erythromycins have not been shown to cause problems in humans, the chance always exists.
- if you have lifer disease.

Treatment

This medication belongs to the general family of medicines called antibiotics. It is used to treat a wide variety of bacterial infections. It is also used to treat infections in persons who are allergic to penicillin. Erythromycins are also used to prevent "strep" infections in patients with a history of rheumatic heart disease. They may also be used in Legionnaires' disease and for other problems as determined by your doctor.

- Keep taking this medicine for the full time of treatment even if you begin to feel better after a few days; do not miss any doses. This is especially important if you have a "strep" infection since serious heart problems could develop later if your infection is not cleared up completely.

- If you do miss a dose of this medicine, take it as soon as possible. This will help to keep a constant amount of medicine in the blood. However, if it is almost time for your next dose, skip the missed dose and go back to your regular dosing schedule.
- This medication has been prescribed for your current infection only. Another infection later on, or one that someone else has, may require a different medicine. You should not give your medicine to other people or use it for other infections, unless your doctor specifically directs you to do so.

Side effects

Along with the needed effects, a medicine may cause some unwanted effects. Side effects that usually do not require medical attention: abdominal cramps, black tongue, cough, diarrhea, fatigue, irritation of the mouth, loss of appetite, nausea, or vomiting. These side effects should disappear as your body adjusts to the medication.

- Other side effects that should be reported to your doctor immediately are:
  Fever
  Hearing loss
  Hives or rash
  Rectal or vaginal itching
  Yellowing of the eyes or skin

Interactions

This medicine may interact with several other drugs such as anticoagulants, theophylline preparations, carbamazepine, etc.

- Be sure to tell your doctor about any medications you are currently taking.

Storage

Tablets, capsules, etc. should be stored at room temperature in tightly closed, light-resistant containers as directed by your pharmacist.

ERYTHROMYCIN

Properties

This medicine contains erythromycin as active ingredient. This antibiotic is prescribed to treat infections caused by bacteria. They will not work for colds, flu, or other virus infections. Erythromycins are available only with your doctor's prescription.

Before using this medicine

Before you use this medicine check with your doctor, or pharmacist:
- if you ever had any unusual or allergic reaction to any of the erythromycins.
- if you are on a low-salt, low-sugar, or any other special diet, or if you are allergic to any substance, such as sulfites or other preservatives or dyes.
- if you are pregnant or inintend to become pregnant while using this medicine. Although erythromycins have not been shown to cause birth defects or other problems in humans, the chance always exists.
- if you are breast-feeding an infant. Most erythromycins pass into the breast milk. Although erythromycins have not been shown to cause problems in humans, the chance always exists.
- if you have lifer disease.

Treatment

This medication belongs to the general family of medicines called antibiotics. It is used to treat a wide variety of bacterial infections. It is also used to treat infections in persons who are allergic to penicillin. Erythromycins are also used to prevent "strep" infections in patients with a history of rheumatic heart disease. They may also be used in Legionnaires' disease and for other problems as determined by your doctor.
- Keep taking this medicine for the full time of treatment even if you begin to feel better after a few days; do not miss any doses. This is especially important if you have a "strep" infection since serious heart problems could develop later if your infection is not cleared up completely.
- If you do miss a dose of this medicine, take it as soon as possible. This will help to keep a constant amount of medicine in the blood. However, if it is almost time for your next dose, skip the missed dose and go back to your regular dosing schedule.
- This medication has been prescribed for your current infection only. Another infection later on, or one that someone else has, may require a different medicine. You should not give your medicine to other people or use it for other infections, unless your doctor specifically directs you to do so.

Side effects

Along with the needed effects, a medicine may cause some unwanted effects. Side effects that usually do not require medical attention: abdominal cramps, black tongue, cough, diarrhea, fatigue, irritation of the mouth, loss of appetite, nausea, or vomiting. These side effects should disappear as your body adjusts to the medication.
- Other side effects that should be reported to your doctor immediately are:
Fever
Hearing loss
Hives or rash
Rectal or vaginal itching
Yellowing of the eyes or skin

Interactions

This medicine may interact with several other drugs such as anticoagulants, theophylline preparations, carbamazepine, etc.
- Be sure to tell your doctor about any medications you are currently taking.

Storage

Tablets, capsules, etc. should be stored at room temperature in tightly closed, light-resistant containers as directed by your pharmacist.

ESIDRIX

Properties
This medicine contains as active ingredient hydrochlorothiazide, a thiazide-like diuretic. Thiazide or thiazide-like diuretics are prescribed to treat high blood pressure (hypertension). They are also used to reduce fluid accumulation in the body caused by conditions such as heart failure, cirrhosis, kidney disease, and the long-term use of some medications. Thiazide diuretics may also be used for other conditions as determined by your doctor.

Before using this medicine
Before you use this medicine check with your doctor, or pharmacist:
- if you ever had any unusual or allergic reaction to sulfonamides (sulfa drugs) or any of the thiazide diuretics.
- if you are on a low-salt, low-sugar, or any other special diet, or if you are allergic to any substance, such as sulfites or other preservatives or dyes.
- if you are pregnant or inintend to become pregnant while using this medicine. When this medicine is used during pregnancy, it may cause side effects including jaundice, blood problems, and low potassium in the newborn.
- if you are breast-feeding an infant. Although this medicine has not been shown to cause problems in humans, the chance always exists since thiazide diuretics pass into breast milk.
- if you have any of the following medical problems:
Diabetes
Gout
Kidney disease
Liver disease
Lupus erythematosus
Pancreas disease

Treatment
This medication is used to treat high blood pressure (hypertension) and also to help reduce the amount of water in the body by increasing the flow of urine. This medicine will not cure your high blood pressure but it does help control it. You must continue to take it - even if you feel well - if you expect to keep your blood pressure down. You may have to take high blood pressure medicine for the rest of your life.

Thiazide diuretics may cause an unusual feeling of tiredness when you begin to take them. You may also notice an increase in urine or in frequency of urination. To keep this from affecting sleep:
- if you are to take a single dose a day, take it in the morning after breakfast;
- if you are to take more than one dose, take the last one not later than 6 p.m.

Side effects
Along with the needed effects, a medicine may cause some unwanted effects. Side effects that usually do not require medical attention: decreased sexual ability; dizziness or lightheadedness when standing up; increased sensitivity of skin to sunlight; loss of appetite; upset stomach.
- Side effects that should be reported to your doctor: black, tarry stools; blood in urine or stools; cough or hoarseness; fever or chills; joint pain; lower back or side pains; painful or difficult urination; pinpoint red spots on skin; skin rash or hives; stomach pain (severe) with nausea; unusual bleeding or bruising; yellow eyes or skin. This medicine may cause a loss of potassium from your body. Signs of too much potassium loss are: dryness of mouth; increased thirst; mood changes; muscle cramps or pain; nausea or vomiting; unusual tiredness or weakness; weak or irregular heartbeat.

Interactions
This medicine may interact with several other drugs.
- Be sure to tell your doctor about any medications you are currently taking.

Storage
Store at room temperature in a tightly closed container.

ESTINYL

Properties
This medicine contains ethinyl estradiol as active ingredient. The medicine is prescribed for treatment of estrogen deficiency; it restores normal estrogen levels in tissues. There is no evidence that this drug is effective for nervous symptoms or depression occurring during menopause. They should not be used to treat this condition; they should be used only to replace the estrogen that is naturally absent after menopause.

Before using this medicine
Before you use this medicine check with your doctor, or pharmacist:
- if you ever had any unusual or allergic reaction to estrogens;
- if you are pregnant or intend to become pregnant within three months;
- if you are breast-feeding an infant;
- if you have any of the following medical problems:
  Diabetes
  Breast cancer
  Fibrocystic breast disease
  Fibroid uterine tumors
  Endometriosis
  Migraine headaches
  Epilepsy
  Porphyria
  High blood pressure
  Asthma
  Congestive heart failure
  Kidney disease
  Gallstones

Treatment
This medication is used to treat estrogen deficiency, specific symptoms of menopause, estrogen-deficiency osteoporosis, atrophic vaginitis, prostate cancer.
  For safe and effective use of this medicine:
♦ Follow your doctor's instructions if this medicine was prescribed.
♦ Follow the manufacturer's package directions if you are treating yourself.
♦ Estrogens have been reported to increase the risk of endometrial carcinoma.

Side effects
Along with the needed effects, a medicine may cause some unwanted effects. Possible side effects include:
  Stomach cramps
  Profuse bleeding
  Appetite loss
  Nausea and vomiting
  Swollen breasts
  Change in menstruation
  Rash, skin blisters
  Depression
  Dizziness

Overdose
The following symptoms may indicate an overdose:
  Nausea and vomiting
  Fluid retention
  Breast enlargement
  Abnormal vaginal bleeding
■ Call a doctor or hospital emergency room for instructions.

Interactions
This medicine may interact with several other drugs such as adrenocorticosteroids, antidepressants, oral antidiabetics, insulin, phenobarbital, primidone.
■ Be sure to tell your doctor about any medications you are currently taking.

Storage
Capsules, tablets, vaginal cream, transdermal patches, etc. should be stored at room temperature; store away from heat and direct light. Keep out of reach of children, since this medicine may be dangerous in children.

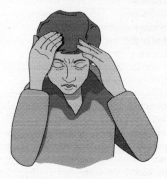

ESTRACE

Properties
This medicine contains estrogen as active ingredient. The medicine is prescribed for treatment of estrogen deficiency; it restores normal estrogen levels in tissues. There is no evidence that this drug is effective for nervous symptoms or depression occurring during menopause. They should not be used to treat this condition; they should be used only to replace the estrogen that is naturally absent after menopause.

Before using this medicine
Before you use this medicine check with your doctor, or pharmacist:
- if you ever had any unusual or allergic reaction to estrogens;
- if you are pregnant or intend to become pregnant within three months;
- if you are breast-feeding an infant;
- if you have any of the following medical problems:
  Diabetes
  Breast cancer
  Fibrocystic breast disease
  Fibroid uterine tumors
  Endometriosis
  Migraine headaches
  Epilepsy
  Porphyria
  High blood pressure
  Asthma
  Congestive heart failure
  Kidney disease
  Gallstones

Treatment
This medication is used to treat estrogen deficiency, specific symptoms of menopause, estrogen-deficiency osteoporosis, atrophic vaginitis, prostate cancer.
   For safe and effective use of this medicine:
- ◆ Follow your doctor's instructions if this medicine was prescribed.
- ◆ Follow the manufacturer's package directions if you are treating yourself.
- ◆ Estrogens have been reported to increase the risk of endometrial carcinoma.

Side effects
Along with the needed effects, a medicine may cause some unwanted effects. Possible side effects include:
   Stomach cramps
   Profuse bleeding
   Appetite loss
   Nausea and vomiting
   Swollen breasts
   Change in menstruation
   Rash, skin blisters
   Depression
   Dizziness

Overdose
The following symptoms may indicate an overdose:
   Nausea and vomiting
   Fluid retention
   Breast enlargement
   Abnormal vaginal bleeding
- ■ Call a doctor or hospital emergency room for instructions.

Interactions
This medicine may interact with several other drugs such as adrenocorticosteroids, antidepressants, oral antidiabetics, insulin, phenobarbital, primidone.
- ■ Be sure to tell your doctor about any medications you are currently taking.

Storage
Capsules, tablets, vaginal cream, transdermal patches, etc. should be stored at room temperature; store away from heat and direct light. Keep out of reach of children, since this medicine may be dangerous in children.

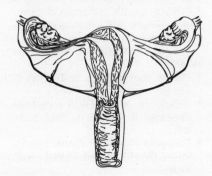

ESTRADERM

Properties

This medicine contains estrogen as active ingredient. The medicine is prescribed for treatment of estrogen deficiency; it restores normal estrogen levels in tissues. There is no evidence that this drug is effective for nervous symptoms or depression occurring during menopause. They should not be used to treat this condition; they should be used only to replace the estrogen that is naturally absent after menopause.

Before using this medicine

Before you use this medicine check with your doctor, or pharmacist:
- if you ever had any unusual or allergic reaction to estrogens;
- if you are pregnant or intend to become pregnant within three months;
- if you are breast-feeding an infant;
- if you have any of the following medical problems:
  Diabetes
  Breast cancer
  Fibrocystic breast disease
  Fibroid uterine tumors
  Endometriosis
  Migraine headaches
  Epilepsy
  Porphyria
  High blood pressure
  Asthma
  Congestive heart failure
  Kidney disease
  Gallstones

Treatment

This medication is used to treat estrogen deficiency, specific symptoms of menopause, estrogen-deficiency osteoporosis, atrophic vaginitis, prostate cancer.

For safe and effective use of this medicine:
- Follow your doctor's instructions if this medicine was prescribed.
- Follow the manufacturer's package directions if you are treating yourself.
- Estrogens have been reported to increase the risk of endometrial carcinoma.

Side effects

Along with the needed effects, a medicine may cause some unwanted effects. Possible side effects include:
  Stomach cramps
  Profuse bleeding
  Appetite loss
  Nausea and vomiting
  Swollen breasts
  Change in menstruation
  Rash, skin blisters
  Depression
  Dizziness

Overdose

The following symptoms may indicate an overdose:
  Nausea and vomiting
  Fluid retention
  Breast enlargement
  Abnormal vaginal bleeding
- Call a doctor or hospital emergency room for instructions.

Interactions

This medicine may interact with several other drugs such as adrenocorticosteroids, antidepressants, oral antidiabetics, insulin, phenobarbital, primidone.
- Be sure to tell your doctor about any medications you are currently taking.

Storage

Capsules, tablets, vaginal cream, transdermal patches, etc. should be stored at room temperature; store away from heat and direct light. Keep out of reach of children, since this medicine may be dangerous in children.

ESTRADIOL

Properties

This medicine contains estradiol as active ingredient. The medicine is prescribed for treatment of estrogen deficiency; it restores normal estrogen levels in tissues. There is no evidence that this drug is effective for nervous symptoms or depression occurring during menopause. They should not be used to treat this condition; they should be used only to replace the estrogen that is naturally absent after menopause.

Before using this medicine

Before you use this medicine check with your doctor, or pharmacist:
- if you ever had any unusual or allergic reaction to estrogens;
- if you are pregnant or intend to become pregnant within three months;
- if you are breast-feeding an infant;
- if you have any of the following medical problems:
  Diabetes
  Breast cancer
  Fibrocystic breast disease
  Fibroid uterine tumors
  Endometriosis
  Migraine headaches
  Epilepsy
  Porphyria
  High blood pressure
  Asthma
  Congestive heart failure
  Kidney disease
  Gallstones

Treatment

This medication is used to treat estrogen deficiency, specific symptoms of menopause, estrogen-deficiency osteoporosis, atrophic vaginitis, prostate cancer.

For safe and effective use of this medicine:
- ◆ Follow your doctor's instructions if this medicine was prescribed.
- ◆ Follow the manufacturer's package directions if you are treating yourself.
- ◆ Estrogens have been reported to increase the risk of endometrial carcinoma.

Side effects

Along with the needed effects, a medicine may cause some unwanted effects. Possible side effects include:
  Stomach cramps
  Profuse bleeding
  Appetite loss
  Nausea and vomiting
  Swollen breasts
  Change in menstruation
  Rash, skin blisters
  Depression
  Dizziness

Overdose

The following symptoms may indicate an overdose:
  Nausea and vomiting
  Fluid retention
  Breast enlargement
  Abnormal vaginal bleeding
- ■ Call a doctor or hospital emergency room for instructions.

Interactions

This medicine may interact with several other drugs such as adrenocorticosteroids, antidepressants, oral antidiabetics, insulin, phenobarbital, primidone.
- ■ Be sure to tell your doctor about any medications you are currently taking.

Storage

Capsules, tablets, vaginal cream, transdermal patches, etc. should be stored at room temperature; store away from heat and direct light. Keep out of reach of children, since this medicine may be dangerous in children.

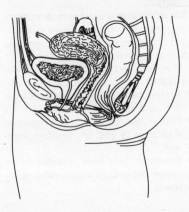

ESTRO-A

Properties
This medicine contains estrone as active ingredient. The medicine is prescribed for treatment of estrogen deficiency; it restores normal estrogen levels in tissues. There is no evidence that this drug is effective for nervous symptoms or depression occurring during menopause. They should not be used to treat this condition; they should be used only to replace the estrogen that is naturally absent after menopause.

Before using this medicine
Before you use this medicine check with your doctor, or pharmacist:
- if you ever had any unusual or allergic reaction to estrogens;
- if you are pregnant or intend to become pregnant within three months;
- if you are breast-feeding an infant;
- if you have any of the following medical problems:
Diabetes
Breast cancer
Fibrocystic breast disease
Fibroid uterine tumors
Endometriosis
Migraine headaches
Epilepsy
Porphyria
High blood pressure
Asthma
Congestive heart failure
Kidney disease
Gallstones

Treatment
This medication is used to treat estrogen deficiency, specific symptoms of menopause, estrogen-deficiency osteoporosis, atrophic vaginitis, prostate cancer.

For safe and effective use of this medicine:
- ◆ Follow your doctor's instructions if this medicine was prescribed.
- ◆ Follow the manufacturer's package directions if you are treating yourself.
- ◆ Estrogens have been reported to increase the risk of endometrial carcinoma.

Side effects
Along with the needed effects, a medicine may cause some unwanted effects. Possible side effects include:
Stomach cramps
Profuse bleeding
Appetite loss
Nausea and vomiting
Swollen breasts
Change in menstruation
Rash, skin blisters
Depression
Dizziness

Overdose
The following symptoms may indicate an overdose:
Nausea and vomiting
Fluid retention
Breast enlargement
Abnormal vaginal bleeding
- Call a doctor or hospital emergency room for instructions.

Interactions
This medicine may interact with several other drugs such as adrenocorticosteroids, antidepressants, oral antidiabetics, insulin, phenobarbital, primidone.
- Be sure to tell your doctor about any medications you are currently taking.

Storage
Capsules, tablets, vaginal cream, transdermal patches, etc. should be stored at room temperature; store away from heat and direct light. Keep out of reach of children, since this medicine may be dangerous in children.

ESTROGEN

Properties

This medicine contains estrogen as active ingredient. The medicine is prescribed for treatment of estrogen deficiency; it restores normal estrogen levels in tissues. There is no evidence that this drug is effective for nervous symptoms or depression occurring during menopause. They should not be used to treat this condition; they should be used only to replace the estrogen that is naturally absent after menopause.

Before using this medicine

Before you use this medicine check with your doctor, or pharmacist:
- if you ever had any unusual or allergic reaction to estrogens;
- if you are pregnant or intend to become pregnant within three months;
- if you are breast-feeding an infant;
- if you have any of the following medical problems:
  Diabetes
  Breast cancer
  Fibrocystic breast disease
  Fibroid uterine tumors
  Endometriosis
  Migraine headaches
  Epilepsy
  Porphyria
  High blood pressure
  Asthma
  Congestive heart failure
  Kidney disease
  Gallstones

Treatment

This medication is used to treat estrogen deficiency, specific symptoms of menopause, estrogen-deficiency osteoporosis, atrophic vaginitis, prostate cancer.

For safe and effective use of this medicine:
- Follow your doctor's instructions if this medicine was prescribed.
- Follow the manufacturer's package directions if you are treating yourself.
- Estrogens have been reported to increase the risk of endometrial carcinoma.

Side effects

Along with the needed effects, a medicine may cause some unwanted effects. Possible side effects include:
  Stomach cramps
  Profuse bleeding
  Appetite loss
  Nausea and vomiting
  Swollen breasts
  Change in menstruation
  Rash, skin blisters
  Depression
  Dizziness

Overdose

The following symptoms may indicate an overdose:
  Nausea and vomiting
  Fluid retention
  Breast enlargement
  Abnormal vaginal bleeding
- Call a doctor or hospital emergency room for instructions.

Interactions

This medicine may interact with several other drugs such as adrenocorticosteroids, antidepressants, oral antidiabetics, insulin, phenobarbital, primidone.
- Be sure to tell your doctor about any medications you are currently taking.

Storage

Capsules, tablets, vaginal cream, transdermal patches, etc. should be stored at room temperature; store away from heat and direct light. Keep out of reach of children, since this medicine may be dangerous in children.

ESTROJECT-L.A.

Properties
This medicine contains estrogen as active ingredient. The medicine is prescribed for treatment of estrogen deficiency; it restores normal estrogen levels in tissues. There is no evidence that this drug is effective for nervous symptoms or depression occurring during menopause. They should not be used to treat this condition; they should be used only to replace the estrogen that is naturally absent after menopause.

Before using this medicine
Before you use this medicine check with your doctor, or pharmacist:
- if you ever had any unusual or allergic reaction to estrogens;
- if you are pregnant or intend to become pregnant within three months;
- if you are breast-feeding an infant;
- if you have any of the following medical problems:
  Diabetes
  Breast cancer
  Fibrocystic breast disease
  Fibroid uterine tumors
  Endometriosis
  Migraine headaches
  Epilepsy
  Porphyria
  High blood pressure
  Asthma
  Congestive heart failure
  Kidney disease
  Gallstones

Treatment
This medication is used to treat estrogen deficiency, specific symptoms of menopause, estrogen-deficiency osteoporosis, atrophic vaginitis, prostate cancer.

For safe and effective use of this medicine:
- Follow your doctor's instructions if this medicine was prescribed.
- Follow the manufacturer's package directions if you are treating yourself.
- Estrogens have been reported to increase the risk of endometrial carcinoma.

Side effects
Along with the needed effects, a medicine may cause some unwanted effects. Possible side effects include:
  Stomach cramps
  Profuse bleeding
  Appetite loss
  Nausea and vomiting
  Swollen breasts
  Change in menstruation
  Rash, skin blisters
  Depression
  Dizziness

Overdose
The following symptoms may indicate an overdose:
  Nausea and vomiting
  Fluid retention
  Breast enlargement
  Abnormal vaginal bleeding
- Call a doctor or hospital emergency room for instructions.

Interactions
This medicine may interact with several other drugs such as adrenocorticosteroids, antidepressants, oral antidiabetics, insulin, phenobarbital, primidone.
- Be sure to tell your doctor about any medications you are currently taking.

Storage
Capsules, tablets, vaginal cream, transdermal patches, etc. should be stored at room temperature; store away from heat and direct light. Keep out of reach of children, since this medicine may be dangerous in children.

ESTRONE

Properties
This medicine contains estrone as active ingredient. The medicine is prescribed for treatment of estrogen deficiency; it restores normal estrogen levels in tissues. There is no evidence that this drug is effective for nervous symptoms or depression occurring during menopause. They should not be used to treat this condition; they should be used only to replace the estrogen that is naturally absent after menopause.

Before using this medicine
Before you use this medicine check with your doctor, or pharmacist:
– if you ever had any unusual or allergic reaction to estrogens;
– if you are pregnant or intend to become pregnant within three months;
– if you are breast-feeding an infant;
– if you have any of the following medical problems:
  Diabetes
  Breast cancer
  Fibrocystic breast disease
  Fibroid uterine tumors
  Endometriosis
  Migraine headaches
  Epilepsy
  Porphyria
  High blood pressure
  Asthma
  Congestive heart failure
  Kidney disease
  Gallstones

Treatment
This medication is used to treat estrogen deficiency, specific symptoms of menopause, estrogen-deficiency osteoporosis, atrophic vaginitis, prostate cancer.
    For safe and effective use of this medicine:
♦ Follow your doctor's instructions if this medicine was prescribed.
♦ Follow the manufacturer's package directions if you are treating yourself.
♦ Estrogens have been reported to increase the risk of endometrial carcinoma.

Side effects
Along with the needed effects, a medicine may cause some unwanted effects. Possible side effects include:
    Stomach cramps
    Profuse bleeding
    Appetite loss
    Nausea and vomiting
    Swollen breasts
    Change in menstruation
    Rash, skin blisters
    Depression
    Dizziness

Overdose
The following symptoms may indicate an overdose:
    Nausea and vomiting
    Fluid retention
    Breast enlargement
    Abnormal vaginal bleeding
■ Call a doctor or hospital emergency room for instructions.

Interactions
This medicine may interact with several other drugs such as adrenocorticosteroids, antidepressants, oral antidiabetics, insulin, phenobarbital, primidone.
■ Be sure to tell your doctor about any medications you are currently taking.

Storage
Capsules, tablets, vaginal cream, transdermal patches, etc. should be stored at room temperature; store away from heat and direct light. Keep out of reach of children, since this medicine may be dangerous in children.

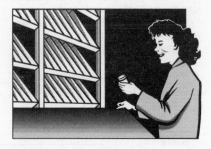

ESTROPIPATE

Properties

This medicine contains estropipate as active ingredient. The medicine is prescribed for treatment of estrogen deficiency; it restores normal estrogen levels in tissues. There is no evidence that this drug is effective for nervous symptoms or depression occurring during menopause. They should not be used to treat this condition; they should be used only to replace the estrogen that is naturally absent after menopause.

Before using this medicine

Before you use this medicine check with your doctor, or pharmacist:
– if you ever had any unusual or allergic reaction to estrogens;
– if you are pregnant or intend to become pregnant within three months;
– if you are breast-feeding an infant;
– if you have any of the following medical problems:
Diabetes
Breast cancer
Fibrocystic breast disease
Fibroid uterine tumors
Endometriosis
Migraine headaches
Epilepsy
Porphyria
High blood pressure
Asthma
Congestive heart failure
Kidney disease
Gallstones

Treatment

This medication is used to treat estrogen deficiency, specific symptoms of menopause, estrogen-deficiency osteoporosis, atrophic vaginitis, prostate cancer.

For safe and effective use of this medicine:
◆ Follow your doctor's instructions if this medicine was prescribed.
◆ Follow the manufacturer's package directions if you are treating yourself.
◆ Estrogens have been reported to increase the risk of endometrial carcinoma.

Side effects

Along with the needed effects, a medicine may cause some unwanted effects. Possible side effects include:
Stomach cramps
Profuse bleeding
Appetite loss
Nausea and vomiting
Swollen breasts
Change in menstruation
Rash, skin blisters
Depression
Dizziness

Overdose

The following symptoms may indicate an overdose:
Nausea and vomiting
Fluid retention
Breast enlargement
Abnormal vaginal bleeding
■ Call a doctor or hospital emergency room for instructions.

Interactions

This medicine may interact with several other drugs such as adrenocorticosteroids, antidepressants, oral antidiabetics, insulin, phenobarbital, primidone.
■ Be sure to tell your doctor about any medications you are currently taking.

Storage

Capsules, tablets, vaginal cream, transdermal patches, etc. should be stored at room temperature; store away from heat and direct light. Keep out of reach of children, since this medicine may be dangerous in children.

ETHON

Properties
This medicine contains as active ingredient methyclothiazide, a thiazide-like diuretic. Thiazide or thiazide-like diuretics are prescribed to treat high blood pressure (hypertension). They are also used to reduce fluid accumulation in the body caused by conditions such as heart failure, cirrhosis, kidney disease, and the long-term use of some medications. Thiazide diuretics may also be used for other conditions as determined by your doctor.

Before using this medicine
Before you use this medicine check with your doctor, or pharmacist:
- if you ever had any unusual or allergic reaction to sulfonamides (sulfa drugs) or any of the thiazide diuretics.
- if you are on a low-salt, low-sugar, or any other special diet, or if you are allergic to any substance, such as sulfites or other preservatives or dyes.
- if you are pregnant or inintend to become pregnant while using this medicine. When this medicine is used during pregnancy, it may cause side effects including jaundice, blood problems, and low potassium in the newborn.
- if you are breast-feeding an infant. Although this medicine has not been shown to cause problems in humans, the chance always exists since thiazide diuretics pass into breast milk.
- if you have any of the following medical problems:
  Diabetes
  Gout
  Kidney disease
  Liver disease
  Lupus erythematosus
  Pancreas disease

Treatment
This medication is used to treat high blood pressure (hypertension) and also to help reduce the amount of water in the body by increasing the flow of urine. This medicine will not cure your high blood pressure but it does help control it. You must continue to take it - even if you feel well - if you expect to keep your blood pressure down. You may have to take high blood pressure medicine for the rest of your life.

Thiazide diuretics may cause an unusual feeling of tiredness when you begin to take them. You may also notice an increase in urine or in frequency of urination. To keep this from affecting sleep:
- if you are to take a single dose a day, take it in the morning after breakfast;
- if you are to take more than one dose, take the last one not later than 6 p.m.

Side effects
Along with the needed effects, a medicine may cause some unwanted effects. Side effects that usually do not require medical attention: decreased sexual ability; dizziness or lightheadedness when standing up; increased sensitivity of skin to sunlight; loss of appetite; upset stomach.
- Side effects that should be reported to your doctor: black, tarry stools; blood in urine or stools; cough or hoarseness; fever or chills; joint pain; lower back or side pains; painful or difficult urination; pinpoint red spots on skin; skin rash or hives; stomach pain (severe) with nausea; unusual bleeding or bruising; yellow eyes or skin. This medicine may cause a loss of potassium from your body. Signs of too much potassium loss are: dryness of mouth; increased thirst; mood changes; muscle cramps or pain; nausea or vomiting; unusual tiredness or weakness; weak or irregular heartbeat.

Interactions
This medicine may interact with several other drugs.
- Be sure to tell your doctor about any medications you are currently taking.

Storage
Store at room temperature in a tightly closed container.

ETHRIL

Properties

This medicine contains erythromycin as active ingredient. This antibiotic is prescribed to treat infections caused by bacteria. They will not work for colds, flu, or other virus infections. Erythromycins are available only with your doctor's prescription.

Before using this medicine

Before you use this medicine check with your doctor, or pharmacist:
- if you ever had any unusual or allergic reaction to any of the erythromycins.
- if you are on a low-salt, low-sugar, or any other special diet, or if you are allergic to any substance, such as sulfites or other preservatives or dyes.
- if you are pregnant or inintend to become pregnant while using this medicine. Although erythromycins have not been shown to cause birth defects or other problems in humans, the chance always exists.
- if you are breast-feeding an infant. Most erythromycins pass into the breast milk. Although erythromycins have not been shown to cause problems in humans, the chance always exists.
- if you have lifer disease.

Treatment

This medication belongs to the general family of medicines called antibiotics. It is used to treat a wide variety of bacterial infections. It is also used to treat infections in persons who are allergic to penicillin. Erythromycins are also used to prevent "strep" infections in patients with a history of rheumatic heart disease. They may also be used in Legionnaires' disease and for other problems as determined by your doctor.
- Keep taking this medicine for the full time of treatment even if you begin to feel better after a few days; do not miss any doses. This is especially important if you have a "strep" infection since serious heart problems could develop later if your infection is not cleared up completely.
- If you do miss a dose of this medicine, take it as soon as possible. This will help to keep a constant amount of medicine in the blood. However, if it is almost time for your next dose, skip the missed dose and go back to your regular dosing schedule.
- This medication has been prescribed for your current infection only. Another infection later on, or one that someone else has, may require a different medicine. You should not give your medicine to other people or use it for other infections, unless your doctor specifically directs you to do so.

Side effects

Along with the needed effects, a medicine may cause some unwanted effects. Side effects that usually do not require medical attention: abdominal cramps, black tongue, cough, diarrhea, fatigue, irritation of the mouth, loss of appetite, nausea, or vomiting. These side effects should disappear as your body adjusts to the medication.
- Other side effects that should be reported to your doctor immediately are:
Fever
Hearing loss
Hives or rash
Rectal or vaginal itching
Yellowing of the eyes or skin

Interactions

This medicine may interact with several other drugs such as anticoagulants, theophylline preparations, carbamazepine, etc.
- Be sure to tell your doctor about any medications you are currently taking.

Storage

Tablets, capsules, etc. should be stored at room temperature in tightly closed, light-resistant containers as directed by your pharmacist.

ETHYLESTRENOL

Properties

This medicine is a member of the androgenic, or male, hormone group, containing an androgenic preparation as active ingredient. It is used in diseases in which male hormone replacement or augmentation is needed and also in so-called male menopause. It is also used to decrease calcium loss in osteoporosis, to block growth of breast cancer cells in females and to reduce breast pain and fullness following childbirth.

Before using this medicine

Before you use this medicine check with your doctor, or pharmacist:
- if you ever had any unusual or allergic reaction to androgens or corticosteroids in general.
- if you are on a low-salt, low-sugar, or any other special diet, or if you are allergic to any substance, such as certain preservatives or dyes.
- if you have any of the following medical problems:
Cancer prostate
Heart disease or atherosclerosis
Kidney or lifer disease
Breast cancer (males)
High blood pressure
High level of blood calcium
Epilepsy

Treatment

This medication is used to relieve or prevent the symptoms of your medical problem. Take them as directed. Do not take more of them and do not take them more often than recommended on the label. One should take the tablets or capsules with food to lessen stomach irritation. Take the medication at the same time each day. If you forget a dose take it as soon as you remember up to two hours late; wait for the next scheduled dose; don't double this dose. The risk to the unborn child outweighs the benefits of the drug.

Side effects

Females taking any androgenic drug should watch for deepening of the voice, oily skin, acne, hairiness, increased libido, and menstrual irregularities.

The following side effects may occur:
Acne or oily skin
Deep voice
Enlarged clitoris in females
Frequent erections in men
Sore mouth
Higher sex drive
Impotence in men
Yellow skin or eyes

These side effects should disappear as your body adjusts to the medication. Tell your doctor about any side effects that are persistent or particularly bothersome.

- Discontinue the use of the medication and seek emergency treatment in the following situations:
Intense itching
Weakness
Loss of consciousness
Depression or confusion
Swollen feet or legs
Shortness of breath
Irregularities of heartbeat
Difficult urination
Vaginal bleeding in women
Scrotum pain in men

Interactions

This medicine interacts with several other drugs such as anticoagulants, oral antidiabetics, cyclosporine, hepatotoxic drugs, oxyphenbutazone, phenobarbital, and phenylbutazone.

- Be sure to tell your doctor about any medications you are currently taking.

Storage

This medicine should be stored at room temperature in closed containers. Store away from heat and direct light. Keep out of reach of children, since overdose may be dangerous in children.

ETHYNIL ESTRADIOL

Properties
This medicine contains ethinyl estradiol as active ingredient. The medicine is prescribed for treatment of estrogen deficiency; it restores normal estrogen levels in tissues. There is no evidence that this drug is effective for nervous symptoms or depression occurring during menopause. They should not be used to treat this condition; they should be used only to replace the estrogen that is naturally absent after menopause.

Before using this medicine
Before you use this medicine check with your doctor, or pharmacist:
- if you ever had any unusual or allergic reaction to estrogens;
- if you are pregnant or intend to become pregnant within three months;
- if you are breast-feeding an infant;
- if you have any of the following medical problems:
  Diabetes
  Breast cancer
  Fibrocystic breast disease
  Fibroid uterine tumors
  Endometriosis
  Migraine headaches
  Epilepsy
  Porphyria
  High blood pressure
  Asthma
  Congestive heart failure
  Kidney disease
  Gallstones

Treatment
This medication is used to treat estrogen deficiency, specific symptoms of menopause, estrogen-deficiency osteoporosis, atrophic vaginitis, prostate cancer.
For safe and effective use of this medicine:
- ◆ Follow your doctor's instructions if this medicine was prescribed.
- ◆ Follow the manufacturer's package directions if you are treating yourself.
- ◆ Estrogens have been reported to increase the risk of endometrial carcinoma.

Side effects
Along with the needed effects, a medicine may cause some unwanted effects. Possible side effects include:
  Stomach cramps
  Profuse bleeding
  Appetite loss
  Nausea and vomiting
  Swollen breasts
  Change in menstruation
  Rash, skin blisters
  Depression
  Dizziness

Overdose
The following symptoms may indicate an overdose:
  Nausea and vomiting
  Fluid retention
  Breast enlargement
  Abnormal vaginal bleeding
- ▪ Call a doctor or hospital emergency room for instructions.

Interactions
This medicine may interact with several other drugs such as adrenocorticosteroids, antidepressants, oral antidiabetics, insulin, phenobarbital, primidone.
- ▪ Be sure to tell your doctor about any medications you are currently taking.

Storage
Capsules, tablets, vaginal cream, transdermal patches, etc. should be stored at room temperature; store away from heat and direct light. Keep out of reach of children, since this medicine may be dangerous in children.

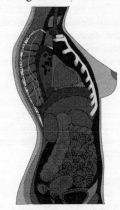

EVERONE

Properties
This medicine is a member of the androgenic, or male, hormone group, containing an androgenic preparation as active ingredient. It is used in diseases in which male hormone replacement or augmentation is needed and also in so-called male menopause. It is also used to decrease calcium loss in osteoporosis, to block growth of breast cancer cells in females and to reduce breast pain and fullness following childbirth.

Before using this medicine
Before you use this medicine check with your doctor, or pharmacist:
- if you ever had any unusual or allergic reaction to androgens or corticosteroids in general.
- if you are on a low-salt, low-sugar, or any other special diet, or if you are allergic to any substance, such as certain preservatives or dyes.
- if you have any of the following medical problems:
Cancer prostate
Heart disease or atherosclerosis
Kidney or lifer disease
Breast cancer (males)
High blood pressure
High level of blood calcium
Epilepsy

Treatment
This medication is used to relieve or prevent the symptoms of your medical problem. Take them as directed. Do not take more of them and do not take them more often than recommended on the label. One should take the tablets or capsules with food to lessen stomach irritation. Take the medication at the same time each day. If you forget a dose take it as soon as you remember up to two hours late; wait for the next scheduled dose; don't double this dose. The risk to the unborn child outweighs the benefits of the drug.

Side effects
Females taking any androgenic drug should watch for deepening of the voice, oily skin, acne, hairiness, increased libido, and menstrual irregularities.

The following side effects may occur:
Acne or oily skin
Deep voice
Enlarged clitoris in females
Frequent erections in men
Sore mouth
Higher sex drive
Impotence in men
Yellow skin or eyes
These side effects should disappear as your body adjusts to the medication. Tell your doctor about any side effects that are persistent or particularly bothersome.
- Discontinue the use of the medication and seek emergency treatment in the following situations:
Intense itching
Weakness
Loss of consciousness
Depression or confusion
Swollen feet or legs
Shortness of breath
Irregularities of heartbeat
Difficult urination
Vaginal bleeding in women
Scrotum pain in men

Interactions
This medicine interacts with several other drugs such as anticoagulants, oral antidiabetics, cyclosporine, hepatotoxic drugs, oxyphenbutazone, phenobarbital, and phenylbutazone.
- Be sure to tell your doctor about any medications you are currently taking.

Storage
This medicine should be stored at room temperature in closed containers. Store away from heat and direct light. Keep out of reach of children, since overdose may be dangerous in children.

FASTIN

Properties
This medicine contains phentermine as active ingredient; it is prescribed for appetite suppression.

Appetite suppressants are used in the short-term (a few weeks) treatment of obesity.

In a few weeks (6 to 12), these medicines in combination with dieting, exercise, and changes in eating habits can help patients lose weight.

However, since their appetite reducing effect is only temporary, they are useful only for the first weeks of dieting until new eating habits are established.

Before using this medicine
Before you use this medicine check with your doctor, or pharmacist:
- if you ever had any unusual or allergic reaction to any of the compounds of this medicine.
- if you are on a low-salt, low-sugar, or any other special diet, or if you are allergic to any substance, such as sulfites or other preservatives or dyes.
- if you are pregnant, inintend to become pregnant or breast-feeding an infant while using this medicine.
- if you have any of the following medical problems:
Diabetes mellitus
Epilepsy
Glaucoma
Heart disease
High blood pressure
Mental illness (severe)

Treatment
This medication is used to relieve or prevent the symptoms of your medical problem. Take them as directed. Do not take more of them and do not take them more often than recommended on the label. If too much of the drug is taken, it may become habit-forming.
- The medicine produces central nervous system stimulation, and it should not be taken by people with heart disease or high blood pressure.
- If you think this medicine is not working as well after you have taken it for a few weeks, do not increase the dose. Instead, check with your doctor.

Side effects
The following minor side effects may occur: irritability, nervousness, restlessness, trouble in sleeping.

These side effects should disappear as your body adjusts to the medication. Tell your doctor about any side effects that are persistent or particularly bothersome. It is especially important to tell your doctor about:
Mental depression
Nausea or vomiting
Stomach cramps or pain
Trembling
Unusual tiredness
- Discontinue use of the drug; call your doctor right away. Adverse reactions and side effects may be more frequent and severe in people over age 60 than in younger persons.

Interactions
This medicine interacts with several other drugs such as antihypertensives, other appetite suppressants, caffeine, central nervous system depressants, central nervous system stimulants, furazolidone, guanethidine, hydralazine, MAO inhibitors, methyldopa, molindone, phenothiazines, rauwolfia alkaloids, sodium bicarbonate. Interaction with alcoholic beverages may produce drowsiness, sleepiness, and/or inability to concentrate.
- Be sure to tell your doctor about any medications you are currently taking.

Storage
This medicine should be stored at room temperature in tightly closed containers. Store away from heat and direct light. Keep out of reach of children, since overdose may be very dangerous in children. Do not store this medicine in the bathroom medicine cabinet because the heat and moisture cause the medicine to break down. Do not keep outdated medicine or medicine no longer needed. Flush the contents of the container down the toilet.

FELODIPINE

Properties
This medicine contains felodipine as active ingredient. It is a so-called calcium channel blocker, working by blocking the passage of calcium into heart and smooth muscle. Since calcium is an essential factor in muscle contraction, any medicine that affects calcium in this way will interfere with the contraction of these muscles.

The medicine works by:
◆ reducing the work that the heart must perform;
◆ reducing the normal arterial blood pressure;
◆ increasing oxygen to the heart muscle.

The medicine is prescribed for the treatment of attacks of angina pectoris, irregular heartbeat, and high blood pressure. In many cases it can be used for the treatment and prevention of migraine.

Before using this medicine
Before you use this medicine check with your doctor, or pharmacist:
– if you ever had any unusual or allergic reaction to this medicine or any calcium channel blocker;
– if you are pregnant or inintend to become pregnant while using this medicine;
– if you have low blood pressure;
– if you have kidney or lifer disease;
– if you are breast-feeding an infant;
– if you easily get a rash or intensity sunburn in areas exposed to sun or ultraviolet light.

Treatment
This medication is used for treatment of heart conditions (for instance, angina pectoris) and high blood pressure. Tablets, capsules or extended-release tablets should be taken with liquid. The usual dose amounts to 30 to 100 milligrams a day.

For safe and effective use of medicine:
◆ Follow your doctor's instructions if this medicine was prescribed.
◆ Follow the manufacturer's package directions if you are treating yourself.

Side effects
Along with the needed effects, a medicine may cause some unwanted effects. Possible side effects include:
Tiredness
Changes in heartbeat
Wheezing
Cough
Shortness of breath
Dizziness
Fainting
Numbness in hands and feet
Tingling in hands and feet
Difficult urination
Constipation

Overdose
The following symptoms may be a sign of overdose:
Unusually fast heartbeat
Unusually slow heartbeat
Loss of consciousness
Cardiac arrest
▪ Call a doctor or hospital emergency room for instructions. If necessary start first aid immediately.

Interactions
The effect of this medicine may cause a blood pressure drop if taken together with antihypertensives. Cimetidine may increase the effect of the calcium blocker.

The simultaneous use of diuretics and calcium channel blockers may cause dangerous blood pressure drop.
▪ Be sure to tell your doctor about any medications you are currently taking.

Storage
Capsules, tablets, etc. should be stored at room temperature; store away from heat and direct light. Keep out of reach of children, since this medicine may be dangerous in children.

FEMOGEX

Properties
This medicine contains estrogen as active ingredient. The medicine is prescribed for treatment of estrogen deficiency; it restores normal estrogen levels in tissues. There is no evidence that this drug is effective for nervous symptoms or depression occurring during menopause. They should not be used to treat this condition; they should be used only to replace the estrogen that is naturally absent after menopause.

Before using this medicine
Before you use this medicine check with your doctor, or pharmacist:
- if you ever had any unusual or allergic reaction to estrogens;
- if you are pregnant or intend to become pregnant within three months;
- if you are breast-feeding an infant;
- if you have any of the following medical problems:
  Diabetes
  Breast cancer
  Fibrocystic breast disease
  Fibroid uterine tumors
  Endometriosis
  Migraine headaches
  Epilepsy
  Porphyria
  High blood pressure
  Asthma
  Congestive heart failure
  Kidney disease
  Gallstones

Treatment
This medication is used to treat estrogen deficiency, specific symptoms of menopause, estrogen-deficiency osteoporosis, atrophic vaginitis, prostate cancer.

For safe and effective use of this medicine:
- Follow your doctor's instructions if this medicine was prescribed.
- Follow the manufacturer's package directions if you are treating yourself.
- Estrogens have been reported to increase the risk of endometrial carcinoma.

Side effects
Along with the needed effects, a medicine may cause some unwanted effects. Possible side effects include:
  Stomach cramps
  Profuse bleeding
  Appetite loss
  Nausea and vomiting
  Swollen breasts
  Change in menstruation
  Rash, skin blisters
  Depression
  Dizziness

Overdose
The following symptoms may indicate an overdose:
  Nausea and vomiting
  Fluid retention
  Breast enlargement
  Abnormal vaginal bleeding
- Call a doctor or hospital emergency room for instructions.

Interactions
This medicine may interact with several other drugs such as adrenocorticosteroids, antidepressants, oral antidiabetics, insulin, phenobarbital, primidone.
- Be sure to tell your doctor about any medications you are currently taking.

Storage
Capsules, tablets, vaginal cream, transdermal patches, etc. should be stored at room temperature; store away from heat and direct light. Keep out of reach of children, since this medicine may be dangerous in children.

FLUNARIZINE

Properties

This medicine contains flunarizine as active ingredient. It is a so-called calcium channel blocker, working by blocking the passage of calcium into heart and smooth muscle. Since calcium is an essential factor in muscle contraction, any medicine that affects calcium in this way will interfere with the contraction of these muscles.

The medicine works by:

♦ reducing the work that the heart must perform;
♦ reducing the normal arterial blood pressure;
♦ increasing oxygen to the heart muscle.

The medicine is prescribed for the treatment of attacks of angina pectoris, irregular heartbeat, and high blood pressure. In many cases it can be used for the treatment and prevention of migraine.

Before using this medicine

Before you use this medicine check with your doctor, or pharmacist:

- if you ever had any unusual or allergic reaction to this medicine or any calcium channel blocker;
- if you are pregnant or inintend to become pregnant while using this medicine;
- if you have low blood pressure;
- if you have kidney or lifer disease;
- if you are breast-feeding an infant;
- if you easily get a rash or intensity sunburn in areas exposed to sun or ultraviolet light.

Treatment

This medication is used for treatment of heart conditions (for instance, angina pectoris) and high blood pressure. Tablets, capsules or extended-release tablets should be taken with liquid. The usual dose amounts to 30 to 100 milligrams a day.

For safe and effective use of medicine:

♦ Follow your doctor's instructions if this medicine was prescribed.
♦ Follow the manufacturer's package directions if you are treating yourself.

Side effects

Along with the needed effects, a medicine may cause some unwanted effects. Possible side effects include:

Tiredness
Changes in heartbeat
Wheezing
Cough
Shortness of breath
Dizziness
Fainting
Numbness in hands and feet
Tingling in hands and feet
Difficult urination
Constipation

Overdose

The following symptoms may be a sign of overdose:

Unusually fast heartbeat
Unusually slow heartbeat
Loss of consciousness
Cardiac arrest

■ Call a doctor or hospital emergency room for instructions. If necessary start first aid immediately.

Interactions

The effect of this medicine may cause a blood pressure drop if taken together with antihypertensives. Cimetidine may increase the effect of the calcium blocker.

The simultaneous use of diuretics and calcium channel blockers may cause dangerous blood pressure drop.

■ Be sure to tell your doctor about any medications you are currently taking.

Storage

Capsules, tablets, etc. should be stored at room temperature; store away from heat and direct light. Keep out of reach of children, since this medicine may be dangerous in children.

FLUOXYMESTERONE

Properties
This medicine is a member of the androgenic, or male, hormone group, containing an androgenic preparation as active ingredient. It is used in diseases in which male hormone replacement or augmentation is needed and also in so-called male menopause. It is also used to decrease calcium loss in osteoporosis, to block growth of breast cancer cells in females and to reduce breast pain and fullness following childbirth.

Before using this medicine
Before you use this medicine check with your doctor, or pharmacist:
– if you ever had any unusual or allergic reaction to androgens or corticosteroids in general.
– if you are on a low-salt, low-sugar, or any other special diet, or if you are allergic to any substance, such as certain preservatives or dyes.
– if you have any of the following medical problems:
Cancer prostate
Heart disease or atherosclerosis
Kidney or lifer disease
Breast cancer (males)
High blood pressure
High level of blood calcium
Epilepsy

Treatment
This medication is used to relieve or prevent the symptoms of your medical problem. Take them as directed. Do not take more of them and do not take them more often than recommended on the label. One should take the tablets or capsules with food to lessen stomach irritation. Take the medication at the same time each day. If you forget a dose take it as soon as you remember up to two hours late; wait for the next scheduled dose; don't double this dose. The risk to the unborn child outweighs the benefits of the drug.

Side effects
Females taking any androgenic drug should watch for deepening of the voice, oily skin, acne, hairiness, increased libido, and menstrual irregularities.

The following side effects may occur:
Acne or oily skin
Deep voice
Enlarged clitoris in females
Frequent erections in men
Sore mouth
Higher sex drive
Impotence in men
Yellow skin or eyes
These side effects should disappear as your body adjusts to the medication. Tell your doctor about any side effects that are persistent or particularly bothersome.
- Discontinue the use of the medication and seek emergency treatment in the following situations:
Intense itching
Weakness
Loss of consciousness
Depression or confusion
Swollen feet or legs
Shortness of breath
Irregularities of heartbeat
Difficult urination
Vaginal bleeding in women
Scrotum pain in men

Interactions
This medicine interacts with several other drugs such as anticoagulants, oral antidiabetics, cyclosporine, hepatotoxic drugs, oxyphenbutazone, phenobarbital, and phenylbutazone.
- Be sure to tell your doctor about any medications you are currently taking.

Storage
This medicine should be stored at room temperature in closed containers. Store away from heat and direct light. Keep out of reach of children, since overdose may be dangerous in children.

FLUPHENAZINE

Properties
This medicine contains as active ingredient fluphenazine, a phenothiazine derivative. Phenothiazines are a family of medicines used to treat nervous, mental, and emotional conditions. Some are used to control anxiety, restlessness, nausea and vomiting, and severe hiccups. This medicine is available only with your doctor's prescription.

Before using this medicine
Before you use this medicine check with your doctor, or pharmacist:
- if you ever had any unusual or allergic reaction to phenothiazine medicines.
- if you are on a low-salt, low-sugar, or any other special diet, or if you are allergic to any substance, such as sulfites or other preservatives or dyes.
- if you are pregnant or intend to become pregnant while using this medicine. Although phenothiazines have not been shown to cause birth defects, some side effects such as jaundice and muscle tremors have occurred in a few newborns whose mothers received phenothiazines during pregnancy.
- if you are breast-feeding an infant. Although this medicine has not been shown to cause problems in humans the chance does exist since some phenothiazines are known to pass into the breast milk.
- if you have any of the following medical problems:
Alcoholism
Blood disease
Difficult urination
Enlarged prostate
Glaucoma
Heart or blood vessel disease
Liver or lung disease
Parkinson's disease
Stomach ulcers

Treatment
This medication is prescribed to treat the symptoms of certain types of mental illness or emotional problems. In order to avoid stomach irritation, you can take the tablet or capsule forms of this medication with a meal or with a glass of water or milk (unless your doctor or pharmacist directs you to do otherwise).

Side effects
Along with the needed effects, a medicine may cause some unwanted effects. Minor side effects are: blurred vision, constipation, decreased sweating, diarrhea, dizziness, drooling, drowsiness, dry mouth, fatigue, jitteriness, menstrual irregularities, nasal congestion, restlessness, tremors, vomiting, or weight gain.
- Tell your doctor about any side effects that are persistent or particularly bothersome. It is especially important to tell your doctor about:
Breast enlargement
Chest pain or convulsions
Darkened skin
Difficulty in swallowing
Fainting or fever
Involuntary movements
Palpitations or sleep disorders
Rash or sore throat
Uncoordinated movements
Unusual bleeding or bruising
Visual disturbances
Yellowing of the eyes or skin

Interactions
This medicine may interact with several other drugs such as barbiturates, sleeping pills, narcotics, other tranquilizers, or any other medication that may produce a sedative effect. Avoid alcohol.

Storage
Store this medication as directed on the label. Keep out of the reach of children.

FLURAZEPAM

Properties

This medicine contains as active ingredient flurazepam, a benzodiazepine preparation. Benzodiazepines belong to the group of psychoactive medicines that influence the activity of the brain. Some are used to relieve nervousness or tension. It is effective for this purpose for short periods. Others are used for sleeplessness or to relax muscles or relieve muscle spasm. The benzodiazepines may also be used for other conditions as determined by your doctor.

Before using this medicine

Before you use this medicine check with your doctor:
- if you ever had any unusual or allergic reaction to benzodiazepines.
- if you are on a low-salt, low-sugar, or any other special diet, or if you are allergic to any substance, such as sulfites or other preservatives or dyes.
- if you are pregnant or inintend to become pregnant while using this medicine. Some benzodiazepines have been reported to increase the chance of birth defects when used during the first 3 months of pregnancy.
- if you are breast-feeding an infant. Benzodiazepines may pass into the breast milk and cause drowsiness, unusually slow heartbeat, shortness of breath, or troubled breathing in infants of mothers taking this medicine.
- if you have any of the following medical problems: asthma, bronchitis, emphysema, or other chronic lung disease; epilepsy or history of convulsions; hyperactivity (in children); kidney or lifer disease; mental depression or illness; myasthania gravis, porphyria.

Treatment

This medication is used to relieve or prevent the symptoms of your medical problem. Benzodiazepines are mainly used as antianxiety agents, anticonvulsants, or sedatives. Take them as directed. Do not take more of them and do not take them more often than recommended on the label, unless otherwise directed by your doctor. Benzodiazepine tranquilizing drugs can be abused if taken for long periods of time and it is possible to develop withdrawal symptoms if you discontinue the therapy abruptly.

Side effects

Along with the needed effects, a medicine may cause some unwanted effects. Minor side effects are: bitter taste in the mouth, dizziness, drowsiness, depression, constipation, dry mouth, excessive salivation, fatigue, flushing, headache, heartburn, loss of appetite, nausea, nervousness, sweating or vomiting. As your body adjusts to the medicine, these side effects should disappear.
- Tell your doctor about any side effects that are persistent or particularly bothersome. It is especially important to tell your doctor about:
  Blurred or double vision
  Chest pain
  Difficulty in urinating
  Fainting or falling
  Fever or hallucinations
  Joint pain
  Mouth sores
  Nightmares
  Palpitations
  Severe depression
  Shortness of breath
  Slurred speech
  Uncoordinated movements
  Unusual tiredness
  Yellowing of the skin

Interactions
- This medicine may interact with several other drugs. This medicine will add to the effects of alcohol, and CNS depressants.
- Be sure to tell your doctor about any medications you are currently taking.

Storage

Store at room temperature in tightly closed, light-resistant-resistant containers. Keep out of the reach of children since overdose may be especially dangerous in children.

FORTAZ

Properties
This medicine contains cephalosporin as active ingredient. Cephalosporins belong to the general family of medicines called antibiotics, used in the treatment of infections caused by bacteria. They work by killing bacteria or preventing their growth. Cephalosporins will not work for colds, fly, or other viral infections.

Before using this medicine
Before you use this medicine check with your doctor:
- if you ever had any unusual or allergic reaction to any of the cephalosporins, penicillins, penicillin-like medicines, or penicillamine.
- if you are on a low-salt, low-sugar, or any other special diet, or if you are allergic to any substance, such as sulfites or other preservatives or dyes.
- if you are pregnant or inintend to become pregnant while using this medicine. Although cephalosporins have not been shown to cause birth defects or other problems in humans, the chance always exists.
- if you are breast-feeding an infant. Most cephalosporins pass into the breast milk, usually in small amounts.
- if you have any of the following medical problems:
Bleeding problem
Kidney or lifer disease

Treatment
This medication belongs to the general family of medicines called antibiotics. It is used to treat a wide variety of bacterial infections. It is also used to treat infections in persons who are allergic to penicillin.
- Keep taking this medicine for the full time of treatment even if you begin to feel better after a few days; do not miss any doses.
- If you do miss a dose of this medicine, take it as soon as possible. This will help to keep a constant amount of medicine in the blood. However, if it is almost time for your next dose, skip the missed dose and go back to your regular dosing schedule.
- This medication has been prescribed for your current infection only. Another infection later on, or one that someone else has, may require a different medicine. You should not give your medicine to other people or use it for other infections, unless your doctor specifically directs you to do so.
- Take the medicine at the same times each day, 1 hour before or 2 hours after eating.

Side effects
Along with the needed effects, a medicine may cause some unwanted effects. Side effects that usually do not require medical attention: rectal itching, oral or vaginal white spots, mild diarrhea. These side effects should disappear as your body adjusts to the medication.
- Other side effects that should be reported to your doctor immediately are:
Hives, rash
Intense itching
Faintness soon after a dose
Difficulty in breathing
Nausea and vomiting
Severe diarrhea
Unusual weakness or tiredness
Bleeding or bruising

Interactions
This medicine may interact with several other drugs such as anticoagulants, theophylline preparations, probenecid, tetracyclines, etc.
- Be sure to tell your doctor about any medications you are currently taking.

Storage
Tablets, capsules, etc. should be stored at room temperature. Store the liquid form in the refrigerator. Keep out of the reach of children. Do not keep outdated medicine or medicine no longer needed.

GAMAZOLE

Properties

This medicine contains sulfamethoxazole, a sulfonamide, as active ingredient. Sulfonamides are prescribed to treat infections caused by bacteria. They will not work for colds, flu, or other virus infections.

Before using this medicine

Before you use this medicine check with your doctor:
- if you ever had any unusual or allergic reaction to any of the compounds of the medicine.
- if you are on a low-salt, low-sugar, or any other special diet, or if you are allergic to any substance, such as sulfites or other preservatives or dyes.
- if you are pregnant or in intend to become pregnant while using this medicine. Although sulfonamides have not been shown to cause defects in humans, the chance may exists.
- if you are breast-feeding an infant. Most sulfonamides pass into the breast milk in small amounts and may cause unwanted effects in infants with some specific conditions.
- if you have any of the following medical problems:
  Kidney disease
  Liver disease
  Porphyria
  Deficiency of enzymes such as G6PD

Treatment

This medication is used to treat an infection caused by bacteria. Most sulfonamides are best taken with a full glass (8 ounces) of water on an empty stomach, either one hour before or two hours after a meal. Follow your doctor's or pharmacist's directions on how to take your medicine.
- Keep taking this medicine for the full time of treatment even if you begin to feel better after a few days; do not miss any doses.
- If you do miss a dose of this medicine, take the missed dose immediately.
- This medication works best when the level of medicine in your bloodstream (and urine) is kept constant. It is best, therefore, to take the doses at evenly spaced intervals day and night. if you take two doses a day, the doses should be spaced 12 hours apart.

Side effects

Along with the needed effects, a medicine may cause some unwanted effects. Side effects that usually do not require medical attention: abdominal pain, diarrhea, dizziness, headache, loss of appetite, nausea, sore mouth, or vomiting. These side effects should disappear as your body adjusts to the medication. Sulfonamides can increase sensitivity to sunlight. It is, therefore, important to avoid prolonged exposure to sunlight and sunlamps.

Tell your doctor about any side effects that are persistent or particularly bothersome. It is especially important to tell your doctor about:
  Bloody urine
  Difficult urination
  Difficulty in breathing
  Difficulty in swallowing
  Fever or hallucinations
  Itching, rash, or pale skin
  Joint pain, lower back pain
  Ringing in the ears
  Sore throat
  Swollen or inflamed tongue
  Tingling in hands or feet
  Unusual bleeding, bruising
  Yellowing of the eyes or skin

Interactions

This medicine may interact with several other drugs such as anticoagulants, oral antidiabetic agents, aspirin, some antibiotics, or anticancer drugs.
- Be sure to tell your doctor about any medications you are currently taking.

Storage

Tablets, capsules, suspension, etc. should be stored at room temperature as directed by your pharmacist or according to instructions on the label.

GANTANOL

Properties

This medicine contains sumfamethoxazole, a sulfonamide, as active ingredient. Sulfonamides are prescribed to treat infections caused by bacteria. They will not work for colds, flu, or other virus infections.

Before using this medicine

Before you use this medicine check with your doctor:
- if you ever had any unusual or allergic reaction to any of the compounds of the medicine.
- if you are on a low-salt, low-sugar, or any other special diet, or if you are allergic to any substance, such as sulfites or other preservatives or dyes.
- if you are pregnant or inintend to become pregnant while using this medicine. Although sulfonamides have not been shown to cause defects in humans, the chance may exists.
- if you are breast-feeding an infant. Most sulfonamides pass into the breast milk in small amounts and may cause unwanted effects in infants with some specific conditions.
- if you have any of the following medical problems:
  Kidney disease
  Liver disease
  Porphyria
  Deficiency of enzymes such as
   G6PD

Treatment

This medication is used to treat an infection caused by bacteria. Most sulfonamides are best taken with a full glass (8 ounces) of water on an empty stomach, either one hour before or two hours after a meal. Follow your doctor's or pharmacist's directions on how to take your medicine.
- Keep taking this medicine for the full time of treatment even if you begin to feel better after a few days; do not miss any doses.
- If you do miss a dose of this medicine, take the missed dose immediately.
- This medication works best when the level of medicine in your bloodstream (and urine) is kept constant. It is best, therefore, to take the doses at evenly spaced intervals day and night. if you take two doses a day, the doses should be spaced 12 hours apart.

Side effects

Along with the needed effects, a medicine may cause some unwanted effects. Side effects that usually do not require medical attention: abdominal pain, diarrhea, dizziness, headache, loss of appetite, nausea, sore mouth, or vomiting. These side effects should disappear as your body adjusts to the medication. Sulfonamides can increase sensitivity to sunlight. It is, therefore, important to avoid prolonged exposure to sunlight and sunlamps.

Tell your doctor about any side effects that are persistent or particularly bothersome. It is especially important to tell your doctor about:
  Bloody urine
  Difficult or painful urination
  Difficulty in breathing
  Difficulty in swallowing
  Fever or hallucinations
  Itching, rash, or pale skin
  Joint pain, lower back pain
  Ringing in the ears
  Sore throat
  Swollen or inflamed tongue
  Tingling in hands or feet
  Unusual bleeding, bruising
  Yellowing of the eyes or skin

Interactions

This medicine may interact with several other drugs such as anticoagulants, oral antidiabetic agents, aspirin, some antibiotics, or anticancer drugs.
- Be sure to tell your doctor about any medications you are currently taking.

Storage

Tablets, capsules, suspension, etc. should be stored at room temperature as directed by your pharmacist or according to instructions on the label.

GANTRISIN

Properties
This medicine contains sulfisoxasole, a sulfonamide, as active ingredient. Sulfonamides are prescribed to treat infections caused by bacteria. They will not work for colds, flu, or other virus infections.

Before using this medicine
Before you use this medicine check with your doctor:
- if you ever had any unusual or allergic reaction to any of the compounds of the medicine.
- if you are on a low-salt, low-sugar, or any other special diet, or if you are allergic to any substance, such as sulfites or other preservatives or dyes.
- if you are pregnant or inintend to become pregnant while using this medicine. Although sulfonamides have not been shown to cause defects in humans, the chance may exists.
- if you are breast-feeding an infant. Most sulfonamides pass into the breast milk in small amounts and may cause unwanted effects in infants with some specific conditions.
- if you have any of the following medical problems:
Kidney disease
Liver disease
Porphyria
Deficiency of enzymes such as G6PD

Treatment
This medication is used to treat an infection caused by bacteria. Most sulfonamides are best taken with a full glass (8 ounces) of water on an empty stomach, either one hour before or two hours after a meal. Follow your doctor's or pharmacist's directions on how to take your medicine.
- Keep taking this medicine for the full time of treatment even if you begin to feel better after a few days; do not miss any doses.
- If you do miss a dose of this medicine, take the missed dose immediately.
- This medication works best when the level of medicine in your bloodstream (and urine) is kept constant. It is best, therefore, to take the doses at evenly spaced intervals day and night. if you take two doses a day, the doses should be spaced 12 hours apart.

Side effects
Along with the needed effects, a medicine may cause some unwanted effects. Side effects that usually do not require medical attention: abdominal pain, diarrhea, dizziness, headache, loss of appetite, nausea, sore mouth, or vomiting. These side effects should disappear as your body adjusts to the medication.
Sulfonamides can increase sensitivity to sunlight. It is, therefore, important to avoid prolonged exposure to sunlight and sunlamps.
Tell your doctor about any side effects that are persistent or particularly bothersome. It is especially important to tell your doctor about:
Bloody urine
Difficult urination
Difficulty in breathing
Difficulty in swallowing
Fever or hallucinations
Itching, rash, or pale skin
Joint pain, lower back pain
Ringing in the ears
Sore throat
Swollen or inflamed tongue
Tingling in hands or feet
Unusual bleeding
Yellowing of the eyes or skin

Interactions
This medicine may interact with several other drugs such as anticoagulants, oral antidiabetic agents, aspirin, some antibiotics, or anticancer drugs.
- Be sure to tell your doctor about any medications you are currently taking.

Storage
Tablets, capsules, suspension, etc. should be stored at room temperature as directed by your pharmacist or according to instructions on the label.

GARDENAL

Properties
This medicine contains as active ingredient the barbiturate phenobarbital. Barbiturates belong to the group of medicines called central nervous system depressants (medicines that slow down the nervous system).

Barbiturates may partially block nerve impulses at nerve-cell connections. They may be used to treat insomnia (sleeplessness) by helping patients fall asleep. Also, they may be used to relieve anxiety or tension. Some of the barbiturates are used as anticonvulsants to help control convulsions in certain disorders or diseases, such as epilepsy. If too much of the drug is used, it may become habit-forming (causing mental or physical dependence).

Before using this medicine
Before you use this medicine check with your doctor, or pharmacist:
- if you ever had any unusual or allergic reaction to this medicine or one of its components.
- if you are on a low-salt, low-sugar, or any other special diet, or if you are allergic to preservatives or dyes.
- if you are pregnant or inintend to become pregnant while using this medicine, since barbiturates have been shown to increase the chance of birth defects in humans. Taking barbiturates regularly during the last 3 months of pregnancy may cause the baby to become dependent on the medicine. This may lead to withdrawal side effects in the baby after birth.
- if you have any of the following medical problems:
  Anemia (severe)
  Diabetes mellitus (sugar disease)
  Hyperactivity (in children)
  Kidney or lifer disease
  Mental depression
  Overactive thyroid

Treatment
This medication is used to treat the symptoms of your medical condition. Barbiturates act in the central nervous system; some of their side effects are also caused by actions in the central nervous system. Use this medicine as directed by your doctor. Do not use more of it, do not use it more often, and do not use it for a longer period of time than your doctor ordered.
- If you are taking this medication on a regular schedule and you miss a dose, take the missed dose as soon as possible, unless it is almost time for your next dose. In that case do not take the missed dose at all.
- If a barbiturate is used for a long time, it may become habit-forming. Physical dependence may lead to withdrawal side effects when you stop taking this medicine.

Side effects
Along with the needed effects, a medicine may cause some unwanted effects. These side effects may go away during treatment as your body adjusts to the medicine. Such minor side effects are: depression, confusion, diarrhea, nausea, vomiting, joint or muscle pain, slurred speech, hallucinations, headache, decreased sex drive.
- Check with your doctor immediately if any of the following side effects occur:
  Rash or hives
  Face, lip or eyelid swelling
  Sore throat, fever
  Agitation
  Slow heartbeat
  Difficult breathing or chest pain

Interactions
This medicine may interact with several other drugs such as medicines acting on the central nervous system (e.g., antihistamines; beta-adrenergic blockers; MAO inhibitors; mind-altering drugs; nabilone; antidepressants; clozapine; anticonvulsants).

Storage
The medicine should be stored at room temperature in a tightly closed, light-resistant container. Keep out of reach of children since overdose is very dangerous in children.

GEMONIL

Properties

This medicine contains as active ingredient the barbiturate metharbital. Barbiturates belong to the group of medicines called central nervous system depressants (medicines that slow down the nervous system).

Barbiturates may partially block nerve impulses at nerve-cell connections. They may be used to treat insomnia (sleeplessness) by helping patients fall asleep. Also, they may be used to relieve anxiety or tension. Some of the barbiturates are used as anticonvulsants to help control convulsions in certain disorders or diseases, such as epilepsy. If too much of the drug is used, it may become habit-forming (causing mental or physical dependence).

Before using this medicine

Before you use this medicine check with your doctor, or pharmacist:
- if you ever had any unusual or allergic reaction to this medicine or one of its components.
- if you are on a low-salt, low-sugar, or any other special diet, or if you are allergic to preservatives or dyes.
- if you are pregnant or inintend to become pregnant while using this medicine, since barbiturates have been shown to increase the chance of birth defects in humans. Taking barbiturates regularly during the last 3 months of pregnancy may cause the baby to become dependent on the medicine. This may lead to withdrawal side effects in the baby after birth.
- if you have any of the following medical problems:
  Anemia (severe)
  Diabetes mellitus (sugar disease)
  Hyperactivity (in children)
  Kidney or lifer disease
  Mental depression
  Overactive thyroid

Treatment

This medication is used to treat the symptoms of your medical condition. Barbiturates act in the central nervous system; some of their side effects are also caused by actions in the central nervous system. Use this medicine as directed by your doctor. Do not use more of it, do not use it more often, and do not use it for a longer period of time than your doctor ordered.

- If you are taking this medication on a regular schedule and you miss a dose, take the missed dose as soon as possible, unless it is almost time for your next dose. In that case do not take the missed dose at all.
- If a barbiturate is used for a long time, it may become habit-forming. Physical dependence may lead to withdrawal side effects when you stop taking this medicine.

Side effects

Along with the needed effects, a medicine may cause some unwanted effects. These side effects may go away during treatment as your body adjusts to the medicine. Such minor side effects are: depression, confusion, diarrhea, nausea, vomiting, joint or muscle pain, slurred speech, hallucinations, headache, decreased sex drive.

- Check with your doctor immediately if any of the following side effects occur:
  Rash or hives
  Face, lip or eyelid swelling
  Sore throat, fever
  Agitation
  Slow heartbeat
  Difficult breathing or chest pain

Interactions

This medicine may interact with several other drugs such as medicines acting on the central nervous system (e.g., antihistamines; beta-adrenergic blockers; MAO inhibitors; mind-altering drugs; nabilone; antidepressants; clozapine; anticonvulsants).

Storage

The medicine should be stored at room temperature in a tightly closed, light-resistant container. Keep out of reach of children since overdose is very dangerous in children.

GENCEPT

Properties
This medicine contains norethindrone and ethinyl estradiol as active ingredients. It is an oral contraceptive prescribed to prevent pregnancy and/or to regulate menstrual periods.

The drug works by altering the mucus at the cervix entrance to prevent the entry of sperm. It also alters the uterus lining to resist implantation of the fertilized egg. Oral contraceptives create the same chemical atmosphere in blood that exists during pregnancy.

Before using this medicine
Before you use this medicine check with your doctor, or pharmacist:
- if you ever had any unusual or allergic reaction to estrogens or progestogen;
- if you are pregnant or want to become pregnant within three months;
- if you are breast-feeding an infant;
- if you have any of the following medical problems:
  Diabetes
  Ailments of the breast
  Disorders of the uterus
  Migraine or epilepsy
  High blood pressure
  Asthma or heart conditions
  Kidney disease
  Gallstones

Treatment
This medication is used to prevent pregnancy or to regulate menstrual periods.

Adverse reactions
Along with the needed effects, a medicine may cause some unwanted effects or adverse reactions.
- *An increased risk of the following adverse reactions has been associated with the use of oral contraceptives:*
  Thrombophlebitis
  Venous thrombosis
  Arterial thromboembolism
  Pulmonary (lung) embolism
  Myocardial infarction
  Cerebral hemorrhage
  Cerebral thrombosis
  Hypertension
  Gallbladder disease
  Hepatic (liver) hepatomas
  Benign lifer tumors
- *The following adverse reactions have been reported in patients receiving oral contraceptives and are believed to be drug-related:*
  Nausea and vomiting
  Abdominal cramps
  Breakthrough bleeding
  Spotting
  Change in menstrual flow
  Amenorrhea
  Temporary infertility
  Edema
  Breast changes
  Weight changes
  Cholestatic jaundice
  Migraine
  Rash (allergic)
  Mental depression
  Vaginal candidiasis

Interactions
This medicine may interact with several other drugs such as antibiotics, anticoagulants, anticonvulsants, antidepressants, oral antidiabetics, antihistamines, barbiturates, oral hypoglycemics, insulin, meperidine.
- Be sure to tell your doctor about any medications you are currently taking.

Storage
Tablets should be stored at room temperature; store away from heat and direct light. Keep out of reach of children, since this medicine may be dangerous in children.

GENORA

Properties

This medicine contains norethindrone and ethinyl estradiol as active ingredients. It is an oral contraceptive prescribed to prevent pregnancy and/or to regulate menstrual periods.

The drug works by altering the mucus at the cervix entrance to prevent the entry of sperm. It also alters the uterus lining to resist implantation of the fertilized egg. Oral contraceptives create the same chemical atmosphere in blood that exists during pregnancy.

Before using this medicine

Before you use this medicine check with your doctor, or pharmacist:
- if you ever had any unusual or allergic reaction to estrogens or progestogen;
- if you are pregnant or want to become pregnant within three months;
- if you are breast-feeding an infant;
- if you have any of the following medical problems:
  Diabetes
  Ailments of the breast
  Disorders of the uterus
  Migraine or epilepsy
  High blood pressure
  Asthma or heart conditions
  Kidney disease
  Gallstones

Treatment

This medication is used to prevent pregnancy or to regulate menstrual periods.

Adverse reactions

Along with the needed effects, a medicine may cause some unwanted effects or adverse reactions.
- *An increased risk of the following adverse reactions has been associated with the use of oral contraceptives:*
  Thrombophlebitis
  Venous thrombosis
  Arterial thromboembolism
  Pulmonary (lung) embolism
  Myocardial infarction
  Cerebral hemorrhage
  Cerebral thrombosis

Hypertension
Gallbladder disease
Hepatic (liver) hepatomas
Benign lifer tumors
- *The following adverse reactions have been reported in patients receiving oral contraceptives and are believed to be drug-related:*
  Nausea and vomiting
  Abdominal cramps
  Breakthrough bleeding
  Spotting
  Change in menstrual flow
  Amenorrhea
  Temporary infertility
  Edema
  Breast changes
  Weight changes
  Cholestatic jaundice
  Migraine
  Rash (allergic)
  Mental depression
  Vaginal candidiasis

Interactions

This medicine may interact with several other drugs such as antibiotics, anticoagulants, anticonvulsants, antidepressants, oral antidiabetics, antihistamines, barbiturates, oral hypoglycemics, insulin, meperidine.
- Be sure to tell your doctor about any medications you are currently taking.

Storage

Tablets should be stored at room temperature; store away from heat and direct light. Keep out of reach of children, since this medicine may be dangerous in children.

GLYCERYL TRINITRATE

Properties
This medicine contains nitroglycerin as active ingredient. Nitrates improve the supply of blood and oxygen to the heart. This medication is for oral use.

Before using this medicine
Before you use this medicine check with your doctor, or pharmacist:
- if you ever had any unusual or allergic reaction to nitrates or nitrites.
- if you are on a low-salt, low-sugar, or any other special diet, or if you are allergic to any substance, such as sulfites or other preservatives or dyes.
- if you are pregnant or intend to become pregnant while using this medicine. Although nitrates have not been shown to cause problems in humans, the chance always exists.
- if you are breast-feeding an infant.
- if you have recently had a heart attack or stroke.
- if you have any of the following medical problems:
  Anemia
  Glaucoma
  Intestinal problems
  Overactive thyroid
- if you are now taking any of the following medicines or types of medicines:
  Antihypertensives
  Asthma or hay fever medicine
  Cold medicine
  Decongestant
  Medicine for appetite control
  Narcotic
  Pain medicine
  Sinus congestion medicine

Treatment
This medication is used to treat and prevent angina (chest pain). Nitroglycerin is a vasodilator, which relaxes the muscles of the blood vessels, causing an increase in the oxygen supply to the heart. The oral tablets, capsules, ointment and patches do not act quickly; they are used to prevent chest pain. The sublingual tablets and oral spray act quickly and can be used to relieve chest pain after it has started.

- Take this medicine exactly as directed by your doctor or pharmacist. It will work only if taken correctly.
- If you are taking this medicine regularly and you miss a dose, take it as soon as possible. However, if your next scheduled dose; is within 2 hours (or within 6 hours for extended-release capsules or tablets), skip the missed dose and go back to your regular dosing schedule.
- If you have been taking this medicine regularly for several weeks or more, do not suddenly stop using it. Stopping suddenly may bring on attacks of angina.

Side effects
There are a number of side effects that usually do not require medical attention. These possible side effects may go away during treatment; however, if they continue or are bothersome, check with your doctor, nurse, or pharmacist. More common are: dizziness, lightheadedness, or fainting when standing up; fast pulse; flushing of face and neck; headache; nausea or vomiting.
Side effects that should be reported to your doctor are: blurred vision; dry mouth; severe or prolonged headache; skin rash.

Interactions
This medicine may interact with several other drugs such as tricyclic antidepressants and cough medicines. Before starting to take or apply nitroglycerin.
- Be sure to tell your doctor about any medications you are currently taking.

Storage
Tablets, capsules, and oral spray should be stored as in a tightly capped bottle in a cool, dry place. Ointment and patches should be stored at room temperature in their original containers. Keep out of reach of children. Do not keep outdated medicine or medicine no longer needed.

GYNOGEN L.A.

Properties

This medicine contains estrogen as active ingredient. The medicine is prescribed for treatment of estrogen deficiency; it restores normal estrogen levels in tissues. There is no evidence that this drug is effective for nervous symptoms or depression occurring during menopause. They should not be used to treat this condition; they should be used only to replace the estrogen that is naturally absent after menopause.

Before using this medicine

Before you use this medicine check with your doctor, or pharmacist:
- if you ever had any unusual or allergic reaction to estrogens;
- if you are pregnant or intend to become pregnant within three months;
- if you are breast-feeding an infant;
- if you have any of the following medical problems:
Diabetes
Breast cancer
Fibrocystic breast disease
Fibroid uterine tumors
Endometriosis
Migraine headaches
Epilepsy
Porphyria
High blood pressure
Asthma
Congestive heart failure
Kidney disease
Gallstones

Treatment

This medication is used to treat estrogen deficiency, specific symptoms of menopause, estrogen-deficiency osteoporosis, atrophic vaginitis, prostate cancer.

For safe and effective use of this medicine:
- ◆ Follow your doctor's instructions if this medicine was prescribed.
- ◆ Follow the manufacturer's package directions if you are treating yourself.
- ◆ Estrogens have been reported to increase the risk of endometrial carcinoma.

Side effects

Along with the needed effects, a medicine may cause some unwanted effects. Possible side effects include:
Stomach cramps
Profuse bleeding
Appetite loss
Nausea and vomiting
Swollen breasts
Change in menstruation
Rash, skin blisters
Depression
Dizziness

Overdose

The following symptoms may indicate an overdose:
Nausea and vomiting
Fluid retention
Breast enlargement
Abnormal vaginal bleeding
- ▪ Call a doctor or hospital emergency room for instructions.

Interactions

This medicine may interact with several other drugs such as adrenocorticosteroids, antidepressants, oral antidiabetics, insulin, phenobarbital, primidone.
- ▪ Be sure to tell your doctor about any medications you are currently taking.

Storage

Capsules, tablets, vaginal cream, transdermal patches, etc. should be stored at room temperature; store away from heat and direct light. Keep out of reach of children, since this medicine may be dangerous in children.

HALAZEPAM

Properties
This medicine contains as active ingredient halazepam, a benzodiazepine preparation. Benzodiazepines belong to the group of psychoactive medicines that influence the activity of the brain. Some are used to relieve nervousness or tension. It is effective for this purpose for short periods. Others are used for sleeplessness or to relax muscles or relieve muscle spasm. The benzodiazepines may also be used for other conditions as determined by your doctor.

Before using this medicine
Before you use this medicine check with your doctor:
- if you ever had any unusual or allergic reaction to benzodiazepines.
- if you are on a low-salt, low-sugar, or any other special diet, or if you are allergic to any substance, such as sulfites or other preservatives or dyes.
- if you are pregnant or intend to become pregnant while using this medicine. Some benzodiazepines have been reported to increase the chance of birth defects when used during the first 3 months of pregnancy.
- if you are breast-feeding an infant. Benzodiazepines may pass into the breast milk and cause drowsiness, unusually slow heartbeat, shortness of breath, or troubled breathing in infants of mothers taking this medicine.
- if you have any of the following medical problems: asthma, bronchitis, emphysema, or other chronic lung disease; epilepsy or history of convulsions; hyperactivity (in children); kidney or lifer disease; mental depression or illness; myasthania gravis, porphyria.

Treatment
This medication is used to relieve or prevent the symptoms of your medical problem. Benzodiazepines are mainly used as antianxiety agents, anticonvulsants, or sedatives. Take them as directed. Do not take more of them and do not take them more often than recommended on the label, unless otherwise directed by your doctor. Benzodiazepine tranquilizing drugs can be abused if taken for long periods of time and it is possible to develop withdrawal symptoms if you discontinue the therapy abruptly.

Side effects
Along with the needed effects, a medicine may cause some unwanted effects. Minor side effects are: bitter taste in the mouth, dizziness, drowsiness, depression, constipation, dry mouth, excessive salivation, fatigue, flushing, headache, heartburn, loss of appetite, nausea, nervousness, sweating or vomiting. As your body adjusts to the medicine, these side effects should disappear.
- Tell your doctor about any side effects that are persistent or particularly bothersome. It is especially important to tell your doctor about:
  Blurred or double vision
  Chest pain
  Difficulty in urinating
  Fainting or falling
  Fever or hallucinations
  Joint pain
  Mouth sores
  Nightmares
  Palpitations
  Severe depression
  Shortness of breath
  Slurred speech
  Uncoordinated movements
  Unusual tiredness
  Yellowing of the skin

Interactions
This medicine may interact with several other drugs. This medicine will add to the effects of alcohol, and CNS depressants.
- Be sure to tell your doctor about any medications you are currently taking.

Storage
Store at room temperature in tightly closed, light-resistant-resistant containers. Keep out of the reach of children since overdose may be especially dangerous in children.

HALCION

Properties
This medicine contains as active ingredient triazolam, a benzodiazepine preparation. Benzodiazepines belong to the group of psychoactive medicines that influence the activity of the brain. Some are used to relieve nervousness or tension. It is effective for this purpose for short periods. Others are used for sleeplessness or to relax muscles or relieve muscle spasm. The benzodiazepines may also be used for other conditions as determined by your doctor.

Before using this medicine
Before you use this medicine check with your doctor:
- if you ever had any unusual or allergic reaction to benzodiazepines.
- if you are on a low-salt, low-sugar, or any other special diet, or if you are allergic to any substance, such as sulfites or other preservatives or dyes.
- if you are pregnant or intend to become pregnant while using this medicine. Some benzodiazepines have been reported to increase the chance of birth defects when used during the first 3 months of pregnancy.
- if you are breast-feeding an infant. Benzodiazepines may pass into the breast milk and cause drowsiness, unusually slow heartbeat, shortness of breath, or troubled breathing in infants of mothers taking this medicine.
- if you have any of the following medical problems: asthma, bronchitis, emphysema, or other chronic lung disease; epilepsy or history of convulsions; hyperactivity (in children); kidney or lifer disease; mental depression or illness; myasthania gravis, porphyria.

Treatment
This medication is used to relieve or prevent the symptoms of your medical problem. Benzodiazepines are mainly used as antianxiety agents, anticonvulsants, or sedatives. Take them as directed. Do not take more of them and do not take them more often than recommended on the label, unless otherwise directed by your doctor. Benzodiazepine tranquilizing drugs can be abused if taken for long periods of time and it is possible to develop withdrawal symptoms if you discontinue the therapy abruptly.

Side effects
Along with the needed effects, a medicine may cause some unwanted effects. Minor side effects are: bitter taste in the mouth, dizziness, drowsiness, depression, constipation, dry mouth, excessive salivation, fatigue, flushing, headache, heartburn, loss of appetite, nausea, nervousness, sweating or vomiting. As your body adjusts to the medicine, these side effects should disappear.
- Tell your doctor about any side effects that are persistent or particularly bothersome. It is especially important to tell your doctor about:
  Blurred or double vision
  Chest pain
  Difficulty in urinating
  Fainting or falling
  Fever or hallucinations
  Joint pain
  Mouth sores
  Nightmares
  Palpitations
  Severe depression
  Shortness of breath
  Slurred speech
  Uncoordinated movements
  Unusual tiredness
  Yellowing of the skin

Interactions
- This medicine may interact with several other drugs. This medicine will add to the effects of alcohol, and CNS depressants.
- Be sure to tell your doctor about any medications you are currently taking.

Storage
Store at room temperature in tightly closed, light-resistant-resistant containers. Keep out of the reach of children since overdose may be especially dangerous in children.

HALOTESTIN

Properties
This medicine is a member of the androgenic, or male, hormone group, containing an androgenic preparation as active ingredient. It is used in diseases in which male hormone replacement or augmentation is needed and also in so-called male menopause. It is also used to decrease calcium loss in osteoporosis, to block growth of breast cancer cells in females and to reduce breast pain and fullness following childbirth.

Before using this medicine
Before you use this medicine check with your doctor, or pharmacist:
- if you ever had any unusual or allergic reaction to androgens or corticosteroids in general.
- if you are on a low-salt, low-sugar, or any other special diet, or if you are allergic to any substance, such as certain preservatives or dyes.
- if you have any of the following medical problems:
Cancer prostate
Heart disease or atherosclerosis
Kidney or lifer disease
Breast cancer (males)
High blood pressure
High level of blood calcium
Epilepsy

Treatment
This medication is used to relieve or prevent the symptoms of your medical problem. Take them as directed. Do not take more of them and do not take them more often than recommended on the label. One should take the tablets or capsules with food to lessen stomach irritation. Take the medication at the same time each day. If you forget a dose take it as soon as you remember up to two hours late; wait for the next scheduled dose; Do not double this dose. The risk to the unborn child outweighs the benefits of the drug.

Side effects
Females taking any androgenic drug should watch for deepening of the voice, oily skin, acne, hairiness, increased libido, and menstrual irregularities.

The following side effects may occur:
Acne or oily skin
Deep voice
Enlarged clitoris in females
Frequent erections in men
Sore mouth
Higher sex drive
Impotence in men
Yellow skin or eyes
These side effects should disappear as your body adjusts to the medication. Tell your doctor about any side effects that are persistent or particularly bothersome.
- Discontinue the use of the medication and seek emergency treatment in the following situations:
Intense itching
Weakness
Loss of consciousness
Depression or confusion
Swollen feet or legs
Shortness of breath
Irregularities of heartbeat
Difficult urination
Vaginal bleeding in women
Scrotum pain in men

Interactions
This medicine interacts with several other drugs such as anticoagulants, oral antidiabetics, cyclosporine, hepatotoxic drugs, oxyphenbutazone, phenobarbital, and phenylbutazone.
- Be sure to tell your doctor about any medications you are currently taking.

Storage
This medicine should be stored at room temperature in closed containers. Store away from heat and direct light. Keep out of reach of children, since overdose may be dangerous in children.

HISTERONE

Properties
This medicine is a member of the androgenic, or male, hormone group, containing an androgenic preparation as active ingredient. It is used in diseases in which male hormone replacement or augmentation is needed and also in so-called male menopause. It is also used to decrease calcium loss in osteoporosis, to block growth of breast cancer cells in females and to reduce breast pain and fullness following childbirth.

Before using this medicine
Before you use this medicine check with your doctor, or pharmacist:
- if you ever had any unusual or allergic reaction to androgens or corticosteroids in general.
- if you are on a low-salt, low-sugar, or any other special diet, or if you are allergic to any substance, such as certain preservatives or dyes.
- if you have any of the following medical problems:
  Cancer prostate
  Heart disease or atherosclerosis
  Kidney or lifer disease
  Breast cancer (males)
  High blood pressure
  High level of blood calcium
  Epilepsy

Treatment
This medication is used to relieve or prevent the symptoms of your medical problem. Take them as directed. Do not take more of them and do not take them more often than recommended on the label. One should take the tablets or capsules with food to lessen stomach irritation. Take the medication at the same time each day. If you forget a dose take it as soon as you remember up to two hours late; wait for the next scheduled dose; Do not double this dose. The risk to the unborn child outweighs the benefits of the drug.

Side effects
Females taking any androgenic drug should watch for deepening of the voice, oily skin, acne, hairiness, increased libido, and menstrual irregularities.

The following side effects may occur:
Acne or oily skin
Deep voice
Enlarged clitoris in females
Frequent erections in men
Sore mouth
Higher sex drive
Impotence in men
Yellow skin or eyes
These side effects should disappear as your body adjusts to the medication. Tell your doctor about any side effects that are persistent or particularly bothersome.
- Discontinue the use of the medication and seek emergency treatment in the following situations:
Intense itching
Weakness
Loss of consciousness
Depression or confusion
Swollen feet or legs
Shortness of breath
Irregularities of heartbeat
Difficult urination
Vaginal bleeding in women
Scrotum pain in men

Interactions
This medicine interacts with several other drugs such as anticoagulants, oral antidiabetics, cyclosporine, hepatotoxic drugs, oxyphenbutazone, phenobarbital, and phenylbutazone.
- Be sure to tell your doctor about any medications you are currently taking.

Storage
This medicine should be stored at room temperature in closed containers. Store away from heat and direct light. Keep out of reach of children, since overdose may be dangerous in children.

HONVOL

Properties
This medicine contains diethylstilbestrol as active ingredient. The medicine is prescribed for treatment of estrogen deficiency; it restores normal estrogen levels in tissues. There is no evidence that this drug is effective for
nervous symptoms or depression occurring during menopause. They should
not be used to treat this condition; they
should be used only to replace the estrogen that is naturally absent after menopause.

Before using this medicine
Before you use this medicine check
with your doctor, or pharmacist:
- if you ever had any unusual or aller-
  gic reaction to estrogens;
- if you are pregnant or intend to be-
  come pregnant within three months;
- if you are breast-feeding an infant;
- if you have any of the following
  medical problems:
  Diabetes
  Breast cancer
  Fibrocystic breast disease
  Fibroid uterine tumors
  Endometriosis
  Migraine headaches
  Epilepsy
  Porphyria
  High blood pressure
  Congestive heart failure
  Kidney disease
  Gallstones

Treatment
This medication is used to treat estrogen
deficiency, specific symptoms of menopause, estrogen-deficiency osteoporosis,
atrophic vaginitis, prostate cancer.

For safe and effective use of this
medicine:
♦ Follow your doctor's instructions if
  this medicine was prescribed.
♦ Follow the manufacturer's package
  directions if you are treating yourself.
♦ Estrogens have been reported to increase the risk of endometrial carcinoma.

Side effects
Along with the needed effects, a medi-
cine may cause some unwanted effects.
Possible side effects include:
  Stomach cramps
  Profuse bleeding
  Appetite loss
  Nausea and vomiting
  Swollen breasts
  Change in menstruation
  Rash, skin blisters
  Depression
  Dizziness

Overdose
The following symptoms may indicate
an overdose:
  Nausea and vomiting
  Fluid retention
  Breast enlargement
  Abnormal vaginal bleeding
- Call a doctor or hospital emergency
  room for instructions.

Interactions
This medicine may interact with several
other drugs such as adrenocorticosteroids, antidepressants, oral antidiabetics, insulin, phenobarbital, primidone.
- Be sure to tell your doctor about any
  medications you are currently taking.

Storage
Capsules, tablets, vaginal cream,
transdermal patches, etc. should be
stored at room temperature; store away
from heat and direct light. Keep out of
reach of children, since this medicine
may be dangerous in children.

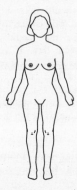

HYBOLIN DECANOATE

Properties
This medicine is a member of the androgenic, or male, hormone group, containing an androgenic preparation as active ingredient. It is used in diseases in which male hormone replacement or augmentation is needed and also in so-called male menopause. It is also used to decrease calcium loss in osteoporosis, to block growth of breast cancer cells in females and to reduce breast pain and fullness following childbirth.

Before using this medicine
Before you use this medicine check with your doctor, or pharmacist:
- if you ever had any unusual or allergic reaction to androgens or corticosteroids in general.
- if you are on a low-salt, low-sugar, or any other special diet, or if you are allergic to any substance, such as certain preservatives or dyes.
- if you have any of the following medical problems:
Cancer prostate
Heart disease or atherosclerosis
Kidney or lifer disease
Breast cancer (males)
High blood pressure
High level of blood calcium
Epilepsy

Treatment
This medication is used to relieve or prevent the symptoms of your medical problem. Take them as directed. Do not take more of them and do not take them more often than recommended on the label. One should take the tablets or capsules with food to lessen stomach irritation. Take the medication at the same time each day. If you forget a dose take it as soon as you remember up to two hours late; wait for the next scheduled dose; Do not double this dose. The risk to the unborn child outweighs the benefits of the drug.

Side effects
Females taking any androgenic drug should watch for deepening of the voice, oily skin, acne, hairiness, increased libido, and menstrual irregularities.

The following side effects may occur:
Acne or oily skin
Deep voice
Enlarged clitoris in females
Frequent erections in men
Sore mouth
Higher sex drive
Impotence in men
Yellow skin or eyes
These side effects should disappear as your body adjusts to the medication. Tell your doctor about any side effects that are persistent or particularly bothersome.
- Discontinue the use of the medication and seek emergency treatment in the following situations:
Intense itching
Weakness
Loss of consciousness
Depression or confusion
Swollen feet or legs
Shortness of breath
Irregularities of heartbeat
Difficult urination
Vaginal bleeding in women
Scrotum pain in men

Interactions
This medicine interacts with several other drugs such as anticoagulants, oral antidiabetics, cyclosporine, hepatotoxic drugs, oxyphenbutazone, phenobarbital, and phenylbutazone.
- Be sure to tell your doctor about any medications you are currently taking.

Storage
This medicine should be stored at room temperature in closed containers. Store away from heat and direct light. Keep out of reach of children, since overdose may be dangerous in children.

HYCODAN

Properties
This medicine contains as active ingredient hydrocodone.

It is a narcotic analgesic that acts directly on the central nervous system (brain and spinal cord). It is used to relieve pain or to suppress coughing.

Before using this medicine
Before you use this medicine check with your doctor, or pharmacist:
- if you ever had any unusual or allergic reaction to this medicine or one of its components.
- if you are on a low-salt, low-sugar, or any other special diet, or if you are allergic to any substance, such as sulfites or other preservatives or dyes.
- if you are pregnant or intend to become pregnant while using this medicine. Studies on birth defects have not been done in humans. Too much use of narcotics during pregnancy may cause the baby to become dependent on the medicine.
- if you are breast-feeding an infant. Although this medicine has not been shown to cause problems in humans, it passes into the breast milk in small amounts.
- if you have any of the following medical problems:
Brain disease or head injury
Colitis
Convulsions
Emphysema, asthma, or chronic lung disease
Enlarged prostate
Gallbladder disease or gallstones
Heart disease
Kidney or lifer disease
Underactive thyroid

Treatment
This medication is used to relieve pain or to suppress coughing. Narcotic analgesics act in the central nervous system; some of their side effects are also caused by actions in the central nervous system.
- If you are taking this medication on a regular schedule and you miss a dose, take the missed dose as soon as possible, unless it is almost time for your next dose. In that case do not take the missed dose at all.
- If a narcotic analgesic is used for a long time, it may become habit-forming (causing mental or physical dependence). Physical dependence may lead to withdrawal side effects when you stop taking this medicine.

Unless otherwise directed by your doctor or pharmacist take this as directed. Do not take more of them and do not take them more often than recommended on the label. Children up to 12 years of age should not take this medicine more than 3 times a day or for more than 5 days in a row.

Side effects
Along with the needed effects, a medicine may cause some unwanted effects. These side effects may go away during treatment as your body adjusts to the medicine. Such minor side effects are: constipation, dizziness, drowsiness, dry mouth, false sense of well-being, flushing, light-headedness, loss of appetite, nausea, painful or difficult urination, or sweating.
- Check with your doctor immediately if any of the following side effects occur:
Anxiety or breathing difficulties
Excitation or restlessness
Fatigue, palpitations
Rash, sore throat and fever
Tremors or weakness

Interactions
This medicine may interact with several other drugs such as medicines acting on the central nervous system (e.g., antidepressants, tranquilizers), cimetidine, nitrates, quinidine, etc.
- Be sure to tell your doctor about any medications you are currently taking.

Storage
Tablets, elixir, suppository etc. should be stored at room temperature in a tightly closed, light-resistant container.

HYDRO-T

Properties

This medicine contains as active ingredient hydrochlorothiazide, a thiazide-like diuretic. Thiazide or thiazide-like diuretics are prescribed to treat high blood pressure (hypertension). They are also used to reduce fluid accumulation in the body caused by conditions such as heart failure, cirrhosis, kidney disease, and the long-term use of some medications. Thiazide diuretics may also be used for other conditions as determined by your doctor.

Before using this medicine

Before you use this medicine check with your doctor, or pharmacist:
- if you ever had any unusual or allergic reaction to sulfonamides (sulfa drugs) or any of the thiazide diuretics.
- if you are on a low-salt, low-sugar, or any other special diet, or if you are allergic to any substance, such as sulfites or other preservatives or dyes.
- if you are pregnant or intend to become pregnant while using this medicine. When this medicine is used during pregnancy, it may cause side effects including jaundice, blood problems, and low potassium in the newborn.
- if you are breast-feeding an infant. Although this medicine has not been shown to cause problems in humans, the chance always exists since thiazide diuretics pass into breast milk.
- if you have any of the following medical problems:
  Diabetes
  Gout
  Kidney disease
  Liver disease
  Lupus erythematosus
  Pancreas disease

Treatment

This medication is used to treat high blood pressure (hypertension) and also to help reduce the amount of water in the body by increasing the flow of urine. This medicine will not cure your high blood pressure but it does help control it. You must continue to take it - even if you feel well - if you expect to keep your blood pressure down. You may have to take high blood pressure medicine for the rest of your life.

Thiazide diuretics may cause an unusual feeling of tiredness when you begin to take them. You may also notice an increase in urine or in frequency of urination. To keep this from affecting sleep:
- if you are to take a single dose a day, take it in the morning after breakfast;
- if you are to take more than one dose, take the last one not later than 6 p.m.

Side effects

Along with the needed effects, a medicine may cause some unwanted effects. Side effects that usually do not require medical attention: decreased sexual ability; dizziness or lightheadedness when standing up; increased sensitivity of skin to sunlight; loss of appetite; upset stomach.
- Side effects that should be reported to your doctor: black, tarry stools; blood in urine or stools; cough or hoarseness; fever or chills; joint pain; lower back or side pains; painful or difficult urination; pinpoint red spots on skin; skin rash or hives; stomach pain (severe) with nausea; unusual bleeding or bruising; yellow eyes or skin. This medicine may cause a loss of potassium from your body. Signs of too much potassium loss are: dryness of mouth; increased thirst; mood changes; muscle cramps or pain; nausea or vomiting; unusual tiredness or weakness; weak or irregular heartbeat.

Interactions

This medicine may interact with several other drugs.
- Be sure to tell your doctor about any medications you are currently taking.

Storage

Store at room temperature in a tightly closed container.

HYDRO-Z-50

Properties
This medicine contains as active ingredient hydrochlorothiazide, a thiazide-like diuretic. Thiazide or thiazide-like diuretics are prescribed to treat high blood pressure (hypertension). They are also used to reduce fluid accumulation in the body caused by conditions such as heart failure, cirrhosis, kidney disease, and the long-term use of some medications. Thiazide diuretics may also be used for other conditions as determined by your doctor.

Before using this medicine
Before you use this medicine check with your doctor, or pharmacist:
- if you ever had any unusual or allergic reaction to sulfonamides (sulfa drugs) or any of the thiazide diuretics.
- if you are on a low-salt, low-sugar, or any other special diet, or if you are allergic to any substance, such as sulfites or other preservatives or dyes.
- if you are pregnant or intend to become pregnant while using this medicine. When this medicine is used during pregnancy, it may cause side effects including jaundice, blood problems, and low potassium in the newborn.
- if you are breast-feeding an infant. Although this medicine has not been shown to cause problems in humans, the chance always exists since thiazide diuretics pass into breast milk.
- if you have any of the following medical problems:
  Diabetes
  Gout
  Kidney disease
  Liver disease
  Lupus erythematosus
  Pancreas disease

Treatment
This medication is used to treat high blood pressure (hypertension) and also to help reduce the amount of water in the body by increasing the flow of urine. This medicine will not cure your high blood pressure but it does help control it. You must continue to take it - even if you feel well - if you expect to keep your blood pressure down. You may have to take high blood pressure medicine for the rest of your life.

Thiazide diuretics may cause an unusual feeling of tiredness when you begin to take them. You may also notice an increase in urine or in frequency of urination. To keep this from affecting sleep:
- if you are to take a single dose a day, take it in the morning after breakfast;
- if you are to take more than one dose, take the last one not later than 6 p.m.

Side effects
Along with the needed effects, a medicine may cause some unwanted effects. Side effects that usually do not require medical attention: decreased sexual ability; dizziness or lightheadedness when standing up; increased sensitivity of skin to sunlight; loss of appetite; upset stomach.
- Side effects that should be reported to your doctor: black, tarry stools; blood in urine or stools; cough or hoarseness; fever or chills; joint pain; lower back or side pains; painful or difficult urination; pinpoint red spots on skin; skin rash or hives; stomach pain (severe) with nausea; unusual bleeding or bruising; yellow eyes or skin. This medicine may cause a loss of potassium from your body. Signs of too much potassium loss are: dryness of mouth; increased thirst; mood changes; muscle cramps or pain; nausea or vomiting; unusual tiredness or weakness; weak or irregular heartbeat.

Interactions
This medicine may interact with several other drugs.
- Be sure to tell your doctor about any medications you are currently taking.

Storage
Store at room temperature in a tightly closed container.

HYDROCHLOROTHIAZIDE IN-TENSOL

Properties

This medicine contains as active ingredient hydrochlorothiazide, a thiazide-like diuretic. Thiazide or thiazide-like diuretics are prescribed to treat high blood pressure (hypertension). They are also used to reduce fluid accumulation in the body caused by conditions such as heart failure, cirrhosis, kidney disease, and the long-term use of some medications. Thiazide diuretics may also be used for other conditions as determined by your doctor.

Before using this medicine

Before you use this medicine check with your doctor, or pharmacist:
- if you ever had any unusual or allergic reaction to sulfonamides (sulfa drugs) or any of the thiazide diuretics.
- if you are on a low-salt, low-sugar, or any other special diet, or if you are allergic to any substance, such as sulfites or other preservatives or dyes.
- if you are pregnant or intend to become pregnant while using this medicine. When this medicine is used during pregnancy, it may cause side effects including jaundice, blood problems, and low potassium in the newborn.
- if you are breast-feeding an infant. Although this medicine has not been shown to cause problems in humans, the chance always exists since thiazide diuretics pass into breast milk.
- if you have any of the following medical problems:
  Diabetes
  Gout
  Kidney disease
  Liver disease
  Lupus erythematosus
  Pancreas disease

Treatment

This medication is used to treat high blood pressure (hypertension) and also to help reduce the amount of water in the body by increasing the flow of urine. This medicine will not cure your high blood pressure but it does help control it. You must continue to take it - even if you feel well - if you expect to keep your blood pressure down. You may have to take high blood pressure medicine for the rest of your life.

Thiazide diuretics may cause an unusual feeling of tiredness when you begin to take them. You may also notice an increase in urine or in frequency of urination. To keep this from affecting sleep:
- if you are to take a single dose a day, take it in the morning after breakfast;
- if you are to take more than one dose, take the last one not later than 6 p.m.

Side effects

Along with the needed effects, a medicine may cause some unwanted effects. Side effects that usually do not require medical attention: decreased sexual ability; dizziness or lightheadedness when standing up; increased sensitivity of skin to sunlight; loss of appetite; upset stomach.
- Side effects that should be reported to your doctor: black, tarry stools; blood in urine or stools; cough or hoarseness; fever or chills; joint pain; lower back or side pains; painful or difficult urination; pinpoint red spots on skin; skin rash or hives; stomach pain (severe) with nausea; unusual bleeding or bruising; yellow eyes or skin. This medicine may cause a loss of potassium from your body. Signs of too much potassium loss are: dryness of mouth; increased thirst; mood changes; muscle cramps or pain; nausea or vomiting; unusual tiredness or weakness; weak or irregular heartbeat.

Interactions

This medicine may interact with several other drugs.
- Be sure to tell your doctor about any medications you are currently taking.

Storage

Store at room temperature in a tightly closed container.

HYDRODIURIL

Properties
This medicine contains as active ingredient hydrochlorothiazide, a thiazide-like diuretic. Thiazide or thiazide-like diuretics are prescribed to treat high blood pressure (hypertension). They are also used to reduce fluid accumulation in the body caused by conditions such as heart failure, cirrhosis, kidney disease, and the long-term use of some medications. Thiazide diuretics may also be used for other conditions as determined by your doctor.

Before using this medicine
Before you use this medicine check with your doctor, or pharmacist:
- if you ever had any unusual or allergic reaction to sulfonamides (sulfa drugs) or any of the thiazide diuretics.
- if you are on a low-salt, low-sugar, or any other special diet, or if you are allergic to any substance, such as sulfites or other preservatives or dyes.
- if you are pregnant or intend to become pregnant while using this medicine. When this medicine is used during pregnancy, it may cause side effects including jaundice, blood problems, and low potassium in the newborn.
- if you are breast-feeding an infant. Although this medicine has not been shown to cause problems in humans, the chance always exists since thiazide diuretics pass into breast milk.
- if you have any of the following medical problems:
Diabetes
Gout
Kidney disease
Liver disease
Lupus erythematosus
Pancreas disease

Treatment
This medication is used to treat high blood pressure (hypertension) and also to help reduce the amount of water in the body by increasing the flow of urine. This medicine will not cure your high blood pressure but it does help

control it. You must continue to take it - even if you feel well - if you expect to keep your blood pressure down. You may have to take high blood pressure medicine for the rest of your life.

Thiazide diuretics may cause an unusual feeling of tiredness when you begin to take them. You may also notice an increase in urine or in frequency of urination. To keep this from affecting sleep:
- if you are to take a single dose a day, take it in the morning after breakfast;
- if you are to take more than one dose, take the last one not later than 6 p.m.

Side effects
Along with the needed effects, a medicine may cause some unwanted effects. Side effects that usually do not require medical attention: decreased sexual ability; dizziness or lightheadedness when standing up; increased sensitivity of skin to sunlight; loss of appetite; upset stomach.
- Side effects that should be reported to your doctor: black, tarry stools; blood in urine or stools; cough or hoarseness; fever or chills; joint pain; lower back or side pains; painful or difficult urination; pinpoint red spots on skin; skin rash or hives; stomach pain (severe) with nausea; unusual bleeding or bruising; yellow eyes or skin. This medicine may cause a loss of potassium from your body. Signs of too much potassium loss are: dryness of mouth; increased thirst; mood changes; muscle cramps or pain; nausea or vomiting; unusual tiredness or weakness; weak or irregular heartbeat.

Interactions
This medicine may interact with several other drugs.
- Be sure to tell your doctor about any medications you are currently taking.

Storage
Store at room temperature in a tightly closed container.

HYDROMAL

Properties
This medicine contains as active ingredient hydrochlorothiazide, a thiazide-like diuretic. Thiazide or thiazide-like diuretics are prescribed to treat high blood pressure (hypertension). They are also used to reduce fluid accumulation in the body caused by conditions such as heart failure, cirrhosis, kidney disease, and the long-term use of some medications. Thiazide diuretics may also be used for other conditions as determined by your doctor.

Before using this medicine
Before you use this medicine check with your doctor, or pharmacist:
- if you ever had any unusual or allergic reaction to sulfonamides (sulfa drugs) or any of the thiazide diuretics.
- if you are on a low-salt, low-sugar, or any other special diet, or if you are allergic to any substance, such as sulfites or other preservatives or dyes.
- if you are pregnant or intend to become pregnant while using this medicine. When this medicine is used during pregnancy, it may cause side effects including jaundice, blood problems, and low potassium in the newborn.
- if you are breast-feeding an infant. Although this medicine has not been shown to cause problems in humans, the chance always exists since thiazide diuretics pass into breast milk.
- if you have any of the following medical problems:
Diabetes
Gout
Kidney disease
Liver disease
Lupus erythematosus
Pancreas disease

Treatment
This medication is used to treat high blood pressure (hypertension) and also to help reduce the amount of water in the body by increasing the flow of urine. This medicine will not cure your high blood pressure but it does help control it. You must continue to take it - even if you feel well - if you expect to keep your blood pressure down. You may have to take high blood pressure medicine for the rest of your life.

Thiazide diuretics may cause an unusual feeling of tiredness when you begin to take them. You may also notice an increase in urine or in frequency of urination. To keep this from affecting sleep:
- if you are to take a single dose a day, take it in the morning after breakfast;
- if you are to take more than one dose, take the last one not later than 6 p.m.

Side effects
Along with the needed effects, a medicine may cause some unwanted effects. Side effects that usually do not require medical attention: decreased sexual ability; dizziness or lightheadedness when standing up; increased sensitivity of skin to sunlight; loss of appetite; upset stomach.
- Side effects that should be reported to your doctor: black, tarry stools; blood in urine or stools; cough or hoarseness; fever or chills; joint pain; lower back or side pains; painful or difficult urination; pinpoint red spots on skin; skin rash or hives; stomach pain (severe) with nausea; unusual bleeding or bruising; yellow eyes or skin. This medicine may cause a loss of potassium from your body. Signs of too much potassium loss are: dryness of mouth; increased thirst; mood changes; muscle cramps or pain; nausea or vomiting; unusual tiredness or weakness; weak or irregular heartbeat.

Interactions
This medicine may interact with several other drugs.
- Be sure to tell your doctor about any medications you are currently taking.

Storage
Store at room temperature in a tightly closed container.

HYDROZIDE-50

Properties
This medicine contains as active ingredient hydrochlorothiazide, a thiazide-like diuretic. Thiazide or thiazide-like diuretics are prescribed to treat high blood pressure (hypertension). They are also used to reduce fluid accumulation in the body caused by conditions such as heart failure, cirrhosis, kidney disease, and the long-term use of some medications. Thiazide diuretics may also be used for other conditions as determined by your doctor.

Before using this medicine
Before you use this medicine check with your doctor, or pharmacist:
- if you ever had any unusual or allergic reaction to sulfonamides (sulfa drugs) or any of the thiazide diuretics.
- if you are on a low-salt, low-sugar, or any other special diet, or if you are allergic to any substance, such as sulfites or other preservatives or dyes.
- if you are pregnant or intend to become pregnant while using this medicine. When this medicine is used during pregnancy, it may cause side effects including jaundice, blood problems, and low potassium in the newborn.
- if you are breast-feeding an infant. Although this medicine has not been shown to cause problems in humans, the chance always exists since thiazide diuretics pass into breast milk.
- if you have any of the following medical problems:
Diabetes
Gout
Kidney disease
Liver disease
Lupus erythematosus
Pancreas disease

Treatment
This medication is used to treat high blood pressure (hypertension) and also to help reduce the amount of water in the body by increasing the flow of urine. This medicine will not cure your high blood pressure but it does help control it. You must continue to take it - even if you feel well - if you expect to keep your blood pressure down. You may have to take high blood pressure medicine for the rest of your life.

Thiazide diuretics may cause an unusual feeling of tiredness when you begin to take them. You may also notice an increase in urine or in frequency of urination. To keep this from affecting sleep:
- if you are to take a single dose a day, take it in the morning after breakfast;
- if you are to take more than one dose, take the last one not later than 6 p.m.

Side effects
Along with the needed effects, a medicine may cause some unwanted effects. Side effects that usually do not require medical attention: decreased sexual ability; dizziness or lightheadedness when standing up; increased sensitivity of skin to sunlight; loss of appetite; upset stomach.
- Side effects that should be reported to your doctor: black, tarry stools; blood in urine or stools; cough or hoarseness; fever or chills; joint pain; lower back or side pains; painful or difficult urination; pinpoint red spots on skin; skin rash or hives; stomach pain (severe) with nausea; unusual bleeding or bruising; yellow eyes or skin. This medicine may cause a loss of potassium from your body. Signs of too much potassium loss are: dryness of mouth; increased thirst; mood changes; muscle cramps or pain; nausea or vomiting; unusual tiredness or weakness; weak or irregular heartbeat.

Interactions
This medicine may interact with several other drugs.
- Be sure to tell your doctor about any medications you are currently taking.

Storage
Store at room temperature in a tightly closed container.

HYREX-105

Properties
This medicine contains phendimetrazine as active ingredient; it is prescribed for appetite suppression.

Appetite suppressants are used in the short-term (a few weeks) treatment of obesity. In a few weeks (6 to 12), these medicines in combination with dieting, exercise, and changes in eating habits can help patients lose weight. However, since their appetite reducing effect is only temporary, they are useful only for the first weeks of dieting until new eating habits are established.

Before using this medicine
Before you use this medicine check with your doctor, or pharmacist:
- if you ever had any unusual or allergic reaction to any of the compounds of this medicine.
- if you are on a low-salt, low-sugar, or any other special diet, or if you are allergic to any substance, such as sulfites or other preservatives or dyes.
- if you are pregnant, intend to become pregnant or breast-feeding an infant while using this medicine.
- if you have any of the following medical problems:
  Diabetes mellitus (sugar diabetes)
  Epilepsy
  Glaucoma
  Heart or blood vessel disease
  High blood pressure
  Mental illness (severe)

Treatment
This medication is used to relieve or prevent the symptoms of your medical problem. Take them as directed. Do not take more of them and do not take them more often than recommended on the label. If too much of the drug is taken, it may become habit-forming.

The medicine produces central nervous system stimulation, and it should not be taken by people with heart disease or high blood pressure.

If you think this medicine is not working as well after you have taken it for a few weeks, do not increase the dose. Instead, check with your doctor.

Side effects
The following minor side effects may occur: irritability, nervousness, restlessness, trouble in sleeping.

These side effects should disappear as your body adjusts to the medication. Tell your doctor about any side effects that are persistent or particularly bothersome. It is especially important to tell your doctor about:
  Mental depression
  Nausea or vomiting
  Stomach cramps or pain
  Trembling
  Unusual tiredness or weakness
- Discontinue use of the drug; call your doctor right away. Adverse reactions and side effects may be more frequent and severe in people over age 60 than in younger persons.

Interactions
This medicine interacts with several other drugs such as antihypertensives, other appetite suppressants, caffeine, central nervous system depressants, central nervous system stimulants, furazolidone, guanethidine, hydralazine, MAO inhibitors, methyldopa, molindone, phenothiazines, rauwolfia alkaloids, sodium bicarbonate. Interaction with alcoholic beverages may produce drowsiness, sleepiness, and/or inability to concentrate.
- Be sure to tell your doctor about any medications you are currently taking.

Storage
This medicine should be stored at room temperature in tightly closed containers. Store away from heat and direct light. Keep out of reach of children, since overdose may be very dangerous in children.

Do not store this medicine in the bathroom medicine cabinet because the heat and moisture cause the medicine to break down. Do not keep outdated medicine or medicine no longer needed. Flush the contents of the container down the toilet.

ILOSONE

Properties

This medicine contains erythromycin as active ingredient. This antibiotic is prescribed to treat infections caused by bacteria. They will not work for colds, flu, or other virus infections. Erythromycins are available only with your doctor's prescription.

Before using this medicine

Before you use this medicine check with your doctor, or pharmacist:
- if you ever had any unusual or allergic reaction to any of the erythromycins.
- if you are on a low-salt, low-sugar, or any other special diet, or if you are allergic to any substance, such as sulfites or other preservatives or dyes.
- if you are pregnant or intend to become pregnant while using this medicine. Although erythromycins have not been shown to cause birth defects or other problems in humans, the chance always exists.
- if you are breast-feeding an infant. Most erythromycins pass into the breast milk. Although erythromycins have not been shown to cause problems in humans, the chance always exists.
- if you have lifer disease.

Treatment

This medication belongs to the general family of medicines called antibiotics. It is used to treat a wide variety of bacterial infections. It is also used to treat infections in persons who are allergic to penicillin. Erythromycins are also used to prevent "strep" infections in patients with a history of rheumatic heart disease. They may also be used in Legionnaires' disease and for other problems as determined by your doctor.
- Keep taking this medicine for the full time of treatment even if you begin to feel better after a few days; do not miss any doses. This is especially important if you have a "strep" infection since serious heart problems could develop later if your infection is not cleared up completely.
- If you do miss a dose of this medicine, take it as soon as possible. This will help to keep a constant amount of medicine in the blood. However, if it is almost time for your next dose, skip the missed dose and go back to your regular dosing schedule.
- This medication has been prescribed for your current infection only. Another infection later on, or one that someone else has, may require a different medicine. You should not give your medicine to other people or use it for other infections, unless your doctor specifically directs you to do so.

Side effects

Along with the needed effects, a medicine may cause some unwanted effects. Side effects that usually do not require medical attention: abdominal cramps, black tongue, cough, diarrhea, fatigue, irritation of the mouth, loss of appetite, nausea, or vomiting. These side effects should disappear as your body adjusts to the medication.
- Other side effects that should be reported to your doctor immediately are:
Fever
Hearing loss
Hives or rash
Rectal or vaginal itching
Yellowing of the eyes or skin

Interactions

This medicine may interact with several other drugs such as anticoagulants, theophylline preparations, carbamazepine, etc.
- Be sure to tell your doctor about any medications you are currently taking.

Storage

Tablets, capsules, etc. should be stored at room temperature in tightly closed, light-resistant containers as directed by your pharmacist.

ILOTYCIN

Properties
This medicine contains erythromycin as active ingredient. This antibiotic is prescribed to treat infections caused by bacteria. They will not work for colds, flu, or other virus infections. Erythromycins are available only with your doctor's prescription.

Before using this medicine
Before you use this medicine check with your doctor, or pharmacist:
- if you ever had any unusual or allergic reaction to any of the erythromycins.
- if you are on a low-salt, low-sugar, or any other special diet, or if you are allergic to any substance, such as sulfites or other preservatives or dyes.
- if you are pregnant or intend to become pregnant while using this medicine. Although erythromycins have not been shown to cause birth defects or other problems in humans, the chance always exists.
- if you are breast-feeding an infant. Most erythromycins pass into the breast milk. Although erythromycins have not been shown to cause problems in humans, the chance always exists.
- if you have lifer disease.

Treatment
This medication belongs to the general family of medicines called antibiotics. It is used to treat a wide variety of bacterial infections. It is also used to treat infections in persons who are allergic to penicillin. Erythromycins are also used to prevent "strep" infections in patients with a history of rheumatic heart disease. They may also be used in Legionnaires' disease and for other problems as determined by your doctor.
- Keep taking this medicine for the full time of treatment even if you begin to feel better after a few days; do not miss any doses. This is especially important if you have a "strep" infection since serious heart problems could develop later if your infection is not cleared up completely.
- If you do miss a dose of this medicine, take it as soon as possible. This will help to keep a constant amount of medicine in the blood. However, if it is almost time for your next dose, skip the missed dose and go back to your regular dosing schedule.
- This medication has been prescribed for your current infection only. Another infection later on, or one that someone else has, may require a different medicine. You should not give your medicine to other people or use it for other infections, unless your doctor specifically directs you to do so.

Side effects
Along with the needed effects, a medicine may cause some unwanted effects. Side effects that usually do not require medical attention: abdominal cramps, black tongue, cough, diarrhea, fatigue, irritation of the mouth, loss of appetite, nausea, or vomiting. These side effects should disappear as your body adjusts to the medication.
- Other side effects that should be reported to your doctor immediately are:
Fever
Hearing loss
Hives or rash
Rectal or vaginal itching
Yellowing of the eyes or skin

Interactions
This medicine may interact with several other drugs such as anticoagulants, theophylline preparations, carbamazepine, etc.
- Be sure to tell your doctor about any medications you are currently taking.

Storage
Tablets, capsules, etc. should be stored at room temperature in tightly closed, light-resistant containers as directed by your pharmacist.

ILOTYCIN

Properties
This medicine contains erythromycin as active ingredient. This antibiotic is prescribed to treat infections caused by bacteria. They will not work for colds, flu, or other virus infections. Erythromycins are available only with your doctor's prescription.

Before using this medicine
Before you use this medicine check with your doctor, or pharmacist:
- if you ever had any unusual or allergic reaction to any of the erythromycins.
- if you are on a low-salt, low-sugar, or any other special diet, or if you are allergic to any substance, such as sulfites or other preservatives or dyes.
- if you are pregnant or intend to become pregnant while using this medicine. Although erythromycins have not been shown to cause birth defects or other problems in humans, the chance always exists.
- if you are breast-feeding an infant. Most erythromycins pass into the breast milk. Although erythromycins have not been shown to cause problems in humans, the chance always exists.
- if you have lifer disease.

Treatment
This medication belongs to the general family of medicines called antibiotics. It is used to treat a wide variety of bacterial infections. It is also used to treat infections in persons who are allergic to penicillin. Erythromycins are also used to prevent "strep" infections in patients with a history of rheumatic heart disease. They may also be used in Legionnaires' disease and for other problems as determined by your doctor.
■ Keep taking this medicine for the full time of treatment even if you begin to feel better after a few days; do not miss any doses. This is especially important if you have a "strep" infection since serious heart problems could develop later if your infection is not cleared up completely.

■ If you do miss a dose of this medicine, take it as soon as possible. This will help to keep a constant amount of medicine in the blood. However, if it is almost time for your next dose, skip the missed dose and go back to your regular dosing schedule.
■ This medication has been prescribed for your current infection only. Another infection later on, or one that someone else has, may require a different medicine. You should not give your medicine to other people or use it for other infections, unless your doctor specifically directs you to do so.

Side effects
Along with the needed effects, a medicine may cause some unwanted effects. Side effects that usually do not require medical attention: abdominal cramps, black tongue, cough, diarrhea, fatigue, irritation of the mouth, loss of appetite, nausea, or vomiting. These side effects should disappear as your body adjusts to the medication.
■ Other side effects that should be reported to your doctor immediately are:
Fever
Hearing loss
Hives or rash
Rectal or vaginal itching
Yellowing of the eyes or skin

Interactions
This medicine may interact with several other drugs such as anticoagulants, theophylline preparations, carbamazepine, etc.
■ Be sure to tell your doctor about any medications you are currently taking.

Storage
Tablets, capsules, etc. should be stored at room temperature in tightly closed, light-resistant containers as directed by your pharmacist.

ILOTYCIN (Ophthalmic)

Properties
This medicine contains an ophthalmic antibacterial, as active ingredient. It helps the body to overcome eye infections on surface tissues of the eye. It is most useful when the infecting organism is one known to be sensitive to the antibacterial drug.

The drug penetrates the bacterial cell membrane and prevents cells from multiplying.

Before using this medicine
Before you use this medicine check with your doctor:
- if you ever had any unusual or allergic reaction to any of the compounds of the medicine.
- if you are on a low-salt, low-sugar, or any other special diet, or if you are allergic to any substance, such as sulfites or other preservatives or dyes.
- if you are pregnant or intend to become pregnant while using this medicine. Although ophthalmic antibacterials have been found to be safe for use during pregnancy, you should check with your doctor before taking any drug if you are pregnant.

Treatment
This medication is used to treat an infection caused by bacteria. The medicine may be used in the form of eye drops or as an eye ointment. Use the medication as directed, Do not miss a dose. If you forget a dose, use it as soon as you remember. Notify your doctor if eye symptoms fail to improve in two to four days.
- ◆ To apply eye drops: Till the head backward when applying the eye drops. Pull the lower eyelid away from the eye to form a pouch. After applying the drop, keep the eye closed for a minute or so. This allows the medication to come in contact with the infection.
- ◆ To apply eye ointment: Pull lower lid down from eye to form a pouch. Squeeze tube to apply thin strip of ointment into pouch. Close eye for 1 to 2 minutes.

Always wash your hands before applying the ointment.

The drug starts to work in about one hour. Treatment may require 7 to 10 days to control infection.

Older adults or seniors may take this medication without special restriction.

Side effects
Along with the needed effects, a medicine may cause some unwanted effects. Side effects that usually do not require medical attention: occasional local irritation after application to the eye. Ointments may cause blurred vision for a few minutes; continue the use of the eye drops or ointment, but tell your doctor at the next visit.
- ■ Discontinue the use of eye drops or eye ointment in the following cases:
  Sore throat
  Aplastic anemia
  Unusual redness of the eye
  Unusual irritation of the eye
  Fever
  Unusual bleeding
  Unusual bruising
- ■ Tell your doctor about any side effects that are persistent or particularly bothersome. In case of prolonged use sensitivity reactions may develop.

Interactions
Clinically significant interactions with oral or injected medicines are unlikely. Do not use the eye drops or ointment with any other eye drops or ointment without checking with your ophthalmologist.

Storage
Keep bottle (with eye drops) or container (containing ointment) lightly closed. Store in a cool place, but Do not freeze. Wash hands immediately after using. Do not store in the bathroom medicine cabinet because the heat or moisture may cause the medicine to break down. Do not keep outdated medicine or medicine no longer needed. Flush the contents of the bottle or tube down the toilet, unless otherwise directed.

IMIPRAMINE

Properties
This medicine contains imipramine as active ingredient. It belongs to the group of medicines known as tricyclic antidepressants or 'mood elevators.' It is used to relieve mental depression and depression that sometimes occurs with anxiety. The medication gradually relieves, but doesn't cure, symptoms of depression. The medication may also be used for the treatment of narcolepsy, bulimia, painic attacks, cocaine withdrawal, attention deficit disorder.

Before using this medicine
Before you use this medicine check with your doctor, or pharmacist:
- if you ever had any unusual or allergic reaction to any tricyclic antidepressant, maprotiline or trazodone.
- if you are on a low-salt, low-sugar, or any other special diet, or if you are allergic to any substance, such as sulfites or other preservatives or dyes.
- if you are pregnant or intend to become pregnant while using this medicine.
  There have been reports of newborns suffering from heart, breathing, and urinary problems when their mothers had taken tricyclic antidepressants before delivery.
- if you are breast-feeding an infant. Some tricyclic antidepressants pass into the breast milk.

Treatment
Take this medicine only as directed by your doctor, to benefit your condition as much as possible. Do not take more of it, do not take it more often, and do not take it for a longer period of time than your doctor ordered.
To lessen stomach upset, take this medicine with food, even for a daily bedtime dose, unless your doctor has told you to take it on an empty stomach. If you forget your once-a-day bedtime dose, Do not take it more than 3 hours late. If more than 3 hours, wait for next scheduled dose;.
Sometimes this medicine must be taken for several weeks before you begin to feel better.

Side effects
Along with the needed effects, a medicine may cause some unwanted effects. Side effects that usually do not require medical attention: difficult or frequent urination; decreased sex drive; muscle aches; abnormal dreams; nasal congestion; weakness and faintness when arising from bed or chair; back pain.
- Other side effects that should be reported to your doctor immediately are:
  Hallucinations
  Shakiness
  Dizziness or fainting
  Blurred vision, eye pain
  Irregular heartbeat or slow pulse
  Inflamed tongue
  Abdominal pain
  Jaundice
  Hair loss, rash
  Fever, chills
  Joint pain
  Palpitations

Interactions
This medicine may interact with several other drugs such as anticoagulants, anticholinergics, cold remedies, oral contraceptives, seizure medicines, sleeping medicines, thyroid medicines, etc.
- Be sure to tell your doctor about any medications you are currently taking.

Storage
Tablets, capsules, etc. should be stored at room temperature in tightly closed, light-resistant containers as directed by your pharmacist. Keep out of reach of children since overdose is especially dangerous in young children. Do not store in the bathroom medicine cabinet because the heat or moisture may cause the medicine to break down. Keep the liquid form of the medicine from freezing.

IMITREX

Properties
This medicine contains sumatriptan as active ingredient and is therefore called an iron supplement. The medicine helps relieve headache pain and associated symptoms of migraine. It was created specifically for the acute treatment of migraine attacks. The tablets do not only relieve the pain but also the nausea and sensitivity to light that often accompany migraine.

Before using this medicine
Before you use this medicine check with your doctor, or pharmacist:
- if you ever had any unusual or allergic reaction to this medicine.
- if you are pregnant or intend to become pregnant while using this medicine. Animal studies have shown an adverse effect on the fetus, but there are no adequate studies in humans. The drug may be used by pregnant women because of its benefits and despite its potential risks;
- if you are breast-feeding an infant;
- if you are suffering from ischemic heart disease;
- if you are suffering from uncontrolled hypertension (high blood pressure).

Treatment
This medication is used to treat acute migraine headaches and cluster headaches. The medicine may be used as self-administered injection or in the form of tablets. The usual oral dose amounts to 140 to 300 mg.

For safe and effective use of this medicine:
♦ Follow your doctor's instructions if this medicine was prescribed.
♦ Follow the manufacturer's package directions if you are treating yourself.

Side effects
Along with the needed effects, a medicine may cause some unwanted effects. Possible side effects include:
Burning at injection site
Pain at injection site
Nausea
Vomiting
Sensation of warmth
Dizziness
Numbness
Drowsiness
Flushing
Lightheadedness
Cramps
Stiffness
Muscle ache
Weakness
Anxiety
Vision changes

Overdose
Significant symptoms of overdose are:
Convulsions
Tremor
Swelling of arms
Swelling of legs
Breathing difficulty
Paralysis
Chest pain
■ Call a doctor or hospital emergency room for instructions. If neccessary, start first aid immediately.

Interactions
This medicine may interact with several other drugs such as propranolol. Ergot-containing drugs have been reported to cause prolonged vasospastic reactions.
■ Be sure to tell your doctor about any medications you are currently taking.

Storage
Tablets and injection vials should be stored at room temperature; store away from heat and direct light. Keep out of reach of children.

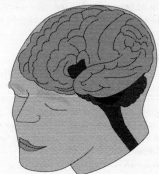

IMPRIL

Properties

This medicine contains imipramine as active ingredient. It belongs to the group of medicines known as tricyclic antidepressants or 'mood elevators.' It is used to relieve mental depression and depression that sometimes occurs with anxiety. The medication gradually relieves, but doesn't cure, symptoms of depression. The medication may also be used for the treatment of narcolepsy, bulimia, painic attacks, cocaine withdrawal, attention deficit disorder.

Before using this medicine

Before you use this medicine check with your doctor, or pharmacist:
- if you ever had any unusual or allergic reaction to any tricyclic antidepressant, maprotiline or trazodone.
- if you are on a low-salt, low-sugar, or any other special diet, or if you are allergic to any substance, such as sulfites or other preservatives or dyes.
- if you are pregnant or intend to become pregnant while using this medicine.
  There have been reports of newborns suffering from heart, breathing, and urinary problems when their mothers had taken tricyclic antidepressants before delivery.
- if you are breast-feeding an infant. Some tricyclic antidepressants pass into the breast milk.

Treatment

Take this medicine only as directed by your doctor, to benefit your condition as much as possible. Do not take more of it, do not take it more often, and do not take it for a longer period of time than your doctor ordered.

To lessen stomach upset, take this medicine with food, even for a daily bedtime dose, unless your doctor has told you to take it on an empty stomach. If you forget your once-a-day bedtime dose, Do not take it more than 3 hours late. If more than 3 hours, wait for next scheduled dose;.

Sometimes this medicine must be taken for several weeks before you begin to feel better.

Side effects

Along with the needed effects, a medicine may cause some unwanted effects. Side effects that usually do not require medical attention: difficult or frequent urination; decreased sex drive; muscle aches; abnormal dreams; nasal congestion; weakness and faintness when arising from bed or chair; back pain.
- Other side effects that should be reported to your doctor immediately are:
  Hallucinations
  Shakiness
  Dizziness or fainting
  Blurred vision, eye pain
  Irregular heartbeat or slow pulse
  Inflamed tongue
  Abdominal pain
  Jaundice
  Hair loss, rash
  Fever, chills
  Joint pain
  Palpitations

Interactions

This medicine may interact with several other drugs such as anticoagulants, anticholinergics, cold remedies, oral contraceptives, seizure medicines, sleeping medicines, thyroid medicines, etc.
- Be sure to tell your doctor about any medications you are currently taking.

Storage

Tablets, capsules, etc. should be stored at room temperature in tightly closed, light-resistant containers as directed by your pharmacist. Keep out of reach of children since overdose is especially dangerous in young children. Do not store in the bathroom medicine cabinet because the heat or moisture may cause the medicine to break down. Keep the liquid form of the medicine from freezing.

IONAMIN

Properties
This medicine contains phentermine as active ingredient; it is prescribed for appetite suppression.

Appetite suppressants are used in the short-term (a few weeks) treatment of obesity. In a few weeks (6 to 12), these medicines in combination with dieting, exercise, and changes in eating habits can help patients lose weight. However, since their appetite reducing effect is only temporary, they are useful only for the first weeks of dieting until new eating habits are established.

Before using this medicine
Before you use this medicine check with your doctor, or pharmacist:
- if you ever had any unusual or allergic reaction to any of the compounds of this medicine.
- if you are on a low-salt, low-sugar, or any other special diet, or if you are allergic to any substance, such as sulfites or other preservatives or dyes.
- if you are pregnant, intend to become pregnant or breast-feeding an infant while using this medicine.
- if you have any of the following medical problems:
  Diabetes mellitus
  Epilepsy
  Glaucoma
  Heart disease
  High blood pressure
  Mental illness (severe)

Treatment
This medication is used to relieve or prevent the symptoms of your medical problem.

Take them as directed. Do not take more of them and do not take them more often than recommended on the label. If too much of the drug is taken, it may become habit-forming.
- The medicine produces central nervous system stimulation, and it should not be taken by people with heart disease or high blood pressure.
- If you think this medicine is not working as well after you have taken it for a few weeks, do not increase the dose. Instead, check with your doctor.

Side effects
The following minor side effects may occur: irritability, nervousness, restlessness, trouble in sleeping.

These side effects should disappear as your body adjusts to the medication. Tell your doctor about any side effects that are persistent or particularly bothersome. It is especially important to tell your doctor about:
  Mental depression
  Nausea or vomiting
  Stomach cramps or pain
  Trembling
  Unusual tiredness
- Discontinue use of the drug; call your doctor right away. Adverse reactions and side effects may be more frequent and severe in people over age 60 than in younger persons.

Interactions
This medicine interacts with several other drugs such as antihypertensives, other appetite suppressants, caffeine, central nervous system depressants, central nervous system stimulants, furazolidone, guanethidine, hydralazine, MAO inhibitors, methyldopa, molindone, phenothiazines, rauwolfia alkaloids, sodium bicarbonate. Interaction with alcoholic beverages may produce drowsiness, sleepiness, and/or inability to concentrate.
- Be sure to tell your doctor about any medications you are currently taking.

Storage
This medicine should be stored at room temperature in tightly closed containers. Store away from heat and direct light. Keep out of reach of children, since overdose may be very dangerous in children. Do not store this medicine in the bathroom medicine cabinet because the heat and moisture cause the medicine to break down. Do not keep outdated medicine or medicine no longer needed. Flush the contents of the container down the toilet.

ISO-BID

Properties
This medicine contains isosorbide dinitrate as active ingredient. Nitrates improve the supply of blood and oxygen to the heart. This medication is for oral use.

Before using this medicine
Before you use this medicine check with your doctor, or pharmacist:
- if you ever had any unusual or allergic reaction to nitrates or nitrites.
- if you are on a low-salt, low-sugar, or any other special diet, or if you are allergic to any substance, such as sulfites or other preservatives or dyes.
- if you are pregnant or intend to become pregnant while using this medicine. Although nitrates have not been shown to cause problems in humans, the chance always exists.
- if you are breast-feeding an infant.
- if you have recently had a heart attack or stroke.
- if you have any of the following medical problems:
  Anemia
  Glaucoma
  Intestinal problems
  Overactive thyroid
- if you are now taking any of the following medicines or types of medicines:
  Antihypertensives
  Asthma or hay fever medicine
  Cold medicine
  Decongestant
  Medicine for appetite control
  Narcotic
  Pain medicine
  Sinus congestion medicine

Treatment
This medication is used to treat and prevent angina (chest pain). Nitroglycerin is a vasodilator, which relaxes the muscles of the blood vessels, causing an increase in the oxygen supply to the heart. The oral tablets, capsules, ointment and patches do not act quickly; they are used to prevent chest pain. The sublingual tablets and oral spray act quickly and can be used to relieve chest pain after it has started.

- Take this medicine exactly as directed by your doctor or pharmacist. It will work only if taken correctly.
- If you are taking this medicine regularly and you miss a dose, take it as soon as possible. However, if your next scheduled dose; is within 2 hours (or within 6 hours for extended-release capsules or tablets), skip the missed dose and go back to your regular dosing schedule.
- If you have been taking this medicine regularly for several weeks or more, do not suddenly stop using it. Stopping suddenly may bring on attacks of angina.

Side effects
There are a number of side effects that usually do not require medical attention. These possible side effects may go away during treatment; however, if they continue or are bothersome, check with your doctor, nurse, or pharmacist. More common are: dizziness, lightheadedness, or fainting when standing up; fast pulse; flushing of face and neck; headache; nausea or vomiting.

Side effects that should be reported to your doctor are: blurred vision; dry mouth; severe or prolonged headache; skin rash.

Interactions
This medicine may interact with several other drugs such as tricyclic antidepressants and cough medicines. Before starting to take or apply nitroglycerin, be sure to tell your doctor about any medications you are currently taking.

Storage
Tablets, capsules, and oral spray should be stored as in a tightly capped bottle in a cool, dry place. Ointment and patches should be stored at room temperature in their original containers. Keep out of reach of children. Do not keep outdated medicine or medicine no longer needed.

ISOCHRON

Properties
This medicine contains isosorbide dinitrate as active ingredient. Nitrates improve the supply of blood and oxygen to the heart. This medication is for oral use.

Before using this medicine
Before you use this medicine check with your doctor, or pharmacist:
- if you ever had any unusual or allergic reaction to nitrates or nitrites.
- if you are on a low-salt, low-sugar, or any other special diet, or if you are allergic to any substance, such as sulfites or other preservatives or dyes.
- if you are pregnant or intend to become pregnant while using this medicine. Although nitrates have not been shown to cause problems in humans, the chance always exists.
- if you are breast-feeding an infant.
- if you have recently had a heart attack or stroke.
- if you have any of the following medical problems:
Anemia
Glaucoma
Intestinal problems
Overactive thyroid
- if you are now taking any of the following medicines or types of medicines:
Antihypertensives
Asthma or hay fever medicine
Cold medicine
Decongestant
Medicine for appetite control
Narcotic
Pain medicine
Sinus congestion medicine

Treatment
This medication is used to treat and prevent angina (chest pain). Nitroglycerin is a vasodilator, which relaxes the muscles of the blood vessels, causing an increase in the oxygen supply to the heart. The oral tablets, capsules, ointment and patches do not act quickly; they are used to prevent chest pain. The sublingual tablets and oral spray act quickly and can be used to relieve chest pain after it has started.
- Take this medicine exactly as directed by your doctor or pharmacist. It will work only if taken correctly.
- If you are taking this medicine regularly and you miss a dose, take it as soon as possible. However, if your next scheduled dose; is within 2 hours (or within 6 hours for extended-release capsules or tablets), skip the missed dose and go back to your regular dosing schedule.
- If you have been taking this medicine regularly for several weeks or more, do not suddenly stop using it. Stopping suddenly may bring on attacks of angina.

Side effects
There are a number of side effects that usually do not require medical attention. These possible side effects may go away during treatment; however, if they continue or are bothersome, check with your doctor, nurse, or pharmacist. More common are: dizziness, lightheadedness, or fainting when standing up; fast pulse; flushing of face and neck; headache; nausea or vomiting.
  Side effects that should be reported to your doctor are: blurred vision; dry mouth; severe or prolonged headache; skin rash.

Interactions
This medicine may interact with several other drugs such as tricyclic antidepressants and cough medicines. Before starting to take or apply nitroglycerin, be sure to tell your doctor about any medications you are currently taking.

Storage
Tablets, capsules, and oral spray should be stored as in a tightly capped bottle in a cool, dry place. Ointment and patches should be stored at room temperature in their original containers. Keep out of reach of children. Do not keep outdated medicine or medicine no longer needed.

ISONATE

Properties
This medicine contains isosorbide dinitrate as active ingredient. Nitrates improve the supply of blood and oxygen to the heart. This medication is for oral use.

Before using this medicine
Before you use this medicine check with your doctor, or pharmacist:
- if you ever had any unusual or allergic reaction to nitrates or nitrites.
- if you are on a low-salt, low-sugar, or any other special diet, or if you are allergic to any substance, such as sulfites or other preservatives or dyes.
- if you are pregnant or intend to become pregnant while using this medicine. Although nitrates have not been shown to cause problems in humans, the chance always exists.
- if you are breast-feeding an infant.
- if you have recently had a heart attack or stroke.
- if you have any of the following medical problems:
  Anemia
  Glaucoma
  Intestinal problems
  Overactive thyroid
- if you are now taking any of the following medicines or types of medicines:
  Antihypertensives
  Asthma or hay fever medicine
  Cold medicine
  Decongestant
  Medicine for appetite control
  Narcotic
  Pain medicine
  Sinus congestion medicine

Treatment
This medication is used to treat and prevent angina (chest pain). Nitroglycerin is a vasodilator, which relaxes the muscles of the blood vessels, causing an increase in the oxygen supply to the heart. The oral tablets, capsules, ointment and patches do not act quickly; they are used to prevent chest pain. The sublingual tablets and oral spray act quickly and can be used to relieve chest pain after it has started.
- Take this medicine exactly as directed by your doctor or pharmacist. It will work only if taken correctly.
- If you are taking this medicine regularly and you miss a dose, take it as soon as possible. However, if your next scheduled dose; is within 2 hours (or within 6 hours for extended-release capsules or tablets), skip the missed dose and go back to your regular dosing schedule.
- If you have been taking this medicine regularly for several weeks or more, do not suddenly stop using it. Stopping suddenly may bring on attacks of angina.

Side effects
There are a number of side effects that usually do not require medical attention. These possible side effects may go away during treatment; however, if they continue or are bothersome, check with your doctor, nurse, or pharmacist. More common are: dizziness, lightheadedness, or fainting when standing up; fast pulse; flushing of face and neck; headache; nausea or vomiting.

Side effects that should be reported to your doctor are: blurred vision; dry mouth; severe or prolonged headache; skin rash.

Interactions
This medicine may interact with several other drugs such as tricyclic antidepressants and cough medicines. Before starting to take or apply nitroglycerin, be sure to tell your doctor about any medications you are currently taking.

Storage
Tablets, capsules, and oral spray should be stored as in a tightly capped bottle in a cool, dry place. Ointment and patches should be stored at room temperature in their original containers. Keep out of reach of children. Do not keep outdated medicine or medicine no longer needed.

ISONATE TR

Properties
This medicine contains isosorbide dinitrate as active ingredient. Nitrates improve the supply of blood and oxygen to the heart. This medication is for oral use.

Before using this medicine
Before you use this medicine check with your doctor, or pharmacist:
- if you ever had any unusual or allergic reaction to nitrates or nitrites.
- if you are on a low-salt, low-sugar, or any other special diet, or if you are allergic to any substance, such as sulfites or other preservatives or dyes.
- if you are pregnant or intend to become pregnant while using this medicine. Although nitrates have not been shown to cause problems in humans, the chance always exists.
- if you are breast-feeding an infant.
- if you have recently had a heart attack or stroke.
- if you have any of the following medical problems:
  Anemia
  Glaucoma
  Intestinal problems
  Overactive thyroid
- if you are now taking any of the following medicines or types of medicines:
  Antihypertensives
  Asthma or hay fever medicine
  Cold medicine
  Decongestant
  Medicine for appetite control
  Narcotic
  Pain medicine
  Sinus congestion medicine

Treatment
This medication is used to treat and prevent angina (chest pain). Nitroglycerin is a vasodilator, which relaxes the muscles of the blood vessels, causing an increase in the oxygen supply to the heart. The oral tablets, capsules, ointment and patches do not act quickly; they are used to prevent chest pain. The sublingual tablets and oral spray act quickly and can be used to relieve chest pain after it has started.

- Take this medicine exactly as directed by your doctor or pharmacist. It will work only if taken correctly.
- If you are taking this medicine regularly and you miss a dose, take it as soon as possible. However, if your next scheduled dose; is within 2 hours (or within 6 hours for extended-release capsules or tablets), skip the missed dose and go back to your regular dosing schedule.
- If you have been taking this medicine regularly for several weeks or more, do not suddenly stop using it. Stopping suddenly may bring on attacks of angina.

Side effects
There are a number of side effects that usually do not require medical attention. These possible side effects may go away during treatment; however, if they continue or are bothersome, check with your doctor, nurse, or pharmacist. More common are: dizziness, lightheadedness, or fainting when standing up; fast pulse; flushing of face and neck; headache; nausea or vomiting.

Side effects that should be reported to your doctor are: blurred vision; dry mouth; severe or prolonged headache; skin rash.

Interactions
This medicine may interact with several other drugs such as tricyclic antidepressants and cough medicines. Before starting to take or apply nitroglycerin, be sure to tell your doctor about any medications you are currently taking.

Storage
Tablets, capsules, and oral spray should be stored as in a tightly capped bottle in a cool, dry place. Ointment and patches should be stored at room temperature in their original containers. Keep out of reach of children. Do not keep outdated medicine or medicine no longer needed.

ISOPTIN

Properties
This medicine contains verapamil as active ingredient. It is a so-called calcium channel blocker, working by blocking the passage of calcium into heart and smooth muscle. Since calcium is an essential factor in muscle contraction, any medicine that affects calcium in this way will interfere with the contraction of these muscles.

The medicine works by:
◆ reducing the work that the heart must perform;
◆ reducing the normal arterial blood pressure;
◆ increasing oxygen to the heart muscle.

The medicine is prescribed for the treatment of attacks of angina pectoris, irregular heartbeat, and high blood pressure. In many cases it can be used for the treatment and prevention of migraine.

Before using this medicine
Before you use this medicine check with your doctor, or pharmacist:
- if you ever had any unusual or allergic reaction to this medicine or any calcium channel blocker;
- if you are pregnant or intend to become pregnant while using this medicine;
- if you have low blood pressure;
- if you have kidney or lifer disease;
- if you are breast-feeding an infant;
- if you easily get a rash or intensity sunburn in areas exposed to sun or ultraviolet light.

Treatment
This medication is used for treatment of heart conditions (for instance, angina pectoris) and high blood pressure. Tablets, capsules or extended-release tablets should be taken with liquid. The usual dose amounts to 30 to 100 milligrams a day.

For safe and effective use of medicine:
◆ Follow your doctor's instructions if this medicine was prescribed.
◆ Follow the manufacturer's package directions if you are treating yourself.

Side effects
Along with the needed effects, a medicine may cause some unwanted effects. Possible side effects include:
Tiredness
Changes in heartbeat
Wheezing
Cough
Shortness of breath
Dizziness
Fainting
Numbness in hands and feet
Tingling in hands and feet
Difficult urination
Constipation

Overdose
The following symptoms may be a sign of overdose:
Unusually fast heartbeat
Unusually slow heartbeat
Loss of consciousness
Cardiac arrest
■ Call a doctor or hospital emergency room for instructions. If necessary start first aid immediately.

Interactions
The effect of this medicine may cause a blood pressure drop if taken together with antihypertensives. Cimetidine may increase the effect of the calcium blocker.

The simultaneous use of diuretics and calcium channel blockers may cause dangerous blood pressure drop.
■ Be sure to tell your doctor about any medications you are currently taking.

Storage
Capsules, tablets, etc. should be stored at room temperature; store away from heat and direct light. Keep out of reach of children, since this medicine may be dangerous in children.

ISOPTO CETAMIDE (Ophthalmic)

Properties

This medicine contains an ophthalmic antibacterial, as active ingredient. It helps the body to overcome eye infections on surface tissues of the eye. It is most useful when the infecting organism is one known to be sensitive to the antibacterial drug. The drug penetrates the bacterial cell membrane and prevents cells from multiplying.

Before using this medicine

Before you use this medicine check with your doctor:
- if you ever had any unusual or allergic reaction to any of the compounds of the medicine.
- if you are on a low-salt, low-sugar, or any other special diet, or if you are allergic to any substance, such as sulfites or other preservatives or dyes.
- if you are pregnant or intend to become pregnant while using this medicine. Although ophthalmic antibacterials have been found to be safe for use during pregnancy, you should check with your doctor before taking any drug if you are pregnant.

Treatment

This medication is used to treat an infection caused by bacteria. The medicine may be used in the form of eye drops or as an eye ointment. Use the medication as directed, Do not miss a dose. If you forget a dose, use it as soon as you remember. Notify your doctor if eye symptoms fail to improve in two to four days.
- ◆ To apply eye drops: Till the head backward when applying the eye drops. Pull the lower eyelid away from the eye to form a pouch. After applying the drop, keep the eye closed for a minute or so. This allows the medication to come in contact with the infection.
- ◆ To apply eye ointment: Pull lower lid down from eye to form a pouch. Squeeze tube to apply thin strip of ointment into pouch. Close eye for 1 to 2 minutes.

Always wash your hands before applying the ointment. The drug starts to work in about one hour. Treatment may require 7 to 10 days to control infection. Older adults or seniors may take this medication without special restriction.

Side effects

Along with the needed effects, a medicine may cause some unwanted effects. Side effects that usually do not require medical attention: occasional local irritation after application to the eye. Ointments may cause blurred vision for a few minutes; continue the use of the eye drops or ointment, but tell your doctor at the next visit.
- ■ Discontinue the use of eye drops or eye ointment in the following cases:
  Sore throat
  Aplastic anemia
  Pale skin
  Unusual redness of the eye
  Unusual irritation of the eye
  Fever
  Unusual bleeding
  Unusual bruising
- ■ Tell your doctor about any side effects that are persistent or particularly bothersome. In case of prolonged use sensitivity reactions may develop.

Interactions

Clinically significant interactions with oral or injected medicines are unlikely. Do not use the eye drops or ointment with any other eye drops or ointment without checking with your ophthalmologist.

Storage

Keep bottle (with eye drops) or container (containing ointment) lightly closed. Store in a cool place, but Do not freeze. Wash hands immediately after using.

Do not store in the bathroom medicine cabinet because the heat or moisture may cause the medicine to break down.

Do not keep outdated medicine or medicine no longer needed. Flush the contents of the bottle or tube down the toilet, unless otherwise directed.

ISOPTO FENICOL (Ophthalmic)

Properties
This medicine contains an ophthalmic antibacterial, as active ingredient. It helps the body to overcome eye infections on surface tissues of the eye. It is most useful when the infecting organism is one known to be sensitive to the antibacterial drug.

The drug penetrates the bacterial cell membrane and prevents cells from multiplying.

Before using this medicine
Before you use this medicine check with your doctor:
- if you ever had any unusual or allergic reaction to any of the compounds of the medicine.
- if you are on a low-salt, low-sugar, or any other special diet, or if you are allergic to any substance, such as sulfites or other preservatives or dyes.
- if you are pregnant or intend to become pregnant while using this medicine. Although ophthalmic antibacterials have been found to be safe for use during pregnancy, you should check with your doctor before taking any drug if you are pregnant.

Treatment
This medication is used to treat an infection caused by bacteria. The medicine may be used in the form of eye drops or as an eye ointment. Use the medication as directed, Do not miss a dose. If you forget a dose, use it as soon as you remember. Notify your doctor if eye symptoms fail to improve in two to four days.
- ◆ To apply eye drops: Till the head backward when applying the eye drops. Pull the lower eyelid away from the eye to form a pouch. After applying the drop, keep the eye closed for a minute or so. This allows the medication to come in contact with the infection.
- ◆ To apply eye ointment: Pull lower lid down from eye to form a pouch. Squeeze tube to apply thin strip of ointment into pouch. Close eye for 1 to 2 minutes.

Always wash your hands before applying the ointment.
The drug starts to work in about one hour. Treatment may require 7 to 10 days to control infection.
Older adults or seniors may take this medication without special restriction.

Side effects
Along with the needed effects, a medicine may cause some unwanted effects. Side effects that usually do not require medical attention: occasional local irritation after application to the eye. Ointments may cause blurred vision for a few minutes; continue the use of the eye drops or ointment, but tell your doctor at the next visit.
- ■ Discontinue the use of eye drops or eye ointment in the following cases:
  Sore throat
  Aplastic anemia
  Pale skin
  Unusual redness of the eye
  Unusual irritation of the eye
  Fever
  Unusual bleeding
  Unusual bruising
- ■ Tell your doctor about any side effects that are persistent or particularly bothersome. In case of prolonged use sensitivity reactions may develop.

Interactions
Clinically significant interactions with oral or injected medicines are unlikely. Do not use the eye drops or ointment with any other eye drops or ointment without checking with your ophthalmologist.

Storage
Keep bottle (with eye drops) or container (containing ointment) lightly closed. Store in a cool place, but Do not freeze. Wash hands immediately after using. Do not store in the bathroom medicine cabinet because the heat or moisture may cause the medicine to break down. Do not keep outdated medicine or medicine no longer needed. Flush the contents of the bottle or tube down the toilet, unless otherwise directed.

ISORDIL

Properties

This medicine contains isosorbide dinitrate as active ingredient. Nitrates improve the supply of blood and oxygen to the heart. This medication is for oral use.

Before using this medicine

Before you use this medicine check with your doctor, or pharmacist:
- if you ever had any unusual or allergic reaction to nitrates or nitrites.
- if you are on a low-salt, low-sugar, or any other special diet, or if you are allergic to any substance, such as sulfites or other preservatives or dyes.
- if you are pregnant or intend to become pregnant while using this medicine. Although nitrates have not been shown to cause problems in humans, the chance always exists.
- if you are breast-feeding an infant.
- if you have recently had a heart attack or stroke.
- if you have any of the following medical problems:
  Anemia
  Glaucoma
  Intestinal problems
  Overactive thyroid
- if you are now taking any of the following medicines or types of medicines:
  Antihypertensives
  Asthma or hay fever medicine
  Cold medicine
  Decongestant
  Medicine for appetite control
  Narcotic
  Pain medicine
  Sinus congestion medicine

Treatment

This medication is used to treat and prevent angina (chest pain). Nitroglycerin is a vasodilator, which relaxes the muscles of the blood vessels, causing an increase in the oxygen supply to the heart. The oral tablets, capsules, ointment and patches do not act quickly; they are used to prevent chest pain. The sublingual tablets and oral spray act quickly and can be used to relieve chest pain after it has started.
- Take this medicine exactly as directed by your doctor or pharmacist. It will work only if taken correctly.
- If you are taking this medicine regularly and you miss a dose, take it as soon as possible. However, if your next scheduled dose; is within 2 hours (or within 6 hours for extended-release capsules or tablets), skip the missed dose and go back to your regular dosing schedule.
- If you have been taking this medicine regularly for several weeks or more, do not suddenly stop using it. Stopping suddenly may bring on attacks of angina.

Side effects

There are a number of side effects that usually do not require medical attention. These possible side effects may go away during treatment; however, if they continue or are bothersome, check with your doctor, nurse, or pharmacist. More common are: dizziness, lightheadedness, or fainting when standing up; fast pulse; flushing of face and neck; headache; nausea or vomiting.

Side effects that should be reported to your doctor are: blurred vision; dry mouth; severe or prolonged headache; skin rash.

Interactions

This medicine may interact with several other drugs such as tricyclic antidepressants and cough medicines. Before starting to take or apply nitroglycerin, be sure to tell your doctor about any medications you are currently taking.

Storage

Tablets, capsules, and oral spray should be stored as in a tightly capped bottle in a cool, dry place. Ointment and patches should be stored at room temperature in their original containers. Keep out of reach of children. Do not keep outdated medicine or medicine no longer needed.

ISOSORBIDE DINITRATE

Properties
This medicine contains isosorbide dinitrate as active ingredient. Nitrates improve the supply of blood and oxygen
to the heart. This medication is for oral
use.

Before using this medicine
Before you use this medicine check
with your doctor, or pharmacist:
- if you ever had any unusual or allergic reaction to nitrates or nitrites.
- if you are on a low-salt, low-sugar,
  or any other special diet, or if you are
  allergic to any substance, such as sulfites or other preservatives or dyes.
- if you are pregnant or intend to become pregnant while using this
  medicine. Although nitrates have not
  been shown to cause problems in humans, the chance always exists.
- if you are breast-feeding an infant.
- if you have recently had a heart attack or stroke.
- if you have any of the following
  medical problems:
  Anemia
  Glaucoma
  Intestinal problems
  Overactive thyroid
- if you are now taking any of the following medicines or types of medicines:
  Antihypertensives
  Asthma or hay fever medicine
  Cold medicine
  Decongestant
  Medicine for appetite control
  Narcotic
  Pain medicine
  Sinus congestion medicine

Treatment
This medication is used to treat and prevent angina (chest pain). Nitroglycerin
is a vasodilator, which relaxes the muscles of the blood vessels, causing an increase in the oxygen supply to the heart.
The oral tablets, capsules, ointment and
patches do not act quickly; they are
used to prevent chest pain. The sublingual tablets and oral spray act quickly
and can be used to relieve chest pain after it has started.
- Take this medicine exactly as directed by your doctor or pharmacist.
  It will work only if taken correctly.
- If you are taking this medicine regularly and you miss a dose, take it as
  soon as possible. However, if your
  next scheduled dose; is within 2
  hours (or within 6 hours for extended-release capsules or tablets),
  skip the missed dose and go back to
  your regular dosing schedule.
- If you have been taking this medicine regularly for several weeks or
  more, do not suddenly stop using it.
  Stopping suddenly may bring on attacks of angina.

Side effects
There are a number of side effects that
usually do not require medical attention. These possible side effects may go
away during treatment; however, if they
continue or are bothersome, check with
your doctor, nurse, or pharmacist. More
common are: dizziness, lightheadedness, or fainting when standing up; fast
pulse; flushing of face and neck; headache; nausea or vomiting.
    Side effects that should be reported
to your doctor are: blurred vision; dry
mouth; severe or prolonged headache;
skin rash.

Interactions
This medicine may interact with several
other drugs such as tricyclic antidepressants and cough medicines. Before
starting to take or apply nitroglycerin,
be sure to tell your doctor about any
medications you are currently taking.

Storage
Tablets, capsules, and oral spray should
be stored as in a tightly capped bottle in
a cool, dry place. Ointment and patches
should be stored at room temperature in
their original containers. Keep out of
reach of children. Do not keep outdated
medicine or medicine no longer needed.

ISOTRATE

Properties
This medicine contains isosorbide dinitrate as active ingredient. Nitrates improve the supply of blood and oxygen to the heart. This medication is for oral use.

Before using this medicine
Before you use this medicine check with your doctor, or pharmacist:
- if you ever had any unusual or allergic reaction to nitrates or nitrites.
- if you are on a low-salt, low-sugar, or any other special diet, or if you are allergic to any substance, such as sulfites or other preservatives or dyes.
- if you are pregnant or intend to become pregnant while using this medicine. Although nitrates have not been shown to cause problems in humans, the chance always exists.
- if you are breast-feeding an infant.
- if you have recently had a heart attack or stroke.
- if you have any of the following medical problems:
  Anemia
  Glaucoma
  Intestinal problems
  Overactive thyroid
- if you are now taking any of the following medicines or types of medicines:
  Antihypertensives
  Asthma or hay fever medicine
  Cold medicine
  Decongestant
  Medicine for appetite control
  Narcotic
  Pain medicine
  Sinus congestion medicine

Treatment
This medication is used to treat and prevent angina (chest pain). Nitroglycerin is a vasodilator, which relaxes the muscles of the blood vessels, causing an increase in the oxygen supply to the heart. The oral tablets, capsules, ointment and patches do not act quickly; they are used to prevent chest pain. The sublingual tablets and oral spray act quickly and can be used to relieve chest pain after it has started.

- Take this medicine exactly as directed by your doctor or pharmacist. It will work only if taken correctly.
- If you are taking this medicine regularly and you miss a dose, take it as soon as possible. However, if your next scheduled dose; is within 2 hours (or within 6 hours for extended-release capsules or tablets), skip the missed dose and go back to your regular dosing schedule.
- If you have been taking this medicine regularly for several weeks or more, do not suddenly stop using it. Stopping suddenly may bring on attacks of angina.

Side effects
There are a number of side effects that usually do not require medical attention. These possible side effects may go away during treatment; however, if they continue or are bothersome, check with your doctor, nurse, or pharmacist. More common are: dizziness, lightheadedness, or fainting when standing up; fast pulse; flushing of face and neck; headache; nausea or vomiting.

Side effects that should be reported to your doctor are: blurred vision; dry mouth; severe or prolonged headache; skin rash.

Interactions
This medicine may interact with several other drugs such as tricyclic antidepressants and cough medicines. Before starting to take or apply nitroglycerin, be sure to tell your doctor about any medications you are currently taking.

Storage
Tablets, capsules, and oral spray should be stored as in a tightly capped bottle in a cool, dry place. Ointment and patches should be stored at room temperature in their original containers. Keep out of reach of children. Do not keep outdated medicine or medicine no longer needed.

ISRADIPINE

Properties

This medicine contains isradipine as active ingredient. It is a so-called calcium channel blocker, working by blocking the passage of calcium into heart and smooth muscle. Since calcium is an essential factor in muscle contraction, any medicine that affects calcium in this way will interfere with the contraction of these muscles.

The medicine works by:
◆ reducing the work that the heart must perform;
◆ reducing the normal arterial blood pressure;
◆ increasing oxygen to the heart muscle.

The medicine is prescribed for the treatment of attacks of angina pectoris, irregular heartbeat, and high blood pressure. In many cases it can be used for the treatment and prevention of migraine.

Before using this medicine

Before you use this medicine check with your doctor, or pharmacist:
- if you ever had any unusual or allergic reaction to this medicine or any calcium channel blocker;
- if you are pregnant or intend to become pregnant while using this medicine;
- if you have low blood pressure;
- if you have kidney or lifer disease;
- if you are breast-feeding an infant;
- if you easily get a rash or intensity sunburn in areas exposed to sun or ultraviolet light.

Treatment

This medication is used for treatment of heart conditions (for instance, angina pectoris) and high blood pressure. Tablets, capsules or extended-release tablets should be taken with liquid. The usual dose amounts to 30 to 100 milligrams a day.

For safe and effective use of medicine:
◆ Follow your doctor's instructions if this medicine was prescribed.
◆ Follow the manufacturer's package directions if you are treating yourself.

Side effects

Along with the needed effects, a medicine may cause some unwanted effects. Possible side effects include:
Tiredness
Changes in heartbeat
Wheezing
Cough
Shortness of breath
Dizziness
Fainting
Numbness in hands and feet
Tingling in hands and feet
Difficult urination
Constipation

Overdose

The following symptoms may be a sign of overdose:
Unusually fast heartbeat
Unusually slow heartbeat
Loss of consciousness
Cardiac arrest
■ Call a doctor or hospital emergency room for instructions. If necessary start first aid immediately.

Interactions

The effect of this medicine may cause a blood pressure drop if taken together with antihypertensives. Cimetidine may increase the effect of the calcium blocker.

The simultaneous use of diuretics and calcium channel blockers may cause dangerous blood pressure drop.
■ Be sure to tell your doctor about any medications you are currently taking.

Storage

Capsules, tablets, etc. should be stored at room temperature; store away from heat and direct light. Keep out of reach of children, since this medicine may be dangerous in children.

JANIMINE

Properties

This medicine contains imipramine as active ingredient. It belongs to the group of medicines known as tricyclic antidepressants or 'mood elevators.' It is used to relieve mental depression and depression that sometimes occurs with anxiety. The medication gradually relieves, but doesn't cure, symptoms of depression. The medication may also be used for the treatment of narcolepsy, bulimia, painic attacks, cocaine withdrawal, attention deficit disorder.

Before using this medicine

Before you use this medicine check with your doctor, or pharmacist:
- if you ever had any unusual or allergic reaction to any tricyclic antidepressant, maprotiline or trazodone.
- if you are on a low-salt, low-sugar, or any other special diet, or if you are allergic to any substance, such as sulfites or other preservatives or dyes.
- if you are pregnant or intend to become pregnant while using this medicine. There have been reports of newborns suffering from heart, breathing, and urinary problems when their mothers had taken tricyclic antidepressants before delivery.
- if you are breast-feeding an infant. Some tricyclic antidepressants pass into the breast milk.

Treatment

Take this medicine only as directed by your doctor, to benefit your condition as much as possible. Do not take more of it, do not take it more often, and do not take it for a longer period of time than your doctor ordered.

To lessen stomach upset, take this medicine with food, even for a daily bedtime dose, unless your doctor has told you to take it on an empty stomach. If you forget your once-a-day bedtime dose, Do not take it more than 3 hours late. If more than 3 hours, wait for next scheduled dose;.

Sometimes this medicine must be taken for several weeks before you begin to feel better.

Side effects

Along with the needed effects, a medicine may cause some unwanted effects. Side effects that usually do not require medical attention: difficult or frequent urination; decreased sex drive; muscle aches; abnormal dreams; nasal congestion; weakness and faintness when arising from bed or chair; back pain.
- Other side effects that should be reported to your doctor immediately are:
  Hallucinations
  Shakiness
  Dizziness or fainting
  Blurred vision, eye pain
  Irregular heartbeat or slow pulse
  Inflamed tongue
  Abdominal pain
  Jaundice
  Hair loss, rash
  Fever, chills
  Joint pain
  Palpitations

Interactions

This medicine may interact with several other drugs such as anticoagulants, anticholinergics, cold remedies, oral contraceptives, seizure medicines, sleeping medicines, thyroid medicines, etc.
- Be sure to tell your doctor about any medications you are currently taking.

Storage

Tablets, capsules, etc. should be stored at room temperature in tightly closed, light-resistant containers as directed by your pharmacist. Keep out of reach of children since overdose is especially dangerous in young children. Do not store in the bathroom medicine cabinet because the heat or moisture may cause the medicine to break down. Keep the liquid form of the medicine from freezing.

JENEST

Properties
This medicine contains norethindrone and ethinyl estradiol as active ingredients. It is an oral contraceptive prescribed to prevent pregnancy and/or to regulate menstrual periods.

The drug works by altering the mucus at the cervix entrance to prevent the entry of sperm. It also alters the uterus lining to resist implantation of the fertilized egg. Oral contraceptives create the same chemical atmosphere in blood that exists during pregnancy.

Before using this medicine
Before you use this medicine check with your doctor, or pharmacist:
- if you ever had any unusual or allergic reaction to estrogens or progestogen;
- if you are pregnant or want to become pregnant within three months;
- if you are breast-feeding an infant;
- if you have any of the following medical problems:
  Diabetes
  Ailments of the breast
  Disorders of the uterus
  Migraine or epilepsy
  High blood pressure
  Asthma or heart conditions
  Kidney disease
  Gallstones

Treatment
This medication is used to prevent pregnancy or to regulate menstrual periods.

Adverse reactions
Along with the needed effects, a medicine may cause some unwanted effects or adverse reactions.
- *An increased risk of the following adverse reactions has been associated with the use of oral contraceptives:*
  Thrombophlebitis
  Venous thrombosis
  Arterial thromboembolism
  Pulmonary (lung) embolism
  Myocardial infarction
  Cerebral hemorrhage
  Cerebral thrombosis
  Hypertension
  Gallbladder disease
  Hepatic (liver) hepatomas
  Benign lifer tumors
- *The following adverse reactions have been reported in patients receiving oral contraceptives and are believed to be drug-related:*
  Nausea and vomiting
  Abdominal cramps
  Breakthrough bleeding
  Spotting
  Change in menstrual flow
  Amenorrhea
  Temporary infertility
  Edema
  Breast changes
  Weight changes
  Cholestatic jaundice
  Migraine
  Rash (allergic)
  Mental depression
  Vaginal candidiasis

Interactions
This medicine may interact with several other drugs such as antibiotics, anticoagulants, anticonvulsants, antidepressants, oral antidiabetics, antihistamines, barbiturates, oral hypoglycemics, insulin, meperidine.
- Be sure to tell your doctor about any medications you are currently taking.

Storage
Tablets should be stored at room temperature; store away from heat and direct light. Keep out of reach of children, since this medicine may be dangerous in chidren.

K-DUR

Properties

This medicine contains potassium chloride as active ingredient; it is used to treat or prevent potassium deficiency, especially potassium deficiency that is caused by the use of diuretics (water pills).

Potassium is needed to maintain good health. Potassium supplements may be needed by patients who do not have enough potassium in their regular diet and by those who have lost too much potassium because of illness or treatment with certain medicines.

Since too much potassium may also cause health problems, most potassium supplements are available only with your doctor's prescription.

Before using this medicine

Before you use this medicine check with your doctor, or pharmacist:
- if you ever had any unusual or allergic reaction to potassium preparations;
- if you are on a low-salt, low-sugar, or any other special diet, or if you are allergic to any substance, such as sulfites or other preservatives or dyes.
- if you are pregnant or intend to become pregnant while using this medicine. Although potassium supplements have not been shown to cause problems in humans, the chance always exists.
- if you are breast-feeding an infant. Although this medicine has not been shown to cause problems in humans, the chance always exists since small amounts of potassium pass into the breast milk.
- if you have any of the following medical problems:
Addison's disease
Heart disease
Diarrhea
Kidney disease
Stomach ulcer

Treatment

This medication is used to relieve or prevent the symptoms of your medical problem. Take them as directed. Do not take more of them and do not take them more often than recommended on the label, unless otherwise directed by your doctor. To do so may increase the chance of side effects.

In order to avoid stomach irritation, you should take potassium supplements with food or immediately after a meal. If you miss a dose of this medication, take the missed dose as soon as possible, unless it is within two hours of the next scheduled dose;.

Side effects

The following minor side effects may occur:
Diarrhea
Nausea
Stomach pains
Vomiting.
These side effects should disappear as your body adjusts to the medication. Tell your doctor about any side effects that are persistent or particularly bothersome. It is especially important to tell your doctor about anxiety; bloody or black, tarry stools; confusion; difficulty in breathing; numbness or tingling in the arms, legs, or feet; palpitations; severe abdominal pain; or unusual weakness.

Interactions

This medicine interacts with several other drugs such as adrenocorticosteroids, antimuscarinics, calcium-containing medicines; heart medicines such as digitalis or digoxin; laxatives; other potassium-containing medicines.
- Be sure to tell your doctor about any medications you are currently taking.

Storage

Tablets, elixir, etc. should be stored at room temperature in tightly closed containers. Store away from heat and direct light. Keep out of reach of children, since overdose may be very dangerous in children. Do not keep outdated medicine or medicine no longer needed. Flush the contents of the container down the toilet, unless otherwise directed.

K-G ELIXIR

Properties
This medicine contains potassium gluconate as active ingredient; it is used to
treat or prevent potassium deficiency,
especially potassium deficiency that is
caused by the use of diuretics (water
pills).

Potassium is needed to maintain
good health. Potassium supplements
may be needed by patients who do not
have enough potassium in their regular
diet and by those who have lost too
much potassium because of illness or
treatment with certain medicines.

Since too much potassium may also
cause health problems, most potassium
supplements are available only with
your doctor's prescription.

Before using this medicine
Before you use this medicine check
with your doctor, or pharmacist:
- if you ever had any unusual or allergic reaction to potassium preparations;
- if you are on a low-salt, low-sugar,
or any other special diet, or if you are
allergic to any substance, such as sulfites or other preservatives or dyes.
- if you are pregnant or intend to become pregnant while using this
medicine. Although potassium supplements have not been shown to
cause problems in humans, the
chance always exists.
- if you are breast-feeding an infant.
Although this medicine has not been
shown to cause problems in humans,
the chance always exists since small
amounts of potassium pass into the
breast milk.
- if you have any of the following
medical problems:
Addison's disease
Heart disease
Diarrhea
Kidney disease
Stomach ulcer

Treatment
This medication is used to relieve or
prevent the symptoms of your medical
problem. Take them as directed. Do not
take more of them and do not take them
more often than recommended on the
label, unless otherwise directed by your
doctor. To do so may increase the
chance of side effects.

In order to avoid stomach irritation,
you should take potassium supplements
with food or immediately after a meal.
If you miss a dose of this medication,
take the missed dose as soon as possible, unless it is within two hours of the
next scheduled dose;.

Side effects
The following minor side effects may
occur:
Diarrhea
Nausea
Stomach pains
Vomiting.
These side effects should disappear as
your body adjusts to the medication.
Tell your doctor about any side effects
that are persistent or particularly bothersome. It is especially important to tell
your doctor about anxiety; bloody or
black, tarry stools; confusion; difficulty
in breathing; numbness or tingling in
the arms, legs, or feet; palpitations; severe abdominal pain; or unusual weakness.

Interactions
This medicine interacts with several
other drugs such as adrenocorticosteroids, antimuscarinics, calcium-containing medicines; heart medicines such
as digitalis or digoxin; laxatives; other
potassium-containing medicines.
- Be sure to tell your doctor about any
medications you are currently taking.

Storage
Tablets, elixir, etc. should be stored at
room temperature in tightly closed containers. Store away from heat and direct
light. Keep out of reach of children,
since overdose may be very dangerous
in children. Do not keep outdated
medicine or medicine no longer needed.
Flush the contents of the container
down the toilet, unless otherwise directed.

K-DUR

Properties

This medicine contains potassium chloride as active ingredient; it is used to treat or prevent potassium deficiency, especially potassium deficiency that is caused by the use of diuretics (water pills).

Potassium is needed to maintain good health. Potassium supplements may be needed by patients who do not have enough potassium in their regular diet and by those who have lost too much potassium because of illness or treatment with certain medicines.

Since too much potassium may also cause health problems, most potassium supplements are available only with your doctor's prescription.

Before using this medicine

Before you use this medicine check with your doctor, or pharmacist:
- if you ever had any unusual or allergic reaction to potassium preparations;
- if you are on a low-salt, low-sugar, or any other special diet, or if you are allergic to any substance, such as sulfites or other preservatives or dyes.
- if you are pregnant or intend to become pregnant while using this medicine. Although potassium supplements have not been shown to cause problems in humans, the chance always exists.
- if you are breast-feeding an infant. Although this medicine has not been shown to cause problems in humans, the chance always exists since small amounts of potassium pass into the breast milk.
- if you have any of the following medical problems:
Addison's disease
Heart disease
Diarrhea
Kidney disease
Stomach ulcer

Treatment

This medication is used to relieve or prevent the symptoms of your medical problem. Take them as directed. Do not take more of them and do not take them more often than recommended on the label, unless otherwise directed by your doctor. To do so may increase the chance of side effects.

In order to avoid stomach irritation, you should take potassium supplements with food or immediately after a meal. If you miss a dose of this medication, take the missed dose as soon as possible, unless it is within two hours of the next scheduled dose;.

Side effects

The following minor side effects may occur:
Diarrhea
Nausea
Stomach pains
Vomiting.

These side effects should disappear as your body adjusts to the medication. Tell your doctor about any side effects that are persistent or particularly bothersome. It is especially important to tell your doctor about anxiety; bloody or black, tarry stools; confusion; difficulty in breathing; numbness or tingling in the arms, legs, or feet; palpitations; severe abdominal pain; or unusual weakness.

Interactions

This medicine interacts with several other drugs such as adrenocorticosteroids, antimuscarinics, calcium-containing medicines; heart medicines such as digitalis or digoxin; laxatives; other potassium-containing medicines.
- Be sure to tell your doctor about any medications you are currently taking.

Storage

Tablets, elixir, etc. should be stored at room temperature in tightly closed containers. Store away from heat and direct light. Keep out of reach of children, since overdose may be very dangerous in children. Do not keep outdated medicine or medicine no longer needed. Flush the contents of the container down the toilet, unless otherwise directed.

K-G ELIXIR

Properties

This medicine contains potassium gluconate as active ingredient; it is used to treat or prevent potassium deficiency, especially potassium deficiency that is caused by the use of diuretics (water pills).

Potassium is needed to maintain good health. Potassium supplements may be needed by patients who do not have enough potassium in their regular diet and by those who have lost too much potassium because of illness or treatment with certain medicines.

Since too much potassium may also cause health problems, most potassium supplements are available only with your doctor's prescription.

Before using this medicine

Before you use this medicine check with your doctor, or pharmacist:

- if you ever had any unusual or allergic reaction to potassium preparations;
- if you are on a low-salt, low-sugar, or any other special diet, or if you are allergic to any substance, such as sulfites or other preservatives or dyes.
- if you are pregnant or intend to become pregnant while using this medicine. Although potassium supplements have not been shown to cause problems in humans, the chance always exists.
- if you are breast-feeding an infant. Although this medicine has not been shown to cause problems in humans, the chance always exists since small amounts of potassium pass into the breast milk.
- if you have any of the following medical problems:
  Addison's disease
  Heart disease
  Diarrhea
  Kidney disease
  Stomach ulcer

Treatment

This medication is used to relieve or prevent the symptoms of your medical problem. Take them as directed. Do not take more of them and do not take them more often than recommended on the label, unless otherwise directed by your doctor. To do so may increase the chance of side effects.

In order to avoid stomach irritation, you should take potassium supplements with food or immediately after a meal. If you miss a dose of this medication, take the missed dose as soon as possible, unless it is within two hours of the next scheduled dose;.

Side effects

The following minor side effects may occur:
  Diarrhea
  Nausea
  Stomach pains
  Vomiting.

These side effects should disappear as your body adjusts to the medication. Tell your doctor about any side effects that are persistent or particularly bothersome. It is especially important to tell your doctor about anxiety; bloody or black, tarry stools; confusion; difficulty in breathing; numbness or tingling in the arms, legs, or feet; palpitations; severe abdominal pain; or unusual weakness.

Interactions

This medicine interacts with several other drugs such as adrenocorticosteroids, antimuscarinics, calcium-containing medicines; heart medicines such as digitalis or digoxin; laxatives; other potassium-containing medicines.

- Be sure to tell your doctor about any medications you are currently taking.

Storage

Tablets, elixir, etc. should be stored at room temperature in tightly closed containers. Store away from heat and direct light. Keep out of reach of children, since overdose may be very dangerous in children. Do not keep outdated medicine or medicine no longer needed. Flush the contents of the container down the toilet, unless otherwise directed.

K-LOR

Properties
This medicine contains potassium chloride as active ingredient; it is used to treat or prevent potassium deficiency, especially potassium deficiency that is caused by the use of diuretics (water pills).

Potassium is needed to maintain good health. Potassium supplements may be needed by patients who do not have enough potassium in their regular diet and by those who have lost too much potassium because of illness or treatment with certain medicines.

Since too much potassium may also cause health problems, most potassium supplements are available only with your doctor's prescription.

Before using this medicine
Before you use this medicine check with your doctor, or pharmacist:
- if you ever had any unusual or allergic reaction to potassium preparations;
- if you are on a low-salt, low-sugar, or any other special diet, or if you are allergic to any substance, such as sulfites or other preservatives or dyes.
- if you are pregnant or intend to become pregnant while using this medicine. Although potassium supplements have not been shown to cause problems in humans, the chance always exists.
- if you are breast-feeding an infant. Although this medicine has not been shown to cause problems in humans, the chance always exists since small amounts of potassium pass into the breast milk.
- if you have any of the following medical problems:
Addison's disease
Heart disease
Diarrhea
Kidney disease
Stomach ulcer

Treatment
This medication is used to relieve or prevent the symptoms of your medical problem. Take them as directed. Do not take more of them and do not take them more often than recommended on the label, unless otherwise directed by your doctor. To do so may increase the chance of side effects.

In order to avoid stomach irritation, you should take potassium supplements with food or immediately after a meal. If you miss a dose of this medication, take the missed dose as soon as possible, unless it is within two hours of the next scheduled dose;.

Side effects
The following minor side effects may occur:
    Diarrhea
    Nausea
    Stomach pains
    Vomiting.
These side effects should disappear as your body adjusts to the medication. Tell your doctor about any side effects that are persistent or particularly bothersome. It is especially important to tell your doctor about anxiety; bloody or black, tarry stools; confusion; difficulty in breathing; numbness or tingling in the arms, legs, or feet; palpitations; severe abdominal pain; or unusual weakness.

Interactions
This medicine interacts with several other drugs such as adrenocorticosteroids, antimuscarinics, calcium-containing medicines; heart medicines such as digitalis or digoxin; laxatives; other potassium-containing medicines.
- Be sure to tell your doctor about any medications you are currently taking.

Storage
Tablets, elixir, etc. should be stored at room temperature in tightly closed containers. Store away from heat and direct light. Keep out of reach of children, since overdose may be very dangerous in children. Do not keep outdated medicine or medicine no longer needed. Flush the contents of the container down the toilet, unless otherwise directed.

K-TAB

Properties
This medicine contains potassium chloride as active ingredient; it is used to treat or prevent potassium deficiency, especially potassium deficiency that is caused by the use of diuretics (water pills).

Potassium is needed to maintain good health. Potassium supplements may be needed by patients who do not have enough potassium in their regular diet and by those who have lost too much potassium because of illness or treatment with certain medicines.

Since too much potassium may also cause health problems, most potassium supplements are available only with your doctor's prescription.

Before using this medicine
Before you use this medicine check with your doctor, or pharmacist:
– if you ever had any unusual or allergic reaction to potassium preparations;
– if you are on a low-salt, low-sugar, or any other special diet, or if you are allergic to any substance, such as sulfites or other preservatives or dyes.
– if you are pregnant or intend to become pregnant while using this medicine. Although potassium supplements have not been shown to cause problems in humans, the chance always exists.
– if you are breast-feeding an infant. Although this medicine has not been shown to cause problems in humans, the chance always exists since small amounts of potassium pass into the breast milk.
– if you have any of the following medical problems:
Addison's disease
Heart disease
Diarrhea
Kidney disease
Stomach ulcer

Treatment
This medication is used to relieve or prevent the symptoms of your medical problem. Take them as directed. Do not take more of them and do not take them more often than recommended on the label, unless otherwise directed by your doctor. To do so may increase the chance of side effects.

In order to avoid stomach irritation, you should take potassium supplements with food or immediately after a meal. If you miss a dose of this medication, take the missed dose as soon as possible, unless it is within two hours of the next scheduled dose;.

Side effects
The following minor side effects may occur:
Diarrhea
Nausea
Stomach pains
Vomiting.
These side effects should disappear as your body adjusts to the medication. Tell your doctor about any side effects that are persistent or particularly bothersome. It is especially important to tell your doctor about anxiety; bloody or black, tarry stools; confusion; difficulty in breathing; numbness or tingling in the arms, legs, or feet; palpitations; severe abdominal pain; or unusual weakness.

Interactions
This medicine interacts with several other drugs such as adrenocorticosteroids, antimuscarinics, calcium-containing medicines; heart medicines such as digitalis or digoxin; laxatives; other potassium-containing medicines.
▪ Be sure to tell your doctor about any medications you are currently taking.

Storage
Tablets, elixir, etc. should be stored at room temperature in tightly closed containers. Store away from heat and direct light. Keep out of reach of children, since overdose may be very dangerous in children. Do not keep outdated medicine or medicine no longer needed. Flush the contents of the container down the toilet, unless otherwise directed.

K-LYTE/Cl

Properties

This medicine contains potassium bicarbonate and potassium chloride as active ingredients; it is used to treat or prevent potassium deficiency, especially potassium deficiency that is caused by the use of diuretics (water pills). Potassium is needed to maintain good health. Potassium supplements may be needed by patients who do not have enough potassium in their regular diet and by those who have lost too much potassium because of illness or treatment with certain medicines.

Since too much potassium may also cause health problems, most potassium supplements are available only with your doctor's prescription.

Before using this medicine

Before you use this medicine check with your doctor, or pharmacist:
- if you ever had any unusual or allergic reaction to potassium preparations;
- if you are on a low-salt, low-sugar, or any other special diet, or if you are allergic to any substance, such as sulfites or other preservatives or dyes.
- if you are pregnant or intend to become pregnant while using this medicine. Although potassium supplements have not been shown to cause problems in humans, the chance always exists.
- if you are breast-feeding an infant. Although this medicine has not been shown to cause problems in humans, the chance always exists since small amounts of potassium pass into the breast milk.
- if you have any of the following medical problems:
Addison's disease
Heart disease
Diarrhea
Kidney disease
Stomach ulcer

Treatment

This medication is used to relieve or prevent the symptoms of your medical problem. Take them as directed. Do not take more of them and do not take them more often than recommended on the label, unless otherwise directed by your doctor. To do so may increase the chance of side effects.

In order to avoid stomach irritation, you should take potassium supplements with food or immediately after a meal. If you miss a dose of this medication, take the missed dose as soon as possible, unless it is within two hours of the next scheduled dose;.

Side effects

The following minor side effects may occur:
Diarrhea
Nausea
Stomach pains
Vomiting.
These side effects should disappear as your body adjusts to the medication. Tell your doctor about any side effects that are persistent or particularly bothersome. It is especially important to tell your doctor about anxiety; bloody or black, tarry stools; confusion; difficulty in breathing; numbness or tingling in the arms, legs, or feet; palpitations; severe abdominal pain; or unusual weakness.

Interactions

This medicine interacts with several other drugs such as adrenocorticosteroids, antimuscarinics, calcium-containing medicines; heart medicines such as digitalis or digoxin; laxatives; other potassium-containing medicines.
- Be sure to tell your doctor about any medications you are currently taking.

Storage

Tablets, elixir, etc. should be stored at room temperature in tightly closed containers. Store away from heat and direct light. Keep out of reach of children, since overdose may be very dangerous in children. Do not keep outdated medicine or medicine no longer needed. Flush the contents of the container down the toilet, unless otherwise directed.

KAO-NOR

Properties

This medicine contains potassium gluconate as active ingredient; it is used to treat or prevent potassium deficiency, especially potassium deficiency that is caused by the use of diuretics (water pills).

Potassium is needed to maintain good health. Potassium supplements may be needed by patients who do not have enough potassium in their regular diet and by those who have lost too much potassium because of illness or treatment with certain medicines.

Since too much potassium may also cause health problems, most potassium supplements are available only with your doctor's prescription.

Before using this medicine

Before you use this medicine check with your doctor, or pharmacist:

- if you ever had any unusual or allergic reaction to potassium preparations;
- if you are on a low-salt, low-sugar, or any other special diet, or if you are allergic to any substance, such as sulfites or other preservatives or dyes.
- if you are pregnant or intend to become pregnant while using this medicine. Although potassium supplements have not been shown to cause problems in humans, the chance always exists.
- if you are breast-feeding an infant. Although this medicine has not been shown to cause problems in humans, the chance always exists since small amounts of potassium pass into the breast milk.
- if you have any of the following medical problems:
Addison's disease
Heart disease
Diarrhea
Kidney disease
Stomach ulcer

Treatment

This medication is used to relieve or prevent the symptoms of your medical problem. Take them as directed. Do not take more of them and do not take them more often than recommended on the label, unless otherwise directed by your doctor. To do so may increase the chance of side effects.

In order to avoid stomach irritation, you should take potassium supplements with food or immediately after a meal. If you miss a dose of this medication, take the missed dose as soon as possible, unless it is within two hours of the next scheduled dose;.

Side effects

The following minor side effects may occur:
Diarrhea
Nausea
Stomach pains
Vomiting.

These side effects should disappear as your body adjusts to the medication. Tell your doctor about any side effects that are persistent or particularly bothersome. It is especially important to tell your doctor about anxiety; bloody or black, tarry stools; confusion; difficulty in breathing; numbness or tingling in the arms, legs, or feet; palpitations; severe abdominal pain; or unusual weakness.

Interactions

This medicine interacts with several other drugs such as adrenocorticosteroids, antimuscarinics, calcium-containing medicines; heart medicines such as digitalis or digoxin; laxatives; other potassium-containing medicines.

- Be sure to tell your doctor about any medications you are currently taking.

Storage

Tablets, elixir, etc. should be stored at room temperature in tightly closed containers. Store away from heat and direct light. Keep out of reach of children, since overdose may be very dangerous in children. Do not keep outdated medicine or medicine no longer needed. Flush the contents of the container down the toilet, unless otherwise directed.

KAOCHLOR

Properties
This medicine contains potassium chloride as active ingredient; it is used to treat or prevent potassium deficiency, especially potassium deficiency that is caused by the use of diuretics (water pills).

Potassium is needed to maintain good health. Potassium supplements may be needed by patients who do not have enough potassium in their regular diet and by those who have lost too much potassium because of illness or treatment with certain medicines.

Since too much potassium may also cause health problems, most potassium supplements are available only with your doctor's prescription.

Before using this medicine
Before you use this medicine check with your doctor, or pharmacist:
- if you ever had any unusual or allergic reaction to potassium preparations;
- if you are on a low-salt, low-sugar, or any other special diet, or if you are allergic to any substance, such as sulfites or other preservatives or dyes.
- if you are pregnant or intend to become pregnant while using this medicine. Although potassium supplements have not been shown to cause problems in humans, the chance always exists.
- if you are breast-feeding an infant. Although this medicine has not been shown to cause problems in humans, the chance always exists since small amounts of potassium pass into the breast milk.
- if you have any of the following medical problems:
Addison's disease
Heart disease
Diarrhea
Kidney disease
Stomach ulcer

Treatment
This medication is used to relieve or prevent the symptoms of your medical problem. Take them as directed. Do not take more of them and do not take them more often than recommended on the label, unless otherwise directed by your doctor. To do so may increase the chance of side effects.

In order to avoid stomach irritation, you should take potassium supplements with food or immediately after a meal. If you miss a dose of this medication, take the missed dose as soon as possible, unless it is within two hours of the next scheduled dose;.

Side effects
The following minor side effects may occur:
Diarrhea
Nausea
Stomach pains
Vomiting.
These side effects should disappear as your body adjusts to the medication. Tell your doctor about any side effects that are persistent or particularly bothersome. It is especially important to tell your doctor about anxiety; bloody or black, tarry stools; confusion; difficulty in breathing; numbness or tingling in the arms, legs, or feet; palpitations; severe abdominal pain; or unusual weakness.

Interactions
This medicine interacts with several other drugs such as adrenocorticosteroids, antimuscarinics, calcium-containing medicines; heart medicines such as digitalis or digoxin; laxatives; other potassium-containing medicines.
- Be sure to tell your doctor about any medications you are currently taking.

Storage
Tablets, elixir, etc. should be stored at room temperature in tightly closed containers. Store away from heat and direct light. Keep out of reach of children, since overdose may be very dangerous in children. Do not keep outdated medicine or medicine no longer needed. Flush the contents of the container down the toilet, unless otherwise directed.

KAON

Properties

This medicine contains potassium gluconate as active ingredient; it is used to treat or prevent potassium deficiency, especially potassium deficiency that is caused by the use of diuretics (water pills).

Potassium is needed to maintain good health. Potassium supplements may be needed by patients who do not have enough potassium in their regular diet and by those who have lost too much potassium because of illness or treatment with certain medicines.

Since too much potassium may also cause health problems, most potassium supplements are available only with your doctor's prescription.

Before using this medicine

Before you use this medicine check with your doctor, or pharmacist:
- if you ever had any unusual or allergic reaction to potassium preparations;
- if you are on a low-salt, low-sugar, or any other special diet, or if you are allergic to any substance, such as sulfites or other preservatives or dyes.
- if you are pregnant or intend to become pregnant while using this medicine. Although potassium supplements have not been shown to cause problems in humans, the chance always exists.
- if you are breast-feeding an infant. Although this medicine has not been shown to cause problems in humans, the chance always exists since small amounts of potassium pass into the breast milk.
- if you have any of the following medical problems:
Addison's disease
Heart disease
Diarrhea
Kidney disease
Stomach ulcer

Treatment

This medication is used to relieve or prevent the symptoms of your medical problem. Take them as directed. Do not take more of them and do not take them more often than recommended on the label, unless otherwise directed by your doctor. To do so may increase the chance of side effects.

In order to avoid stomach irritation, you should take potassium supplements with food or immediately after a meal. If you miss a dose of this medication, take the missed dose as soon as possible, unless it is within two hours of the next scheduled dose;.

Side effects

The following minor side effects may occur:
    Diarrhea
    Nausea
    Stomach pains
    Vomiting.
These side effects should disappear as your body adjusts to the medication. Tell your doctor about any side effects that are persistent or particularly bothersome. It is especially important to tell your doctor about anxiety; bloody or black, tarry stools; confusion; difficulty in breathing; numbness or tingling in the arms, legs, or feet; palpitations; severe abdominal pain; or unusual weakness.

Interactions

This medicine interacts with several other drugs such as adrenocorticosteroids, antimuscarinics, calcium-containing medicines; heart medicines such as digitalis or digoxin; laxatives; other potassium-containing medicines.
- Be sure to tell your doctor about any medications you are currently taking.

Storage

Tablets, elixir, etc. should be stored at room temperature in tightly closed containers. Store away from heat and direct light. Keep out of reach of children, since overdose may be very dangerous in children. Do not keep outdated medicine or medicine no longer needed. Flush the contents of the container down the toilet, unless otherwise directed.

KATO

Properties

This medicine contains potassium chloride as active ingredient; it is used to treat or prevent potassium deficiency, especially potassium deficiency that is caused by the use of diuretics (water pills).

Potassium is needed to maintain good health. Potassium supplements may be needed by patients who do not have enough potassium in their regular diet and by those who have lost too much potassium because of illness or treatment with certain medicines.

Since too much potassium may also cause health problems, most potassium supplements are available only with your doctor's prescription.

Before using this medicine

Before you use this medicine check with your doctor, or pharmacist:

- if you ever had any unusual or allergic reaction to potassium preparations;
- if you are on a low-salt, low-sugar, or any other special diet, or if you are allergic to any substance, such as sulfites or other preservatives or dyes.
- if you are pregnant or intend to become pregnant while using this medicine. Although potassium supplements have not been shown to cause problems in humans, the chance always exists.
- if you are breast-feeding an infant. Although this medicine has not been shown to cause problems in humans, the chance always exists since small amounts of potassium pass into the breast milk.
- if you have any of the following medical problems:
Addison's disease
Heart disease
Diarrhea
Kidney disease
Stomach ulcer

Treatment

This medication is used to relieve or prevent the symptoms of your medical problem. Take them as directed. Do not take more of them and do not take them more often than recommended on the label, unless otherwise directed by your doctor. To do so may increase the chance of side effects.

In order to avoid stomach irritation, you should take potassium supplements with food or immediately after a meal. If you miss a dose of this medication, take the missed dose as soon as possible, unless it is within two hours of the next scheduled dose;.

Side effects

The following minor side effects may occur:

Diarrhea
Nausea
Stomach pains
Vomiting.

These side effects should disappear as your body adjusts to the medication. Tell your doctor about any side effects that are persistent or particularly bothersome. It is especially important to tell your doctor about anxiety; bloody or black, tarry stools; confusion; difficulty in breathing; numbness or tingling in the arms, legs, or feet; palpitations; severe abdominal pain; or unusual weakness.

Interactions

This medicine interacts with several other drugs such as adrenocorticosteroids, antimuscarinics, calcium-containing medicines; heart medicines such as digitalis or digoxin; laxatives; other potassium-containing medicines.

- Be sure to tell your doctor about any medications you are currently taking.

Storage

Tablets, elixir, etc. should be stored at room temperature in tightly closed containers. Store away from heat and direct light. Keep out of reach of children, since overdose may be very dangerous in children. Do not keep outdated medicine or medicine no longer needed. Flush the contents of the container down the toilet, unless otherwise directed.

KAY CIEL

Properties

This medicine contains potassium chloride as active ingredient; it is used to treat or prevent potassium deficiency, especially potassium deficiency that is caused by the use of diuretics (water pills).

Potassium is needed to maintain good health. Potassium supplements may be needed by patients who do not have enough potassium in their regular diet and by those who have lost too much potassium because of illness or treatment with certain medicines.

Since too much potassium may also cause health problems, most potassium supplements are available only with your doctor's prescription.

Before using this medicine

Before you use this medicine check with your doctor, or pharmacist:
- if you ever had any unusual or allergic reaction to potassium preparations;
- if you are on a low-salt, low-sugar, or any other special diet, or if you are allergic to any substance, such as sulfites or other preservatives or dyes.
- if you are pregnant or intend to become pregnant while using this medicine. Although potassium supplements have not been shown to cause problems in humans, the chance always exists.
- if you are breast-feeding an infant. Although this medicine has not been shown to cause problems in humans, the chance always exists since small amounts of potassium pass into the breast milk.
- if you have any of the following medical problems:
  Addison's disease
  Heart disease
  Diarrhea
  Kidney disease
  Stomach ulcer

Treatment

This medication is used to relieve or prevent the symptoms of your medical problem. Take them as directed. Do not take more of them and do not take them more often than recommended on the label, unless otherwise directed by your doctor. To do so may increase the chance of side effects.

In order to avoid stomach irritation, you should take potassium supplements with food or immediately after a meal. If you miss a dose of this medication, take the missed dose as soon as possible, unless it is within two hours of the next scheduled dose;.

Side effects

The following minor side effects may occur:
  Diarrhea
  Nausea
  Stomach pains
  Vomiting.

These side effects should disappear as your body adjusts to the medication. Tell your doctor about any side effects that are persistent or particularly bothersome. It is especially important to tell your doctor about anxiety; bloody or black, tarry stools; confusion; difficulty in breathing; numbness or tingling in the arms, legs, or feet; palpitations; severe abdominal pain; or unusual weakness.

Interactions

This medicine interacts with several other drugs such as adrenocorticosteroids, antimuscarinics, calcium-containing medicines; heart medicines such as digitalis or digoxin; laxatives; other potassium-containing medicines.
- Be sure to tell your doctor about any medications you are currently taking.

Storage

Tablets, elixir, etc. should be stored at room temperature in tightly closed containers. Store away from heat and direct light. Keep out of reach of children, since overdose may be very dangerous in children. Do not keep outdated medicine or medicine no longer needed. Flush the contents of the container down the toilet, unless otherwise directed.

KAYLIXIR

Properties

This medicine contains potassium gluconate as active ingredient; it is used to treat or prevent potassium deficiency, especially potassium deficiency that is caused by the use of diuretics (water pills).

Potassium is needed to maintain good health. Potassium supplements may be needed by patients who do not have enough potassium in their regular diet and by those who have lost too much potassium because of illness or treatment with certain medicines.

Since too much potassium may also cause health problems, most potassium supplements are available only with your doctor's prescription.

Before using this medicine

Before you use this medicine check with your doctor, or pharmacist:

- if you ever had any unusual or allergic reaction to potassium preparations;
- if you are on a low-salt, low-sugar, or any other special diet, or if you are allergic to any substance, such as sulfites or other preservatives or dyes.
- if you are pregnant or intend to become pregnant while using this medicine. Although potassium supplements have not been shown to cause problems in humans, the chance always exists.
- if you are breast-feeding an infant. Although this medicine has not been shown to cause problems in humans, the chance always exists since small amounts of potassium pass into the breast milk.
- if you have any of the following medical problems:
  Addison's disease
  Heart disease
  Diarrhea
  Kidney disease
  Stomach ulcer

Treatment

This medication is used to relieve or prevent the symptoms of your medical problem. Take them as directed. Do not take more of them and do not take them more often than recommended on the label, unless otherwise directed by your doctor. To do so may increase the chance of side effects.

In order to avoid stomach irritation, you should take potassium supplements with food or immediately after a meal. If you miss a dose of this medication, take the missed dose as soon as possible, unless it is within two hours of the next scheduled dose;.

Side effects

The following minor side effects may occur:

Diarrhea
Nausea
Stomach pains
Vomiting.

These side effects should disappear as your body adjusts to the medication. Tell your doctor about any side effects that are persistent or particularly bothersome. It is especially important to tell your doctor about anxiety; bloody or black, tarry stools; confusion; difficulty in breathing; numbness or tingling in the arms, legs, or feet; palpitations; severe abdominal pain; or unusual weakness.

Interactions

This medicine interacts with several other drugs such as adrenocorticosteroids, antimuscarinics, calcium-containing medicines; heart medicines such as digitalis or digoxin; laxatives; other potassium-containing medicines.

- Be sure to tell your doctor about any medications you are currently taking.

Storage

Tablets, elixir, etc. should be stored at room temperature in tightly closed containers. Store away from heat and direct light. Keep out of reach of children, since overdose may be very dangerous in children. Do not keep outdated medicine or medicine no longer needed. Flush the contents of the container down the toilet, unless otherwise directed.

KEACHLOR-EFF

Properties
This medicine contains potassium chloride, potassium bicarbonate and potassium citrate as active ingredients; it is used to treat or prevent potassium deficiency, especially potassium deficiency that is caused by the use of diuretics (water pills). Potassium is needed to maintain good health. Potassium supplements may be needed by patients who do not have enough potassium in their regular diet and by those who have lost too much potassium because of illness or treatment with certain medicines. Since too much potassium may also cause health problems, most potassium supplements are available only with your doctor's prescription.

Before using this medicine
Before you use this medicine check with your doctor, or pharmacist:
- if you ever had any unusual or allergic reaction to potassium preparations;
- if you are on a low-salt, low-sugar, or any other special diet, or if you are allergic to any substance, such as sulfites or other preservatives or dyes.
- if you are pregnant or intend to become pregnant while using this medicine. Although potassium supplements have not been shown to cause problems in humans, the chance always exists.
- if you are breast-feeding an infant. Although this medicine has not been shown to cause problems in humans, the chance always exists since small amounts of potassium pass into the breast milk.
- if you have any of the following medical problems:
  Addison's disease
  Heart disease
  Diarrhea
  Kidney disease
  Stomach ulcer

Treatment
This medication is used to relieve or prevent the symptoms of your medical problem. Take them as directed. Do not take more of them and do not take them more often than recommended on the label, unless otherwise directed by your doctor. To do so may increase the chance of side effects.

In order to avoid stomach irritation, you should take potassium supplements with food or immediately after a meal. If you miss a dose of this medication, take the missed dose as soon as possible, unless it is within two hours of the next scheduled dose;.

Side effects
The following minor side effects may occur:
  Diarrhea
  Nausea
  Stomach pains
  Vomiting.
These side effects should disappear as your body adjusts to the medication. Tell your doctor about any side effects that are persistent or particularly bothersome. It is especially important to tell your doctor about anxiety; bloody or black, tarry stools; confusion; difficulty in breathing; numbness or tingling in the arms, legs, or feet; palpitations; severe abdominal pain; or unusual weakness.

Interactions
This medicine interacts with several other drugs such as adrenocorticosteroids, antimuscarinics, calcium-containing medicines; heart medicines such as digitalis or digoxin; laxatives; other potassium-containing medicines.
- Be sure to tell your doctor about any medications you are currently taking.

Storage
Tablets, elixir, etc. should be stored at room temperature in tightly closed containers. Store away from heat and direct light. Keep out of reach of children, since overdose may be very dangerous in children. Do not keep outdated medicine or medicine no longer needed. Flush the contents of the container down the toilet, unless otherwise directed.

KEFLET

Properties

This medicine contains cephalosporin as active ingredient. Cephalosporins belong to the general family of medicines called antibiotics, used in the treatment of infections caused by bacteria. They work by killing bacteria or preventing their growth. Cephalosporins will not work for colds, flu, or other viral infections.

Before using this medicine

Before you use this medicine check with your doctor:

- if you ever had any unusual or allergic reaction to any of the cephalosporins, penicillins, penicillin-like medicines, or penicillamine.
- if you are on a low-salt, low-sugar, or any other special diet, or if you are allergic to any substance, such as sulfites or other preservatives or dyes.
- if you are pregnant or intend to become pregnant while using this medicine. Although cephalosporins have not been shown to cause birth defects or other problems in humans, the chance always exists.
- if you are breast-feeding an infant. Most cephalosporins pass into the breast milk, usually in small amounts.
- if you have any of the following medical problems:
Bleeding problem
Kidney or lifer disease

Treatment

This medication belongs to the general family of medicines called antibiotics. It is used to treat a wide variety of bacterial infections. It is also used to treat infections in persons who are allergic to penicillin.

- Keep taking this medicine for the full time of treatment even if you begin to feel better after a few days; do not miss any doses.
- If you do miss a dose of this medicine, take it as soon as possible. This will help to keep a constant amount of medicine in the blood. However, if it is almost time for your next dose, skip the missed dose and go back to your regular dosing schedule.
- This medication has been prescribed for your current infection only. Another infection later on, or one that someone else has, may require a different medicine. You should not give your medicine to other people or use it for other infections, unless your doctor specifically directs you to do so.
- Take the medicine at the same times each day, 1 hour before or 2 hours after eating.

Side effects

Along with the needed effects, a medicine may cause some unwanted effects. Side effects that usually do not require medical attention: rectal itching, oral or vaginal white spots, mild diarrhea. These side effects should disappear as your body adjusts to the medication.

- Other side effects that should be reported to your doctor immediately are:
Hives, rash
Intense itching
Faintness soon after a dose
Difficulty in breathing
Nausea and vomiting
Severe diarrhea
Unusual weakness or tiredness
Bleeding or bruising

Interactions

This medicine may interact with several other drugs such as anticoagulants, theophylline preparations, probenecid, tetracyclines, etc.

- Be sure to tell your doctor about any medications you are currently taking.

Storage

Tablets, capsules, etc. should be stored at room temperature. Store the liquid form in the refrigerator. Keep out of the reach of children. Do not keep outdated medicine or medicine no longer needed.

KEFTAB

Properties

This medicine contains cephalosporin as active ingredient. Cephalosporins belong to the general family of medicines called antibiotics, used in the treatment of infections caused by bacteria. They work by killing bacteria or preventing their growth. Cephalosporins will not work for colds, flu, or other viral infections.

Before using this medicine

Before you use this medicine check with your doctor:
- if you ever had any unusual or allergic reaction to any of the cephalosporins, penicillins, penicillin-like medicines, or penicillamine.
- if you are on a low-salt, low-sugar, or any other special diet, or if you are allergic to any substance, such as sulfites or other preservatives or dyes.
- if you are pregnant or intend to become pregnant while using this medicine. Although cephalosporins have not been shown to cause birth defects or other problems in humans, the chance always exists.
- if you are breast-feeding an infant. Most cephalosporins pass into the breast milk, usually in small amounts.
- if you have any of the following medical problems:
  Bleeding problem
  Kidney or lifer disease

Treatment

This medication belongs to the general family of medicines called antibiotics. It is used to treat a wide variety of bacterial infections. It is also used to treat infections in persons who are allergic to penicillin.
- Keep taking this medicine for the full time of treatment even if you begin to feel better after a few days; do not miss any doses.
- If you do miss a dose of this medicine, take it as soon as possible. This will help to keep a constant amount of medicine in the blood. However, if it is almost time for your next dose, skip the missed dose and go back to your regular dosing schedule.
- This medication has been prescribed for your current infection only. Another infection later on, or one that someone else has, may require a different medicine. You should not give your medicine to other people or use it for other infections, unless your doctor specifically directs you to do so.
- Take the medicine at the same times each day, 1 hour before or 2 hours after eating.

Side effects

Along with the needed effects, a medicine may cause some unwanted effects. Side effects that usually do not require medical attention: rectal itching, oral or vaginal white spots, mild diarrhea. These side effects should disappear as your body adjusts to the medication.
- Other side effects that should be reported to your doctor immediately are:
  Hives, rash
  Intense itching
  Faintness soon after a dose
  Difficulty in breathing
  Nausea and vomiting
  Severe diarrhea
  Unusual weakness or tiredness
  Bleeding or bruising

Interactions

This medicine may interact with several other drugs such as anticoagulants, theophylline preparations, probenecid, tetracyclines, etc.
- Be sure to tell your doctor about any medications you are currently taking.

Storage

Tablets, capsules, etc. should be stored at room temperature. Store the liquid form in the refrigerator. Keep out of the reach of children. Do not keep outdated medicine or medicine no longer needed.

KEFZOL

Properties

This medicine contains cephalosporin as active ingredient. Cephalosporins belong to the general family of medicines called antibiotics, used in the treatment of infections caused by bacteria. They work by killing bacteria or preventing their growth. Cephalosporins will not work for colds, flu, or other viral infections.

Before using this medicine

Before you use this medicine check with your doctor:
- if you ever had any unusual or allergic reaction to any of the cephalosporins, penicillins, penicillin-like medicines, or penicillamine.
- if you are on a low-salt, low-sugar, or any other special diet, or if you are allergic to any substance, such as sulfites or other preservatives or dyes.
- if you are pregnant or intend to become pregnant while using this medicine. Although cephalosporins have not been shown to cause birth defects or other problems in humans, the chance always exists.
- if you are breast-feeding an infant. Most cephalosporins pass into the breast milk, usually in small amounts.
- if you have any of the following medical problems:
  Bleeding problem
  Kidney or lifer disease

Treatment

This medication belongs to the general family of medicines called antibiotics. It is used to treat a wide variety of bacterial infections. It is also used to treat infections in persons who are allergic to penicillin.
- Keep taking this medicine for the full time of treatment even if you begin to feel better after a few days; do not miss any doses.
- If you do miss a dose of this medicine, take it as soon as possible. This will help to keep a constant amount of medicine in the blood. However, if it is almost time for your next dose, skip the missed dose and go back to your regular dosing schedule.
- This medication has been prescribed for your current infection only. Another infection later on, or one that someone else has, may require a different medicine. You should not give your medicine to other people or use it for other infections, unless your doctor specifically directs you to do so.
- Take the medicine at the same times each day, 1 hour before or 2 hours after eating.

Side effects

Along with the needed effects, a medicine may cause some unwanted effects. Side effects that usually do not require medical attention: rectal itching, oral or vaginal white spots, mild diarrhea. These side effects should disappear as your body adjusts to the medication.
- Other side effects that should be reported to your doctor immediately are:
  Hives, rash
  Intense itching
  Faintness soon after a dose
  Difficulty in breathing
  Nausea and vomiting
  Severe diarrhea
  Unusual weakness or tiredness
  Bleeding or bruising

Interactions

This medicine may interact with several other drugs such as anticoagulants, theophylline preparations, probenecid, tetracyclines, etc.
- Be sure to tell your doctor about any medications you are currently taking.

Storage

Tablets, capsules, etc. should be stored at room temperature. Store the liquid form in the refrigerator. Keep out of the reach of children. Do not keep outdated medicine or medicine no longer needed.

KESTRONE-5

Properties
This medicine contains estrone as active ingredient. The medicine is prescribed for treatment of estrogen deficiency; it restores normal estrogen levels in tissues. There is no evidence that this drug is effective for nervous symptoms or depression occurring during menopause. They should not be used to treat this condition; they should be used only to replace the estrogen that is naturally absent after menopause.

Before using this medicine
Before you use this medicine check with your doctor, or pharmacist:
- if you ever had any unusual or allergic reaction to estrogens;
- if you are pregnant or intend to become pregnant within three months;
- if you are breast-feeding an infant;
- if you have any of the following medical problems:
  Diabetes
  Breast cancer
  Fibrocystic breast disease
  Fibroid uterine tumors
  Endometriosis
  Migraine headaches
  Epilepsy
  Porphyria
  High blood pressure
  Asthma
  Congestive heart failure
  Kidney disease
  Gallstones

Treatment
This medication is used to treat estrogen deficiency, specific symptoms of menopause, estrogen-deficiency osteoporosis, atrophic vaginitis, prostate cancer.

For safe and effective use of this medicine:
- ◆ Follow your doctor's instructions if this medicine was prescribed.
- ◆ Follow the manufacturer's package directions if you are treating yourself.
- ◆ Estrogens have been reported to increase the risk of endometrial carcinoma.

Side effects
Along with the needed effects, a medicine may cause some unwanted effects. Possible side effects include:
  Stomach cramps
  Profuse bleeding
  Appetite loss
  Nausea and vomiting
  Swollen breasts
  Change in menstruation
  Rash, skin blisters
  Depression
  Dizziness

Overdose
The following symptoms may indicate an overdose:
  Nausea and vomiting
  Fluid retention
  Breast enlargement
  Abnormal vaginal bleeding
- ■ Call a doctor or hospital emergency room for instructions.

Interactions
This medicine may interact with several other drugs such as adrenocorticosteroids, antidepressants, oral antidiabetics, insulin, phenobarbital, primidone.
- ■ Be sure to tell your doctor about any medications you are currently taking.

Storage
Capsules, tablets, vaginal cream, transdermal patches, etc. should be stored at room temperature; store away from heat and direct light. Keep out of reach of children, since this medicine may be dangerous in children.

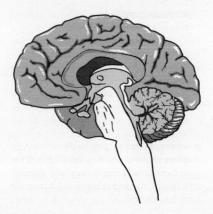

KLAVIKORDAL

Properties

This medicine contains nitroglycerin as active ingredient. Nitrates improve the supply of blood and oxygen to the heart. This medication is for oral use.

Before using this medicine

Before you use this medicine check with your doctor, or pharmacist:
- if you ever had any unusual or allergic reaction to nitrates or nitrites.
- if you are on a low-salt, low-sugar, or any other special diet, or if you are allergic to any substance, such as sulfites or other preservatives or dyes.
- if you are pregnant or intend to become pregnant while using this medicine. Although nitrates have not been shown to cause problems in humans, the chance always exists.
- if you are breast-feeding an infant.
- if you have recently had a heart attack or stroke.
- if you have any of the following medical problems:
  Anemia
  Glaucoma
  Intestinal problems
  Overactive thyroid
- if you are now taking any of the following medicines or types of medicines:
  Antihypertensives
  Asthma or hay fever medicine
  Cold medicine
  Decongestant
  Medicine for appetite control
  Narcotic
  Pain medicine
  Sinus congestion medicine

Treatment

This medication is used to treat and prevent angina (chest pain). Nitroglycerin is a vasodilator, which relaxes the muscles of the blood vessels, causing an increase in the oxygen supply to the heart. The oral tablets, capsules, ointment and patches do not act quickly; they are used to prevent chest pain. The sublingual tablets and oral spray act quickly and can be used to relieve chest pain after it has started.

- Take this medicine exactly as directed by your doctor or pharmacist. It will work only if taken correctly.
- If you are taking this medicine regularly and you miss a dose, take it as soon as possible. However, if your next scheduled dose; is within 2 hours (or within 6 hours for extended-release capsules or tablets), skip the missed dose and go back to your regular dosing schedule.
- If you have been taking this medicine regularly for several weeks or more, do not suddenly stop using it. Stopping suddenly may bring on attacks of angina.

Side effects

There are a number of side effects that usually do not require medical attention. These possible side effects may go away during treatment; however, if they continue or are bothersome, check with your doctor, nurse, or pharmacist. More common are: dizziness, lightheadedness, or fainting when standing up; fast pulse; flushing of face and neck; headache; nausea or vomiting.

Side effects that should be reported to your doctor are: blurred vision; dry mouth; severe or prolonged headache; skin rash.

Interactions

This medicine may interact with several other drugs such as tricyclic antidepressants and cough medicines. Before starting to take or apply nitroglycerin, be sure to tell your doctor about any medications you are currently taking.

Storage

Tablets, capsules, and oral spray should be stored as in a tightly capped bottle in a cool, dry place. Ointment and patches should be stored at room temperature in their original containers. Keep out of reach of children. Do not keep outdated medicine or medicine no longer needed.

KLOR-CON

Properties

This medicine contains potassium chloride as active ingredient; it is used to treat or prevent potassium deficiency, especially potassium deficiency that is caused by the use of diuretics (water pills).

Potassium is needed to maintain good health. Potassium supplements may be needed by patients who do not have enough potassium in their regular diet and by those who have lost too much potassium because of illness or treatment with certain medicines.

Since too much potassium may also cause health problems, most potassium supplements are available only with your doctor's prescription.

Before using this medicine

Before you use this medicine check with your doctor, or pharmacist:

- if you ever had any unusual or allergic reaction to potassium preparations;
- if you are on a low-salt, low-sugar, or any other special diet, or if you are allergic to any substance, such as sulfites or other preservatives or dyes.
- if you are pregnant or intend to become pregnant while using this medicine. Although potassium supplements have not been shown to cause problems in humans, the chance always exists.
- if you are breast-feeding an infant. Although this medicine has not been shown to cause problems in humans, the chance always exists since small amounts of potassium pass into the breast milk.
- if you have any of the following medical problems:
Addison's disease
Heart disease
Diarrhea
Kidney disease
Stomach ulcer

Treatment

This medication is used to relieve or prevent the symptoms of your medical problem. Take them as directed. Do not take more of them and do not take them more often than recommended on the label, unless otherwise directed by your doctor. To do so may increase the chance of side effects.

In order to avoid stomach irritation, you should take potassium supplements with food or immediately after a meal. If you miss a dose of this medication, take the missed dose as soon as possible, unless it is within two hours of the next scheduled dose;.

Side effects

The following minor side effects may occur:
Diarrhea
Nausea
Stomach pains
Vomiting.

These side effects should disappear as your body adjusts to the medication. Tell your doctor about any side effects that are persistent or particularly bothersome. It is especially important to tell your doctor about anxiety; bloody or black, tarry stools; confusion; difficulty in breathing; numbness or tingling in the arms, legs, or feet; palpitations; severe abdominal pain; or unusual weakness.

Interactions

This medicine interacts with several other drugs such as adrenocorticosteroids, antimuscarinics, calcium-containing medicines; heart medicines such as digitalis or digoxin; laxatives; other potassium-containing medicines.

- Be sure to tell your doctor about any medications you are currently taking.

Storage

Tablets, elixir, etc. should be stored at room temperature in tightly closed containers. Store away from heat and direct light. Keep out of reach of children, since overdose may be very dangerous in children. Do not keep outdated medicine or medicine no longer needed. Flush the contents of the container down the toilet, unless otherwise directed.

KLORVESS

Properties

This medicine contains potassium bicarbonate and potassium chloride as active ingredients; it is used to treat or prevent potassium deficiency, especially potassium deficiency that is caused by the use of diuretics (water pills). Potassium is needed to maintain good health.

Potassium supplements may be needed by patients who do not have enough potassium in their regular diet and by those who have lost too much potassium because of illness or treatment with certain medicines.

Since too much potassium may also cause health problems, most potassium supplements are available only with your doctor's prescription.

Before using this medicine

Before you use this medicine check with your doctor, or pharmacist:

- if you ever had any unusual or allergic reaction to potassium preparations;
- if you are on a low-salt, low-sugar, or any other special diet, or if you are allergic to any substance, such as sulfites or other preservatives or dyes.
- if you are pregnant or intend to become pregnant while using this medicine. Although potassium supplements have not been shown to cause problems in humans, the chance always exists.
- if you are breast-feeding an infant. Although this medicine has not been shown to cause problems in humans, the chance always exists since small amounts of potassium pass into the breast milk.
- if you have any of the following medical problems:
  Addison's disease
  Heart disease
  Diarrhea
  Kidney disease
  Stomach ulcer

Treatment

This medication is used to relieve or prevent the symptoms of your medical problem. Take them as directed. Do not take more of them and do not take them more often than recommended on the label, unless otherwise directed by your doctor. To do so may increase the chance of side effects.

In order to avoid stomach irritation, you should take potassium supplements with food or immediately after a meal. If you miss a dose of this medication, take the missed dose as soon as possible, unless it is within two hours of the next scheduled dose;.

Side effects

The following minor side effects may occur:

Diarrhea
Nausea
Stomach pains
Vomiting.

These side effects should disappear as your body adjusts to the medication. Tell your doctor about any side effects that are persistent or particularly bothersome. It is especially important to tell your doctor about anxiety; bloody or black, tarry stools; confusion; difficulty in breathing; numbness or tingling in the arms, legs, or feet; palpitations; severe abdominal pain; or unusual weakness.

Interactions

This medicine interacts with several other drugs such as adrenocorticosteroids, antimuscarinics, calcium-containing medicines; heart medicines such as digitalis or digoxin; laxatives; other potassium-containing medicines.

- Be sure to tell your doctor about any medications you are currently taking.

Storage

Tablets, elixir, etc. should be stored at room temperature in tightly closed containers. Store away from heat and direct light. Keep out of reach of children, since overdose may be very dangerous in children. Do not keep outdated medicine or medicine no longer needed. Flush the contents of the container down the toilet, unless otherwise directed.

KLORVESS 10%

Properties
This medicine contains potassium chloride as active ingredient; it is used to treat or prevent potassium deficiency, especially potassium deficiency that is caused by the use of diuretics (water pills).

Potassium is needed to maintain good health. Potassium supplements may be needed by patients who do not have enough potassium in their regular diet and by those who have lost too much potassium because of illness or treatment with certain medicines.

Since too much potassium may also cause health problems, most potassium supplements are available only with your doctor's prescription.

Before using this medicine
Before you use this medicine check with your doctor, or pharmacist:
- if you ever had any unusual or allergic reaction to potassium preparations;
- if you are on a low-salt, low-sugar, or any other special diet, or if you are allergic to any substance, such as sulfites or other preservatives or dyes.
- if you are pregnant or intend to become pregnant while using this medicine. Although potassium supplements have not been shown to cause problems in humans, the chance always exists.
- if you are breast-feeding an infant. Although this medicine has not been shown to cause problems in humans, the chance always exists since small amounts of potassium pass into the breast milk.
- if you have any of the following medical problems:
Addison's disease
Heart disease
Diarrhea
Kidney disease
Stomach ulcer

Treatment
This medication is used to relieve or prevent the symptoms of your medical problem. Take them as directed. Do not take more of them and do not take them more often than recommended on the label, unless otherwise directed by your doctor. To do so may increase the chance of side effects.

In order to avoid stomach irritation, you should take potassium supplements with food or immediately after a meal. If you miss a dose of this medication, take the missed dose as soon as possible, unless it is within two hours of the next scheduled dose;.

Side effects
The following minor side effects may occur:
Diarrhea
Nausea
Stomach pains
Vomiting.

These side effects should disappear as your body adjusts to the medication. Tell your doctor about any side effects that are persistent or particularly bothersome. It is especially important to tell your doctor about anxiety; bloody or black, tarry stools; confusion; difficulty in breathing; numbness or tingling in the arms, legs, or feet; palpitations; severe abdominal pain; or unusual weakness.

Interactions
This medicine interacts with several other drugs such as adrenocorticosteroids, antimuscarinics, calcium-containing medicines; heart medicines such as digitalis or digoxin; laxatives; other potassium-containing medicines.
- Be sure to tell your doctor about any medications you are currently taking.

Storage
Tablets, elixir, etc. should be stored at room temperature in tightly closed containers. Store away from heat and direct light. Keep out of reach of children, since overdose may be very dangerous in children. Do not keep outdated medicine or medicine no longer needed. Flush the contents of the container down the toilet, unless otherwise directed.

KLOTRIX

Properties

This medicine contains potassium chloride as active ingredient; it is used to treat or prevent potassium deficiency, especially potassium deficiency that is caused by the use of diuretics (water pills).

Potassium is needed to maintain good health. Potassium supplements may be needed by patients who do not have enough potassium in their regular diet and by those who have lost too much potassium because of illness or treatment with certain medicines.

Since too much potassium may also cause health problems, most potassium supplements are available only with your doctor's prescription.

Before using this medicine

Before you use this medicine check with your doctor, or pharmacist:

- if you ever had any unusual or allergic reaction to potassium preparations;
- if you are on a low-salt, low-sugar, or any other special diet, or if you are allergic to any substance, such as sulfites or other preservatives or dyes.
- if you are pregnant or intend to become pregnant while using this medicine. Although potassium supplements have not been shown to cause problems in humans, the chance always exists.
- if you are breast-feeding an infant. Although this medicine has not been shown to cause problems in humans, the chance always exists since small amounts of potassium pass into the breast milk.
- if you have any of the following medical problems:
Addison's disease
Heart disease
Diarrhea
Kidney disease
Stomach ulcer

Treatment

This medication is used to relieve or prevent the symptoms of your medical problem. Take them as directed. Do not take more of them and do not take them more often than recommended on the label, unless otherwise directed by your doctor. To do so may increase the chance of side effects.

In order to avoid stomach irritation, you should take potassium supplements with food or immediately after a meal. If you miss a dose of this medication, take the missed dose as soon as possible, unless it is within two hours of the next scheduled dose;.

Side effects

The following minor side effects may occur:

Diarrhea
Nausea
Stomach pains
Vomiting.

These side effects should disappear as your body adjusts to the medication. Tell your doctor about any side effects that are persistent or particularly bothersome. It is especially important to tell your doctor about anxiety; bloody or black, tarry stools; confusion; difficulty in breathing; numbness or tingling in the arms, legs, or feet; palpitations; severe abdominal pain; or unusual weakness.

Interactions

This medicine interacts with several other drugs such as adrenocorticosteroids, antimuscarinics, calcium-containing medicines; heart medicines such as digitalis or digoxin; laxatives; other potassium-containing medicines.

- Be sure to tell your doctor about any medications you are currently taking.

Storage

Tablets, elixir, etc. should be stored at room temperature in tightly closed containers. Store away from heat and direct light. Keep out of reach of children, since overdose may be very dangerous in children. Do not keep outdated medicine or medicine no longer needed. Flush the contents of the container down the toilet, unless otherwise directed.

KOLYUM

Properties
This medicine contains potassium gluconate and potassium chloride as active ingredients; it is used to treat or prevent potassium deficiency, especially potassium deficiency that is caused by the use of diuretics (water pills). Potassium is needed to maintain good health.

Potassium supplements may be needed by patients who do not have enough potassium in their regular diet and by those who have lost too much potassium because of illness or treatment with certain medicines.

Since too much potassium may also cause health problems, most potassium supplements are available only with your doctor's prescription.

Before using this medicine
Before you use this medicine check with your doctor, or pharmacist:
- if you ever had any unusual or allergic reaction to potassium preparations;
- if you are on a low-salt, low-sugar, or any other special diet, or if you are allergic to any substance, such as sulfites or other preservatives or dyes.
- if you are pregnant or intend to become pregnant while using this medicine. Although potassium supplements have not been shown to cause problems in humans, the chance always exists.
- if you are breast-feeding an infant. Although this medicine has not been shown to cause problems in humans, the chance always exists since small amounts of potassium pass into the breast milk.
- if you have any of the following medical problems:
Addison's disease
Heart disease
Diarrhea
Kidney disease
Stomach ulcer

Treatment
This medication is used to relieve or prevent the symptoms of your medical problem. Take them as directed. Do not take more of them and do not take them more often than recommended on the label, unless otherwise directed by your doctor. To do so may increase the chance of side effects.

In order to avoid stomach irritation, you should take potassium supplements with food or immediately after a meal. If you miss a dose of this medication, take the missed dose as soon as possible, unless it is within two hours of the next scheduled dose;.

Side effects
The following minor side effects may occur:
Diarrhea
Nausea
Stomach pains
Vomiting.
These side effects should disappear as your body adjusts to the medication. Tell your doctor about any side effects that are persistent or particularly bothersome. It is especially important to tell your doctor about anxiety; bloody or black, tarry stools; confusion; difficulty in breathing; numbness or tingling in the arms, legs, or feet; palpitations; severe abdominal pain; or unusual weakness.

Interactions
This medicine interacts with several other drugs such as adrenocorticosteroids, antimuscarinics, calcium-containing medicines; heart medicines such as digitalis or digoxin; laxatives; other potassium-containing medicines.
- Be sure to tell your doctor about any medications you are currently taking.

Storage
Tablets, elixir, etc. should be stored at room temperature in tightly closed containers. Store away from heat and direct light. Keep out of reach of children, since overdose may be very dangerous in children. Do not keep outdated medicine or medicine no longer needed. Flush the contents of the container down the toilet, unless otherwise directed.

LABID

Properties
This medicine contains theophylline as active ingredient; it is used to treat or prevent breathing problems (wheezing and shortness of breath) caused by asthma, bronchitis, or emphysema. This medication belongs to a group known as xanthine-derivative bronchodilators. They work by opening up the bronchial tubes or air passages of the lungs and increasing the flow of air through them. These medicines are available only with your doctor's prescription.

Before using this medicine
Before you use this medicine check with your doctor, or pharmacist:
- if you ever had any unusual or allergic reaction to xanthine-derivative bronchodilators.
- if you are on a low-salt, low-sugar, or any other special diet, or if you are allergic to any substance, such as sulfites or other preservatives or dyes.
- if you are pregnant or intend to become pregnant while using this medicine.
- if you are breast-feeding an infant. Theophylline passes into the breast milk and may cause irritability, fretfulness, or trouble in sleeping in infants of mothers taking this medicine.
- if you have any of the following medical problems:
Diarrhea
Enlarged prostate
Fibrocystic breast disease
Heart disease
Stomach ulcer

Treatment
This medication is used to relieve or prevent the symptoms of your medical problem. Take them as directed. Do not take more of them and do not take them more often than recommended on the label, unless otherwise directed by your doctor. To do so may increase the chance of side effects. The medicine should be taken on an empty stomach 30 to 60 minutes before a meal or two hours after a meal. Try not to miss any doses of this medication. If you do miss a dose, take the missed dose as soon as possible, unless it is almost time for the next dose. Do not double the next dose. It works best when taken with a glass of water.

Side effects
The following minor side effects may occur:
    Dizziness or flushing
    Headache
    Diarrhea
    Heartburn
    Increased urination
    Insomnia
    Nervousness or irritability
    Loss of appetite
    Nausea or stomach upset
    Stomach pain.
These side effects should disappear as your body adjusts to the medication. Tell your doctor about any side effects that are persistent or particularly bothersome. It is especially important to tell your doctor about black, tarry stools; confusion; convulsions; difficulty in breathing; fainting; muscle twitching; palpitations; rash; severe abdominal pain; or unusual weakness.

Interactions
This medicine interacts with several other drugs such as diuretics, reserpine, beta blockers, phenytoin, lithium, phenobarbital, birth control pills, and other medications.
- Be sure to tell your doctor about any medications you are currently taking.

Storage
Tablets, capsules, liquid and suspension should be stored at room temperature in tightly closed containers. Store away from heat and direct light. Keep out of reach of children, since overdose may be very dangerous in children. Discard any outdated medication.

LANOPHYLLIN

Properties
This medicine contains theophylline as active ingredient; it is used to treat or prevent breathing problems (wheezing and shortness of breath) caused by asthma, bronchitis, or emphysema. This medication belongs to a group known as xanthine-derivative bronchodilators. They work by opening up the bronchial tubes or air passages of the lungs and increasing the flow of air through them. These medicines are available only with your doctor's prescription.

Before using this medicine
Before you use this medicine check with your doctor, or pharmacist:
- if you ever had any unusual or allergic reaction to xanthine-derivative bronchodilators.
- if you are on a low-salt, low-sugar, or any other special diet, or if you are allergic to any substance, such as sulfites or other preservatives or dyes.
- if you are pregnant or intend to become pregnant while using this medicine.
- if you are breast-feeding an infant. Theophylline passes into the breast milk and may cause irritability, fretfulness, or trouble in sleeping in infants of mothers taking this medicine.
- if you have any of the following medical problems:
Diarrhea
Enlarged prostate
Fibrocystic breast disease
Heart disease
Stomach ulcer

Treatment
This medication is used to relieve or prevent the symptoms of your medical problem. Take them as directed. Do not take more of them and do not take them more often than recommended on the label, unless otherwise directed by your doctor. To do so may increase the chance of side effects. The medicine should be taken on an empty stomach 30 to 60 minutes before a meal or two hours after a meal. Try not to miss any doses of this medication. If you do miss a dose, take the missed dose as soon as possible, unless it is almost time for the next dose. Do not double the next dose. It works best when taken with a glass of water.

Side effects
The following minor side effects may occur:
Dizziness or flushing
Headache
Diarrhea
Heartburn
Increased urination
Insomnia
Nervousness or irritability
Loss of appetite
Nausea or stomach upset
Stomach pain.
These side effects should disappear as your body adjusts to the medication. Tell your doctor about any side effects that are persistent or particularly bothersome. It is especially important to tell your doctor about black, tarry stools; confusion; convulsions; difficulty in breathing; fainting; muscle twitching; palpitations; rash; severe abdominal pain; or unusual weakness.

Interactions
This medicine interacts with several other drugs such as diuretics, reserpine, beta blockers, phenytoin, lithium, phenobarbital, birth control pills, and other medications.
- Be sure to tell your doctor about any medications you are currently taking.

Storage
Tablets, capsules, liquid and suspension should be stored at room temperature in tightly closed containers. Store away from heat and direct light. Keep out of reach of children, since overdose may be very dangerous in children. Discard any outdated medication.

LANSPORAZOLE

Properties

This medicine contains lansporazole as active ingredient. It is a so-called proton pump inhibitor, a medicine that inhibits the production and secretion of hydrochloric acid from the cells in the mucosal lining of the stomach.

The medicine is prescribed for the short-term treatment of duodenal (intestinal) and gastric (stomach) ulcers. It is also prescribed for gastroesophageal reflex, that is the splashing of stomach acid from the stomach up onto the lower end of the esophagus.

Before using this medicine

Before you use this medicine check with your doctor, or pharmacist:
- if you ever had any unusual or allergic reaction to this medicine or any proton pump inhibitor;
- if you are allergic to any medicines, foods or other substances;
- if you are pregnant or intend to become pregnant while using this medicine (animal studies have shown toxic effects to developing fetuses);
- if you are breast-feeding an infant.

Treatment

This medication is used for treatment of peptic ulcers (duodenal or gastric ulcers), and certain ailments of the esophagus. The usual dose amounts to 20 to 80 milligrams a day. If you forget to take a dose of this medicine, take it as soon as you remember.

The medicine should be taken immediately before a meal or with an antacid if it upsets the stomach.

For safe and effective use of medicine:
- ◆ Follow your doctor's instructions if this medicine was prescribed.
- ◆ Follow the manufacturer's package directions if you are treating yourself.

Side effects

Along with the needed effects, a medicine may cause some unwanted effects. Possible side effects include:
Abdominal pain
Headache
Diarrhea
Nausea
Sore throat
Vomiting
Dizziness
Constipation
Back pain
Urinary infections
Skin rash
Heartburn
Drowsiness
Unusual bleeding
Unusual bruising
Muscle cramps
Appetite loss

Overdose

The following symptoms may be a sign of overdose:
Seizures
Breathing difficulty
Severe drowsiness
- ■ Call a doctor or hospital emergency room for instructions. If necessary, give first aid immediately.

Interactions

The effect of this medicine may be reduced if it is taken together with sucralfate. Taken together with anticoagulants it may increase the effect of the latter.
- ■ Be sure to tell your doctor about any medications you are currently taking.

Storage

Delayed-release and extended-release capsules should be stored at room temperature; store away from heat and direct light. Keep out of reach of children, since overdose may be dangerous in children.

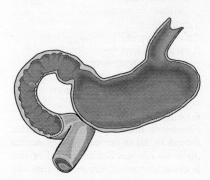

LARGACTIL

Properties
This medicine contains as active ingredient chlorpromazine, a phenothiazine derivative. Phenothiazines are a family of medicines used to treat nervous, mental, and emotional conditions. Some are used to control anxiety, restlessness, nausea and vomiting, and severe hiccups. This medicine is available only with your doctor's prescription.

Before using this medicine
Before you use this medicine check with your doctor, or pharmacist:
- if you ever had any unusual or allergic reaction to phenothiazine medicines.
- if you are on a low-salt, low-sugar, or any other special diet, or if you are allergic to any substance, such as sulfites or other preservatives or dyes.
- if you are pregnant or intend to become pregnant while using this medicine. Although phenothiazines have not been shown to cause birth defects, some side effects such as jaundice and muscle tremors have occurred in a few newborns whose mothers received phenothiazines during pregnancy.
- if you are breast-feeding an infant. Although this medicine has not been shown to cause problems in humans the chance does exist since some phenothiazines are known to pass into the breast milk.
- if you have any of the following medical problems:
Alcoholism
Blood disease
Difficult urination
Enlarged prostate
Glaucoma
Heart or blood vessel disease
Liver or lung disease
Parkinson's disease
Stomach ulcers

Treatment
This medication is prescribed to treat the symptoms of certain types of mental illness or emotional problems. In order to avoid stomach irritation, you can take the tablet or capsule forms of this medication with a meal or with a glass of water or milk (unless your doctor or pharmacist directs you to do otherwise).

Side effects
Along with the needed effects, a medicine may cause some unwanted effects. Minor side effects are: blurred vision, constipation, decreased sweating, diarrhea, dizziness, drooling, drowsiness, dry mouth, fatigue, jitteriness, menstrual irregularities, nasal congestion, restlessness, tremors, vomiting, or weight gain.
- Tell your doctor about any side effects that are persistent or particularly bothersome. It is especially important to tell your doctor about:
Breast enlargement
Chest pain or convulsions
Darkened skin
Difficulty in swallowing
Fainting or fever
Involuntary movements
Palpitations or sleep disorders
Rash or sore throat
Uncoordinated movements
Unusual bleeding or bruising
Visual disturbances
Yellowing of the eyes or skin

Interactions
This medicine may interact with several other drugs such as barbiturates, sleeping pills, narcotics, other tranquilizers, or any other medication that may produce a sedative effect. Avoid alcohol.

Storage
Store this medication as directed on the label. Keep out of the reach of children.

LEVLEN

Properties

This medicine contains levonorgestrel and ethinyl estradiol as active ingredients. It is an oral contraceptive prescribed to prevent pregnancy and/or to regulate menstrual periods.

The drug works by altering the mucus at the cervix entrance to prevent the entry of sperm. It also alters the uterus lining to resist implantation of the fertilized egg. Oral contraceptives create the same chemical atmosphere in blood that exists during pregnancy.

Before using this medicine

Before you use this medicine check with your doctor, or pharmacist:

- if you ever had any unusual or allergic reaction to estrogens or progestogen;
- if you are pregnant or want to become pregnant within three months;
- if you are breast-feeding an infant;
- if you have any of the following medical problems:
  Diabetes
  Ailments of the breast
  Disorders of the uterus
  Migraine or epilepsy
  High blood pressure
  Asthma or heart conditions
  Kidney disease
  Gallstones

Treatment

This medication is used to prevent pregnancy or to regulate menstrual periods.

Adverse reactions

Along with the needed effects, a medicine may cause some unwanted effects or adverse reactions.

- *An increased risk of the following adverse reactions has been associated with the use of oral contraceptives:*
  Thrombophlebitis
  Venous thrombosis
  Arterial thromboembolism
  Pulmonary (lung) embolism
  Myocardial infarction
  Cerebral hemorrhage
  Cerebral thrombosis
  Hypertension
  Gallbladder disease
  Hepatic (liver) hepatomas
  Benign lifer tumors
- *The following adverse reactions have been reported in patients receiving oral contraceptives and are believed to be drug-related:*
  Nausea and vomiting
  Abdominal cramps
  Breakthrough bleeding
  Spotting
  Change in menstrual flow
  Amenorrhea
  Temporary infertility
  Edema
  Breast changes
  Weight changes
  Cholestatic jaundice
  Migraine
  Rash (allergic)
  Mental depression
  Vaginal candidiasis

Interactions

This medicine may interact with several other drugs such as antibiotics, anticoagulants, anticonvulsants, antidepressants, oral antidiabetics, antihistamines, barbiturates, oral hypoglycemics, insulin, meperidine.

- Be sure to tell your doctor about any medications you are currently taking.

Storage

Tablets should be stored at room temperature; store away from heat and direct light. Keep out of reach of children, since this medicine may be dangerous in chidren.

LEVO-DROMORAN

Properties
This medicine contains as active ingredient

It is a narcotic analgesic that acts directly on the central nervous system (brain and spinal cord). It is used to relieve pain or to suppress coughing.

Before using this medicine
Before you use this medicine check with your doctor, or pharmacist:
- if you ever had any unusual or allergic reaction to this medicine or one of its components.
- if you are on a low-salt, low-sugar, or any other special diet, or if you are allergic to any substance, such as sulfites or other preservatives or dyes.
- if you are pregnant or intend to become pregnant while using this medicine. Studies on birth defects have not been done in humans. Too much use of narcotics during pregnancy may cause the baby to become dependent on the medicine.
- if you are breast-feeding an infant. Although this medicine has not been shown to cause problems in humans, it passes into the breast milk in small amounts.
- if you have any of the following medical problems:
  Brain disease or head injury
  Colitis
  Convulsions
  Emphysema, asthma, or chronic lung disease
  Enlarged prostate
  Gallbladder disease or gallstones
  Heart disease
  Kidney or lifer disease
  Underactive thyroid

Treatment
This medication is used to relieve pain or to suppress coughing. Narcotic analgesics act in the central nervous system; some of their side effects are also caused by actions in the central nervous system.
- If you are taking this medication on a regular schedule and you miss a dose, take the missed dose as soon as possible, unless it is almost time for your next dose. In that case do not take the missed dose at all.
- If a narcotic analgesic is used for a long time, it may become habit-forming (causing mental or physical dependence). Physical dependence may lead to withdrawal side effects when you stop taking this medicine.

Unless otherwise directed by your doctor or pharmacist take this as directed. Do not take more of them and do not take them more often than recommended on the label. Children up to 12 years of age should not take this medicine more than 3 times a day or for more than 5 days in a row.

Side effects
Along with the needed effects, a medicine may cause some unwanted effects. These side effects may go away during treatment as your body adjusts to the medicine. Such minor side effects are: constipation, dizziness, drowsiness, dry mouth, false sense of well-being, flushing, light-headedness, loss of appetite, nausea, painful or difficult urination, or sweating.
- Check with your doctor immediately if any of the following side effects occur:
  Anxiety or breathing difficulties
  Excitation or restlessness
  Fatigue, palpitations
  Rash, sore throat and fever
  Tremors or weakness

Interactions
This medicine may interact with several other drugs such as medicines acting on the central nervous system (e.g., antidepressants, tranquilizers), cimetidine, nitrates, quinidine, etc.
- Be sure to tell your doctor about any medications you are currently taking.

Storage
Tablets, elixir, suppository etc. should be stored at room temperature in a tightly closed, light-resistant container.

LEVORA

Properties
This medicine contains levonorgestrel and ethinyl estradiol as active ingredients. It is an oral contraceptive prescribed to prevent pregnancy and/or to regulate menstrual periods.

The drug works by altering the mucus at the cervix entrance to prevent the entry of sperm. It also alters the uterus lining to resist implantation of the fertilized egg. Oral contraceptives create the same chemical atmosphere in blood that exists during pregnancy.

Before using this medicine
Before you use this medicine check with your doctor, or pharmacist:
- if you ever had any unusual or allergic reaction to estrogens or progestogen;
- if you are pregnant or want to become pregnant within three months;
- if you are breast-feeding an infant;
- if you have any of the following medical problems:
  Diabetes
  Ailments of the breast
  Disorders of the uterus
  Migraine or epilepsy
  High blood pressure
  Asthma or heart conditions
  Kidney disease
  Gallstones

Treatment
This medication is used to prevent pregnancy or to regulate menstrual periods.

Adverse reactions
Along with the needed effects, a medicine may cause some unwanted effects or adverse reactions.
- *An increased risk of the following adverse reactions has been associated with the use of oral contraceptives:*
  Thrombophlebitis
  Venous thrombosis
  Arterial thromboembolism
  Pulmonary (lung) embolism
  Myocardial infarction
  Cerebral hemorrhage
  Cerebral thrombosis
  Hypertension
  Gallbladder disease
  Hepatic (liver) hepatomas
  Benign lifer tumors
- *The following adverse reactions have been reported in patients receiving oral contraceptives and are believed to be drug-related:*
  Nausea and vomiting
  Abdominal cramps
  Breakthrough bleeding
  Spotting
  Change in menstrual flow
  Amenorrhea
  Temporary infertility
  Edema
  Breast changes
  Weight changes
  Cholestatic jaundice
  Migraine
  Rash (allergic)
  Mental depression
  Vaginal candidiasis

Interactions
This medicine may interact with several other drugs such as antibiotics, anticoagulants, anticonvulsants, antidepressants, oral antidiabetics, antihistamines, barbiturates, oral hypoglycemics, insulin, meperidine.
- Be sure to tell your doctor about any medications you are currently taking.

Storage
Tablets should be stored at room temperature; store away from heat and direct light. Keep out of reach of children, since this medicine may be dangerous in chidren.

LEVORPHANOL

Properties
This medicine contains as active ingredient levorphanol.

It is a narcotic analgesic that acts directly on the central nervous system (brain and spinal cord). It is used to relieve pain or to suppress coughing.

Before using this medicine
Before you use this medicine check with your doctor, or pharmacist:
- if you ever had any unusual or allergic reaction to this medicine or one of its components.
- if you are on a low-salt, low-sugar, or any other special diet, or if you are allergic to any substance, such as sulfites or other preservatives or dyes.
- if you are pregnant or intend to become pregnant while using this medicine. Studies on birth defects have not been done in humans. Too much use of narcotics during pregnancy may cause the baby to become dependent on the medicine.
- if you are breast-feeding an infant. Although this medicine has not been shown to cause problems in humans, it passes into the breast milk in small amounts.
- if you have any of the following medical problems:
  Brain disease or head injury
  Colitis
  Convulsions
  Emphysema, asthma, or chronic lung disease
  Enlarged prostate
  Gallbladder disease or gallstones
  Heart disease
  Kidney or lifer disease
  Underactive thyroid

Treatment
This medication is used to relieve pain or to suppress coughing. Narcotic analgesics act in the central nervous system; some of their side effects are also caused by actions in the central nervous system.
- If you are taking this medication on a regular schedule and you miss a dose, take the missed dose as soon as possible, unless it is almost time for your next dose. In that case do not take the missed dose at all.
- If a narcotic analgesic is used for a long time, it may become habit-forming (causing mental or physical dependence). Physical dependence may lead to withdrawal side effects when you stop taking this medicine.

Unless otherwise directed by your doctor or pharmacist take this as directed. Do not take more of them and do not take them more often than recommended on the label. Children up to 12 years of age should not take this medicine more than 3 times a day or for more than 5 days in a row.

Side effects
Along with the needed effects, a medicine may cause some unwanted effects. These side effects may go away during treatment as your body adjusts to the medicine. Such minor side effects are: constipation, dizziness, drowsiness, dry mouth, false sense of well-being, flushing, light-headedness, loss of appetite, nausea, painful or difficult urination, or sweating.
- Check with your doctor immediately if any of the following side effects occur:
  Anxiety or breathing difficulties
  Excitation or restlessness
  Fatigue, palpitations
  Rash, sore throat and fever
  Tremors or weakness

Interactions
This medicine may interact with several other drugs such as medicines acting on the central nervous system (e.g., antidepressants, tranquilizers), cimetidine, nitrates, quinidine, etc.
- Be sure to tell your doctor about any medications you are currently taking.

Storage
Tablets, elixir, suppository etc. should be stored at room temperature in a tightly closed, light-resistant container.

LIPO-GANTRISIN

Properties
This medicine contains sulfisoxasole, a sulfonamide, as active ingredient. Sulfonamides are prescribed to treat infections caused by bacteria. They will not work for colds, flu, or other virus infections.

Before using this medicine
Before you use this medicine check with your doctor:
- if you ever had any unusual or allergic reaction to any of the compounds of the medicine.
- if you are on a low-salt, low-sugar, or any other special diet, or if you are allergic to any substance, such as sulfites or other preservatives or dyes.
- if you are pregnant or intend to become pregnant while using this medicine. Although sulfonamides have not been shown to cause defects in humans, the chance may exists.
- if you are breast-feeding an infant. Most sulfonamides pass into the breast milk in small amounts and may cause unwanted effects in infants with some specific conditions.
- if you have any of the following medical problems:
Kidney disease
Liver disease
Porphyria
Deficiency of enzymes such as G6PD

Treatment
This medication is used to treat an infection caused by bacteria. Most sulfonamides are best taken with a full glass (8 ounces) of water on an empty stomach, either one hour before or two hours after a meal. Follow your doctor's or pharmacist's directions on how to take your medicine.
- Keep taking this medicine for the full time of treatment even if you begin to feel better after a few days; do not miss any doses.
- If you do miss a dose of this medicine, take the missed dose immediately.
- This medication works best when the level of medicine in your bloodstream (and urine) is kept constant. It is best, therefore, to take the doses at evenly spaced intervals day and night. if you take two doses a day, the doses should be spaced 12 hours apart.

Side effects
Along with the needed effects, a medicine may cause some unwanted effects. Side effects that usually do not require medical attention: abdominal pain, diarrhea, dizziness, headache, loss of appetite, nausea, sore mouth, or vomiting. These side effects should disappear as your body adjusts to the medication.

Sulfonamides can increase sensitivity to sunlight. It is, therefore, important to avoid prolonged exposure to sunlight and sunlamps.

Tell your doctor about any side effects that are persistent or particularly bothersome. It is especially important to tell your doctor about:
Bloody urine
Difficult urination
Difficulty in breathing
Difficulty in swallowing
Fever or hallucinations
Itching, rash, or pale skin
Joint pain, lower back pain
Ringing in the ears
Sore throat
Swollen or inflamed tongue
Tingling in hands or feet
Unusual bleeding
Yellowing of the eyes or skin

Interactions
This medicine may interact with several other drugs such as anticoagulants, oral antidiabetic agents, aspirin, some antibiotics, or anticancer drugs.

Be sure to tell your doctor about any medications you are currently taking.

Storage
Tablets, capsules, suspension, etc. should be stored at room temperature as directed by your pharmacist or according to instructions on the label.

LIQUIFILM (Ophthalmic)

Properties
This medicine contains an ophthalmic antibacterial, as active ingredient. It helps the body to overcome eye infections on surface tissues of the eye. It is most useful when the infecting organism is one known to be sensitive to the antibacterial drug. The drug penetrates the bacterial cell membrane and prevents cells from multiplying.

Before using this medicine
Before you use this medicine check with your doctor:
- if you ever had any unusual or allergic reaction to any of the compounds of the medicine.
- if you are on a low-salt, low-sugar, or any other special diet, or if you are allergic to any substance, such as sulfites or other preservatives or dyes.
- if you are pregnant or intend to become pregnant while using this medicine. Although ophthalmic antibacterials have been found to be safe for use during pregnancy, you should check with your doctor before taking any drug if you are pregnant.

Treatment
This medication is used to treat an infection caused by bacteria. The medicine may be used in the form of eye drops or as an eye ointment. Use the medication as directed, Do not miss a dose. If you forget a dose, use it as soon as you remember. Notify your doctor if eye symptoms fail to improve in two to four days.
- ◆ To apply eye drops: Till the head backward when applying the eye drops. Pull the lower eyelid away from the eye to form a pouch. After applying the drop, keep the eye closed for a minute or so. This allows the medication to come in contact with the infection.
- ◆ To apply eye ointment: Pull lower lid down from eye to form a pouch. Squeeze tube to apply thin strip of ointment into pouch. Close eye for 1 to 2 minutes.

Always wash your hands before applying the ointment.The drug starts to work in about one hour. Treatment may require 7 to 10 days to control infection.Older adults or seniors may take this medication without special restriction.

Side effects
Along with the needed effects, a medicine may cause some unwanted effects. Side effects that usually do not require medical attention: occasional local irritation after application to the eye. Ointments may cause blurred vision for a few minutes; continue the use of the eye drops or ointment, but tell your doctor at the next visit.
- ▪ Discontinue the use of eye drops or eye ointment in the following cases:
  Sore throat
  Aplastic anemia
  Pale skin
  Unusual redness of the eye
  Unusual irritation of the eye
  Fever
  Unusual bleeding
  Unusual bruising
- ▪ Tell your doctor about any side effects that are persistent or particularly bothersome. In case of prolonged use sensitivity reactions may develop.

Interactions
Clinically significant interactions with oral or injected medicines are unlikely. Do not use the eye drops or ointment with any other eye drops or ointment without checking with your ophthalmologist.

Storage
Keep bottle (with eye drops) or container (containing ointment) lightly closed. Store in a cool place, but Do not freeze. Wash hands immediately after using. Do not store in the bathroom medicine cabinet because the heat or moisture may cause the medicine to break down.

Do not keep outdated medicine or medicine no longer needed. Flush the contents of the bottle or tube down the toilet, unless otherwise directed.

LIQUOPHYLLINE

Properties
This medicine contains theophylline as active ingredient; it is used to treat or prevent breathing problems (wheezing and shortness of breath) caused by asthma, bronchitis, or emphysema. This medication belongs to a group known as xanthine-derivative bronchodilators. They work by opening up the bronchial tubes or air passages of the lungs and increasing the flow of air through them. These medicines are available only with your doctor's prescription.

Before using this medicine
Before you use this medicine check with your doctor, or pharmacist:
- if you ever had any unusual or allergic reaction to xanthine-derivative bronchodilators.
- if you are on a low-salt, low-sugar, or any other special diet, or if you are allergic to any substance, such as sulfites or other preservatives or dyes.
- if you are pregnant or intend to become pregnant while using this medicine.
- if you are breast-feeding an infant. Theophylline passes into the breast milk and may cause irritability, fretfulness, or trouble in sleeping in infants of mothers taking this medicine.
- if you have any of the following medical problems:
Diarrhea
Enlarged prostate
Fibrocystic breast disease
Heart disease
Stomach ulcer

Treatment
This medication is used to relieve or prevent the symptoms of your medical problem. Take them as directed. Do not take more of them and do not take them more often than recommended on the label, unless otherwise directed by your doctor. To do so may increase the chance of side effects. The medicine should be taken on an empty stomach 30 to 60 minutes before a meal or two hours after a meal. Try not to miss any doses of this medication. If you do miss a dose, take the missed dose as soon as possible, unless it is almost time for the next dose. Do not double the next dose. It works best when taken with a glass of water.

Side effects
The following minor side effects may occur:
Dizziness or flushing
Headache
Diarrhea
Heartburn
Increased urination
Insomnia
Nervousness or irritability
Loss of appetite
Nausea or stomach upset
Stomach pain.
These side effects should disappear as your body adjusts to the medication. Tell your doctor about any side effects that are persistent or particularly bothersome. It is especially important to tell your doctor about black, tarry stools; confusion; convulsions; difficulty in breathing; fainting; muscle twitching; palpitations; rash; severe abdominal pain; or unusual weakness.

Interactions
This medicine interacts with several other drugs such as diuretics, reserpine, beta blockers, phenytoin, lithium, phenobarbital, birth control pills, and other medications.
- Be sure to tell your doctor about any medications you are currently taking.

Storage
Tablets, capsules, liquid and suspension should be stored at room temperature in tightly closed containers. Store away from heat and direct light. Keep out of reach of children, since overdose may be very dangerous in children. Discard any outdated medication.

LIXOLIN

Properties
This medicine contains theophylline as active ingredient; it is used to treat or prevent breathing problems (wheezing and shortness of breath) caused by asthma, bronchitis, or emphysema. This medication belongs to a group known as xanthine-derivative bronchodilators. They work by opening up the bronchial tubes or air passages of the lungs and increasing the flow of air through them. These medicines are available only with your doctor's prescription.

Before using this medicine
Before you use this medicine check with your doctor, or pharmacist:
- if you ever had any unusual or allergic reaction to xanthine-derivative bronchodilators.
- if you are on a low-salt, low-sugar, or any other special diet, or if you are allergic to any substance, such as sulfites or other preservatives or dyes.
- if you are pregnant or intend to become pregnant while using this medicine.
- if you are breast-feeding an infant. Theophylline passes into the breast milk and may cause irritability, fretfulness, or trouble in sleeping in infants of mothers taking this medicine.
- if you have any of the following medical problems:
  Diarrhea
  Enlarged prostate
  Fibrocystic breast disease
  Heart disease
  Stomach ulcer

Treatment
This medication is used to relieve or prevent the symptoms of your medical problem. Take them as directed. Do not take more of them and do not take them more often than recommended on the label, unless otherwise directed by your doctor. To do so may increase the chance of side effects. The medicine should be taken on an empty stomach 30 to 60 minutes before a meal or two hours after a meal. Try not to miss any doses of this medication. If you do miss a dose, take the missed dose as soon as possible, unless it is almost time for the next dose. Do not double the next dose. It works best when taken with a glass of water.

Side effects
The following minor side effects may occur:
  Dizziness or flushing
  Headache
  Diarrhea
  Heartburn
  Increased urination
  Insomnia
  Nervousness or irritability
  Loss of appetite
  Nausea or stomach upset
  Stomach pain.
These side effects should disappear as your body adjusts to the medication. Tell your doctor about any side effects that are persistent or particularly bothersome. It is especially important to tell your doctor about black, tarry stools; confusion; convulsions; difficulty in breathing; fainting; muscle twitching; palpitations; rash; severe abdominal pain; or unusual weakness.

Interactions
This medicine interacts with several other drugs such as diuretics, reserpine, beta blockers, phenytoin, lithium, phenobarbital, birth control pills, and other medications.
- Be sure to tell your doctor about any medications you are currently taking.

Storage
Tablets, capsules, liquid and suspension should be stored at room temperature in tightly closed containers. Store away from heat and direct light. Keep out of reach of children, since overdose may be very dangerous in children. Discard any outdated medication.

LO/OVRAL

Properties

This medicine contains norgestrel and ethinyl estradiol as active ingredients. It is an oral contraceptive prescribed to prevent pregnancy and/or to regulate menstrual periods.

The drug works by altering the mucus at the cervix entrance to prevent the entry of sperm. It also alters the uterus lining to resist implantation of the fertilized egg. Oral contraceptives create the same chemical atmosphere in blood that exists during pregnancy.

Before using this medicine

Before you use this medicine check with your doctor, or pharmacist:
- if you ever had any unusual or allergic reaction to estrogens or progestogen;
- if you are pregnant or want to become pregnant within three months;
- if you are breast-feeding an infant;
- if you have any of the following medical problems:
  Diabetes
  Ailments of the breast
  Disorders of the uterus
  Migraine or epilepsy
  High blood pressure
  Asthma or heart conditions
  Kidney disease
  Gallstones

Treatment

This medication is used to prevent pregnancy or to regulate menstrual periods.

Adverse reactions

Along with the needed effects, a medicine may cause some unwanted effects or adverse reactions.
- *An increased risk of the following adverse reactions has been associated with the use of oral contraceptives:*
  Thrombophlebitis
  Venous thrombosis
  Arterial thromboembolism
  Pulmonary (lung) embolism
  Myocardial infarction
  Cerebral hemorrhage
  Cerebral thrombosis
  Hypertension
  Gallbladder disease
  Hepatic (liver) hepatomas
  Benign lifer tumors
- *The following adverse reactions have been reported in patients receiving oral contraceptives and are believed to be drug-related:*
  Nausea and vomiting
  Abdominal cramps
  Breakthrough bleeding
  Spotting
  Change in menstrual flow
  Amenorrhea
  Temporary infertility
  Edema
  Breast changes
  Weight changes
  Cholestatic jaundice
  Migraine
  Rash (allergic)
  Mental depression
  Vaginal candidiasis

Interactions

This medicine may interact with several other drugs such as antibiotics, anticoagulants, anticonvulsants, antidepressants, oral antidiabetics, antihistamines, barbiturates, oral hypoglycemics, insulin, meperidine.
- Be sure to tell your doctor about any medications you are currently taking.

Storage

Tablets should be stored at room temperature; store away from heat and direct light. Keep out of reach of children, since this medicine may be dangerous in chidren.

LODRANE

Properties

This medicine contains theophylline as active ingredient; it is used to treat or prevent breathing problems (wheezing and shortness of breath) caused by asthma, bronchitis, or emphysema. This medication belongs to a group known as xanthine-derivative bronchodilators. They work by opening up the bronchial tubes or air passages of the lungs and increasing the flow of air through them. These medicines are available only with your doctor's prescription.

Before using this medicine

Before you use this medicine check with your doctor, or pharmacist:
- if you ever had any unusual or allergic reaction to xanthine-derivative bronchodilators.
- if you are on a low-salt, low-sugar, or any other special diet, or if you are allergic to any substance, such as sulfites or other preservatives or dyes.
- if you are pregnant or intend to become pregnant while using this medicine.
- if you are breast-feeding an infant. Theophylline passes into the breast milk and may cause irritability, fretfulness, or trouble in sleeping in infants of mothers taking this medicine.
- if you have any of the following medical problems:
Diarrhea
Enlarged prostate
Fibrocystic breast disease
Heart disease
Stomach ulcer

Treatment

This medication is used to relieve or prevent the symptoms of your medical problem. Take them as directed. Do not take more of them and do not take them more often than recommended on the label, unless otherwise directed by your doctor. To do so may increase the chance of side effects. The medicine should be taken on an empty stomach 30 to 60 minutes before a meal or two hours after a meal. Try not to miss any doses of this medication. If you do miss a dose, take the missed dose as soon as possible, unless it is almost time for the next dose. Do not double the next dose. It works best when taken with a glass of water.

Side effects

The following minor side effects may occur:
    Dizziness or flushing
    Headache
    Diarrhea
    Heartburn
    Increased urination
    Insomnia
    Nervousness or irritability
    Loss of appetite
    Nausea or stomach upset
    Stomach pain.
These side effects should disappear as your body adjusts to the medication. Tell your doctor about any side effects that are persistent or particularly bothersome. It is especially important to tell your doctor about black, tarry stools; confusion; convulsions; difficulty in breathing; fainting; muscle twitching; palpitations; rash; severe abdominal pain; or unusual weakness.

Interactions

This medicine interacts with several other drugs such as diuretics, reserpine, beta blockers, phenytoin, lithium, phenobarbital, birth control pills, and other medications.
- Be sure to tell your doctor about any medications you are currently taking.

Storage

Tablets, capsules, liquid and suspension should be stored at room temperature in tightly closed containers. Store away from heat and direct light. Keep out of reach of children, since overdose may be very dangerous in children. Discard any outdated medication.

LOESTRIN

Properties

This medicine contains norethindrone and ethinyl estradiol as active ingredients. It is an oral contraceptive prescribed to prevent pregnancy and/or to regulate menstrual periods.

The drug works by altering the mucus at the cervix entrance to prevent the entry of sperm. It also alters the uterus lining to resist implantation of the fertilized egg. Oral contraceptives create the same chemical atmosphere in blood that exists during pregnancy.

Before using this medicine

Before you use this medicine check with your doctor, or pharmacist:
- if you ever had any unusual or allergic reaction to estrogens or progestogen;
- if you are pregnant or want to become pregnant within three months;
- if you are breast-feeding an infant;
- if you have any of the following medical problems:
  Diabetes
  Ailments of the breast
  Disorders of the uterus
  Migraine or epilepsy
  High blood pressure
  Asthma or heart conditions
  Kidney disease
  Gallstones

Treatment

This medication is used to prevent pregnancy or to regulate menstrual periods.

Adverse reactions

Along with the needed effects, a medicine may cause some unwanted effects or adverse reactions.
- *An increased risk of the following adverse reactions has been associated with the use of oral contraceptives:*
  Thrombophlebitis
  Venous thrombosis
  Arterial thromboembolism
  Pulmonary (lung) embolism
  Myocardial infarction
  Cerebral hemorrhage
  Cerebral thrombosis
  Hypertension
  Gallbladder disease
  Hepatic (liver) hepatomas
  Benign lifer tumors
- *The following adverse reactions have been reported in patients receiving oral contraceptives and are believed to be drug-related:*
  Nausea and vomiting
  Abdominal cramps
  Breakthrough bleeding
  Spotting
  Change in menstrual flow
  Amenorrhea
  Temporary infertility
  Edema
  Breast changes
  Weight changes
  Cholestatic jaundice
  Migraine
  Rash (allergic)
  Mental depression
  Vaginal candidiasis

Interactions

This medicine may interact with several other drugs such as antibiotics, anticoagulants, anticonvulsants, antidepressants, oral antidiabetics, antihistamines, barbiturates, oral hypoglycemics, insulin, meperidine.
- Be sure to tell your doctor about any medications you are currently taking.

Storage

Tablets should be stored at room temperature; store away from heat and direct light. Keep out of reach of children, since this medicine may be dangerous in chidren.

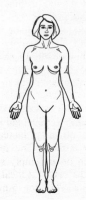

LORAZEPAM

Properties
This medicine contains as active ingredient lorazepam, a benzodiazepine preparation. Benzodiazepines belong to the group of psychoactive medicines that influence the activity of the brain. Some are used to relieve nervousness or tension. It is effective for this purpose for short periods. Others are used for sleeplessness or to relax muscles or relieve muscle spasm. The benzodiazepines may also be used for other conditions as determined by your doctor.

Before using this medicine
Before you use this medicine check with your doctor:
- if you ever had any unusual or allergic reaction to benzodiazepines.
- if you are on a low-salt, low-sugar, or any other special diet, or if you are allergic to any substance, such as sulfites or other preservatives or dyes.
- if you are pregnant or intend to become pregnant while using this medicine. Some benzodiazepines have been reported to increase the chance of birth defects when used during the first 3 months of pregnancy.
- if you are breast-feeding an infant. Benzodiazepines may pass into the breast milk and cause drowsiness, unusually slow heartbeat, shortness of breath, or troubled breathing in infants of mothers taking this medicine.
- if you have any of the following medical problems: asthma, bronchitis, emphysema, or other chronic lung disease; epilepsy or history of convulsions; hyperactivity (in children); kidney or lifer disease; mental depression or illness; myasthania gravis, porphyria.

Treatment
This medication is used to relieve or prevent the symptoms of your medical problem. Benzodiazepines are mainly used as antianxiety agents, anticonvulsants, or sedatives. Take them as directed. Do not take more of them and rected. Do not take more of them and do not take them more often than recommended on the label, unless otherwise directed by your doctor. Benzodiazepine tranquilizing drugs can be abused if taken for long periods of time and it is possible to develop withdrawal symptoms if you discontinue the therapy abruptly.

Side effects
Along with the needed effects, a medicine may cause some unwanted effects. Minor side effects are: bitter taste in the mouth, dizziness, drowsiness, depression, constipation, dry mouth, excessive salivation, fatigue, flushing, headache, heartburn, loss of appetite, nausea, nervousness, sweating or vomiting. As your body adjusts to the medicine, these side effects should disappear.
- Tell your doctor about any side effects that are persistent or particularly bothersome. It is especially important to tell your doctor about:
Blurred or double vision
Chest pain
Difficulty in urinating
Fainting or falling
Fever or hallucinations
Joint pain
Mouth sores
Nightmares
Palpitations
Severe depression
Shortness of breath
Slurred speech
Uncoordinated movements
Unusual tiredness
Yellowing of the skin

Interactions
- This medicine may interact with several other drugs. This medicine will add to the effects of alcohol, and CNS depressants.
- Be sure to tell your doctor about any medications you are currently taking.

Storage
Store at room temperature in tightly closed, light-resistant-resistant containers. Keep out of the reach of children since overdose may be especially dangerous in children.

LOSEC

Properties

This medicine contains omeprazole as active ingredient. It is a so-called proton pump inhibitor, a medicine that inhibits the production and secretion of hydrochloric acid from the cells in the mucosal lining of the stomach.

The medicine is prescribed for the short-term treatment of duodenal (intestinal) and gastric (stomach) ulcers. It is also prescribed for gastroesophageal reflex, that is the splashing of stomach acid from the stomach up onto the lower end of the esophagus.

Before using this medicine

Before you use this medicine check with your doctor, or pharmacist:
- if you ever had any unusual or allergic reaction to this medicine or any proton pump inhibitor;
- if you are allergic to any medicines, foods or other substances;
- if you are pregnant or intend to become pregnant while using this medicine (animal studies have shown toxic effects to developing fetuses);
- if you are breast-feeding an infant.

Treatment

This medication is used for treatment of peptic ulcers (duodenal or gastric ulcers), and certain ailments of the esophagus. The usual dose amounts to 20 to 80 milligrams a day. If you forget to take a dose of this medicine, take it as soon as you remember.

The medicine should be taken immediately before a meal or with an antacid if it upsets the stomach.

For safe and effective use of medicine:
- ◆ Follow your doctor's instructions if this medicine was prescribed.
- ◆ Follow the manufacturer's package directions if you are treating yourself.

Side effects

Along with the needed effects, a medicine may cause some unwanted effects. Possible side effects include:
Abdominal pain
Headache
Diarrhea
Nausea
Sore throat
Vomiting
Dizziness
Constipation
Back pain
Urinary infections
Skin rash
Heartburn
Drowsiness
Unusual bleeding
Unusual bruising
Muscle cramps
Appetite loss

Overdose

The following symptoms may be a sign of overdose:
Seizures
Breathing difficulty
Severe drowsiness
- ▪ Call a doctor or hospital emergency room for instructions. If necessary, give first aid immediately.

Interactions

The effect of this medicine may be reduced if it is taken together with sucralfate. Taken together with anticoagulants it may increase the effect of the latter.
- ▪ Be sure to tell your doctor about any medications you are currently taking.

Storage

Delayed-release and extended-release capsules should be stored at room temperature; store away from heat and direct light. Keep out of reach of children, since overdose may be dangerous in children.

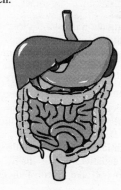

LOTREL

Properties
This medicine contains amlodipine as active ingredient. It is a so-called calcium channel blocker, working by blocking the passage of calcium into heart and smooth muscle. Since calcium is an essential factor in muscle contraction, any medicine that affects calcium in this way will interfere with the contraction of these muscles.

The medicine works by:
◆ reducing the work that the heart must perform;
◆ reducing the normal arterial blood pressure;
◆ increasing oxygen to the heart muscle.

The medicine is prescribed for the treatment of attacks of angina pectoris, irregular heartbeat, and high blood pressure. In many cases it can be used for the treatment and prevention of migraine.

Before using this medicine
Before you use this medicine check with your doctor, or pharmacist:
– if you ever had any unusual or allergic reaction to this medicine or any calcium channel blocker;
– if you are pregnant or intend to become pregnant while using this medicine;
– if you have low blood pressure;
– if you have kidney or lifer disease;
– if you are breast-feeding an infant;
– if you easily get a rash or intensity sunburn in areas exposed to sun or ultraviolet light.

Treatment
This medication is used for treatment of heart conditions (for instance, angina pectoris) and high blood pressure. Tablets, capsules or extended-release tablets should be taken with liquid. The usual dose amounts to 30 to 100 milligrams a day.

For safe and effective use of medicine:
◆ Follow your doctor's instructions if this medicine was prescribed.
◆ Follow the manufacturer's package directions if you are treating yourself.

Side effects
Along with the needed effects, a medicine may cause some unwanted effects. Possible side effects include:
Tiredness
Changes in heartbeat
Wheezing
Cough
Shortness of breath
Dizziness
Fainting
Numbness in hands and feet
Tingling in hands and feet
Difficult urination
Constipation

Overdose
The following symptoms may be a sign of overdose:
Unusually fast heartbeat
Unusually slow heartbeat
Loss of consciousness
Cardiac arrest
■ Call a doctor or hospital emergency room for instructions. If necessary start first aid immediately.

Interactions
The effect of this medicine may cause a blood pressure drop if taken together with antihypertensives. Cimetidine may increase the effect of the calcium blocker.

The simultaneous use of diuretics and calcium channel blockers may cause dangerous blood pressure drop.
■ Be sure to tell your doctor about any medications you are currently taking.

Storage
Capsules, tablets, etc. should be stored at room temperature; store away from heat and direct light. Keep out of reach of children, since this medicine may be dangerous in children.

LOTUSATE

Properties

This medicine contains as active ingredient the barbiturate talbutal. Barbiturates belong to the group of medicines called central nervous system depressants (medicines that slow down the nervous system).

Barbiturates may partially block nerve impulses at nerve-cell connections. They may be used to treat insomnia (sleeplessness) by helping patients fall asleep. Also, they may be used to relieve anxiety or tension. Some of the barbiturates are used as anticonvulsants to help control convulsions in certain disorders or diseases, such as epilepsy. If too much of the drug is used, it may become habit-forming (causing mental or physical dependence).

Before using this medicine

Before you use this medicine check with your doctor, or pharmacist:
- if you ever had any unusual or allergic reaction to this medicine or one of its components.
- if you are on a low-salt, low-sugar, or any other special diet, or if you are allergic to preservatives or dyes.
- if you are pregnant or intend to become pregnant while using this medicine, since barbiturates have been shown to increase the chance of birth defects in humans. Taking barbiturates regularly during the last 3 months of pregnancy may cause the baby to become dependent on the medicine. This may lead to withdrawal side effects in the baby after birth.
- if you have any of the following medical problems:
Anemia (severe)
Diabetes mellitus (sugar disease)
Hyperactivity (in children)
Kidney or lifer disease
Mental depression
Overactive thyroid

Treatment

This medication is used to treat the symptoms of your medical condition. Barbiturates act in the central nervous system; some of their side effects are also caused by actions in the central nervous system. Use this medicine as directed by your doctor. Do not use more of it, do not use it more often, and do not use it for a longer period of time than your doctor ordered.
- If you are taking this medication on a regular schedule and you miss a dose, take the missed dose as soon as possible, unless it is almost time for your next dose. In that case do not take the missed dose at all.
- If a barbiturate is used for a long time, it may become habit-forming. Physical dependence may lead to withdrawal side effects when you stop taking this medicine.

Side effects

Along with the needed effects, a medicine may cause some unwanted effects. These side effects may go away during treatment as your body adjusts to the medicine. Such minor side effects are: depression, confusion, diarrhea, nausea, vomiting, joint or muscle pain, slurred speech, hallucinations, headache, decreased sex drive.
- Check with your doctor immediately if any of the following side effects occur:
Rash or hives
Face, lip or eyelid swelling
Sore throat, fever
Agitation
Slow heartbeat
Difficult breathing or chest pain

Interactions

This medicine may interact with several other drugs such as medicines acting on the central nervous system (e.g., antihistamines; beta-adrenergic blockers; MAO inhibitors; mind-altering drugs; nabilone; antidepressants; clozapine; anticonvulsants).

Storage

The medicine should be stored at room temperature in a tightly closed, light-resistant container. Keep out of reach of children since overdose is very dangerous in children.

LUMINAL

Properties
This medicine contains as active ingredient the barbiturate phenobarbital. Barbiturates belong to the group of medicines called central nervous system depressants (medicines that slow down the nervous system).

Barbiturates may partially block nerve impulses at nerve-cell connections. They may be used to treat insomnia (sleeplessness) by helping patients fall asleep. Also, they may be used to relieve anxiety or tension. Some of the barbiturates are used as anticonvulsants to help control convulsions in certain disorders or diseases, such as epilepsy. If too much of the drug is used, it may become habit-forming (causing mental or physical dependence).

Before using this medicine
Before you use this medicine check with your doctor, or pharmacist:
- if you ever had any unusual or allergic reaction to this medicine or one of its components.
- if you are on a low-salt, low-sugar, or any other special diet, or if you are allergic to preservatives or dyes.
- if you are pregnant or intend to become pregnant while using this medicine, since barbiturates have been shown to increase the chance of birth defects in humans. Taking barbiturates regularly during the last 3 months of pregnancy may cause the baby to become dependent on the medicine. This may lead to withdrawal side effects in the baby after birth.
- if you have any of the following medical problems:
Anemia (severe)
Diabetes mellitus (sugar disease)
Hyperactivity (in children)
Kidney or lifer disease
Mental depression
Overactive thyroid

Treatment
This medication is used to treat the symptoms of your medical condition. Barbiturates act in the central nervous system; some of their side effects are also caused by actions in the central nervous system. Use this medicine as directed by your doctor. Do not use more of it, do not use it more often, and do not use it for a longer period of time than your doctor ordered.
- If you are taking this medication on a regular schedule and you miss a dose, take the missed dose as soon as possible, unless it is almost time for your next dose. In that case do not take the missed dose at all.
- If a barbiturate is used for a long time, it may become habit-forming. Physical dependence may lead to withdrawal side effects when you stop taking this medicine.

Side effects
Along with the needed effects, a medicine may cause some unwanted effects. These side effects may go away during treatment as your body adjusts to the medicine. Such minor side effects are: depression, confusion, diarrhea, nausea, vomiting, joint or muscle pain, slurred speech, hallucinations, headache, decreased sex drive.
- Check with your doctor immediately if any of the following side effects occur:
Rash or hives
Face, lip or eyelid swelling
Sore throat, fever
Agitation
Slow heartbeat
Difficult breathing or chest pain

Interactions
This medicine may interact with several other drugs such as medicines acting on the central nervous system (e.g., antihistamines; beta-adrenergic blockers; MAO inhibitors; mind-altering drugs; nabilone; antidepressants; clozapine; anticonvulsants).

Storage
The medicine should be stored at room temperature in a tightly closed, light-resistant container. Keep out of reach of children since overdose is very dangerous in children.

M S CONTIN

Properties
This medicine contains as active ingredient morphine.

It is a narcotic analgesic that acts directly on the central nervous system (brain and spinal cord). It is used to relieve pain or to suppress coughing.

Before using this medicine
Before you use this medicine check with your doctor, or pharmacist:
- if you ever had any unusual or allergic reaction to this medicine or one of its components.
- if you are on a low-salt, low-sugar, or any other special diet, or if you are allergic to any substance, such as sulfites or other preservatives or dyes.
- if you are pregnant or intend to become pregnant while using this medicine. Studies on birth defects have not been done in humans. Too much use of narcotics during pregnancy may cause the baby to become dependent on the medicine.
- if you are breast-feeding an infant. Although this medicine has not been shown to cause problems in humans, it passes into the breast milk in small amounts.
- if you have any of the following medical problems:
Brain disease or head injury
Colitis
Convulsions
Emphysema, asthma, or chronic lung disease
Enlarged prostate
Gallbladder disease or gallstones
Heart disease
Kidney or lifer disease
Underactive thyroid

Treatment
This medication is used to relieve pain or to suppress coughing. Narcotic analgesics act in the central nervous system; some of their side effects are also caused by actions in the central nervous system.
- If you are taking this medication on a regular schedule and you miss a dose, take the missed dose as soon as possible, unless it is almost time for your next dose. In that case do not take the missed dose at all.
- If a narcotic analgesic is used for a long time, it may become habit-forming (causing mental or physical dependence). Physical dependence may lead to withdrawal side effects when you stop taking this medicine.

Unless otherwise directed by your doctor or pharmacist take this as directed. Do not take more of them and do not take them more often than recommended on the label. Children up to 12 years of age should not take this medicine more than 3 times a day or for more than 5 days in a row.

Side effects
Along with the needed effects, a medicine may cause some unwanted effects. These side effects may go away during treatment as your body adjusts to the medicine. Such minor side effects are: constipation, dizziness, drowsiness, dry mouth, false sense of well-being, flushing, light-headedness, loss of appetite, nausea, painful or difficult urination, or sweating.
- Check with your doctor immediately if any of the following side effects occur:
Anxiety or breathing difficulties
Excitation or restlessness
Fatigue, palpitations
Rash, sore throat and fever
Tremors or weakness

Interactions
This medicine may interact with several other drugs such as medicines acting on the central nervous system (e.g., antidepressants, tranquilizers), cimetidine, nitrates, quinidine, etc.
- Be sure to tell your doctor about any medications you are currently taking.

Storage
Tablets, elixir, suppository etc. should be stored at room temperature in a tightly closed, light-resistant container.

M.O.S.

Properties
This medicine contains as active ingredient morphine.

It is a narcotic analgesic that acts directly on the central nervous system (brain and spinal cord). It is used to relieve pain or to suppress coughing.

Before using this medicine
Before you use this medicine check with your doctor, or pharmacist:
- if you ever had any unusual or allergic reaction to this medicine or one of its components.
- if you are on a low-salt, low-sugar, or any other special diet, or if you are allergic to any substance, such as sulfites or other preservatives or dyes.
- if you are pregnant or intend to become pregnant while using this medicine. Studies on birth defects have not been done in humans. Too much use of narcotics during pregnancy may cause the baby to become dependent on the medicine.
- if you are breast-feeding an infant. Although this medicine has not been shown to cause problems in humans, it passes into the breast milk in small amounts.
- if you have any of the following medical problems:
  Brain disease or head injury
  Colitis
  Convulsions
  Emphysema, asthma, or chronic lung disease
  Enlarged prostate
  Gallbladder disease or gallstones
  Heart disease
  Kidney or lifer disease
  Underactive thyroid

Treatment
This medication is used to relieve pain or to suppress coughing. Narcotic analgesics act in the central nervous system; some of their side effects are also caused by actions in the central nervous system.
- If you are taking this medication on a regular schedule and you miss a dose, take the missed dose as soon as possible, unless it is almost time for your next dose. In that case do not take the missed dose at all.
- If a narcotic analgesic is used for a long time, it may become habit-forming (causing mental or physical dependence). Physical dependence may lead to withdrawal side effects when you stop taking this medicine.

Unless otherwise directed by your doctor or pharmacist take this as directed. Do not take more of them and do not take them more often than recommended on the label. Children up to 12 years of age should not take this medicine more than 3 times a day or for more than 5 days in a row.

Side effects
Along with the needed effects, a medicine may cause some unwanted effects. These side effects may go away during treatment as your body adjusts to the medicine. Such minor side effects are: constipation, dizziness, drowsiness, dry mouth, false sense of well-being, flushing, light-headedness, loss of appetite, nausea, painful or difficult urination, or sweating.
- Check with your doctor immediately if any of the following side effects occur:
  Anxiety or breathing difficulties
  Excitation or restlessness
  Fatigue, palpitations
  Rash, sore throat and fever
  Tremors or weakness

Interactions
This medicine may interact with several other drugs such as medicines acting on the central nervous system (e.g., antidepressants, tranquilizers), cimetidine, nitrates, quinidine, etc.
- Be sure to tell your doctor about any medications you are currently taking.

Storage
Tablets, elixir, suppository etc. should be stored at room temperature in a tightly closed, light-resistant container.

MANDOL

Properties
This medicine contains cephalosporin as active ingredient. Cephalosporins belong to the general family of medicines called antibiotics, used in the treatment of infections caused by bacteria. They work by killing bacteria or preventing their growth. Cephalosporins will not work for colds, flu, or other viral infections.

Before using this medicine
Before you use this medicine check with your doctor:
- if you ever had any unusual or allergic reaction to any of the cephalosporins, penicillins, penicillin-like medicines, or penicillamine.
- if you are on a low-salt, low-sugar, or any other special diet, or if you are allergic to any substance, such as sulfites or other preservatives or dyes.
- if you are pregnant or intend to become pregnant while using this medicine. Although cephalosporins have not been shown to cause birth defects or other problems in humans, the chance always exists.
- if you are breast-feeding an infant. Most cephalosporins pass into the breast milk, usually in small amounts.
- if you have any of the following medical problems:
  Bleeding problem
  Kidney or lifer disease

Treatment
This medication belongs to the general family of medicines called antibiotics. It is used to treat a wide variety of bacterial infections. It is also used to treat infections in persons who are allergic to penicillin.
- Keep taking this medicine for the full time of treatment even if you begin to feel better after a few days; do not miss any doses.
- If you do miss a dose of this medicine, take it as soon as possible. This will help to keep a constant amount of medicine in the blood. However, if it is almost time for your next dose, skip the missed dose and go back to your regular dosing schedule.
- This medication has been prescribed for your current infection only. Another infection later on, or one that someone else has, may require a different medicine. You should not give your medicine to other people or use it for other infections, unless your doctor specifically directs you to do so.
- Take the medicine at the same times each day, 1 hour before or 2 hours after eating.

Side effects
Along with the needed effects, a medicine may cause some unwanted effects. Side effects that usually do not require medical attention: rectal itching, oral or vaginal white spots, mild diarrhea. These side effects should disappear as your body adjusts to the medication.
- Other side effects that should be reported to your doctor immediately are:
  Hives, rash
  Intense itching
  Faintness soon after a dose
  Difficulty in breathing
  Nausea and vomiting
  Severe diarrhea
  Unusual weakness or tiredness
  Bleeding or bruising

Interactions
This medicine may interact with several other drugs such as anticoagulants, theophylline preparations, probenecid, tetracyclines, etc.
- Be sure to tell your doctor about any medications you are currently taking.

Storage
Tablets, capsules, etc. should be stored at room temperature. Store the liquid form in the refrigerator. Keep out of the reach of children. Do not keep outdated medicine or medicine no longer needed.

MANNEST

Properties
This medicine contains conjugated estrogens as active ingredients. The medicine is prescribed for treatment of estrogen deficiency; it restores normal estrogen levels in tissues. There is no evidence that this drug is effective for nervous symptoms or depression occurring during menopause. They should not be used to treat this condition; they should be used only to replace the estrogen that is naturally absent after menopause.

Before using this medicine
Before you use this medicine check with your doctor, or pharmacist:
- if you ever had any unusual or allergic reaction to estrogens;
- if you are pregnant or intend to become pregnant within three months;
- if you are breast-feeding an infant;
- if you have any of the following medical problems:
  Diabetes
  Breast cancer
  Fibrocystic breast disease
  Fibroid uterine tumors
  Endometriosis
  Migraine headaches
  Epilepsy
  Porphyria
  High blood pressure
  Asthma
  Congestive heart failure
  Kidney disease
  Gallstones

Treatment
This medication is used to treat estrogen deficiency, specific symptoms of menopause, estrogen-deficiency osteoporosis, atrophic vaginitis, prostate cancer. For safe and effective use of this medicine:
- ◆ Follow your doctor's instructions if this medicine was prescribed.
- ◆ Follow the manufacturer's package directions if you are treating yourself.
- ◆ Estrogens have been reported to increase the risk of endometrial carcinoma.

Side effects
Along with the needed effects, a medicine may cause some unwanted effects. Possible side effects include:
  Stomach cramps
  Profuse bleeding
  Appetite loss
  Nausea and vomiting
  Swollen breasts
  Change in menstruation
  Rash, skin blisters
  Depression
  Dizziness

Overdose
The following symptoms may indicate an overdose:
  Nausea and vomiting
  Fluid retention
  Breast enlargement
  Abnormal vaginal bleeding
- ■ Call a doctor or hospital emergency room for instructions.

Interactions
This medicine may interact with several other drugs such as adrenocorticosteroids, antidepressants, oral antidiabetics, insulin, phenobarbital, primidone.
- ■ Be sure to tell your doctor about any medications you are currently taking.

Storage
Capsules, tablets, vaginal cream, transdermal patches, etc. should be stored at room temperature; store away from heat and direct light. Keep out of reach of children, since this medicine may be dangerous in children.

MARVELON

Properties

This medicine contains desogestrel and ethinyl estradiol as active ingredients. It is an oral contraceptive prescribed to prevent pregnancy and/or to regulate menstrual periods.

The drug works by altering the mucus at the cervix entrance to prevent the entry of sperm. It also alters the uterus lining to resist implantation of the fertilized egg. Oral contraceptives create the same chemical atmosphere in blood that exists during pregnancy.

Before using this medicine

Before you use this medicine check with your doctor, or pharmacist:
- if you ever had any unusual or allergic reaction to estrogens or progestogen;
- if you are pregnant or want to become pregnant within three months;
- if you are breast-feeding an infant;
- if you have any of the following medical problems:
Diabetes
Ailments of the breast
Disorders of the uterus
Migraine or epilepsy
High blood pressure
Asthma or heart conditions
Kidney disease
Gallstones

Treatment

This medication is used to prevent pregnancy or to regulate menstrual periods.

Adverse reactions

Along with the needed effects, a medicine may cause some unwanted effects or adverse reactions.
- *An increased risk of the following adverse reactions has been associated with the use of oral contraceptives:*
Thrombophlebitis
Venous thrombosis
Arterial thromboembolism
Pulmonary (lung) embolism
Myocardial infarction
Cerebral hemorrhage
Cerebral thrombosis
Hypertension
Gallbladder disease
Hepatic (liver) hepatomas
Benign lifer tumors
- *The following adverse reactions have been reported in patients receiving oral contraceptives and are believed to be drug-related:*
Nausea and vomiting
Abdominal cramps
Breakthrough bleeding
Spotting
Change in menstrual flow
Amenorrhea
Temporary infertility
Edema
Breast changes
Weight changes
Cholestatic jaundice
Migraine
Rash (allergic)
Mental depression
Vaginal candidiasis

Interactions

This medicine may interact with several other drugs such as antibiotics, anticoagulants, anticonvulsants, antidepressants, oral antidiabetics, antihistamines, barbiturates, oral hypoglycemics, insulin, meperidine.
- Be sure to tell your doctor about any medications you are currently taking.

Storage

Tablets should be stored at room temperature; store away from heat and direct light. Keep out of reach of children, since this medicine may be dangerous in children.

MAXIVATE

Properties
This medicine contains betamethasone, a corticosteroid, as active ingredient. Corticosteroids are used to help relieve redness, swelling, itching, inflammation, and discomfort of many skin problems. They exert this effect by interfering with natural body mechanisms that produce the rash, itching, or inflammation. They do not cure the underlying cause of the skin problem. This medication is applied to the skin.

Before using this medicine
Before you use this medicine check with your doctor, or pharmacist:
- if you ever had any unusual or allergic reaction to corticosteroids.
- if you are allergic to any substance, such as sulfites or other preservatives or dyes.
- if you are pregnant or intend to become pregnant while using this medicine. Studies have shown that corticosteroids applied to the skin in large amounts or over long periods of time can be the cause of birth defects.
- if you are breast-feeding an infant. Some corticosteroids pass into breast milk and may interfere with the infant's growth.

Treatment
Do not use this medicine more often or for a longer time than ordered. To do so may increase absorption through the skin and the chance of side effects. In addition, too much use, especially on areas with thinner skin (for example, face, armpits, groin), may result in thinning of the skin and stretch marks.

Before applying this medication, wash your hands. than, unless your doctor or pharmacist gives you different instructions, gently wash the area where the medication is to be applied. With a clean towel pat the area dry. Apply a small amount of the medication to the affected area in a thin layer. Do not bandage the area unless your doctor tells you to do so.

If you miss a dose of this medication, apply the dose as soon as possible, unless it is almost time for the next application.

◆ Do not use this medicine for other skin problems without first checking with your doctor. You should not use a topical corticosteroid if you have a virus disease (such as herpes), fungal infection of the skin (such as athlete's foot), or tuberculosis of the skin.

Side effects
There are a number of side effects that usually do not require medical attention. Minor side effects are:

Acne
Burning sensations
Itching
Rash
Skin dryness

These possible side effects may go away during treatment; however, if they continue or are bothersome, check with your doctor, nurse, or pharmacist. Tell your doctor about any side effects that are persistent or particularly bothersome, such as:

Blistering
Increased hair growth
Irritation of the affected area
Loss of skin
Secondary infection in the area being treated
Thinning of the skin with easy bruising

Interactions
None known as long as it is used according to the directions given to you by your doctor or pharmacist.

Storage
Cream, ointment, lotion, gel, spray, and aerosol should be stored at room temperature in tightly closed containers. This medication should never be frozen.

MAZANOR

Properties

This medicine contains mazindolas active ingredient; it is prescribed for appetite suppression.

Appetite suppressants are used in the short-term (a few weeks) treatment of obesity. In a few weeks (6 to 12), these medicines in combination with dieting, exercise, and changes in eating habits can help patients lose weight. However, since their appetite reducing effect is only temporary, they are useful only for the first weeks of dieting until new eating habits are established.

Before using this medicine

Before you use this medicine check with your doctor, or pharmacist:

- if you ever had any unusual or allergic reaction to any of the compounds of this medicine.
- if you are on a low-salt, low-sugar, or any other special diet, or if you are allergic to any substance, such as sulfites or other preservatives or dyes.
- if you are pregnant, intend to become pregnant or breast-feeding an infant while using this medicine.
- if you have any of the following medical problems:
  Diabetes mellitus
  Epilepsy
  Glaucoma
  Heart disease
  High blood pressure
  Mental illness (severe)

Treatment

This medication is used to relieve or prevent the symptoms of your medical problem.

Take them as directed. Do not take more of them and do not take them more often than recommended on the label. If too much of the drug is taken, it may become habit-forming.

- The medicine produces central nervous system stimulation, and it should not be taken by people with heart disease or high blood pressure.
- If you think this medicine is not working as well after you have taken it for a few weeks, do not increase the dose. Instead, check with your doctor.

Side effects

The following minor side effects may occur: irritability, nervousness, restlessness, trouble in sleeping.

These side effects should disappear as your body adjusts to the medication. Tell your doctor about any side effects that are persistent or particularly bothersome. It is especially important to tell your doctor about:

  Mental depression
  Nausea or vomiting
  Stomach cramps or pain
  Trembling
  Unusual tiredness

- Discontinue use of the drug; call your doctor right away. Adverse reactions and side effects may be more frequent and severe in people over age 60 than in younger persons.

Interactions

This medicine interacts with several other drugs such as antihypertensives, other appetite suppressants, caffeine, central nervous system depressants, central nervous system stimulants, furazolidone, guanethidine, hydralazine, MAO inhibitors, methyldopa, molindone, phenothiazines, rauwolfia alkaloids, sodium bicarbonate. Interaction with alcoholic beverages may produce drowsiness, sleepiness, and/or inability to concentrate.

- Be sure to tell your doctor about any medications you are currently taking.

Storage

This medicine should be stored at room temperature in tightly closed containers. Store away from heat and direct light. Keep out of reach of children, since overdose may be very dangerous in children.

Do not store this medicine in the bathroom medicine cabinet because the heat and moisture cause the medicine to break down. Do not keep outdated medicine or medicine no longer needed. Flush the contents of the container down the toilet.

MAZINDOL

Properties

This medicine contains mazindol as active ingredient; it is prescribed for appetite suppression.

Appetite suppressants are used in the short-term (a few weeks) treatment of obesity. In a few weeks (6 to 12), these medicines in combination with dieting, exercise, and changes in eating habits can help patients lose weight. However, since their appetite reducing effect is only temporary, they are useful only for the first weeks of dieting until new eating habits are established.

Before using this medicine

Before you use this medicine check with your doctor, or pharmacist:
- if you ever had any unusual or allergic reaction to any of the compounds of this medicine.
- if you are on a low-salt, low-sugar, or any other special diet, or if you are allergic to any substance, such as sulfites or other preservatives or dyes.
- if you are pregnant, intend to become pregnant or breast-feeding an infant while using this medicine.
- if you have any of the following medical problems:
  Diabetes mellitus
  Epilepsy
  Glaucoma
  Heart disease
  High blood pressure
  Mental illness (severe)

Treatment

This medication is used to relieve or prevent the symptoms of your medical problem.

Take them as directed. Do not take more of them and do not take them more often than recommended on the label. If too much of the drug is taken, it may become habit-forming.
- The medicine produces central nervous system stimulation, and it should not be taken by people with heart disease or high blood pressure.
- If you think this medicine is not working as well after you have taken it for a few weeks, do not increase the dose. Instead, check with your doctor.

Side effects

The following minor side effects may occur: irritability, nervousness, restlessness, trouble in sleeping.

These side effects should disappear as your body adjusts to the medication. Tell your doctor about any side effects that are persistent or particularly bothersome. It is especially important to tell your doctor about:
  Mental depression
  Nausea or vomiting
  Stomach cramps or pain
  Trembling
  Unusual tiredness
- Discontinue use of the drug; call your doctor right away. Adverse reactions and side effects may be more frequent and severe in people over age 60 than in younger persons.

Interactions

This medicine interacts with several other drugs such as antihypertensives, other appetite suppressants, caffeine, central nervous system depressants, central nervous system stimulants, furazolidone, guanethidine, hydralazine, MAO inhibitors, methyldopa, molindone, phenothiazines, rauwolfia alkaloids, sodium bicarbonate. Interaction with alcoholic beverages may produce drowsiness, sleepiness, and/or inability to concentrate.
- Be sure to tell your doctor about any medications you are currently taking.

Storage

This medicine should be stored at room temperature in tightly closed containers. Store away from heat and direct light. Keep out of reach of children, since overdose may be very dangerous in children.

Do not store this medicine in the bathroom medicine cabinet because the heat and moisture cause the medicine to break down. Do not keep outdated medicine or medicine no longer needed. Flush the contents of the container down the toilet.

MEBARAL

Properties
This medicine contains as active ingredient the barbiturate mephobarbital. Barbiturates belong to the group of medicines called central nervous system depressants (medicines that slow down the nervous system).

Barbiturates may partially block nerve impulses at nerve-cell connections. They may be used to treat insomnia (sleeplessness) by helping patients fall asleep. Also, they may be used to relieve anxiety or tension. Some of the barbiturates are used as anticonvulsants to help control convulsions in certain disorders or diseases, such as epilepsy. If too much of the drug is used, it may become habit-forming (causing mental or physical dependence).

Before using this medicine
Before you use this medicine check with your doctor, or pharmacist:
- if you ever had any unusual or allergic reaction to this medicine or one of its components.
- if you are on a low-salt, low-sugar, or any other special diet, or if you are allergic to preservatives or dyes.
- if you are pregnant or intend to become pregnant while using this medicine, since barbiturates have been shown to increase the chance of birth defects in humans. Taking barbiturates regularly during the last 3 months of pregnancy may cause the baby to become dependent on the medicine. This may lead to withdrawal side effects in the baby after birth.
- if you have any of the following medical problems:
  Anemia (severe)
  Diabetes mellitus (sugar disease)
  Hyperactivity (in children)
  Kidney or lifer disease
  Mental depression
  Overactive thyroid

Treatment
This medication is used to treat the symptoms of your medical condition. Barbiturates act in the central nervous system; some of their side effects are also caused by actions in the central nervous system. Use this medicine as directed by your doctor. Do not use more of it, do not use it more often, and do not use it for a longer period of time than your doctor ordered.
- If you are taking this medication on a regular schedule and you miss a dose, take the missed dose as soon as possible, unless it is almost time for your next dose. In that case do not take the missed dose at all.
- If a barbiturate is used for a long time, it may become habit-forming. Physical dependence may lead to withdrawal side effects when you stop taking this medicine.

Side effects
Along with the needed effects, a medicine may cause some unwanted effects. These side effects may go away during treatment as your body adjusts to the medicine. Such minor side effects are: depression, confusion, diarrhea, nausea, vomiting, joint or muscle pain, slurred speech, hallucinations, headache, decreased sex drive.
- Check with your doctor immediately if any of the following side effects occur:
  Rash or hives
  Face, lip or eyelid swelling
  Sore throat, fever
  Agitation
  Slow heartbeat
  Difficult breathing or chest pain

Interactions
This medicine may interact with several other drugs such as medicines acting on the central nervous system (e.g., antihistamines; beta-adrenergic blockers; MAO inhibitors; mind-altering drugs; nabilone; antidepressants; clozapine; anticonvulsants).

Storage
The medicine should be stored at room temperature in a tightly closed, light-resistant container. Keep out of reach of children since overdose is very dangerous in children.

MEFOXIN

Properties
This medicine contains cephalosporin as active ingredient. Cephalosporins belong to the general family of medicines called antibiotics, used in the treatment of infections caused by bacteria. They work by killing bacteria or preventing their growth. Cephalosporins will not work for colds, flu, or other viral infections.

Before using this medicine
Before you use this medicine check with your doctor:
- if you ever had any unusual or allergic reaction to any of the cephalosporins, penicillins, penicillin-like medicines, or penicillamine.
- if you are on a low-salt, low-sugar, or any other special diet, or if you are allergic to any substance, such as sulfites or other preservatives or dyes.
- if you are pregnant or intend to become pregnant while using this medicine. Although cephalosporins have not been shown to cause birth defects or other problems in humans, the chance always exists.
- if you are breast-feeding an infant. Most cephalosporins pass into the breast milk, usually in small amounts.
- if you have any of the following medical problems:
  Bleeding problem
  Kidney or lifer disease

Treatment
This medication belongs to the general family of medicines called antibiotics. It is used to treat a wide variety of bacterial infections. It is also used to treat infections in persons who are allergic to penicillin.
- Keep taking this medicine for the full time of treatment even if you begin to feel better after a few days; do not miss any doses.
- If you do miss a dose of this medicine, take it as soon as possible. This will help to keep a constant amount of medicine in the blood. However, if it is almost time for your next dose, skip the missed dose and go back to your regular dosing schedule.
- This medication has been prescribed for your current infection only. Another infection later on, or one that someone else has, may require a different medicine. You should not give your medicine to other people or use it for other infections, unless your doctor specifically directs you to do so.
- Take the medicine at the same times each day, 1 hour before or 2 hours after eating.

Side effects
Along with the needed effects, a medicine may cause some unwanted effects. Side effects that usually do not require medical attention: rectal itching, oral or vaginal white spots, mild diarrhea. These side effects should disappear as your body adjusts to the medication.
- Other side effects that should be reported to your doctor immediately are:
  Hives, rash
  Intense itching
  Faintness soon after a dose
  Difficulty in breathing
  Nausea and vomiting
  Severe diarrhea
  Unusual weakness or tiredness
  Bleeding or bruising

Interactions
This medicine may interact with several other drugs such as anticoagulants, theophylline preparations, probenecid, tetracyclines, etc.
- Be sure to tell your doctor about any medications you are currently taking.

Storage
Tablets, capsules, etc. should be stored at room temperature. Store the liquid form in the refrigerator. Keep out of the reach of children. Do not keep outdated medicine or medicine no longer needed.

MEGACILLIN

Properties

This medicine contains penicillin G as active ingredient. Penicillins are prescribed to treat infections caused by bacteria. They will not work for colds, flu, or other virus infections. There are several different kinds of penicillins. Each is used to treat different kinds of infections.

Before using this medicine

Before you use this medicine check with your doctor, or pharmacist:

- if you ever had any unusual or allergic reaction to any of the penicillins, cefalosporins, griseofulvin, or penicillamine. Serious reactions may occur in patients who are allergic to penicillins.
- if you are on a low-salt, low-sugar, or any other special diet, or if you are allergic to any substance, such as sulfites or other preservatives or dyes.
- if you are pregnant or intend to become pregnant while using this medicine. Although penicillins have not been shown to cause problems in humans, the chance always exists.
- if you are breast-feeding an infant. Most penicillins (except amdinocillin) pass into the breast milk. Even though only small amounts may pass, allergic reaction, diarrhea, fungal infection, and skin rash may occur in the infant.
- if you have any of the following medical problems:
  Allergy
  Asthma
  Bleeding problems
  Eczema
  Hay fever, hives
  Kidney disease
  Liver disease
  Mononucleosis
  Stomach or intestinal disease

Treatment

This medication is used to treat an infection caused by bacteria. Most penicillins are best taken with a full glass (8 ounces) of water on an empty stomach, some are best taken with a snack or meal. Follow your doctor's or pharmacist's directions on how to take your medicine.

- Keep taking this medicine for the full time of treatment even if you begin to feel better after a few days; do not miss any doses. This is especially important if you have a "strep" infection since serious heart problems could develop later if your infection is not cleared up completely.
- If you do miss a dose of this medicine, take it as soon as possible. However, if it is almost time for your next dose, skip the missed dose and go back to your regular dosing schedule.

Side effects

Along with the needed effects, a medicine may cause some unwanted effects. Side effects that usually do not require medical attention: diarrhea; nausea or vomiting; sore mouth or tongue.

- Stop taking this medicine and get emergency help immediately if you notice: difficulty in breathing; light-headedness; skin rash, hives, itching; wheezing.

Other side effects that should be reported to your doctor immediately are: abdominal bloating; blood in urine; convulsions (seizures); decreased amount of urine; diarrhea (watery and severe) which may also be bloody; fever; joint pain; sore throat and fever; stomach or abdominal cramps and pain; unusual bleeding or bruising.

Interactions

This medicine may interact with several other drugs such as anticoagulants, diarrhea medicines, heparin, ibuprofen, oral contraceptives, potassium-containing medicines, etc.

- Be sure to tell your doctor about any medications you are currently taking.

Storage

Tablets, capsules, etc. should be stored as directed by your pharmacist or according to instructions on the label.

MELFIAT

Properties

This medicine contains phendi-metrazine as active ingredient; it is pre-scribed for appetite suppression.

Appetite suppressants are used in the short-term (a few weeks) treatment of obesity. In a few weeks (6 to 12), these medicines in combination with dieting, exercise, and changes in eating habits can help patients lose weight. However, since their appetite reducing effect is only temporary, they are useful only for the first weeks of dieting until new eat-ing habits are established.

Before using this medicine

Before you use this medicine check with your doctor, or pharmacist:

- if you ever had any unusual or aller-gic reaction to any of the compounds of this medicine.
- if you are on a low-salt, low-sugar, or any other special diet, or if you are allergic to any substance, such as sul-fites or other preservatives or dyes.
- if you are pregnant, intend to become pregnant or breast-feeding an infant while using this medicine.
- if you have any of the following medical problems:
  Diabetes mellitus (sugar diabetes)
  Epilepsy
  Glaucoma
  Heart or blood vessel disease
  High blood pressure
  Mental illness (severe)

Treatment

This medication is used to relieve or prevent the symptoms of your medical problem. Take them as directed. Do not take more of them and do not take them more often than recommended on the label. If too much of the drug is taken, it may become habit-forming.

The medicine produces central nerv-ous system stimulation, and it should not be taken by people with heart dis-ease or high blood pressure.

If you think this medicine is not working as well after you have taken it for a few weeks, do not increase the dose. Instead, check with your doctor.

Side effects

The following minor side effects may occur: irritability, nervousness, restless-ness, trouble in sleeping.

These side effects should disappear as your body adjusts to the medication. Tell your doctor about any side effects that are persistent or particularly bother-some. It is especially important to tell your doctor about:
  Mental depression
  Nausea or vomiting
  Stomach cramps or pain
  Trembling
  Unusual tiredness or weakness
- Discontinue use of the drug; call your doctor right away. Adverse re-actions and side effects may be more frequent and severe in people over age 60 than in younger persons.

Interactions

This medicine interacts with several other drugs such as antihypertensives, other appetite suppressants, caffeine, central nervous system depressants, central nervous system stimulants, fura-zolidone, guanethidine, hydralazine, MAO inhibitors, methyldopa, molin-done, phenothiazines, rauwolfia alka-loids, sodium bicarbonate.
- Be sure to tell your doctor about any medications you are currently taking.
Interaction with alcoholic beverages may produce drowsiness, sleepiness, and/or inability to concentrate.

Storage

This medicine should be stored at room temperature in tightly closed containers. Store away from heat and direct light. Keep out of reach of children, since overdose may be very dangerous in children.

Do not store this medicine in the bathroom medicine cabinet because the heat and moisture cause the medicine to break down. Do not keep outdated medicine or medicine no longer needed. Flush the contents of the container down the toilet.

MELLARIL

Properties
This medicine contains as active ingredient thioridazine, a phenothiazine derivative. Phenothiazines are a family of medicines used to treat nervous, mental, and emotional conditions. Some are used to control anxiety, restlessness, nausea and vomiting, and severe hiccups. This medicine is available only with your doctor's prescription.

Before using this medicine
Before you use this medicine check with your doctor, or pharmacist:
- if you ever had any unusual or allergic reaction to phenothiazine medicines.
- if you are on a low-salt, low-sugar, or any other special diet, or if you are allergic to any substance, such as sulfites or other preservatives or dyes.
- if you are pregnant or intend to become pregnant while using this medicine. Although phenothiazines have not been shown to cause birth defects, some side effects such as jaundice and muscle tremors have occurred in a few newborns whose mothers received phenothiazines during pregnancy.
- if you are breast-feeding an infant. Although this medicine has not been shown to cause problems in humans the chance does exist since some phenothiazines are known to pass into the breast milk.
- if you have any of the following medical problems:
Alcoholism
Blood disease
Difficult urination
Enlarged prostate
Glaucoma
Heart or blood vessel disease
Liver or lung disease
Parkinson's disease
Stomach ulcers

Treatment
This medication is prescribed to treat the symptoms of certain types of mental illness or emotional problems. In order to avoid stomach irritation, you can take the tablet or capsule forms of this medication with a meal or with a glass of water or milk (unless your doctor or pharmacist directs you to do otherwise).

Side effects
Along with the needed effects, a medicine may cause some unwanted effects. Minor side effects are: blurred vision, constipation, decreased sweating, diarrhea, dizziness, drooling, drowsiness, dry mouth, fatigue, jitteriness, menstrual irregularities, nasal congestion, restlessness, tremors, vomiting, or weight gain.
- Tell your doctor about any side effects that are persistent or particularly bothersome. It is especially important to tell your doctor about:
Breast enlargement
Chest pain or convulsions
Darkened skin
Difficulty in swallowing
Fainting or fever
Involuntary movements
Palpitations or sleep disorders
Rash or sore throat
Uncoordinated movements
Unusual bleeding or bruising
Visual disturbances
Yellowing of the eyes or skin

Interactions
This medicine may interact with several other drugs such as barbiturates, sleeping pills, narcotics, other tranquilizers, or any other medication that may produce a sedative effect. Avoid alcohol.

Storage
Store this medication as directed on the label. Keep out of the reach of children.

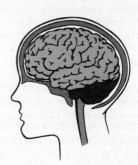

MENAVAL-20

Properties
This medicine contains estrogen as active ingredient. The medicine is prescribed for treatment of estrogen deficiency; it restores normal estrogen levels in tissues. There is no evidence that this drug is effective for nervous symptoms or depression occurring during menopause. They should not be used to treat this condition; they should be used only to replace the estrogen that is naturally absent after menopause.

Before using this medicine
Before you use this medicine check with your doctor, or pharmacist:
- if you ever had any unusual or allergic reaction to estrogens;
- if you are pregnant or intend to become pregnant within three months;
- if you are breast-feeding an infant;
- if you have any of the following medical problems:
  Diabetes
  Breast cancer
  Fibrocystic breast disease
  Fibroid uterine tumors
  Endometriosis
  Migraine headaches
  Epilepsy
  Porphyria
  High blood pressure
  Asthma
  Congestive heart failure
  Kidney disease
  Gallstones

Treatment
This medication is used to treat estrogen deficiency, specific symptoms of menopause, estrogen-deficiency osteoporosis, atrophic vaginitis, prostate cancer.

For safe and effective use of this medicine:
- Follow your doctor's instructions if this medicine was prescribed.
- Follow the manufacturer's package directions if you are treating yourself.
- Estrogens have been reported to increase the risk of endometrial carcinoma.

Side effects
Along with the needed effects, a medicine may cause some unwanted effects. Possible side effects include:
  Stomach cramps
  Profuse bleeding
  Appetite loss
  Nausea and vomiting
  Swollen breasts
  Change in menstruation
  Rash, skin blisters
  Depression
  Dizziness

Overdose
The following symptoms may indicate an overdose:
  Nausea and vomiting
  Fluid retention
  Breast enlargement
  Abnormal vaginal bleeding
- Call a doctor or hospital emergency room for instructions.

Interactions
This medicine may interact with several other drugs such as adrenocorticosteroids, antidepressants, oral antidiabetics, insulin, phenobarbital, primidone.
- Be sure to tell your doctor about any medications you are currently taking.

Storage
Capsules, tablets, vaginal cream, transdermal patches, etc. should be stored at room temperature; store away from heat and direct light. Keep out of reach of children, since this medicine may be dangerous in children.

MENEST

Properties
This medicine contains conjugated estrogens as active ingredients. The medicine is prescribed for treatment of estrogen deficiency; it restores normal estrogen levels in tissues. There is no evidence that this drug is effective for nervous symptoms or depression occurring during menopause. They should not be used to treat this condition; they should be used only to replace the estrogen that is naturally absent after menopause.

Before using this medicine
Before you use this medicine check with your doctor, or pharmacist:
- if you ever had any unusual or allergic reaction to estrogens;
- if you are pregnant or intend to become pregnant within three months;
- if you are breast-feeding an infant;
- if you have any of the following medical problems:
  Diabetes
  Breast cancer
  Fibrocystic breast disease
  Fibroid uterine tumors
  Endometriosis
  Migraine headaches
  Epilepsy
  Porphyria
  High blood pressure
  Asthma
  Congestive heart failure
  Kidney disease
  Gallstones

Treatment
This medication is used to treat estrogen deficiency, specific symptoms of menopause, estrogen-deficiency osteoporosis, atrophic vaginitis, prostate cancer.

For safe and effective use of this medicine:
- Follow your doctor's instructions if this medicine was prescribed.
- Follow the manufacturer's package directions if you are treating yourself.
- Estrogens have been reported to increase the risk of endometrial carcinoma.

Side effects
Along with the needed effects, a medicine may cause some unwanted effects. Possible side effects include:
  Stomach cramps
  Profuse bleeding
  Appetite loss
  Nausea and vomiting
  Swollen breasts
  Change in menstruation
  Rash, skin blisters
  Depression
  Dizziness

Overdose
The following symptoms may indicate an overdose:
  Nausea and vomiting
  Fluid retention
  Breast enlargement
  Abnormal vaginal bleeding
- Call a doctor or hospital emergency room for instructions.

Interactions
This medicine may interact with several other drugs such as adrenocorticosteroids, antidepressants, oral antidiabetics, insulin, phenobarbital, primidone.
- Be sure to tell your doctor about any medications you are currently taking.

Storage
Capsules, tablets, vaginal cream, transdermal patches, etc. should be stored at room temperature; store away from heat and direct light. Keep out of reach of children, since this medicine may be dangerous in children.

MEPERIDINE

Properties
This medicine contains as active ingredient meperidine.

It is a narcotic analgesic that acts directly on the central nervous system (brain and spinal cord). It is used to relieve pain or to suppress coughing.

Before using this medicine
Before you use this medicine check with your doctor, or pharmacist:
- if you ever had any unusual or allergic reaction to this medicine or one of its components.
- if you are on a low-salt, low-sugar, or any other special diet, or if you are allergic to any substance, such as sulfites or other preservatives or dyes.
- if you are pregnant or intend to become pregnant while using this medicine. Studies on birth defects have not been done in humans. Too much use of narcotics during pregnancy may cause the baby to become dependent on the medicine.
- if you are breast-feeding an infant. Although this medicine has not been shown to cause problems in humans, it passes into the breast milk in small amounts.
- if you have any of the following medical problems:
  Brain disease or head injury
  Colitis
  Convulsions
  Emphysema, asthma, or chronic lung disease
  Enlarged prostate
  Gallbladder disease or gallstones
  Heart disease
  Kidney or lifer disease
  Underactive thyroid

Treatment
This medication is used to relieve pain or to suppress coughing. Narcotic analgesics act in the central nervous system; some of their side effects are also caused by actions in the central nervous system.
- If you are taking this medication on a regular schedule and you miss a dose, take the missed dose as soon as possible, unless it is almost time for your next dose. In that case do not take the missed dose at all.
- If a narcotic analgesic is used for a long time, it may become habit-forming (causing mental or physical dependence). Physical dependence may lead to withdrawal side effects when you stop taking this medicine.

Unless otherwise directed by your doctor or pharmacist take this as directed. Do not take more of them and do not take them more often than recommended on the label. Children up to 12 years of age should not take this medicine more than 3 times a day or for more than 5 days in a row.

Side effects
Along with the needed effects, a medicine may cause some unwanted effects. These side effects may go away during treatment as your body adjusts to the medicine. Such minor side effects are: constipation, dizziness, drowsiness, dry mouth, false sense of well-being, flushing, light-headedness, loss of appetite, nausea, painful or difficult urination, or sweating.
- Check with your doctor immediately if any of the following side effects occur:
  Anxiety or breathing difficulties
  Excitation or restlessness
  Fatigue, palpitations
  Rash, sore throat and fever
  Tremors or weakness

Interactions
This medicine may interact with several other drugs such as medicines acting on the central nervous system (e.g., antidepressants, tranquilizers), cimetidine, nitrates, quinidine, etc.
- Be sure to tell your doctor about any medications you are currently taking.

Storage
Tablets, elixir, suppository etc. should be stored at room temperature in a tightly closed, light-resistant container.

MEPHOBARBITAL

Properties
This medicine contains as active ingredient the barbiturate   mephobarbital. Barbiturates belong to the group of medicines called central nervous system depressants (medicines that slow down the nervous system).

Barbiturates may partially block nerve impulses at nerve-cell connections. They may be used to treat insomnia (sleeplessness) by helping patients fall asleep. Also, they may be used to relieve anxiety or tension. Some of the barbiturates are used as anticonvulsants to help control convulsions in certain disorders or diseases, such as epilepsy. If too much of the drug is used, it may become habit-forming (causing mental or physical dependence).

Before using this medicine
Before you use this medicine check with your doctor, or pharmacist:
- if you ever had any unusual or allergic reaction to this medicine or one of its components.
- if you are on a low-salt, low-sugar, or any other special diet, or if you are allergic to preservatives or dyes.
- if you are pregnant or intend to become pregnant while using this medicine, since barbiturates have been shown to increase the chance of birth defects in humans. Taking barbiturates regularly during the last 3 months of pregnancy may cause the baby to become dependent on the medicine. This may lead to withdrawal side effects in the baby after birth.
- if you have any of the following medical problems:
  Anemia (severe)
  Diabetes mellitus (sugar disease)
  Hyperactivity (in children)
  Kidney or lifer disease
  Mental depression
  Overactive thyroid

Treatment
This medication is used to treat the symptoms of your medical condition. Barbiturates act in the central nervous system; some of their side effects are also caused by actions in the central nervous system. Use this medicine as directed by your doctor. Do not use more of it, do not use it more often, and do not use it for a longer period of time than your doctor ordered.
- If you are taking this medication on a regular schedule and you miss a dose, take the missed dose as soon as possible, unless it is almost time for your next dose. In that case do not take the missed dose at all.
- If a barbiturate is used for a long time, it may become habit-forming. Physical dependence may lead to withdrawal side effects when you stop taking this medicine.

Side effects
Along with the needed effects, a medicine may cause some unwanted effects. These side effects may go away during treatment as your body adjusts to the medicine. Such minor side effects are: depression, confusion, diarrhea, nausea, vomiting, joint or muscle pain, slurred speech, hallucinations, headache, decreased sex drive.
- Check with your doctor immediately if any of the following side effects occur:
  Rash or hives
  Face, lip or eyelid swelling
  Sore throat, fever
  Agitation
  Slow heartbeat
  Difficult breathing or chest pain

Interactions
This medicine may interact with several other drugs such as medicines acting on the central nervous system (e.g., antihistamines; beta-adrenergic blockers; MAO inhibitors; mind-altering drugs; nabilone; antidepressants; clozapine; anticonvulsants).

Storage
The medicine should be stored at room temperature in a tightly closed, light-resistant container. Keep out of reach of children since overdose is very dangerous in children.

MESORIDAZINE

Properties
This medicine contains as active ingredient mesoridazine, a phenothiazine derivative. Phenothiazines are a family of medicines used to treat nervous, mental, and emotional conditions. Some are used to control anxiety, restlessness, nausea and vomiting, and severe hiccups. This medicine is available only with your doctor's prescription.

Before using this medicine
Before you use this medicine check with your doctor, or pharmacist:
- if you ever had any unusual or allergic reaction to phenothiazine medicines.
- if you are on a low-salt, low-sugar, or any other special diet, or if you are allergic to any substance, such as sulfites or other preservatives or dyes.
- if you are pregnant or intend to become pregnant while using this medicine. Although phenothiazines have not been shown to cause birth defects, some side effects such as jaundice and muscle tremors have occurred in a few newborns whose mothers received phenothiazines during pregnancy.
- if you are breast-feeding an infant. Although this medicine has not been shown to cause problems in humans the chance does exist since some phenothiazines are known to pass into the breast milk.
- if you have any of the following medical problems:
Alcoholism
Blood disease
Difficult urination
Enlarged prostate
Glaucoma
Heart or blood vessel disease
Liver or lung disease
Parkinson's disease
Stomach ulcers

Treatment
This medication is prescribed to treat the symptoms of certain types of mental illness or emotional problems. In order to avoid stomach irritation, you can take the tablet or capsule forms of this medication with a meal or with a glass of water or milk (unless your doctor or pharmacist directs you to do otherwise).

Side effects
Along with the needed effects, a medicine may cause some unwanted effects. Minor side effects are: blurred vision, constipation, decreased sweating, diarrhea, dizziness, drooling, drowsiness, dry mouth, fatigue, jitteriness, menstrual irregularities, nasal congestion, restlessness, tremors, vomiting, or weight gain.
- Tell your doctor about any side effects that are persistent or particularly bothersome. It is especially important to tell your doctor about:
Breast enlargement
Chest pain or convulsions
Darkened skin
Difficulty in swallowing
Fainting or fever
Involuntary movements
Palpitations or sleep disorders
Rash or sore throat
Uncoordinated movements
Unusual bleeding or bruising
Visual disturbances
Yellowing of the eyes or skin

Interactions
This medicine may interact with several other drugs such as barbiturates, sleeping pills, narcotics, other tranquilizers, or any other medication that may produce a sedative effect. Avoid alcohol.

Storage
Store this medication as directed on the label. Keep out of the reach of children.

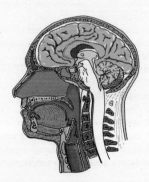

METADERM

Properties
This medicine contains betamethasone, a corticosteroid, as active ingredient. Corticosteroids are used to help relieve redness, swelling, itching, inflammation, and discomfort of many skin problems. They exert this effect by interfering with natural body mechanisms that produce the rash, itching, or inflammation. They do not cure the underlying cause of the skin problem. This medication is applied to the skin.

Before using this medicine
Before you use this medicine check with your doctor, or pharmacist:
- if you ever had any unusual or allergic reaction to corticosteroids.
- if you are allergic to any substance, such as sulfites or other preservatives or dyes.
- if you are pregnant or intend to become pregnant while using this medicine. Studies have shown that corticosteroids applied to the skin in large amounts or over long periods of time can be the cause of birth defects.
- if you are breast-feeding an infant. Some corticosteroids pass into breast milk and may interfere with the infant's growth.

Treatment
Do not use this medicine more often or for a longer time than ordered. To do so may increase absorption through the skin and the chance of side effects. In addition, too much use, especially on areas with thinner skin (for example, face, armpits, groin), may result in thinning of the skin and stretch marks.

Before applying this medication, wash your hands. than, unless your doctor or pharmacist gives you different instructions, gently wash the area where the medication is to be applied. With a clean towel pat the area dry. Apply a small amount of the medication to the affected area in a thin layer. Do not bandage the area unless your doctor tells you to do so.

If you miss a dose of this medication, apply the dose as soon as possible, unless it is almost time for the next application.

- Do not use this medicine for other skin problems without first checking with your doctor. You should not use a topical corticosteroid if you have a virus disease (such as herpes), fungal infection of the skin (such as athlete's foot), or tuberculosis of the skin.

Side effects
There are a number of side effects that usually do not require medical attention. Minor side effects are:

Acne
Burning sensations
Itching
Rash
Skin dryness

These possible side effects may go away during treatment; however, if they continue or are bothersome, check with your doctor, nurse, or pharmacist. Tell your doctor about any side effects that are persistent or particularly bothersome, such as:

Blistering
Increased hair growth
Irritation of the affected area
Loss of skin
Secondary infection in the area being treated
Thinning of the skin with easy bruising

Interactions
None known as long as it is used according to the directions given to you by your doctor or pharmacist.

Storage
Cream, ointment, lotion, gel, spray, and aerosol should be stored at room temperature in tightly closed containers. This medication should never be frozen.

METAHYDRIN

Properties

This medicine contains as active ingredient trichlormethiazide, a thiazide-like diuretic. Thiazide or thiazide-like diuretics are prescribed to treat high blood pressure (hypertension). They are also used to reduce fluid accumulation in the body caused by conditions such as heart failure, cirrhosis, kidney disease, and the long-term use of some medications. Thiazide diuretics may also be used for other conditions as determined by your doctor.

Before using this medicine

Before you use this medicine check with your doctor, or pharmacist:

- if you ever had any unusual or allergic reaction to sulfonamides (sulfa drugs) or any of the thiazide diuretics.
- if you are on a low-salt, low-sugar, or any other special diet, or if you are allergic to any substance, such as sulfites or other preservatives or dyes.
- if you are pregnant or intend to become pregnant while using this medicine. When this medicine is used during pregnancy, it may cause side effects including jaundice, blood problems, and low potassium in the newborn.
- if you are breast-feeding an infant. Although this medicine has not been shown to cause problems in humans, the chance always exists since thiazide diuretics pass into breast milk.
- if you have any of the following medical problems:
  Diabetes
  Gout
  Kidney disease
  Liver disease
  Lupus erythematosus
  Pancreas disease

Treatment

This medication is used to treat high blood pressure (hypertension) and also to help reduce the amount of water in the body by increasing the flow of urine. This medicine will not cure your high blood pressure but it does help control it. You must continue to take it - even if you feel well - if you expect to keep your blood pressure down. You may have to take high blood pressure medicine for the rest of your life.

Thiazide diuretics may cause an unusual feeling of tiredness when you begin to take them. You may also notice an increase in urine or in frequency of urination. To keep this from affecting sleep:

- if you are to take a single dose a day, take it in the morning after breakfast;
- if you are to take more than one dose, take the last one not later than 6 p.m.

Side effects

Along with the needed effects, a medicine may cause some unwanted effects. Side effects that usually do not require medical attention: decreased sexual ability; dizziness or lightheadedness when standing up; increased sensitivity of skin to sunlight; loss of appetite; upset stomach.

- Side effects that should be reported to your doctor: black, tarry stools; blood in urine or stools; cough or hoarseness; fever or chills; joint pain; lower back or side pains; painful or difficult urination; pinpoint red spots on skin; skin rash or hives; stomach pain (severe) with nausea; unusual bleeding or bruising; yellow eyes or skin. This medicine may cause a loss of potassium from your body. Signs of too much potassium loss are: dryness of mouth; increased thirst; mood changes; muscle cramps or pain; nausea or vomiting; unusual tiredness or weakness; weak or irregular heartbeat.

Interactions

This medicine may interact with several other drugs.

- Be sure to tell your doctor about any medications you are currently taking.

Storage

Store at room temperature in a tightly closed container.

METHADONE

Properties
This medicine contains as active ingredient methadone.

It is a narcotic analgesic that acts directly on the central nervous system (brain and spinal cord). It is used to relieve pain or to suppress coughing.

Before using this medicine
Before you use this medicine check with your doctor, or pharmacist:
- if you ever had any unusual or allergic reaction to this medicine or one of its components.
- if you are on a low-salt, low-sugar, or any other special diet, or if you are allergic to any substance, such as sulfites or other preservatives or dyes.
- if you are pregnant or intend to become pregnant while using this medicine. Studies on birth defects have not been done in humans. Too much use of narcotics during pregnancy may cause the baby to become dependent on the medicine.
- if you are breast-feeding an infant. Although this medicine has not been shown to cause problems in humans, it passes into the breast milk in small amounts.
- if you have any of the following medical problems:
  Brain disease or head injury
  Colitis
  Convulsions
  Emphysema, asthma, or chronic lung disease
  Enlarged prostate
  Gallbladder disease or gallstones
  Heart disease
  Kidney or lifer disease
  Underactive thyroid

Treatment
This medication is used to relieve pain or to suppress coughing. Narcotic analgesics act in the central nervous system; some of their side effects are also caused by actions in the central nervous system.
- If you are taking this medication on a regular schedule and you miss a dose, take the missed dose as soon as possible, unless it is almost time for your next dose. In that case do not take the missed dose at all.
- If a narcotic analgesic is used for a long time, it may become habit-forming (causing mental or physical dependence). Physical dependence may lead to withdrawal side effects when you stop taking this medicine.

Unless otherwise directed by your doctor or pharmacist take this as directed. Do not take more of them and do not take them more often than recommended on the label. Children up to 12 years of age should not take this medicine more than 3 times a day or for more than 5 days in a row.

Side effects
Along with the needed effects, a medicine may cause some unwanted effects. These side effects may go away during treatment as your body adjusts to the medicine. Such minor side effects are: constipation, dizziness, drowsiness, dry mouth, false sense of well-being, flushing, light-headedness, loss of appetite, nausea, painful or difficult urination, or sweating.
- Check with your doctor immediately if any of the following side effects occur:
  Anxiety or breathing difficulties
  Excitation or restlessness
  Fatigue, palpitations
  Rash, sore throat and fever
  Tremors or weakness

Interactions
This medicine may interact with several other drugs such as medicines acting on the central nervous system (e.g., antidepressants, tranquilizers), cimetidine, nitrates, quinidine, etc.
- Be sure to tell your doctor about any medications you are currently taking.

Storage
Tablets, elixir, suppository etc. should be stored at room temperature in a tightly closed, light-resistant container.

METHADOSE

Properties

This medicine contains as active ingredient methadone.

It is a narcotic analgesic that acts directly on the central nervous system (brain and spinal cord). It is used to relieve pain or to suppress coughing.

Before using this medicine

Before you use this medicine check with your doctor, or pharmacist:
- if you ever had any unusual or allergic reaction to this medicine or one of its components.
- if you are on a low-salt, low-sugar, or any other special diet, or if you are allergic to any substance, such as sulfites or other preservatives or dyes.
- if you are pregnant or intend to become pregnant while using this medicine. Studies on birth defects have not been done in humans. Too much use of narcotics during pregnancy may cause the baby to become dependent on the medicine.
- if you are breast-feeding an infant. Although this medicine has not been shown to cause problems in humans, it passes into the breast milk in small amounts.
- if you have any of the following medical problems:
Brain disease or head injury
Colitis
Convulsions
Emphysema, asthma, or chronic lung disease
Enlarged prostate
Gallbladder disease or gallstones
Heart disease
Kidney or lifer disease
Underactive thyroid

Treatment

This medication is used to relieve pain or to suppress coughing. Narcotic analgesics act in the central nervous system; some of their side effects are also caused by actions in the central nervous system.
- If you are taking this medication on a regular schedule and you miss a dose, take the missed dose as soon as possible, unless it is almost time for your next dose. In that case do not take the missed dose at all.
- If a narcotic analgesic is used for a long time, it may become habit-forming (causing mental or physical dependence). Physical dependence may lead to withdrawal side effects when you stop taking this medicine.

Unless otherwise directed by your doctor or pharmacist take this as directed. Do not take more of them and do not take them more often than recommended on the label. Children up to 12 years of age should not take this medicine more than 3 times a day or for more than 5 days in a row.

Side effects

Along with the needed effects, a medicine may cause some unwanted effects. These side effects may go away during treatment as your body adjusts to the medicine. Such minor side effects are: constipation, dizziness, drowsiness, dry mouth, false sense of well-being, flushing, light-headedness, loss of appetite, nausea, painful or difficult urination, or sweating.
- Check with your doctor immediately if any of the following side effects occur:
Anxiety or breathing difficulties
Excitation or restlessness
Fatigue, palpitations
Rash, sore throat and fever
Tremors or weakness

Interactions

This medicine may interact with several other drugs such as medicines acting on the central nervous system (e.g., antidepressants, tranquilizers), cimetidine, nitrates, quinidine, etc.
- Be sure to tell your doctor about any medications you are currently taking.

Storage

Tablets, elixir, suppository etc. should be stored at room temperature in a tightly closed, light-resistant container.

METHARBITAL

Properties
This medicine contains as active ingredient the barbiturate   phenobarbital. Barbiturates belong to the group of medicines called central nervous system depressants (medicines that slow down the nervous system).

Barbiturates may partially block nerve impulses at nerve-cell connections. They may be used to treat insomnia (sleeplessness) by helping patients fall asleep. Also, they may be used to relieve anxiety or tension. Some of the barbiturates are used as anticonvulsants to help control convulsions in certain disorders or diseases, such as epilepsy. If too much of the drug is used, it may become habit-forming (causing mental or physical dependence).

Before using this medicine
Before you use this medicine check with your doctor, or pharmacist:
- if you ever had any unusual or allergic reaction to this medicine or one of its components.
- if you are on a low-salt, low-sugar, or any other special diet, or if you are allergic to preservatives or dyes.
- if you are pregnant or intend to become pregnant while using this medicine, since barbiturates have been shown to increase the chance of birth defects in humans. Taking barbiturates regularly during the last 3 months of pregnancy may cause the baby to become dependent on the medicine. This may lead to withdrawal side effects in the baby after birth.
- if you have any of the following medical problems:
  Anemia (severe)
  Diabetes mellitus (sugar disease)
  Hyperactivity (in children)
  Kidney or lifer disease
  Mental depression
  Overactive thyroid

Treatment
This medication is used to treat the symptoms of your medical condition. Barbiturates act in the central nervous system; some of their side effects are also caused by actions in the central nervous system. Use this medicine as directed by your doctor. Do not use more of it, do not use it more often, and do not use it for a longer period of time than your doctor ordered.
- If you are taking this medication on a regular schedule and you miss a dose, take the missed dose as soon as possible, unless it is almost time for your next dose. In that case do not take the missed dose at all.
- If a barbiturate is used for a long time, it may become habit-forming. Physical dependence may lead to withdrawal side effects when you stop taking this medicine.

Side effects
Along with the needed effects, a medicine may cause some unwanted effects. These side effects may go away during treatment as your body adjusts to the medicine. Such minor side effects are: depression, confusion,
diarrhea, nausea, vomiting, joint or muscle pain, slurred speech, hallucinations, headache, decreased sex drive.
- Check with your doctor immediately if any of the following side effects occur:
  Rash or hives
  Face, lip or eyelid swelling
  Sore throat, fever
  Agitation
  Slow heartbeat
  Difficult breathing or chest pain

Interactions
This medicine may interact with several other drugs such as medicines acting on the central nervous system (e.g., antihistamines; beta-adrenergic blockers; MAO inhibitors; mind-altering drugs; nabilone; antidepressants; clozapine; anticonvulsants).

Storage
The medicine should be stored at room temperature in a tightly closed, light-resistant container. Keep out of reach of children since overdose is very dangerous in children.

METHOXANOL

Properties
This medicine contains sulfamethoxa-zole, a sulfonamide, as active ingredi-ent. Sulfonamides are prescribed to treat infections caused by bacteria. They will not work for colds, flu, or other virus infections.

Before using this medicine
Before you use this medicine check with your doctor:
- if you ever had any unusual or aller-gic reaction to any of the compounds of the medicine.
- if you are on a low-salt, low-sugar, or any other special diet, or if you are allergic to any substance, such as sul-fites or other preservatives or dyes.
- if you are pregnant or intend to be-come pregnant while using this medicine. Although sulfonamides have not been shown to cause defects in humans, the chance may exists.
- if you are breast-feeding an infant. Most sulfonamides pass into the breast milk in small amounts and may cause unwanted effects in in-fants with some specific conditions.
- if you have any of the following medical problems:
Kidney disease
Liver disease
Porphyria
Deficiency of enzymes such as G6PD

Treatment
This medication is used to treat an in-fection caused by bacteria. Most sul-fonamides are best taken with a full glass (8 ounces) of water on an empty stomach, either one hour before or two hours after a meal. Follow your doctor's or pharmacist's directions on how to take your medicine.
- Keep taking this medicine for the full time of treatment even if you begin to feel better after a few days; do not miss any doses.
- If you do miss a dose of this medi-cine, take the missed dose immedia-tely.
- This medication works best when the level of medicine in your blood-stream (and urine) is kept constant. It is best, therefore, to take the doses at evenly spaced intervals day and night. if you take two doses a day, the doses should be spaced 12 hours apart.

Side effects
Along with the needed effects, a medi-cine may cause some unwanted effects. Side effects that usually do not require medical attention: abdominal pain, diar-rhea, dizziness, headache, loss of appe-tite, nausea, sore mouth, or vomiting. These side effects should disappear as your body adjusts to the medication.
Sulfonamides can increase sensitivity to sunlight. It is, therefore, important to avoid prolonged exposure to sunlight and sunlamps.

Tell your doctor about any side ef-fects that are persistent or particularly bothersome. It is especially important to tell your doctor about:
Bloody urine
Difficult urination
Difficulty in breathing
Difficulty in swallowing
Fever or hallucinations
Itching, rash, or pale skin
Joint pain, lower back pain
Ringing in the ears
Sore throat
Swollen or inflamed tongue
Tingling in hands or feet
Unusual bleeding, bruising
Yellowing of the eyes or skin

Interactions
This medicine may interact with several other drugs such as anticoagulants, oral antidiabetic agents, aspirin, some antibi-otics, or anticancer drugs.
- Be sure to tell your doctor about any medications you are currently taking.

Storage
Tablets, capsules, suspension, etc. should be stored at room temperature as directed by your pharmacist or ac-cording to instructions on the label.

METHYCLOTHIAZIDE

Properties

This medicine contains as active ingredient methyclothiazide, a thiazide-like diuretic. Thiazide or thiazide-like diuretics are prescribed to treat high blood pressure (hypertension). They are also used to reduce fluid accumulation in the body caused by conditions such as heart failure, cirrhosis, kidney disease, and the long-term use of some medications. Thiazide diuretics may also be used for other conditions as determined by your doctor.

Before using this medicine

Before you use this medicine check with your doctor, or pharmacist:

- if you ever had any unusual or allergic reaction to sulfonamides (sulfa drugs) or any of the thiazide diuretics.
- if you are on a low-salt, low-sugar, or any other special diet, or if you are allergic to any substance, such as sulfites or other preservatives or dyes.
- if you are pregnant or intend to become pregnant while using this medicine. When this medicine is used during pregnancy, it may cause side effects including jaundice, blood problems, and low potassium in the newborn.
- if you are breast-feeding an infant. Although this medicine has not been shown to cause problems in humans, the chance always exists since thiazide diuretics pass into breast milk.
- if you have any of the following medical problems:
Diabetes
Gout
Kidney disease
Liver disease
Lupus erythematosus
Pancreas disease

Treatment

This medication is used to treat high blood pressure (hypertension) and also to help reduce the amount of water in the body by increasing the flow of urine. This medicine will not cure your high blood pressure but it does help control it. You must continue to take it - even if you feel well - if you expect to keep your blood pressure down. You may have to take high blood pressure medicine for the rest of your life.

Thiazide diuretics may cause an unusual feeling of tiredness when you begin to take them. You may also notice an increase in urine or in frequency of urination. To keep this from affecting sleep:

- if you are to take a single dose a day, take it in the morning after breakfast;
- if you are to take more than one dose, take the last one not later than 6 p.m.

Side effects

Along with the needed effects, a medicine may cause some unwanted effects. Side effects that usually do not require medical attention: decreased sexual ability; dizziness or lightheadedness when standing up; increased sensitivity of skin to sunlight; loss of appetite; upset stomach.

- Side effects that should be reported to your doctor: black, tarry stools; blood in urine or stools; cough or hoarseness; fever or chills; joint pain; lower back or side pains; painful or difficult urination; pinpoint red spots on skin; skin rash or hives; stomach pain (severe) with nausea; unusual bleeding or bruising; yellow eyes or skin. This medicine may cause a loss of potassium from your body. Signs of too much potassium loss are: dryness of mouth; increased thirst; mood changes; muscle cramps or pain; nausea or vomiting; unusual tiredness or weakness; weak or irregular heartbeat.

Interactions

This medicine may interact with several other drugs.

- Be sure to tell your doctor about any medications you are currently taking.

Storage

Store at room temperature in a tightly closed container.

METOLAZONE

Properties
This medicine contains as active ingredient metolazone, a thiazide-like diuretic. Thiazide or thiazide-like diuretics are prescribed to treat high blood pressure (hypertension). They are also used to reduce fluid accumulation in the body caused by conditions such as heart failure, cirrhosis, kidney disease, and the long-term use of some medications. Thiazide diuretics may also be used for other conditions as determined by your doctor.

Before using this medicine
Before you use this medicine check with your doctor, or pharmacist:
- if you ever had any unusual or allergic reaction to sulfonamides (sulfa drugs) or any of the thiazide diuretics.
- if you are on a low-salt, low-sugar, or any other special diet, or if you are allergic to any substance, such as sulfites or other preservatives or dyes.
- if you are pregnant or intend to become pregnant while using this medicine. When this medicine is used during pregnancy, it may cause side effects including jaundice, blood problems, and low potassium in the newborn.
- if you are breast-feeding an infant. Although this medicine has not been shown to cause problems in humans, the chance always exists since thiazide diuretics pass into breast milk.
- if you have any of the following medical problems:
Diabetes
Gout
Kidney disease
Liver disease
Lupus erythematosus
Pancreas disease

Treatment
This medication is used to treat high blood pressure (hypertension) and also to help reduce the amount of water in the body by increasing the flow of urine. This medicine will not cure your high blood pressure but it does help control it. You must continue to take it - even if you feel well - if you expect to keep your blood pressure down. You may have to take high blood pressure medicine for the rest of your life.

Thiazide diuretics may cause an unusual feeling of tiredness when you begin to take them. You may also notice an increase in urine or in frequency of urination. To keep this from affecting sleep:
- if you are to take a single dose a day, take it in the morning after breakfast;
- if you are to take more than one dose, take the last one not later than 6 p.m.

Side effects
Along with the needed effects, a medicine may cause some unwanted effects. Side effects that usually do not require medical attention: decreased sexual ability; dizziness or lightheadedness when standing up; increased sensitivity of skin to sunlight; loss of appetite; upset stomach.
- Side effects that should be reported to your doctor: black, tarry stools; blood in urine or stools; cough or hoarseness; fever or chills; joint pain; lower back or side pains; painful or difficult urination; pinpoint red spots on skin; skin rash or hives; stomach pain (severe) with nausea; unusual bleeding or bruising; yellow eyes or skin. This medicine may cause a loss of potassium from your body. Signs of too much potassium loss are: dryness of mouth; increased thirst; mood changes; muscle cramps or pain; nausea or vomiting; unusual tiredness or weakness; weak or irregular heartbeat.

Interactions
This medicine may interact with several other drugs.
- Be sure to tell your doctor about any medications you are currently taking.

Storage
Store at room temperature in a tightly closed container.

METRA

Properties

This medicine contains phendimetrazine as active ingredient; it is prescribed for appetite suppression.

Appetite suppressants are used in the short-term (a few weeks) treatment of obesity. In a few weeks (6 to 12), these medicines in combination with dieting, exercise, and changes in eating habits can help patients lose weight. However, since their appetite reducing effect is only temporary, they are useful only for the first weeks of dieting until new eating habits are established.

Before using this medicine

Before you use this medicine check with your doctor, or pharmacist:
- if you ever had any unusual or allergic reaction to any of the compounds of this medicine.
- if you are on a low-salt, low-sugar, or any other special diet, or if you are allergic to any substance, such as sulfites or other preservatives or dyes.
- if you are pregnant, intend to become pregnant or breast-feeding an infant while using this medicine.
- if you have any of the following medical problems:
  Diabetes mellitus (sugar diabetes)
  Epilepsy
  Glaucoma
  Heart or blood vessel disease
  High blood pressure
  Mental illness (severe)

Treatment

This medication is used to relieve or prevent the symptoms of your medical problem. Take them as directed. Do not take more of them and do not take them more often than recommended on the label. If too much of the drug is taken, it may become habit-forming.

The medicine produces central nervous system stimulation, and it should not be taken by people with heart disease or high blood pressure.

If you think this medicine is not working as well after you have taken it for a few weeks, do not increase the dose. Instead, check with your doctor.

Side effects

The following minor side effects may occur: irritability, nervousness, restlessness, trouble in sleeping.

These side effects should disappear as your body adjusts to the medication. Tell your doctor about any side effects that are persistent or particularly bothersome. It is especially important to tell your doctor about:
  Mental depression
  Nausea or vomiting
  Stomach cramps or pain
  Trembling
  Unusual tiredness or weakness
- Discontinue use of the drug; call your doctor right away. Adverse reactions and side effects may be more frequent and severe in people over age 60 than in younger persons.

Interactions

This medicine interacts with several other drugs such as antihypertensives, other appetite suppressants, caffeine, central nervous system depressants, central nervous system stimulants, furazolidone, guanethidine, hydralazine, MAO inhibitors, methyldopa, molindone, phenothiazines, rauwolfia alkaloids, sodium bicarbonate.
- Be sure to tell your doctor about any medications you are currently taking.
Interaction with alcoholic beverages may produce drowsiness, sleepiness, and/or inability to concentrate.

Storage

This medicine should be stored at room temperature in tightly closed containers. Store away from heat and direct light. Keep out of reach of children, since overdose may be very dangerous in children.

Do not store this medicine in the bathroom medicine cabinet because the heat and moisture cause the medicine to break down. Do not keep outdated medicine or medicine no longer needed. Flush the contents of the container down the toilet.

MICRO EXTENCAPS K 10

Properties

This medicine contains potassium chloride as active ingredient; it is used to treat or prevent potassium deficiency, especially potassium deficiency that is caused by the use of diuretics (water pills).

Potassium is needed to maintain good health. Potassium supplements may be needed by patients who do not have enough potassium in their regular diet and by those who have lost too much potassium because of illness or treatment with certain medicines.

Since too much potassium may also cause health problems, most potassium supplements are available only with your doctor's prescription.

Before using this medicine

Before you use this medicine check with your doctor, or pharmacist:

- if you ever had any unusual or allergic reaction to potassium preparations;
- if you are on a low-salt, low-sugar, or any other special diet, or if you are allergic to any substance, such as sulfites or other preservatives or dyes.
- if you are pregnant or intend to become pregnant while using this medicine. Although potassium supplements have not been shown to cause problems in humans, the chance always exists.
- if you are breast-feeding an infant. Although this medicine has not been shown to cause problems in humans, the chance always exists since small amounts of potassium pass into the breast milk.
- if you have any of the following medical problems:
Addison's disease
Heart disease
Diarrhea
Kidney disease
Stomach ulcer

Treatment

This medication is used to relieve or prevent the symptoms of your medical problem. Take them as directed. Do not take more of them and do not take them more often than recommended on the label, unless otherwise directed by your doctor. To do so may increase the chance of side effects.

In order to avoid stomach irritation, you should take potassium supplements with food or immediately after a meal. If you miss a dose of this medication, take the missed dose as soon as possible, unless it is within two hours of the next scheduled dose;.

Side effects

The following minor side effects may occur:
Diarrhea
Nausea
Stomach pains
Vomiting.

These side effects should disappear as your body adjusts to the medication. Tell your doctor about any side effects that are persistent or particularly bothersome. It is especially important to tell your doctor about anxiety; bloody or black, tarry stools; confusion; difficulty in breathing; numbness or tingling in the arms, legs, or feet; palpitations; severe abdominal pain; or unusual weakness.

Interactions

This medicine interacts with several other drugs such as adrenocorticosteroids, antimuscarinics, calcium-containing medicines; heart medicines such as digitalis or digoxin; laxatives; other potassium-containing medicines.

- Be sure to tell your doctor about any medications you are currently taking.

Storage

Tablets, elixir, etc. should be stored at room temperature in tightly closed containers. Store away from heat and direct light. Keep out of reach of children, since overdose may be very dangerous in children. Do not keep outdated medicine or medicine no longer needed. Flush the contents of the container down the toilet, unless otherwise directed.

MICRO-K

Properties

This medicine contains potassium chloride as active ingredient; it is used to treat or prevent potassium deficiency, especially potassium deficiency that is caused by the use of diuretics (water pills).

Potassium is needed to maintain good health. Potassium supplements may be needed by patients who do not have enough potassium in their regular diet and by those who have lost too much potassium because of illness or treatment with certain medicines.

Since too much potassium may also cause health problems, most potassium supplements are available only with your doctor's prescription.

Before using this medicine

Before you use this medicine check with your doctor, or pharmacist:
- if you ever had any unusual or allergic reaction to potassium preparations;
- if you are on a low-salt, low-sugar, or any other special diet, or if you are allergic to any substance, such as sulfites or other preservatives or dyes.
- if you are pregnant or intend to become pregnant while using this medicine. Although potassium supplements have not been shown to cause problems in humans, the chance always exists.
- if you are breast-feeding an infant. Although this medicine has not been shown to cause problems in humans, the chance always exists since small amounts of potassium pass into the breast milk.
- if you have any of the following medical problems:
  Addison's disease
  Heart disease
  Diarrhea
  Kidney disease
  Stomach ulcer

Treatment

This medication is used to relieve or prevent the symptoms of your medical problem. Take them as directed. Do not take more of them and do not take them more often than recommended on the label, unless otherwise directed by your doctor. To do so may increase the chance of side effects.

In order to avoid stomach irritation, you should take potassium supplements with food or immediately after a meal. If you miss a dose of this medication, take the missed dose as soon as possible, unless it is within two hours of the next scheduled dose;.

Side effects

The following minor side effects may occur:
  Diarrhea
  Nausea
  Stomach pains
  Vomiting.
These side effects should disappear as your body adjusts to the medication. Tell your doctor about any side effects that are persistent or particularly bothersome. It is especially important to tell your doctor about anxiety; bloody or black, tarry stools; confusion; difficulty in breathing; numbness or tingling in the arms, legs, or feet; palpitations; severe abdominal pain; or unusual weakness.

Interactions

This medicine interacts with several other drugs such as adrenocorticosteroids, antimuscarinics, calcium-containing medicines; heart medicines such as digitalis or digoxin; laxatives; other potassium-containing medicines.
- Be sure to tell your doctor about any medications you are currently taking.

Storage

Tablets, elixir, etc. should be stored at room temperature in tightly closed containers. Store away from heat and direct light. Keep out of reach of children, since overdose may be very dangerous in children. Do not keep outdated medicine or medicine no longer needed. Flush the contents of the container down the toilet, unless otherwise directed.

MICROSULFON

Properties
This medicine contains sulfadiazine, a sulfonamide, as active ingredient. Sulfonamides are prescribed to treat infections caused by bacteria. They will not work for colds, flu, or other virus infections.

Before using this medicine
Before you use this medicine check with your doctor:
- if you ever had any unusual or allergic reaction to any of the compounds of the medicine.
- if you are on a low-salt, low-sugar, or any other special diet, or if you are allergic to any substance, such as sulfites or other preservatives or dyes.
- if you are pregnant or intend to become pregnant while using this medicine. Although sulfonamides have not been shown to cause defects in humans, the chance may exists.
- if you are breast-feeding an infant. Most sulfonamides pass into the breast milk in small amounts and may cause unwanted effects in infants with some specific conditions.
- if you have any of the following medical problems:
Kidney disease
Liver disease
Porphyria
Deficiency of enzymes such as G6PD

Treatment
This medication is used to treat an infection caused by bacteria. Most sulfonamides are best taken with a full glass (8 ounces) of water on an empty stomach, either one hour before or two hours after a meal. Follow your doctor's or pharmacist's directions on how to take your medicine.
- Keep taking this medicine for the full time of treatment even if you begin to feel better after a few days; do not miss any doses.
- If you do miss a dose of this medicine, take the missed dose immediately.
- This medication works best when the level of medicine in your bloodstream (and urine) is kept constant. It is best, therefore, to take the doses at evenly spaced intervals day and night. if you take two doses a day, the doses should be spaced 12 hours apart.

Side effects
Along with the needed effects, a medicine may cause some unwanted effects. Side effects that usually do not require medical attention: abdominal pain, diarrhea, dizziness, headache, loss of appetite, nausea, sore mouth, or vomiting. These side effects should disappear as your body adjusts to the medication.
Sulfonamides can increase sensitivity to sunlight. It is, therefore, important to avoid prolonged exposure to sunlight and sunlamps.

Tell your doctor about any side effects that are persistent or particularly bothersome. It is especially important to tell your doctor about:
Bloody urine
Difficult urination
Difficulty in breathing
Difficulty in swallowing
Fever or hallucinations
Itching, rash, or pale skin
Joint pain, lower back pain
Ringing in the ears
Sore throat
Swollen or inflamed tongue
Tingling in hands or feet
Unusual bleeding
Yellowing of the eyes or skin

Interactions
This medicine may interact with several other drugs such as anticoagulants, oral antidiabetic agents, aspirin, some antibiotics, or anticancer drugs.
- Be sure to tell your doctor about any medications you are currently taking.

Storage
Tablets, capsules, suspension, etc. should be stored at room temperature as directed by your pharmacist or according to instructions on the label.

MICROX

Properties

This medicine contains as active ingredient metolazone, a thiazide-like diuretic. Thiazide or thiazide-like diuretics are prescribed to treat high blood pressure (hypertension). They are also used to reduce fluid accumulation in the body caused by conditions such as heart failure, cirrhosis, kidney disease, and the long-term use of some medications. Thiazide diuretics may also be used for other conditions as determined by your doctor.

Before using this medicine

Before you use this medicine check with your doctor, or pharmacist:
- if you ever had any unusual or allergic reaction to sulfonamides (sulfa drugs) or any of the thiazide diuretics.
- if you are on a low-salt, low-sugar, or any other special diet, or if you are allergic to any substance, such as sulfites or other preservatives or dyes.
- if you are pregnant or intend to become pregnant while using this medicine. When this medicine is used during pregnancy, it may cause side effects including jaundice, blood problems, and low potassium in the newborn.
- if you are breast-feeding an infant. Although this medicine has not been shown to cause problems in humans, the chance always exists since thiazide diuretics pass into breast milk.
- if you have any of the following medical problems:
Diabetes
Gout
Kidney disease
Liver disease
Lupus erythematosus
Pancreas disease

Treatment

This medication is used to treat high blood pressure (hypertension) and also to help reduce the amount of water in the body by increasing the flow of urine. This medicine will not cure your high blood pressure but it does help control it. You must continue to take it - even if you feel well - if you expect to keep your blood pressure down. You may have to take high blood pressure medicine for the rest of your life.

Thiazide diuretics may cause an unusual feeling of tiredness when you begin to take them. You may also notice an increase in urine or in frequency of urination. To keep this from affecting sleep:
- if you are to take a single dose a day, take it in the morning after breakfast;
- if you are to take more than one dose, take the last one not later than 6 p.m.

Side effects

Along with the needed effects, a medicine may cause some unwanted effects. Side effects that usually do not require medical attention: decreased sexual ability; dizziness or lightheadedness when standing up; increased sensitivity of skin to sunlight; loss of appetite; upset stomach.
- Side effects that should be reported to your doctor: black, tarry stools; blood in urine or stools; cough or hoarseness; fever or chills; joint pain; lower back or side pains; painful or difficult urination; pinpoint red spots on skin; skin rash or hives; stomach pain (severe) with nausea; unusual bleeding or bruising; yellow eyes or skin. This medicine may cause a loss of potassium from your body. Signs of too much potassium loss are: dryness of mouth; increased thirst; mood changes; muscle cramps or pain; nausea or vomiting; unusual tiredness or weakness; weak or irregular heartbeat.

Interactions

This medicine may interact with several other drugs.
- Be sure to tell your doctor about any medications you are currently taking.

Storage

Store at room temperature in a tightly closed container.

MICTRIN

Properties

This medicine contains as active ingredient hydrochlorothiazide, a thiazide-like diuretic. Thiazide or thiazide-like diuretics are prescribed to treat high blood pressure (hypertension). They are also used to reduce fluid accumulation in the body caused by conditions such as heart failure, cirrhosis, kidney disease, and the long-term use of some medications. Thiazide diuretics may also be used for other conditions as determined by your doctor.

Before using this medicine

Before you use this medicine check with your doctor, or pharmacist:
- if you ever had any unusual or allergic reaction to sulfonamides (sulfa drugs) or any of the thiazide diuretics.
- if you are on a low-salt, low-sugar, or any other special diet, or if you are allergic to any substance, such as sulfites or other preservatives or dyes.
- if you are pregnant or intend to become pregnant while using this medicine. When this medicine is used during pregnancy, it may cause side effects including jaundice, blood problems, and low potassium in the newborn.
- if you are breast-feeding an infant. Although this medicine has not been shown to cause problems in humans, the chance always exists since thiazide diuretics pass into breast milk.
- if you have any of the following medical problems:
  Diabetes
  Gout
  Kidney disease
  Liver disease
  Lupus erythematosus
  Pancreas disease

Treatment

This medication is used to treat high blood pressure (hypertension) and also to help reduce the amount of water in the body by increasing the flow of urine. This medicine will not cure your high blood pressure but it does help control it. You must continue to take it - even if you feel well - if you expect to keep your blood pressure down. You may have to take high blood pressure medicine for the rest of your life.

Thiazide diuretics may cause an unusual feeling of tiredness when you begin to take them. You may also notice an increase in urine or in frequency of urination. To keep this from affecting sleep:
- if you are to take a single dose a day, take it in the morning after breakfast;
- if you are to take more than one dose, take the last one not later than 6 p.m.

Side effects

Along with the needed effects, a medicine may cause some unwanted effects. Side effects that usually do not require medical attention: decreased sexual ability; dizziness or lightheadedness when standing up; increased sensitivity of skin to sunlight; loss of appetite; upset stomach.
- Side effects that should be reported to your doctor: black, tarry stools; blood in urine or stools; cough or hoarseness; fever or chills; joint pain; lower back or side pains; painful or difficult urination; pinpoint red spots on skin; skin rash or hives; stomach pain (severe) with nausea; unusual bleeding or bruising; yellow eyes or skin. This medicine may cause a loss of potassium from your body. Signs of too much potassium loss are: dryness of mouth; increased thirst; mood changes; muscle cramps or pain; nausea or vomiting; unusual tiredness or weakness; weak or irregular heartbeat.

Interactions

This medicine may interact with several other drugs.
- Be sure to tell your doctor about any medications you are currently taking.

Storage

Store at room temperature in a tightly closed container.

MILLAZINE

Properties
This medicine contains as active ingredient thioridazine, a phenothiazine derivative. Phenothiazines are a family of medicines used to treat nervous, mental, and emotional conditions. Some are used to control anxiety, restlessness, nausea and vomiting, and severe hiccups. This medicine is available only with your doctor's prescription.

Before using this medicine
Before you use this medicine check with your doctor, or pharmacist:
- if you ever had any unusual or allergic reaction to phenothiazine medicines.
- if you are on a low-salt, low-sugar, or any other special diet, or if you are allergic to any substance, such as sulfites or other preservatives or dyes.
- if you are pregnant or intend to become pregnant while using this medicine. Although phenothiazines have not been shown to cause birth defects, some side effects such as jaundice and muscle tremors have occurred in a few newborns whose mothers received phenothiazines during pregnancy.
- if you are breast-feeding an infant. Although this medicine has not been shown to cause problems in humans the chance does exist since some phenothiazines are known to pass into the breast milk.
- if you have any of the following medical problems:
Alcoholism
Blood disease
Difficult urination
Enlarged prostate
Glaucoma
Heart or blood vessel disease
Liver or lung disease
Parkinson's disease
Stomach ulcers

Treatment
This medication is prescribed to treat the symptoms of certain types of mental illness or emotional problems. In order to avoid stomach irritation, you can take the tablet or capsule forms of this medication with a meal or with a glass of water or milk (unless your doctor or pharmacist directs you to do otherwise).

Side effects
Along with the needed effects, a medicine may cause some unwanted effects. Minor side effects are: blurred vision, constipation, decreased sweating, diarrhea, dizziness, drooling, drowsiness, dry mouth, fatigue, jitteriness, menstrual irregularities, nasal congestion, restlessness, tremors, vomiting, or weight gain.
- Tell your doctor about any side effects that are persistent or particularly bothersome. It is especially important to tell your doctor about:
Breast enlargement
Chest pain or convulsions
Darkened skin
Difficulty in swallowing
Fainting or fever
Involuntary movements
Palpitations or sleep disorders
Rash or sore throat
Uncoordinated movements
Unusual bleeding or bruising
Visual disturbances
Yellowing of the eyes or skin

Interactions
This medicine may interact with several other drugs such as barbiturates, sleeping pills, narcotics, other tranquilizers, or any other medication that may produce a sedative effect. Avoid alcohol.

Storage
Store this medication as directed on the label. Keep out of the reach of children.

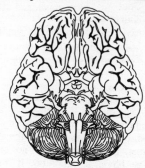

MIN-OVRAL

Properties
This medicine contains levonorgestrel and ethinyl estradiol as active ingredients. It is an oral contraceptive prescribed to prevent pregnancy and/or to regulate menstrual periods.

The drug works by altering the mucus at the cervix entrance to prevent the entry of sperm. It also alters the uterus lining to resist implantation of the fertilized egg. Oral contraceptives create the same chemical atmosphere in blood that exists during pregnancy.

Before using this medicine
Before you use this medicine check with your doctor, or pharmacist:
- if you ever had any unusual or allergic reaction to estrogens or progestogen;
- if you are pregnant or want to become pregnant within three months;
- if you are breast-feeding an infant;
- if you have any of the following medical problems:
  Diabetes
  Ailments of the breast
  Disorders of the uterus
  Migraine or epilepsy
  High blood pressure
  Asthma or heart conditions
  Kidney disease
  Gallstones

Treatment
This medication is used to prevent pregnancy or to regulate menstrual periods.

Adverse reactions
Along with the needed effects, a medicine may cause some unwanted effects or adverse reactions.
- *An increased risk of the following adverse reactions has been associated with the use of oral contraceptives:*
  Thrombophlebitis
  Venous thrombosis
  Arterial thromboembolism
  Pulmonary (lung) embolism
  Myocardial infarction
  Cerebral hemorrhage
  Cerebral thrombosis
  Hypertension
  Gallbladder disease
  Hepatic (liver) hepatomas
  Benign lifer tumors
- *The following adverse reactions have been reported in patients receiving oral contraceptives and are believed to be drug-related:*
  Nausea and vomiting
  Abdominal cramps
  Breakthrough bleeding
  Spotting
  Change in menstrual flow
  Amenorrhea
  Temporary infertility
  Edema
  Breast changes
  Weight changes
  Cholestatic jaundice
  Migraine
  Rash (allergic)
  Mental depression
  Vaginal candidiasis

Interactions
This medicine may interact with several other drugs such as antibiotics, anticoagulants, anticonvulsants, antidepressants, oral antidiabetics, antihistamines, barbiturates, oral hypoglycemics, insulin, meperidine.
- Be sure to tell your doctor about any medications you are currently taking.

Storage
Tablets should be stored at room temperature; store away from heat and direct light. Keep out of reach of children, since this medicine may be dangerous in children.

MINESTRIN

Properties
This medicine contains norethindrone and ethinyl estradiol as active ingredients. It is an oral contraceptive prescribed to prevent pregnancy and/or to regulate menstrual periods.

The drug works by altering the mucus at the cervix entrance to prevent the entry of sperm. It also alters the uterus lining to resist implantation of the fertilized egg. Oral contraceptives create the same chemical atmosphere in blood that exists during pregnancy.

Before using this medicine
Before you use this medicine check with your doctor, or pharmacist:
- if you ever had any unusual or allergic reaction to estrogens or progestogen;
- if you are pregnant or want to become pregnant within three months;
- if you are breast-feeding an infant;
- if you have any of the following medical problems:
  Diabetes
  Ailments of the breast
  Disorders of the uterus
  Migraine or epilepsy
  High blood pressure
  Asthma or heart conditions
  Kidney disease
  Gallstones

Treatment
This medication is used to prevent pregnancy or to regulate menstrual periods.

Adverse reactions
Along with the needed effects, a medicine may cause some unwanted effects or adverse reactions.
- *An increased risk of the following adverse reactions has been associated with the use of oral contraceptives:*
  Thrombophlebitis
  Venous thrombosis
  Arterial thromboembolism
  Pulmonary (lung) embolism
  Myocardial infarction
  Cerebral hemorrhage
  Cerebral thrombosis
  Hypertension
  Gallbladder disease
  Hepatic (liver) hepatomas
  Benign lifer tumors
- *The following adverse reactions have been reported in patients receiving oral contraceptives and are believed to be drug-related:*
  Nausea and vomiting
  Abdominal cramps
  Breakthrough bleeding
  Spotting
  Change in menstrual flow
  Amenorrhea
  Temporary infertility
  Edema
  Breast changes
  Weight changes
  Cholestatic jaundice
  Migraine
  Rash (allergic)
  Mental depression
  Vaginal candidiasis

Interactions
This medicine may interact with several other drugs such as antibiotics, anticoagulants, anticonvulsants, antidepressants, oral antidiabetics, antihistamines, barbiturates, oral hypoglycemics, insulin, meperidine.
- Be sure to tell your doctor about any medications you are currently taking.

Storage
Tablets should be stored at room temperature; store away from heat and direct light. Keep out of reach of children, since this medicine may be dangerous in children.

MODECATE

Properties

This medicine contains as active ingredient fluphenazine, a phenothiazine derivative. Phenothiazines are a family of medicines used to treat nervous, mental, and emotional conditions. Some are used to control anxiety, restlessness, nausea and vomiting, and severe hiccups. This medicine is available only with your doctor's prescription.

Before using this medicine

Before you use this medicine check with your doctor, or pharmacist:
- if you ever had any unusual or allergic reaction to phenothiazine medicines.
- if you are on a low-salt, low-sugar, or any other special diet, or if you are allergic to any substance, such as sulfites or other preservatives or dyes.
- if you are pregnant or intend to become pregnant while using this medicine. Although phenothiazines have not been shown to cause birth defects, some side effects such as jaundice and muscle tremors have occurred in a few newborns whose mothers received phenothiazines during pregnancy.
- if you are breast-feeding an infant. Although this medicine has not been shown to cause problems in humans the chance does exist since some phenothiazines are known to pass into the breast milk.
- if you have any of the following medical problems:
Alcoholism
Blood disease
Difficult urination
Enlarged prostate
Glaucoma
Heart or blood vessel disease
Liver or lung disease
Parkinson's disease
Stomach ulcers

Treatment

This medication is prescribed to treat the symptoms of certain types of mental illness or emotional problems. In order to avoid stomach irritation, you can take the tablet or capsule forms of this medication with a meal or with a glass of water or milk (unless your doctor or pharmacist directs you to do otherwise).

Side effects

Along with the needed effects, a medicine may cause some unwanted effects. Minor side effects are: blurred vision, constipation, decreased sweating, diarrhea, dizziness, drooling, drowsiness, dry mouth, fatigue, jitteriness, menstrual irregularities, nasal congestion, restlessness, tremors, vomiting, or weight gain.
- Tell your doctor about any side effects that are persistent or particularly bothersome. It is especially important to tell your doctor about:
Breast enlargement
Chest pain or convulsions
Darkened skin
Difficulty in swallowing
Fainting or fever
Involuntary movements
Palpitations or sleep disorders
Rash or sore throat
Uncoordinated movements
Unusual bleeding or bruising
Visual disturbances
Yellowing of the eyes or skin

Interactions

This medicine may interact with several other drugs such as barbiturates, sleeping pills, narcotics, other tranquilizers, or any other medication that may produce a sedative effect. Avoid alcohol.

Storage

Store this medication as directed on the label. Keep out of the reach of children.

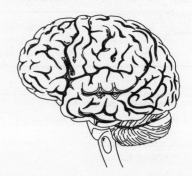

MODICON

Properties

This medicine contains norethindrone and ethinyl estradiol as active ingredients. It is an oral contraceptive prescribed to prevent pregnancy and/or to regulate menstrual periods.

The drug works by altering the mucus at the cervix entrance to prevent the entry of sperm. It also alters the uterus lining to resist implantation of the fertilized egg. Oral contraceptives create the same chemical atmosphere in blood that exists during pregnancy.

Before using this medicine

Before you use this medicine check with your doctor, or pharmacist:
- if you ever had any unusual or allergic reaction to estrogens or progestogen;
- if you are pregnant or want to become pregnant within three months;
- if you are breast-feeding an infant;
- if you have any of the following medical problems:
  Diabetes
  Ailments of the breast
  Disorders of the uterus
  Migraine or epilepsy
  High blood pressure
  Asthma or heart conditions
  Kidney disease
  Gallstones

Treatment

This medication is used to prevent pregnancy or to regulate menstrual periods.

Adverse reactions

Along with the needed effects, a medicine may cause some unwanted effects or adverse reactions.
- *An increased risk of the following adverse reactions has been associated with the use of oral contraceptives:*
  Thrombophlebitis
  Venous thrombosis
  Arterial thromboembolism
  Pulmonary (lung) embolism
  Myocardial infarction
  Cerebral hemorrhage
  Cerebral thrombosis
  Hypertension
  Gallbladder disease
  Hepatic (liver) hepatomas
  Benign lifer tumors
- *The following adverse reactions have been reported in patients receiving oral contraceptives and are believed to be drug-related:*
  Nausea and vomiting
  Abdominal cramps
  Breakthrough bleeding
  Spotting
  Change in menstrual flow
  Amenorrhea
  Temporary infertility
  Edema
  Breast changes
  Weight changes
  Cholestatic jaundice
  Migraine
  Rash (allergic)
  Mental depression
  Vaginal candidiasis

Interactions

This medicine may interact with several other drugs such as antibiotics, anticoagulants, anticonvulsants, antidepressants, oral antidiabetics, antihistamines, barbiturates, oral hypoglycemics, insulin, meperidine.
- Be sure to tell your doctor about any medications you are currently taking.

Storage

Tablets should be stored at room temperature; store away from heat and direct light. Keep out of reach of children, since this medicine may be dangerous in children.

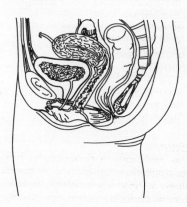

MODITEN

Properties
This medicine contains as active ingredient fluphenazine, a phenothiazine derivative. Phenothiazines are a family of medicines used to treat nervous, mental, and emotional conditions. Some are used to control anxiety, restlessness, nausea and vomiting, and severe hiccups. This medicine is available only with your doctor's prescription.

Before using this medicine
Before you use this medicine check with your doctor, or pharmacist:
- if you ever had any unusual or allergic reaction to phenothiazine medicines.
- if you are on a low-salt, low-sugar, or any other special diet, or if you are allergic to any substance, such as sulfites or other preservatives or dyes.
- if you are pregnant or intend to become pregnant while using this medicine. Although phenothiazines have not been shown to cause birth defects, some side effects such as jaundice and muscle tremors have occurred in a few newborns whose mothers received phenothiazines during pregnancy.
- if you are breast-feeding an infant. Although this medicine has not been shown to cause problems in humans the chance does exist since some phenothiazines are known to pass into the breast milk.
- if you have any of the following medical problems:
  Alcoholism
  Blood disease
  Difficult urination
  Enlarged prostate
  Glaucoma
  Heart or blood vessel disease
  Liver or lung disease
  Parkinson's disease
  Stomach ulcers

Treatment
This medication is prescribed to treat the symptoms of certain types of mental illness or emotional problems. In order to avoid stomach irritation, you can take the tablet or capsule forms of this medication with a meal or with a glass of water or milk (unless your doctor or pharmacist directs you to do otherwise).

Side effects
Along with the needed effects, a medicine may cause some unwanted effects. Minor side effects are: blurred vision, constipation, decreased sweating, diarrhea, dizziness, drooling, drowsiness, dry mouth, fatigue, jitteriness, menstrual irregularities, nasal congestion, restlessness, tremors, vomiting, or weight gain.
- Tell your doctor about any side effects that are persistent or particularly bothersome. It is especially important to tell your doctor about:
  Breast enlargement
  Chest pain or convulsions
  Darkened skin
  Difficulty in swallowing
  Fainting or fever
  Involuntary movements
  Palpitations or sleep disorders
  Rash or sore throat
  Uncoordinated movements
  Unusual bleeding or bruising
  Visual disturbances
  Yellowing of the eyes or skin

Interactions
This medicine may interact with several other drugs such as barbiturates, sleeping pills, narcotics, other tranquilizers, or any other medication that may produce a sedative effect. Avoid alcohol.

Storage
Store this medication as directed on the label. Keep out of the reach of children.

MONOCID

Properties

This medicine contains cephalosporin as active ingredient. Cephalosporins belong to the general family of medicines called antibiotics, used in the treatment of infections caused by bacteria. They work by killing bacteria or preventing their growth. Cephalosporins will not work for colds, flu, or other viral infections.

Before using this medicine

Before you use this medicine check with your doctor:

– if you ever had any unusual or allergic reaction to any of the cephalosporins, penicillins, penicillin-like medicines, or penicillamine.
– if you are on a low-salt, low-sugar, or any other special diet, or if you are allergic to any substance, such as sulfites or other preservatives or dyes.
– if you are pregnant or intend to become pregnant while using this medicine. Although cephalosporins have not been shown to cause birth defects or other problems in humans, the chance always exists.
– if you are breast-feeding an infant. Most cephalosporins pass into the breast milk, usually in small amounts.
– if you have any of the following medical problems:
Bleeding problem
Kidney or lifer disease

Treatment

This medication belongs to the general family of medicines called antibiotics. It is used to treat a wide variety of bacterial infections. It is also used to treat infections in persons who are allergic to penicillin.

■ Keep taking this medicine for the full time of treatment even if you begin to feel better after a few days; do not miss any doses.
■ If you do miss a dose of this medicine, take it as soon as possible. This will help to keep a constant amount of medicine in the blood. However, if it is almost time for your next dose, skip the missed dose and go back to your regular dosing schedule.
■ This medication has been prescribed for your current infection only. Another infection later on, or one that someone else has, may require a different medicine. You should not give your medicine to other people or use it for other infections, unless your doctor specifically directs you to do so.
■ Take the medicine at the same times each day, 1 hour before or 2 hours after eating.

Side effects

Along with the needed effects, a medicine may cause some unwanted effects. Side effects that usually do not require medical attention: rectal itching, oral or vaginal white spots, mild diarrhea. These side effects should disappear as your body adjusts to the medication.

■ Other side effects that should be reported to your doctor immediately are:
Hives, rash
Intense itching
Faintness soon after a dose
Difficulty in breathing
Nausea and vomiting
Severe diarrhea
Unusual weakness or tiredness
Bleeding or bruising

Interactions

This medicine may interact with several other drugs such as anticoagulants, theophylline preparations, probenecid, tetracyclines, etc.

■ Be sure to tell your doctor about any medications you are currently taking.

Storage

Tablets, capsules, etc. should be stored at room temperature. Store the liquid form in the refrigerator. Keep out of the reach of children. Do not keep outdated medicine or medicine no longer needed.

MORPHINE

Properties
This medicine contains as active ingredient morphine.

It is a narcotic analgesic that acts directly on the central nervous system (brain and spinal cord). It is used to relieve pain or to suppress coughing.

Before using this medicine
Before you use this medicine check with your doctor, or pharmacist:
- if you ever had any unusual or allergic reaction to this medicine or one of its components.
- if you are on a low-salt, low-sugar, or any other special diet, or if you are allergic to any substance, such as sulfites or other preservatives or dyes.
- if you are pregnant or intend to become pregnant while using this medicine. Studies on birth defects have not been done in humans. Too much use of narcotics during pregnancy may cause the baby to become dependent on the medicine.
- if you are breast-feeding an infant. Although this medicine has not been shown to cause problems in humans, it passes into the breast milk in small amounts.
- if you have any of the following medical problems:
  Brain disease or head injury
  Colitis
  Convulsions
  Emphysema, asthma, or chronic lung disease
  Enlarged prostate
  Gallbladder disease or gallstones
  Heart disease
  Kidney or lifer disease
  Underactive thyroid

Treatment
This medication is used to relieve pain or to suppress coughing. Narcotic analgesics act in the central nervous system; some of their side effects are also caused by actions in the central nervous system.
- If you are taking this medication on a regular schedule and you miss a dose, take the missed dose as soon as possible, unless it is almost time for your next dose. In that case do not take the missed dose at all.
- If a narcotic analgesic is used for a long time, it may become habit-forming (causing mental or physical dependence). Physical dependence may lead to withdrawal side effects when you stop taking this medicine.

Unless otherwise directed by your doctor or pharmacist take this as directed. Do not take more of them and do not take them more often than recommended on the label. Children up to 12 years of age should not take this medicine more than 3 times a day or for more than 5 days in a row.

Side effects
Along with the needed effects, a medicine may cause some unwanted effects. These side effects may go away during treatment as your body adjusts to the medicine. Such minor side effects are: constipation, dizziness, drowsiness, dry mouth, false sense of well-being, flushing, light-headedness, loss of appetite, nausea, painful or difficult urination, or sweating.
- Check with your doctor immediately if any of the following side effects occur:
  Anxiety or breathing difficulties
  Excitation or restlessness
  Fatigue, palpitations
  Rash, sore throat and fever
  Tremors or weakness

Interactions
This medicine may interact with several other drugs such as medicines acting on the central nervous system (e.g., antidepressants, tranquilizers), cimetidine, nitrates, quinidine, etc.
- Be sure to tell your doctor about any medications you are currently taking.

Storage
Tablets, elixir, suppository etc. should be stored at room temperature in a tightly closed, light-resistant container.

MORPHITEC

Properties
This medicine contains as active ingredient morphine.

It is a narcotic analgesic that acts directly on the central nervous system (brain and spinal cord). It is used to relieve pain or to suppress coughing.

Before using this medicine
Before you use this medicine check with your doctor, or pharmacist:
- if you ever had any unusual or allergic reaction to this medicine or one of its components.
- if you are on a low-salt, low-sugar, or any other special diet, or if you are allergic to any substance, such as sulfites or other preservatives or dyes.
- if you are pregnant or intend to become pregnant while using this medicine. Studies on birth defects have not been done in humans. Too much use of narcotics during pregnancy may cause the baby to become dependent on the medicine.
- if you are breast-feeding an infant. Although this medicine has not been shown to cause problems in humans, it passes into the breast milk in small amounts.
- if you have any of the following medical problems:
Brain disease or head injury
Colitis
Convulsions
Emphysema, asthma, or chronic lung disease
Enlarged prostate
Gallbladder disease or gallstones
Heart disease
Kidney or lifer disease
Underactive thyroid

Treatment
This medication is used to relieve pain or to suppress coughing. Narcotic analgesics act in the central nervous system; some of their side effects are also caused by actions in the central nervous system.
- If you are taking this medication on a regular schedule and you miss a dose, take the missed dose as soon as possible, unless it is almost time for your next dose. In that case do not take the missed dose at all.
- If a narcotic analgesic is used for a long time, it may become habit-forming (causing mental or physical dependence). Physical dependence may lead to withdrawal side effects when you stop taking this medicine.

Unless otherwise directed by your doctor or pharmacist take this as directed. Do not take more of them and do not take them more often than recommended on the label. Children up to 12 years of age should not take this medicine more than 3 times a day or for more than 5 days in a row.

Side effects
Along with the needed effects, a medicine may cause some unwanted effects. These side effects may go away during treatment as your body adjusts to the medicine. Such minor side effects are: constipation, dizziness, drowsiness, dry mouth, false sense of well-being, flushing, light-headedness, loss of appetite, nausea, painful or difficult urination, or sweating.
- Check with your doctor immediately if any of the following side effects occur:
Anxiety or breathing difficulties
Excitation or restlessness
Fatigue, palpitations
Rash, sore throat and fever
Tremors or weakness

Interactions
This medicine may interact with several other drugs such as medicines acting on the central nervous system (e.g., antidepressants, tranquilizers), cimetidine, nitrates, quinidine, etc.
- Be sure to tell your doctor about any medications you are currently taking.

Storage
Tablets, elixir, suppository etc. should be stored at room temperature in a tightly closed, light-resistant container.

MYCITRACIN (Ophthalmic)

Properties
This medicine contains an ophthalmic antibacterial, as active ingredient. It helps the body to overcome eye infections on surface tissues of the eye. It is most useful when the infecting organism is one known to be sensitive to the antibacterial drug.

The drug penetrates the bacterial cell membrane and prevents cells from multiplying.

Before using this medicine
Before you use this medicine check with your doctor:
- if you ever had any unusual or allergic reaction to any of the compounds of the medicine.
- if you are on a low-salt, low-sugar, or any other special diet, or if you are allergic to any substance, such as sulfites or other preservatives or dyes.
- if you are pregnant or intend to become pregnant while using this medicine. Although ophthalmic antibacterials have been found to be safe for use during pregnancy, you should check with your doctor before taking any drug if you are pregnant.

Treatment
This medication is used to treat an infection caused by bacteria. The medicine may be used in the form of eye drops or as an eye ointment. Use the medication as directed, Do not miss a dose. If you forget a dose, use it as soon as you remember. Notify your doctor if eye symptoms fail to improve in two to four days.
- ◆ To apply eye drops: Till the head backward when applying the eye drops. Pull the lower eyelid away from the eye to form a pouch. After applying the drop, keep the eye closed for a minute or so. This allows the medication to come in contact with the infection.
- ◆ To apply eye ointment: Pull lower lid down from eye to form a pouch. Squeeze tube to apply thin strip of ointment into pouch. Close eye for 1 to 2 minutes.

Always wash your hands before applying the ointment. The drug starts to work in about one hour. Treatment may require 7 to 10 days to control infection.

Older adults or seniors may take this medication without special restriction.

Side effects
Along with the needed effects, a medicine may cause some unwanted effects. Side effects that usually do not require medical attention: occasional local irritation after application to the eye. Ointments may cause blurred vision for a few minutes; continue the use of the eye drops or ointment, but tell your doctor at the next visit.
- ■ Discontinue the use of eye drops or eye ointment in the following cases:
  Sore throat
  Aplastic anemia
  Pale skin
  Unusual redness of the eye
  Unusual irritation of the eye
  Fever
  Unusual bleeding
  Unusual bruising
- ■ Tell your doctor about any side effects that are persistent or particularly bothersome. In case of prolonged use sensitivity reactions may develop.

Interactions
Clinically significant interactions with oral or injected medicines are unlikely. Do not use the eye drops or ointment with any other eye drops or ointment without checking with your ophthalmologist.

Storage
Keep bottle (with eye drops) or container (containing ointment) lightly closed. Store in a cool place, but Do not freeze. Wash hands immediately after using. Do not store in the bathroom medicine cabinet because the heat or moisture may cause the medicine to break down. Do not keep outdated medicine or medicine no longer needed. Flush the contents of the bottle or tube down the toilet, unless otherwise directed.

N.E.E.

Properties

This medicine contains norethindrone and ethinyl estradiol as active ingredients. It is an oral contraceptive prescribed to prevent pregnancy and/or to regulate menstrual periods.

The drug works by altering the mucus at the cervix entrance to prevent the entry of sperm. It also alters the uterus lining to resist implantation of the fertilized egg. Oral contraceptives create the same chemical atmosphere in blood that exists during pregnancy.

Before using this medicine

Before you use this medicine check with your doctor, or pharmacist:
- if you ever had any unusual or allergic reaction to estrogens or progestogen;
- if you are pregnant or want to become pregnant within three months;
- if you are breast-feeding an infant;
- if you have any of the following medical problems:
  Diabetes
  Ailments of the breast
  Disorders of the uterus
  Migraine or epilepsy
  High blood pressure
  Asthma or heart conditions
  Kidney disease
  Gallstones

Treatment

This medication is used to prevent pregnancy or to regulate menstrual periods.

Adverse reactions

Along with the needed effects, a medicine may cause some unwanted effects or adverse reactions.
- *An increased risk of the following adverse reactions has been associated with the use of oral contraceptives:*
  Thrombophlebitis
  Venous thrombosis
  Arterial thromboembolism
  Pulmonary (lung) embolism
  Myocardial infarction
  Cerebral hemorrhage
  Cerebral thrombosis
  Hypertension
  Gallbladder disease
  Hepatic (liver) hepatomas
  Benign lifer tumors
- *The following adverse reactions have been reported in patients receiving oral contraceptives and are believed to be drug-related:*
  Nausea and vomiting
  Abdominal cramps
  Breakthrough bleeding
  Spotting
  Change in menstrual flow
  Amenorrhea
  Temporary infertility
  Edema
  Breast changes
  Weight changes
  Cholestatic jaundice
  Migraine
  Rash (allergic)
  Mental depression
  Vaginal candidiasis

Interactions

This medicine may interact with several other drugs such as antibiotics, anticoagulants, anticonvulsants, antidepressants, oral antidiabetics, antihistamines, barbiturates, oral hypoglycemics, insulin, meperidine.
- Be sure to tell your doctor about any medications you are currently taking.

Storage

Tablets should be stored at room temperature; store away from heat and direct light. Keep out of reach of children, since this medicine may be dangerous in children.

N-G-C

Properties
This medicine contains nitroglycerin as active ingredient. Nitrates improve the supply of blood and oxygen to the heart. This medication is for oral use.

Before using this medicine
Before you use this medicine check with your doctor, or pharmacist:
- if you ever had any unusual or allergic reaction to nitrates or nitrites.
- if you are on a low-salt, low-sugar, or any other special diet, or if you are allergic to any substance, such as sulfites or other preservatives or dyes.
- if you are pregnant or intend to become pregnant while using this medicine. Although nitrates have not been shown to cause problems in humans, the chance always exists.
- if you are breast-feeding an infant.
- if you have recently had a heart attack or stroke.
- if you have any of the following medical problems:
  Anemia
  Glaucoma
  Intestinal problems
  Overactive thyroid
- if you are now taking any of the following medicines or types of medicines:
  Antihypertensives
  Asthma or hay fever medicine
  Cold medicine
  Decongestant
  Medicine for appetite control
  Narcotic
  Pain medicine
  Sinus congestion medicine

Treatment
This medication is used to treat and prevent angina (chest pain). Nitroglycerin is a vasodilator, which relaxes the muscles of the blood vessels, causing an increase in the oxygen supply to the heart. The oral tablets, capsules, ointment and patches do not act quickly; they are used to prevent chest pain. The sublingual tablets and oral spray act quickly and can be used to relieve chest pain after it has started.

- Take this medicine exactly as directed by your doctor or pharmacist. It will work only if taken correctly.
- If you are taking this medicine regularly and you miss a dose, take it as soon as possible. However, if your next scheduled dose; is within 2 hours (or within 6 hours for extended-release capsules or tablets), skip the missed dose and go back to your regular dosing schedule.
- If you have been taking this medicine regularly for several weeks or more, do not suddenly stop using it. Stopping suddenly may bring on attacks of angina.

Side effects
There are a number of side effects that usually do not require medical attention. These possible side effects may go away during treatment; however, if they continue or are bothersome, check with your doctor, nurse, or pharmacist. More common are: dizziness, lightheadedness, or fainting when standing up; fast pulse; flushing of face and neck; headache; nausea or vomiting.

Side effects that should be reported to your doctor are: blurred vision; dry mouth; severe or prolonged headache; skin rash.

Interactions
This medicine may interact with several other drugs such as tricyclic antidepressants and cough medicines. Before starting to take or apply nitroglycerin, be sure to tell your doctor about any medications you are currently taking.

Storage
Tablets, capsules, and oral spray should be stored as in a tightly capped bottle in a cool, dry place. Ointment and patches should be stored at room temperature in their original containers. Keep out of reach of children. Do not keep outdated medicine or medicine no longer needed.

NADOPEN-V

Properties
This medicine contains penicillin V as active ingredient. Penicillins are prescribed to treat infections caused by bacteria. They will not work for colds, flu, or other virus infections. There are several different kinds of penicillins. Each is used to treat different kinds of infections.

Before using this medicine
Before you use this medicine check with your doctor, or pharmacist:
- if you ever had any unusual or allergic reaction to any of the penicillins, cefalosporins, griseofulvin, or penicillamine. Serious reactions may occur in patients who are allergic to penicillins.
- if you are on a low-salt, low-sugar, or any other special diet, or if you are allergic to any substance, such as sulfites or other preservatives or dyes.
- if you are pregnant or intend to become pregnant while using this medicine. Although penicillins have not been shown to cause problems in humans, the chance always exists.
- if you are breast-feeding an infant. Most penicillins (except amdinocillin) pass into the breast milk. Even though only small amounts may pass, allergic reaction, diarrhea, fungal infection, and skin rash may occur in the infant.
- if you have any of the following medical problems:
  Allergy
  Asthma
  Bleeding problems
  Eczema
  Hay fever, hives
  Kidney disease
  Liver disease
  Mononucleosis
  Stomach or intestinal disease

Treatment
This medication is used to treat an infection caused by bacteria. Most penicillins are best taken with a full glass (8 ounces) of water on an empty stomach, some are best taken with a snack or meal. Follow your doctor's or pharmacist's directions on how to take your medicine.
- Keep taking this medicine for the full time of treatment even if you begin to feel better after a few days; do not miss any doses. This is especially important if you have a "strep" infection since serious heart problems could develop later if your infection is not cleared up completely.
- If you do miss a dose of this medicine, take it as soon as possible. However, if it is almost time for your next dose, skip the missed dose and go back to your regular dosing schedule.

Side effects
Along with the needed effects, a medicine may cause some unwanted effects. Side effects that usually do not require medical attention: diarrhea; nausea or vomiting; sore mouth or tongue.
- Stop taking this medicine and get emergency help immediately if you notice: difficulty in breathing; lightheadedness; skin rash, hives, itching; wheezing.

Other side effects that should be reported to your doctor immediately are: abdominal bloating; blood in urine; convulsions (seizures); decreased amount of urine; diarrhea (watery and severe) which may also be bloody; fever; joint pain; sore throat and fever; stomach or abdominal cramps and pain; unusual bleeding or bruising.

Interactions
This medicine may interact with several other drugs such as anticoagulants, diarrhea medicines, heparin, ibuprofen, oral contraceptives, potassium-containing medicines, etc.
- Be sure to tell your doctor about any medications you are currently taking.

Storage
Tablets, capsules, etc. should be stored as directed by your pharmacist or according to instructions on the label.

NALBUPHINE

Properties
This medicine contains as active ingredient nalbuphine.

It is a narcotic analgesic that acts directly on the central nervous system (brain and spinal cord). It is used to relieve pain or to suppress coughing.

Before using this medicine
Before you use this medicine check with your doctor, or pharmacist:
- if you ever had any unusual or allergic reaction to this medicine or one of its components.
- if you are on a low-salt, low-sugar, or any other special diet, or if you are allergic to any substance, such as sulfites or other preservatives or dyes.
- if you are pregnant or intend to become pregnant while using this medicine. Studies on birth defects have not been done in humans. Too much use of narcotics during pregnancy may cause the baby to become dependent on the medicine.
- if you are breast-feeding an infant. Although this medicine has not been shown to cause problems in humans, it passes into the breast milk in small amounts.
- if you have any of the following medical problems:
Brain disease or head injury
Colitis
Convulsions
Emphysema, asthma, or chronic lung disease
Enlarged prostate
Gallbladder disease or gallstones
Heart disease
Kidney or lifer disease
Underactive thyroid

Treatment
This medication is used to relieve pain or to suppress coughing. Narcotic analgesics act in the central nervous system; some of their side effects are also caused by actions in the central nervous system.
- If you are taking this medication on a regular schedule and you miss a dose, take the missed dose as soon as possible, unless it is almost time for your next dose. In that case do not take the missed dose at all.
- If a narcotic analgesic is used for a long time, it may become habit-forming (causing mental or physical dependence). Physical dependence may lead to withdrawal side effects when you stop taking this medicine.

Unless otherwise directed by your doctor or pharmacist take this as directed. Do not take more of them and do not take them more often than recommended on the label. Children up to 12 years of age should not take this medicine more than 3 times a day or for more than 5 days in a row.

Side effects
Along with the needed effects, a medicine may cause some unwanted effects. These side effects may go away during treatment as your body adjusts to the medicine. Such minor side effects are: constipation, dizziness, drowsiness, dry mouth, false sense of well-being, flushing, light-headedness, loss of appetite, nausea, painful or difficult urination, or sweating.
- Check with your doctor immediately if any of the following side effects occur:
Anxiety or breathing difficulties
Excitation or restlessness
Fatigue, palpitations
Rash, sore throat and fever
Tremors or weakness

Interactions
This medicine may interact with several other drugs such as medicines acting on the central nervous system (e.g., antidepressants, tranquilizers), cimetidine, nitrates, quinidine, etc.
- Be sure to tell your doctor about any medications you are currently taking.

Storage
Tablets, elixir, suppository etc. should be stored at room temperature in a tightly closed, light-resistant container.

NAQUA

Properties

This medicine contains as active ingredient trichlormethiazide, a thiazide-like diuretic. Thiazide or thiazide-like diuretics are prescribed to treat high blood pressure (hypertension). They are also used to reduce fluid accumulation in the body caused by conditions such as heart failure, cirrhosis, kidney disease, and the long-term use of some medications. Thiazide diuretics may also be used for other conditions as determined by your doctor.

Before using this medicine

Before you use this medicine check with your doctor, or pharmacist:

- if you ever had any unusual or allergic reaction to sulfonamides (sulfa drugs) or any of the thiazide diuretics.
- if you are on a low-salt, low-sugar, or any other special diet, or if you are allergic to any substance, such as sulfites or other preservatives or dyes.
- if you are pregnant or intend to become pregnant while using this medicine. When this medicine is used during pregnancy, it may cause side effects including jaundice, blood problems, and low potassium in the newborn.
- if you are breast-feeding an infant. Although this medicine has not been shown to cause problems in humans, the chance always exists since thiazide diuretics pass into breast milk.
- if you have any of the following medical problems:
  Diabetes
  Gout
  Kidney disease
  Liver disease
  Lupus erythematosus
  Pancreas disease

Treatment

This medication is used to treat high blood pressure (hypertension) and also to help reduce the amount of water in the body by increasing the flow of urine. This medicine will not cure your high blood pressure but it does help control it. You must continue to take it - even if you feel well -if you expect to keep your blood pressure down. You may have to take high blood pressure medicine for the rest of your life.

Thiazide diuretics may cause an unusual feeling of tiredness when you begin to take them. You may also notice an increase in urine or in frequency of urination. To keep this from affecting sleep:

- if you are to take a single dose a day, take it in the morning after breakfast;
- if you are to take more than one dose, take the last one not later than 6 p.m.

Side effects

Along with the needed effects, a medicine may cause some unwanted effects. Side effects that usually do not require medical attention: decreased sexual ability; dizziness or lightheadedness when standing up; increased sensitivity of skin to sunlight; loss of appetite; upset stomach.

- Side effects that should be reported to your doctor: black, tarry stools; blood in urine or stools; cough or hoarseness; fever or chills; joint pain; lower back or side pains; painful or difficult urination; pinpoint red spots on skin; skin rash or hives; stomach pain (severe) with nausea; unusual bleeding or bruising; yellow eyes or skin. This medicine may cause a loss of potassium from your body. Signs of too much potassium loss are: dryness of mouth; increased thirst; mood changes; muscle cramps or pain; nausea or vomiting; unusual tiredness or weakness; weak or irregular heartbeat.

Interactions

This medicine may interact with several other drugs.

- Be sure to tell your doctor about any medications you are currently taking.

Storage

Store at room temperature in a tightly closed container.

NECON

Properties

This medicine contains norethindrone and ethinyl estradiol as active ingredients. It is an oral contraceptive prescribed to prevent pregnancy and/or to regulate menstrual periods.

The drug works by altering the mucus at the cervix entrance to prevent the entry of sperm. It also alters the uterus lining to resist implantation of the fertilized egg. Oral contraceptives create the same chemical atmosphere in blood that exists during pregnancy.

Before using this medicine

Before you use this medicine check with your doctor, or pharmacist:
- if you ever had any unusual or allergic reaction to estrogens or progestogen;
- if you are pregnant or want to become pregnant within three months;
- if you are breast-feeding an infant;
- if you have any of the following medical problems:
  Diabetes
  Ailments of the breast
  Disorders of the uterus
  Migraine or epilepsy
  High blood pressure
  Asthma or heart conditions
  Kidney disease
  Gallstones

Treatment

This medication is used to prevent pregnancy or to regulate menstrual periods.

Adverse reactions

Along with the needed effects, a medicine may cause some unwanted effects or adverse reactions.
- *An increased risk of the following adverse reactions has been associated with the use of oral contraceptives:*
  Thrombophlebitis
  Venous thrombosis
  Arterial thromboembolism
  Pulmonary (lung) embolism
  Myocardial infarction
  Cerebral hemorrhage
  Cerebral thrombosis
  Hypertension
  Gallbladder disease
  Hepatic (liver) hepatomas
  Benign lifer tumors
- *The following adverse reactions have been reported in patients receiving oral contraceptives and are believed to be drug-related:*
  Nausea and vomiting
  Abdominal cramps
  Breakthrough bleeding
  Spotting
  Change in menstrual flow
  Amenorrhea
  Temporary infertility
  Edema
  Breast changes
  Weight changes
  Cholestatic jaundice
  Migraine
  Rash (allergic)
  Mental depression
  Vaginal candidiasis

Interactions

This medicine may interact with several other drugs such as antibiotics, anticoagulants, anticonvulsants, antidepressants, oral antidiabetics, antihistamines, barbiturates, oral hypoglycemics, insulin, meperidine.
- Be sure to tell your doctor about any medications you are currently taking.

Storage

Tablets should be stored at room temperature; store away from heat and direct light. Keep out of reach of children, since this medicine may be dangerous in children.

NEFEDIPINE

Properties
This medicine contains nefedipine as active ingredient. It is a so-called calcium channel blocker, working by blocking the passage of calcium into heart and smooth muscle. Since calcium is an essential factor in muscle contraction, any medicine that affects calcium in this way will interfere with the contraction of these muscles.

The medicine works by:
- reducing the work that the heart must perform;
- reducing the normal arterial blood pressure;
- increasing oxygen to the heart muscle.

The medicine is prescribed for the treatment of attacks of angina pectoris, irregular heartbeat, and high blood pressure. In many cases it can be used for the treatment and prevention of migraine.

Before using this medicine
Before you use this medicine check with your doctor, or pharmacist:
- if you ever had any unusual or allergic reaction to this medicine or any calcium channel blocker;
- if you are pregnant or intend to become pregnant while using this medicine;
- if you have low blood pressure;
- if you have kidney or lifer disease;
- if you are breast-feeding an infant;
- if you easily get a rash or intensity sunburn in areas exposed to sun or ultraviolet light.

Treatment
This medication is used for treatment of heart conditions (for instance, angina pectoris) and high blood pressure. Tablets, capsules or extended-release tablets should be taken with liquid. The usual dose amounts to 30 to 100 milligrams a day.

For safe and effective use of medicine:
- Follow your doctor's instructions if this medicine was prescribed.
- Follow the manufacturer's package directions if you are treating yourself.

Side effects
Along with the needed effects, a medicine may cause some unwanted effects. Possible side effects include:
Tiredness
Changes in heartbeat
Wheezing
Cough
Shortness of breath
Dizziness
Fainting
Numbness in hands and feet
Tingling in hands and feet
Difficult urination
Constipation

Overdose
The following symptoms may be a sign of overdose:
Unusually fast heartbeat
Unusually slow heartbeat
Loss of consciousness
Cardiac arrest
- Call a doctor or hospital emergency room for instructions. If necessary start first aid immediately.

Interactions
The effect of this medicine may cause a blood pressure drop if taken together with antihypertensives. Cimetidine may increase the effect of the calcium blocker.

The simultaneous use of diuretics and calcium channel blockers may cause dangerous blood pressure drop.
- Be sure to tell your doctor about any medications you are currently taking.

Storage
Capsules, tablets, etc. should be stored at room temperature; store away from heat and direct light. Keep out of reach of children, since this medicine may be dangerous in children.

NELOVA

Properties
This medicine contains norethindrone and ethinyl estradiol as active ingredients. It is an oral contraceptive prescribed to prevent pregnancy and/or to regulate menstrual periods.

The drug works by altering the mucus at the cervix entrance to prevent the entry of sperm. It also alters the uterus lining to resist implantation of the fertilized egg. Oral contraceptives create the same chemical atmosphere in blood that exists during pregnancy.

Before using this medicine
Before you use this medicine check with your doctor, or pharmacist:
- if you ever had any unusual or allergic reaction to estrogens or progestogen;
- if you are pregnant or want to become pregnant within three months;
- if you are breast-feeding an infant;
- if you have any of the following medical problems:
  Diabetes
  Ailments of the breast
  Disorders of the uterus
  Migraine or epilepsy
  High blood pressure
  Asthma or heart conditions
  Kidney disease
  Gallstones

Treatment
This medication is used to prevent pregnancy or to regulate menstrual periods.

Adverse reactions
Along with the needed effects, a medicine may cause some unwanted effects or adverse reactions.
- *An increased risk of the following adverse reactions has been associated with the use of oral contraceptives:*
  Thrombophlebitis
  Venous thrombosis
  Arterial thromboembolism
  Pulmonary (lung) embolism
  Myocardial infarction
  Cerebral hemorrhage
  Cerebral thrombosis
  Hypertension
  Gallbladder disease
  Hepatic (liver) hepatomas
  Benign lifer tumors
- *The following adverse reactions have been reported in patients receiving oral contraceptives and are believed to be drug-related:*
  Nausea and vomiting
  Abdominal cramps
  Breakthrough bleeding
  Spotting
  Change in menstrual flow
  Amenorrhea
  Temporary infertility
  Edema
  Breast changes
  Weight changes
  Cholestatic jaundice
  Migraine
  Rash (allergic)
  Mental depression
  Vaginal candidiasis

Interactions
This medicine may interact with several other drugs such as antibiotics, anticoagulants, anticonvulsants, antidepressants, oral antidiabetics, antihistamines, barbiturates, oral hypoglycemics, insulin, meperidine.
- Be sure to tell your doctor about any medications you are currently taking.

Storage
Tablets should be stored at room temperature; store away from heat and direct light. Keep out of reach of children, since this medicine may be dangerous in children.

NELULEN

Properties
This medicine contains ethynodiol and ethinyl estradiol as active ingredients. It is an oral contraceptive prescribed to prevent pregnancy and/or to regulate menstrual periods.

The drug works by altering the mucus at the cervix entrance to prevent the entry of sperm. It also alters the uterus lining to resist implantation of the fertilized egg. Oral contraceptives create the same chemical atmosphere in blood that exists during pregnancy.

Before using this medicine
Before you use this medicine check with your doctor, or pharmacist:
- if you ever had any unusual or allergic reaction to estrogens or progestogen;
- if you are pregnant or want to become pregnant within three months;
- if you are breast-feeding an infant;
- if you have any of the following medical problems:
Diabetes
Ailments of the breast
Disorders of the uterus
Migraine or epilepsy
High blood pressure
Asthma or heart conditions
Kidney disease
Gallstones

Treatment
This medication is used to prevent pregnancy or to regulate menstrual periods.

Adverse reactions
Along with the needed effects, a medicine may cause some unwanted effects or adverse reactions.
- *An increased risk of the following adverse reactions has been associated with the use of oral contraceptives:*
Thrombophlebitis
Venous thrombosis
Arterial thromboembolism
Pulmonary (lung) embolism
Myocardial infarction
Cerebral hemorrhage
Cerebral thrombosis
Hypertension
Gallbladder disease
Hepatic (liver) hepatomas
Benign lifer tumors
- *The following adverse reactions have been reported in patients receiving oral contraceptives and are believed to be drug-related:*
Nausea and vomiting
Abdominal cramps
Breakthrough bleeding
Spotting
Change in menstrual flow
Amenorrhea
Temporary infertility
Edema
Breast changes
Weight changes
Cholestatic jaundice
Migraine
Rash (allergic)
Mental depression
Vaginal candidiasis

Interactions
This medicine may interact with several other drugs such as antibiotics, anticoagulants, anticonvulsants, antidepressants, oral antidiabetics, antihistamines, barbiturates, oral hypoglycemics, insulin, meperidine.
- Be sure to tell your doctor about any medications you are currently taking.

Storage
Tablets should be stored at room temperature; store away from heat and direct light. Keep out of reach of children, since this medicine may be dangerous in children.

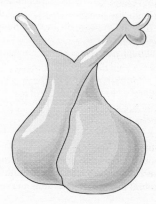

NEMBUTAL

Properties

This medicine contains as active ingredient the barbiturate pentobarbital. Barbiturates belong to the group of medicines called central nervous system depressants (medicines that slow down the nervous system).

Barbiturates may partially block nerve impulses at nerve-cell connections. They may be used to treat insomnia (sleeplessness) by helping patients fall asleep. Also, they may be used to relieve anxiety or tension. Some of the barbiturates are used as anticonvulsants to help control convulsions in certain disorders or diseases, such as epilepsy. If too much of the drug is used, it may become habit-forming (causing mental or physical dependence).

Before using this medicine

Before you use this medicine check with your doctor, or pharmacist:

- if you ever had any unusual or allergic reaction to this medicine or one of its components.
- if you are on a low-salt, low-sugar, or any other special diet, or if you are allergic to preservatives or dyes.
- if you are pregnant or intend to become pregnant while using this medicine, since barbiturates have been shown to increase the chance of birth defects in humans. Taking barbiturates regularly during the last 3 months of pregnancy may cause the baby to become dependent on the medicine. This may lead to withdrawal side effects in the baby after birth.
- if you have any of the following medical problems:
  Anemia (severe)
  Diabetes mellitus (sugar disease)
  Hyperactivity (in children)
  Kidney or lifer disease
  Mental depression
  Overactive thyroid

Treatment

This medication is used to treat the symptoms of your medical condition. Barbiturates act in the central nervous system; some of their side effects are also caused by actions in the central nervous system. Use this medicine as directed by your doctor. Do not use more of it, do not use it more often, and do not use it for a longer period of time than your doctor ordered.

- If you are taking this medication on a regular schedule and you miss a dose, take the missed dose as soon as possible, unless it is almost time for your next dose. In that case do not take the missed dose at all.
- If a barbiturate is used for a long time, it may become habit-forming. Physical dependence may lead to withdrawal side effects when you stop taking this medicine.

Side effects

Along with the needed effects, a medicine may cause some unwanted effects. These side effects may go away during treatment as your body adjusts to the medicine. Such minor side effects are: depression, confusion, diarrhea, nausea, vomiting, joint or muscle pain, slurred speech, hallucinations, headache, decreased sex drive.

- Check with your doctor immediately if any of the following side effects occur:
  Rash or hives
  Face, lip or eyelid swelling
  Sore throat, fever
  Agitation
  Slow heartbeat
  Difficult breathing or chest pain

Interactions

This medicine may interact with several other drugs such as medicines acting on the central nervous system (e.g., antihistamines; beta-adrenergic blockers; MAO inhibitors; mind-altering drugs; nabilone; antidepressants; clozapine; anticonvulsants).

Storage

The medicine should be stored at room temperature in a tightly closed, light-resistant container. Keep out of reach of children since overdose is very dangerous in children.

NEO-BARB

Properties

This medicine contains as active ingredient the barbiturate butabarbital. Barbiturates belong to the group of medicines called central nervous system depressants (medicines that slow down the nervous system).

Barbiturates may partially block nerve impulses at nerve-cell connections. They may be used to treat insomnia (sleeplessness) by helping patients fall asleep. Also, they may be used to relieve anxiety or tension. Some of the barbiturates are used as anticonvulsants to help control convulsions in certain disorders or diseases, such as epilepsy. If too much of the drug is used, it may become habit-forming (causing mental or physical dependence).

Before using this medicine

Before you use this medicine check with your doctor, or pharmacist:
- if you ever had any unusual or allergic reaction to this medicine or one of its components.
- if you are on a low-salt, low-sugar, or any other special diet, or if you are allergic to preservatives or dyes.
- if you are pregnant or intend to become pregnant while using this medicine, since barbiturates have been shown to increase the chance of birth defects in humans. Taking barbiturates regularly during the last 3 months of pregnancy may cause the baby to become dependent on the medicine. This may lead to withdrawal side effects in the baby after birth.
- if you have any of the following medical problems:
  Anemia (severe)
  Diabetes mellitus (sugar disease)
  Hyperactivity (in children)
  Kidney or lifer disease
  Mental depression
  Overactive thyroid

Treatment

This medication is used to treat the symptoms of your medical condition. Barbiturates act in the central nervous system; some of their side effects are also caused by actions in the central nervous system. Use this medicine as directed by your doctor. Do not use more of it, do not use it more often, and do not use it for a longer period of time than your doctor ordered.

- If you are taking this medication on a regular schedule and you miss a dose, take the missed dose as soon as possible, unless it is almost time for your next dose. In that case do not take the missed dose at all.
- If a barbiturate is used for a long time, it may become habit-forming. Physical dependence may lead to withdrawal side effects when you stop taking this medicine.

Side effects

Along with the needed effects, a medicine may cause some unwanted effects. These side effects may go away during treatment as your body adjusts to the medicine. Such minor side effects are: depression, confusion, diarrhea, nausea, vomiting, joint or muscle pain, slurred speech, hallucinations, headache, decreased sex drive.

- Check with your doctor immediately if any of the following side effects occur:
  Rash or hives
  Face, lip or eyelid swelling
  Sore throat, fever
  Agitation
  Slow heartbeat
  Difficult breathing or chest pain

Interactions

This medicine may interact with several other drugs such as medicines acting on the central nervous system (e.g., antihistamines; beta-adrenergic blockers; MAO inhibitors; mind-altering drugs; nabilone; antidepressants; clozapine; anticonvulsants).

Storage

The medicine should be stored at room temperature in a tightly closed, light-resistant container. Keep out of reach of children since overdose is very dangerous in children.

NEO-ESTRONE

Properties
This medicine contains esterified estrogens as active ingredients. The medicine is prescribed for treatment of estrogen deficiency; it restores normal estrogen levels in tissues. There is no evidence that this drug is effective for nervous symptoms or depression occurring during menopause. They should not be used to treat this condition; they should be used only to replace the estrogen that is naturally absent after menopause.

Before using this medicine
Before you use this medicine check with your doctor, or pharmacist:
- if you ever had any unusual or allergic reaction to estrogens;
- if you are pregnant or intend to become pregnant within three months;
- if you are breast-feeding an infant;
- if you have any of the following medical problems:
  Diabetes
  Breast cancer
  Fibrocystic breast disease
  Fibroid uterine tumors
  Endometriosis
  Migraine headaches
  Epilepsy
  Porphyria
  High blood pressure
  Asthma
  Congestive heart failure
  Kidney disease
  Gallstones

Treatment
This medication is used to treat estrogen deficiency, specific symptoms of menopause, estrogen-deficiency osteoporosis, atrophic vaginitis, prostate cancer. For safe and effective use of this medicine:
- ◆ Follow your doctor's instructions if this medicine was prescribed.
- ◆ Follow the manufacturer's package directions if you are treating yourself.
- ◆ Estrogens have been reported to increase the risk of endometrial carcinoma.

Side effects
Along with the needed effects, a medicine may cause some unwanted effects. Possible side effects include:
  Stomach cramps
  Profuse bleeding
  Appetite loss
  Nausea and vomiting
  Swollen breasts
  Change in menstruation
  Rash, skin blisters
  Depression
  Dizziness

Overdose
The following symptoms may indicate an overdose:
  Nausea and vomiting
  Fluid retention
  Breast enlargement
  Abnormal vaginal bleeding
- ■ Call a doctor or hospital emergency room for instructions.

Interactions
This medicine may interact with several other drugs such as adrenocorticosteroids, antidepressants, oral antidiabetics, insulin, phenobarbital, primidone.
- ■ Be sure to tell your doctor about any medications you are currently taking.

Storage
Capsules, tablets, vaginal cream, transdermal patches, etc. should be stored at room temperature; store away from heat and direct light. Keep out of reach of children, since this medicine may be dangerous in children.

NEOCIDEN (Ophthalmic)

Properties
This medicine contains an ophthalmic antibacterial, as active ingredient. It helps the body to overcome eye infections on surface tissues of the eye. It is most useful when the infecting organism is one known to be sensitive to the antibacterial drug.

The drug penetrates the bacterial cell membrane and prevents cells from multiplying.

Before using this medicine
Before you use this medicine check with your doctor:
– if you ever had any unusual or allergic reaction to any of the compounds of the medicine.
– if you are on a low-salt, low-sugar, or any other special diet, or if you are allergic to any substance, such as sulfites or other preservatives or dyes.
– if you are pregnant or intend to become pregnant while using this medicine. Although ophthalmic antibacterials have been found to be safe for use during pregnancy, you should check with your doctor before taking any drug if you are pregnant.

Treatment
This medication is used to treat an infection caused by bacteria. The medicine may be used in the form of eye drops or as an eye ointment. Use the medication as directed, Do not miss a dose. If you forget a dose, use it as soon as you remember. Notify your doctor if eye symptoms fail to improve in two to four days.
◆ To apply eye drops: Till the head backward when applying the eye drops. Pull the lower eyelid away from the eye to form a pouch. After applying the drop, keep the eye closed for a minute or so. This allows the medication to come in contact with the infection.
◆ To apply eye ointment: Pull lower lid down from eye to form a pouch. Squeeze tube to apply thin strip of ointment into pouch. Close eye for 1 to 2 minutes.

Always wash your hands before applying the ointment.

The drug starts to work in about one hour. Treatment may require 7 to 10 days to control infection.

Older adults or seniors may take this medication without special restriction.

Side effects
Along with the needed effects, a medicine may cause some unwanted effects. Side effects that usually do not require medical attention: occasional local irritation after application to the eye. Ointments may cause blurred vision for a few minutes; continue the use of the eye drops or ointment, but tell your doctor at the next visit.
■ Discontinue the use of eye drops or eye ointment in the following cases:
Sore throat
Aplastic anemia
Pale skin
Unusual redness of the eye
Unusual irritation of the eye
Fever
Unusual bleeding
Unusual bruising
■ Tell your doctor about any side effects that are persistent or particularly bothersome. In case of prolonged use sensitivity reactions may develop.

Interactions
Clinically significant interactions with oral or injected medicines are unlikely. Do not use the eye drops or ointment with any other eye drops or ointment without checking with your ophthalmologist.

Storage
Keep bottle (with eye drops) or container (containing ointment) lightly closed. Store in a cool place, but Do not freeze. Wash hands immediately after using. Do not store in the bathroom medicine cabinet because the heat or moisture may cause the medicine to break down. Do not keep outdated medicine or medicine no longer needed. Flush the contents of the bottle or tube down the toilet, unless otherwise directed.

NEOMYCIN (Ophthalmic)

Properties
This medicine contains an ophthalmic antibacterial, as active ingredient. It helps the body to overcome eye infections on surface tissues of the eye. It is most useful when the infecting organism is one known to be sensitive to the antibacterial drug.

The drug penetrates the bacterial cell membrane and prevents cells from multiplying.

Before using this medicine
Before you use this medicine check with your doctor:
- if you ever had any unusual or allergic reaction to any of the compounds of the medicine.
- if you are on a low-salt, low-sugar, or any other special diet, or if you are allergic to any substance, such as sulfites or other preservatives or dyes.
- if you are pregnant or intend to become pregnant while using this medicine. Although ophthalmic antibacterials have been found to be safe for use during pregnancy, you should check with your doctor before taking any drug if you are pregnant.

Treatment
This medication is used to treat an infection caused by bacteria. The medicine may be used in the form of eye drops or as an eye ointment. Use the medication as directed, Do not miss a dose. If you forget a dose, use it as soon as you remember. Notify your doctor if eye symptoms fail to improve in two to four days.
- ◆ To apply eye drops: Till the head backward when applying the eye drops. Pull the lower eyelid away from the eye to form a pouch. After applying the drop, keep the eye closed for a minute or so. This allows the medication to come in contact with the infection.
- ◆ To apply eye ointment: Pull lower lid down from eye to form a pouch. Squeeze tube to apply thin strip of ointment into pouch. Close eye for 1 to 2 minutes.

Always wash your hands before applying the ointment.

The drug starts to work in about one hour. Treatment may require 7 to 10 days to control infection.

Older adults or seniors may take this medication without special restriction.

Side effects
Along with the needed effects, a medicine may cause some unwanted effects. Side effects that usually do not require medical attention: occasional local irritation after application to the eye. Ointments may cause blurred vision for a few minutes; continue the use of the eye drops or ointment, but tell your doctor at the next visit.
- ■ Discontinue the use of eye drops or eye ointment in the following cases:
  Sore throat
  Aplastic anemia
  Pale skin
  Unusual redness of the eye
  Unusual irritation of the eye
  Fever
  Unusual bleeding
  Unusual bruising
- ■ Tell your doctor about any side effects that are persistent or particularly bothersome. In case of prolonged use sensitivity reactions may develop.

Interactions
Clinically significant interactions with oral or injected medicines are unlikely. Do not use the eye drops or ointment with any other eye drops or ointment without checking with your ophthalmologist.

Storage
Keep bottle (with eye drops) or container (containing ointment) lightly closed. Store in a cool place, but Do not freeze. Wash hands immediately after using. Do not store in the bathroom medicine cabinet because the heat or moisture may cause the medicine to break down. Do not keep outdated medicine or medicine no longer needed. Flush the contents of the bottle or tube down the toilet, unless otherwise directed.

NEOSPORIN (Ophthalmic)

Properties
This medicine contains an ophthalmic antibacterial, as active ingredient. It helps the body to overcome eye infections on surface tissues of the eye. It is most useful when the infecting organism is one known to be sensitive to the antibacterial drug.

The drug penetrates the bacterial cell membrane and prevents cells from multiplying.

Before using this medicine
Before you use this medicine check with your doctor:
- if you ever had any unusual or allergic reaction to any of the compounds of the medicine.
- if you are on a low-salt, low-sugar, or any other special diet, or if you are allergic to any substance, such as sulfites or other preservatives or dyes.
- if you are pregnant or intend to become pregnant while using this medicine. Although ophthalmic antibacterials have been found to be safe for use during pregnancy, you should check with your doctor before taking any drug if you are pregnant.

Treatment
This medication is used to treat an infection caused by bacteria. The medicine may be used in the form of eye drops or as an eye ointment. Use the medication as directed, Do not miss a dose. If you forget a dose, use it as soon as you remember. Notify your doctor if eye symptoms fail to improve in two to four days.
- To apply eye drops: Till the head backward when applying the eye drops. Pull the lower eyelid away from the eye to form a pouch. After applying the drop, keep the eye closed for a minute or so. This allows the medication to come in contact with the infection.
- To apply eye ointment: Pull lower lid down from eye to form a pouch. Squeeze tube to apply thin strip of ointment into pouch. Close eye for 1 to 2 minutes.

Always wash your hands before applying the ointment. The drug starts to work in about one hour. Treatment may require 7 to 10 days to control infection. Older adults or seniors may take this medication without special restriction.

Side effects
Along with the needed effects, a medicine may cause some unwanted effects. Side effects that usually do not require medical attention: occasional local irritation after application to the eye. Ointments may cause blurred vision for a few minutes; continue the use of the eye drops or ointment, but tell your doctor at the next visit.
- Discontinue the use of eye drops or eye ointment in the following cases:
  Sore throat
  Aplastic anemia
  Pale skin
  Unusual redness of the eye
  Unusual irritation of the eye
  Fever
  Unusual bleeding
  Unusual bruising
- Tell your doctor about any side effects that are persistent or particularly bothersome. In case of prolonged use sensitivity reactions may develop.

Interactions
Clinically significant interactions with oral or injected medicines are unlikely. Do not use the eye drops or ointment with any other eye drops or ointment without checking with your ophthalmologist.

Storage
Keep bottle (with eye drops) or container (containing ointment) lightly closed. Store in a cool place, but Do not freeze. Wash hands immediately after using. Do not store in the bathroom medicine cabinet because the heat or moisture may cause the medicine to break down.

Do not keep outdated medicine or medicine no longer needed. Flush the contents of the bottle or tube down the toilet, unless otherwise directed.

NEOTAL (Ophthalmic)

Properties

This medicine contains an ophthalmic antibacterial, as active ingredient. It helps the body to overcome eye infections on surface tissues of the eye. It is most useful when the infecting organism is one known to be sensitive to the antibacterial drug.

The drug penetrates the bacterial cell membrane and prevents cells from multiplying.

Before using this medicine

Before you use this medicine check with your doctor:

– if you ever had any unusual or allergic reaction to any of the compounds of the medicine.

– if you are on a low-salt, low-sugar, or any other special diet, or if you are allergic to any substance, such as sulfites or other preservatives or dyes.

– if you are pregnant or intend to become pregnant while using this medicine. Although ophthalmic antibacterials have been found to be safe for use during pregnancy, you should check with your doctor before taking any drug if you are pregnant.

Treatment

This medication is used to treat an infection caused by bacteria. The medicine may be used in the form of eye drops or as an eye ointment. Use the medication as directed, Do not miss a dose. If you forget a dose, use it as soon as you remember. Notify your doctor if eye symptoms fail to improve in two to four days.

◆ To apply eye drops: Till the head backward when applying the eye drops. Pull the lower eyelid away from the eye to form a pouch. After applying the drop, keep the eye closed for a minute or so. This allows the medication to come in contact with the infection.

◆ To apply eye ointment: Pull lower lid down from eye to form a pouch. Squeeze tube to apply thin strip of ointment into pouch. Close eye for 1 to 2 minutes.

Always wash your hands before applying the ointment. The drug starts to work in about one hour. Treatment may require 7 to 10 days to control infection. Older adults or seniors may take this medication without special restriction.

Side effects

Along with the needed effects, a medicine may cause some unwanted effects. Side effects that usually do not require medical attention: occasional local irritation after application to the eye. Ointments may cause blurred vision for a few minutes; continue the use of the eye drops or ointment, but tell your doctor at the next visit.

■ Discontinue the use of eye drops or eye ointment in the following cases:
Sore throat
Aplastic anemia
Pale skin
Unusual redness of the eye
Unusual irritation of the eye
Fever
Unusual bleeding
Unusual bruising

■ Tell your doctor about any side effects that are persistent or particularly bothersome. In case of prolonged use sensitivity reactions may develop.

Interactions

Clinically significant interactions with oral or injected medicines are unlikely. Do not use the eye drops or ointment with any other eye drops or ointment without checking with your ophthalmologist.

Storage

Keep bottle (with eye drops) or container (containing ointment) lightly closed. Store in a cool place, but Do not freeze. Wash hands immediately after using.

Do not store in the bathroom medicine cabinet because the heat or moisture may cause the medicine to break down.

Do not keep outdated medicine or medicine no longer needed. Flush the contents of the bottle or tube down the toilet, unless otherwise directed.

NEOTRICIN (Ophthalmic)

Properties
This medicine contains an ophthalmic antibacterial, as active ingredient. It helps the body to overcome eye infections on surface tissues of the eye. It is most useful when the infecting organism is one known to be sensitive to the antibacterial drug.

The drug penetrates the bacterial cell membrane and prevents cells from multiplying.

Before using this medicine
Before you use this medicine check with your doctor:
- if you ever had any unusual or allergic reaction to any of the compounds of the medicine.
- if you are on a low-salt, low-sugar, or any other special diet, or if you are allergic to any substance, such as sulfites or other preservatives or dyes.
- if you are pregnant or intend to become pregnant while using this medicine. Although ophthalmic antibacterials have been found to be safe for use during pregnancy, you should check with your doctor before taking any drug if you are pregnant.

Treatment
This medication is used to treat an infection caused by bacteria. The medicine may be used in the form of eye drops or as an eye ointment. Use the medication as directed, Do not miss a dose. If you forget a dose, use it as soon as you remember. Notify your doctor if eye symptoms fail to improve in two to four days.

◆ To apply eye drops: Till the head backward when applying the eye drops. Pull the lower eyelid away from the eye to form a pouch. After applying the drop, keep the eye closed for a minute or so. This allows the medication to come in contact with the infection.

◆ To apply eye ointment: Pull lower lid down from eye to form a pouch. Squeeze tube to apply thin strip of ointment into pouch. Close eye for 1 to 2 minutes.

Always wash your hands before applying the ointment. The drug starts to work in about one hour. Treatment may require 7 to 10 days to control infection. Older adults or seniors may take this medication without special restriction.

Side effects
Along with the needed effects, a medicine may cause some unwanted effects. Side effects that usually do not require medical attention: occasional local irritation after application to the eye. Ointments may cause blurred vision for a few minutes; continue the use of the eye drops or ointment, but tell your doctor at the next visit.

■ Discontinue the use of eye drops or eye ointment in the following cases:
Sore throat
Aplastic anemia
Pale skin
Unusual redness of the eye
Unusual irritation of the eye
Fever
Unusual bleeding
Unusual bruising

■ Tell your doctor about any side effects that are persistent or particularly bothersome. In case of prolonged use sensitivity reactions may develop.

Interactions
Clinically significant interactions with oral or injected medicines are unlikely. Do not use the eye drops or ointment with any other eye drops or ointment without checking with your ophthalmologist.

Storage
Keep bottle (with eye drops) or container (containing ointment) lightly closed. Store in a cool place, but Do not freeze. Wash hands immediately after using.

Do not store in the bathroom medicine cabinet because the heat or moisture may cause the medicine to break down.

Do not keep outdated medicine or medicine no longer needed. Flush the contents of the bottle or tube down the toilet, unless otherwise directed.

NICARDIPINE

Properties
This medicine contains nicardipine as active ingredient. It is a so-called calcium channel blocker, working by blocking the passage of calcium into heart and smooth muscle. Since calcium is an essential factor in muscle contraction, any medicine that affects calcium in this way will interfere with the contraction of these muscles.

The medicine works by:
♦ reducing the work that the heart must perform;
♦ reducing the normal arterial blood pressure;
♦ increasing oxygen to the heart muscle.

The medicine is prescribed for the treatment of attacks of angina pectoris, irregular heartbeat, and high blood pressure. In many cases it can be used for the treatment and prevention of migraine.

Before using this medicine
Before you use this medicine check with your doctor, or pharmacist:
− if you ever had any unusual or allergic reaction to this medicine or any calcium channel blocker;
− if you are pregnant or intend to become pregnant while using this medicine;
− if you have low blood pressure;
− if you have kidney or lifer disease;
− if you are breast-feeding an infant;
− if you easily get a rash or intensity sunburn in areas exposed to sun or ultraviolet light.

Treatment
This medication is used for treatment of heart conditions (for instance, angina pectoris) and high blood pressure. Tablets, capsules or extended-release tablets should be taken with liquid. The usual dose amounts to 30 to 100 milligrams a day.

For safe and effective use of medicine:
♦ Follow your doctor's instructions if this medicine was prescribed.
♦ Follow the manufacturer's package directions if you are treating yourself.

Side effects
Along with the needed effects, a medicine may cause some unwanted effects. Possible side effects include:
Tiredness
Changes in heartbeat
Wheezing
Cough
Shortness of breath
Dizziness
Fainting
Numbness in hands and feet
Tingling in hands and feet
Difficult urination
Constipation

Overdose
The following symptoms may be a sign of overdose:
Unusually fast heartbeat
Unusually slow heartbeat
Loss of consciousness
Cardiac arrest
▪ Call a doctor or hospital emergency room for instructions. If necessary start first aid immediately.

Interactions
The effect of this medicine may cause a blood pressure drop if taken together with antihypertensives. Cimetidine may increase the effect of the calcium blocker.

The simultaneous use of diuretics and calcium channel blockers may cause dangerous blood pressure drop.
▪ Be sure to tell your doctor about any medications you are currently taking.

Storage
Capsules, tablets, etc. should be stored at room temperature; store away from heat and direct light. Keep out of reach of children, since this medicine may be dangerous in children.

NIONG

Properties
This medicine contains nitroglycerin as active ingredient. Nitrates improve the supply of blood and oxygen to the heart. This medication is for oral use.

Before using this medicine
Before you use this medicine check with your doctor, or pharmacist:
- if you ever had any unusual or allergic reaction to nitrates or nitrites.
- if you are on a low-salt, low-sugar, or any other special diet, or if you are allergic to any substance, such as sulfites or other preservatives or dyes.
- if you are pregnant or intend to become pregnant while using this medicine. Although nitrates have not been shown to cause problems in humans, the chance always exists.
- if you are breast-feeding an infant.
- if you have recently had a heart attack or stroke.
- if you have any of the following medical problems:
  Anemia
  Glaucoma
  Intestinal problems
  Overactive thyroid
- if you are now taking any of the following medicines or types of medicines:
  Antihypertensives
  Asthma or hay fever medicine
  Cold medicine
  Decongestant
  Medicine for appetite control
  Narcotic
  Pain medicine
  Sinus congestion medicine

Treatment
This medication is used to treat and prevent angina (chest pain). Nitroglycerin is a vasodilator, which relaxes the muscles of the blood vessels, causing an increase in the oxygen supply to the heart. The oral tablets, capsules, ointment and patches do not act quickly; they are used to prevent chest pain. The sublingual tablets and oral spray act quickly and can be used to relieve chest pain after it has started.

- Take this medicine exactly as directed by your doctor or pharmacist. It will work only if taken correctly.
- If you are taking this medicine regularly and you miss a dose, take it as soon as possible. However, if your next scheduled dose; is within 2 hours (or within 6 hours for extended-release capsules or tablets), skip the missed dose and go back to your regular dosing schedule.
- If you have been taking this medicine regularly for several weeks or more, do not suddenly stop using it. Stopping suddenly may bring on attacks of angina.

Side effects
There are a number of side effects that usually do not require medical attention. These possible side effects may go away during treatment; however, if they continue or are bothersome, check with your doctor, nurse, or pharmacist. More common are: dizziness, lightheadedness, or fainting when standing up; fast pulse; flushing of face and neck; headache; nausea or vomiting.
Side effects that should be reported to your doctor are: blurred vision; dry mouth; severe or prolonged headache; skin rash.

Interactions
This medicine may interact with several other drugs such as tricyclic antidepressants and cough medicines. Before starting to take or apply nitroglycerin, be sure to tell your doctor about any medications you are currently taking.

Storage
Tablets, capsules, and oral spray should be stored as in a tightly capped bottle in a cool, dry place. Ointment and patches should be stored at room temperature in their original containers. Keep out of reach of children. Do not keep outdated medicine or medicine no longer needed.

NISOLDIPINE

Properties

This medicine contains nisoldipine as active ingredient. It is a so-called calcium channel blocker, working by blocking the passage of calcium into heart and smooth muscle. Since calcium is an essential factor in muscle contraction, any medicine that affects calcium in this way will interfere with the contraction of these muscles.

The medicine works by:
♦ reducing the work that the heart must perform;
♦ reducing the normal arterial blood pressure;
♦ increasing oxygen to the heart muscle.

The medicine is prescribed for the treatment of attacks of angina pectoris, irregular heartbeat, and high blood pressure. In many cases it can be used for the treatment and prevention of migraine.

Before using this medicine

Before you use this medicine check with your doctor, or pharmacist:
- if you ever had any unusual or allergic reaction to this medicine or any calcium channel blocker;
- if you are pregnant or intend to become pregnant while using this medicine;
- if you have low blood pressure;
- if you have kidney or lifer disease;
- if you are breast-feeding an infant;
- if you easily get a rash or intensity sunburn in areas exposed to sun or ultraviolet light.

Treatment

This medication is used for treatment of heart conditions (for instance, angina pectoris) and high blood pressure. Tablets, capsules or extended-release tablets should be taken with liquid. The usual dose amounts to 30 to 100 milligrams a day.

For safe and effective use of medicine:
♦ Follow your doctor's instructions if this medicine was prescribed.
♦ Follow the manufacturer's package directions if you are treating yourself.

Side effects

Along with the needed effects, a medicine may cause some unwanted effects. Possible side effects include:
Tiredness
Changes in heartbeat
Wheezing
Cough
Shortness of breath
Dizziness
Fainting
Numbness in hands and feet
Tingling in hands and feet
Difficult urination
Constipation

Overdose

The following symptoms may be a sign of overdose:
Unusually fast heartbeat
Unusually slow heartbeat
Loss of consciousness
Cardiac arrest
■ Call a doctor or hospital emergency room for instructions. If necessary start first aid immediately.

Interactions

The effect of this medicine may cause a blood pressure drop if taken together with antihypertensives. Cimetidine may increase the effect of the calcium blocker.

The simultaneous use of diuretics and calcium channel blockers may cause dangerous blood pressure drop.
■ Be sure to tell your doctor about any medications you are currently taking.

Storage

Capsules, tablets, etc. should be stored at room temperature; store away from heat and direct light. Keep out of reach of children, since this medicine may be dangerous in children.

NITRO-BID

Properties

This medicine contains nitroglycerin as active ingredient. Nitrates improve the supply of blood and oxygen to the heart. This medication is for oral use.

Before using this medicine

Before you use this medicine check with your doctor, or pharmacist:
- if you ever had any unusual or allergic reaction to nitrates or nitrites.
- if you are on a low-salt, low-sugar, or any other special diet, or if you are allergic to any substance, such as sulfites or other preservatives or dyes.
- if you are pregnant or intend to become pregnant while using this medicine. Although nitrates have not been shown to cause problems in humans, the chance always exists.
- if you are breast-feeding an infant.
- if you have recently had a heart attack or stroke.
- if you have any of the following medical problems:
  Anemia
  Glaucoma
  Intestinal problems
  Overactive thyroid
- if you are now taking any of the following medicines or types of medicines:
  Antihypertensives
  Asthma or hay fever medicine
  Cold medicine
  Decongestant
  Medicine for appetite control
  Narcotic
  Pain medicine
  Sinus congestion medicine

Treatment

This medication is used to treat and prevent angina (chest pain). Nitroglycerin is a vasodilator, which relaxes the muscles of the blood vessels, causing an increase in the oxygen supply to the heart. The oral tablets, capsules, ointment and patches do not act quickly; they are used to prevent chest pain. The sublingual tablets and oral spray act quickly and can be used to relieve chest pain after it has started.

- Take this medicine exactly as directed by your doctor or pharmacist. It will work only if taken correctly.
- If you are taking this medicine regularly and you miss a dose, take it as soon as possible. However, if your next scheduled dose; is within 2 hours (or within 6 hours for extended-release capsules or tablets), skip the missed dose and go back to your regular dosing schedule.
- If you have been taking this medicine regularly for several weeks or more, do not suddenly stop using it. Stopping suddenly may bring on attacks of angina.

Side effects

There are a number of side effects that usually do not require medical attention. These possible side effects may go away during treatment; however, if they continue or are bothersome, check with your doctor, nurse, or pharmacist. More common are: dizziness, lightheadedness, or fainting when standing up; fast pulse; flushing of face and neck; headache; nausea or vomiting.

Side effects that should be reported to your doctor are: blurred vision; dry mouth; severe or prolonged headache; skin rash.

Interactions

This medicine may interact with several other drugs such as tricyclic antidepressants and cough medicines. Before starting to take or apply nitroglycerin, be sure to tell your doctor about any medications you are currently taking.

Storage

Tablets, capsules, and oral spray should be stored as in a tightly capped bottle in a cool, dry place. Ointment and patches should be stored at room temperature in their original containers. Keep out of reach of children. Do not keep outdated medicine or medicine no longer needed.

NITROBON

Properties
This medicine contains nitroglycerin as active ingredient. Nitrates improve the supply of blood and oxygen to the heart. This medication is for oral use.

Before using this medicine
Before you use this medicine check with your doctor, or pharmacist:
- if you ever had any unusual or allergic reaction to nitrates or nitrites.
- if you are on a low-salt, low-sugar, or any other special diet, or if you are allergic to any substance, such as sulfites or other preservatives or dyes.
- if you are pregnant or intend to become pregnant while using this medicine. Although nitrates have not been shown to cause problems in humans, the chance always exists.
- if you are breast-feeding an infant.
- if you have recently had a heart attack or stroke.
- if you have any of the following medical problems:
  Anemia
  Glaucoma
  Intestinal problems
  Overactive thyroid
- if you are now taking any of the following medicines or types of medicines:
  Antihypertensives
  Asthma or hay fever medicine
  Cold medicine
  Decongestant
  Medicine for appetite control
  Narcotic
  Pain medicine
  Sinus congestion medicine

Treatment
This medication is used to treat and prevent angina (chest pain). Nitroglycerin is a vasodilator, which relaxes the muscles of the blood vessels, causing an increase in the oxygen supply to the heart. The oral tablets, capsules, ointment and patches do not act quickly; they are used to prevent chest pain. The sublingual tablets and oral spray act quickly and can be used to relieve chest pain after it has started.

- Take this medicine exactly as directed by your doctor or pharmacist. It will work only if taken correctly.
- If you are taking this medicine regularly and you miss a dose, take it as soon as possible. However, if your next scheduled dose; is within 2 hours (or within 6 hours for extended-release capsules or tablets), skip the missed dose and go back to your regular dosing schedule.
- If you have been taking this medicine regularly for several weeks or more, do not suddenly stop using it. Stopping suddenly may bring on attacks of angina.

Side effects
There are a number of side effects that usually do not require medical attention. These possible side effects may go away during treatment; however, if they continue or are bothersome, check with your doctor, nurse, or pharmacist. More common are: dizziness, lightheadedness, or fainting when standing up; fast pulse; flushing of face and neck; headache; nausea or vomiting.

Side effects that should be reported to your doctor are: blurred vision; dry mouth; severe or prolonged headache; skin rash.

Interactions
This medicine may interact with several other drugs such as tricyclic antidepressants and cough medicines. Before starting to take or apply nitroglycerin, be sure to tell your doctor about any medications you are currently taking.

Storage
Tablets, capsules, and oral spray should be stored as in a tightly capped bottle in a cool, dry place. Ointment and patches should be stored at room temperature in their original containers. Keep out of reach of children. Do not keep outdated medicine or medicine no longer needed.

NITROCAP

Properties
This medicine contains nitroglycerin as active ingredient. Nitrates improve the supply of blood and oxygen to the heart. This medication is for oral use.

Before using this medicine
Before you use this medicine check with your doctor, or pharmacist:
- if you ever had any unusual or allergic reaction to nitrates or nitrites.
- if you are on a low-salt, low-sugar, or any other special diet, or if you are allergic to any substance, such as sulfites or other preservatives or dyes.
- if you are pregnant or intend to become pregnant while using this medicine. Although nitrates have not been shown to cause problems in humans, the chance always exists.
- if you are breast-feeding an infant.
- if you have recently had a heart attack or stroke.
- if you have any of the following medical problems:
  Anemia
  Glaucoma
  Intestinal problems
  Overactive thyroid
- if you are now taking any of the following medicines or types of medicines:
  Antihypertensives
  Asthma or hay fever medicine
  Cold medicine
  Decongestant
  Medicine for appetite control
  Narcotic
  Pain medicine
  Sinus congestion medicine

Treatment
This medication is used to treat and prevent angina (chest pain). Nitroglycerin is a vasodilator, which relaxes the muscles of the blood vessels, causing an increase in the oxygen supply to the heart. The oral tablets, capsules, ointment and patches do not act quickly; they are used to prevent chest pain. The sublingual tablets and oral spray act quickly and can be used to relieve chest pain after it has started.

- Take this medicine exactly as directed by your doctor or pharmacist. It will work only if taken correctly.
- If you are taking this medicine regularly and you miss a dose, take it as soon as possible. However, if your next scheduled dose; is within 2 hours (or within 6 hours for extended-release capsules or tablets), skip the missed dose and go back to your regular dosing schedule.
- If you have been taking this medicine regularly for several weeks or more, do not suddenly stop using it. Stopping suddenly may bring on attacks of angina.

Side effects
There are a number of side effects that usually do not require medical attention. These possible side effects may go away during treatment; however, if they continue or are bothersome, check with your doctor, nurse, or pharmacist. More common are: dizziness, lightheadedness, or fainting when standing up; fast pulse; flushing of face and neck; headache; nausea or vomiting.

Side effects that should be reported to your doctor are: blurred vision; dry mouth; severe or prolonged headache; skin rash.

Interactions
This medicine may interact with several other drugs such as tricyclic antidepressants and cough medicines. Before starting to take or apply nitroglycerin, be sure to tell your doctor about any medications you are currently taking.

Storage
Tablets, capsules, and oral spray should be stored as in a tightly capped bottle in a cool, dry place. Ointment and patches should be stored at room temperature in their original containers. Keep out of reach of children. Do not keep outdated medicine or medicine no longer needed.

NITROGLYCERINE

Properties
This medicine contains nitroglycerin as active ingredient. Nitrates improve the supply of blood and oxygen to the heart. This medication is for oral use.

Before using this medicine
Before you use this medicine check with your doctor, or pharmacist:
- if you ever had any unusual or allergic reaction to nitrates or nitrites.
- if you are on a low-salt, low-sugar, or any other special diet, or if you are allergic to any substance, such as sulfites or other preservatives or dyes.
- if you are pregnant or intend to become pregnant while using this medicine. Although nitrates have not been shown to cause problems in humans, the chance always exists.
- if you are breast-feeding an infant.
- if you have recently had a heart attack or stroke.
- if you have any of the following medical problems:
  Anemia
  Glaucoma
  Intestinal problems
  Overactive thyroid
- if you are now taking any of the following medicines or types of medicines:
  Antihypertensives
  Asthma or hay fever medicine
  Cold medicine
  Decongestant
  Medicine for appetite control
  Narcotic
  Pain medicine
  Sinus congestion medicine

Treatment
This medication is used to treat and prevent angina (chest pain). Nitroglycerin is a vasodilator, which relaxes the muscles of the blood vessels, causing an increase in the oxygen supply to the heart. The oral tablets, capsules, ointment and patches do not act quickly; they are used to prevent chest pain. The sublingual tablets and oral spray act quickly and can be used to relieve chest pain after it has started.

- Take this medicine exactly as directed by your doctor or pharmacist. It will work only if taken correctly.
- If you are taking this medicine regularly and you miss a dose, take it as soon as possible. However, if your next scheduled dose; is within 2 hours (or within 6 hours for extended-release capsules or tablets), skip the missed dose and go back to your regular dosing schedule.
- If you have been taking this medicine regularly for several weeks or more, do not suddenly stop using it. Stopping suddenly may bring on attacks of angina.

Side effects
There are a number of side effects that usually do not require medical attention. These possible side effects may go away during treatment; however, if they continue or are bothersome, check with your doctor, nurse, or pharmacist. More common are: dizziness, lightheadedness, or fainting when standing up; fast pulse; flushing of face and neck; headache; nausea or vomiting.

Side effects that should be reported to your doctor are: blurred vision; dry mouth; severe or prolonged headache; skin rash.

Interactions
This medicine may interact with several other drugs such as tricyclic antidepressants and cough medicines. Before starting to take or apply nitroglycerin, be sure to tell your doctor about any medications you are currently taking.

Storage
Tablets, capsules, and oral spray should be stored as in a tightly capped bottle in a cool, dry place. Ointment and patches should be stored at room temperature in their original containers. Keep out of reach of children. Do not keep outdated medicine or medicine no longer needed.

NITROGLYN

Properties
This medicine contains nitroglycerin as active ingredient. Nitrates improve the supply of blood and oxygen to the heart. This medication is for oral use.

Before using this medicine
Before you use this medicine check with your doctor, or pharmacist:
- if you ever had any unusual or allergic reaction to nitrates or nitrites.
- if you are on a low-salt, low-sugar, or any other special diet, or if you are allergic to any substance, such as sulfites or other preservatives or dyes.
- if you are pregnant or intend to become pregnant while using this medicine. Although nitrates have not been shown to cause problems in humans, the chance always exists.
- if you are breast-feeding an infant.
- if you have recently had a heart attack or stroke.
- if you have any of the following medical problems:
Anemia
Glaucoma
Intestinal problems
Overactive thyroid
- if you are now taking any of the following medicines or types of medicines:
Antihypertensives
Asthma or hay fever medicine
Cold medicine
Decongestant
Medicine for appetite control
Narcotic
Pain medicine
Sinus congestion medicine

Treatment
This medication is used to treat and prevent angina (chest pain). Nitroglycerin is a vasodilator, which relaxes the muscles of the blood vessels, causing an increase in the oxygen supply to the heart. The oral tablets, capsules, ointment and patches do not act quickly; they are used to prevent chest pain. The sublingual tablets and oral spray act quickly and can be used to relieve chest pain after it has started.

- Take this medicine exactly as directed by your doctor or pharmacist. It will work only if taken correctly.
- If you are taking this medicine regularly and you miss a dose, take it as soon as possible. However, if your next scheduled dose; is within 2 hours (or within 6 hours for extended-release capsules or tablets), skip the missed dose and go back to your regular dosing schedule.
- If you have been taking this medicine regularly for several weeks or more, do not suddenly stop using it. Stopping suddenly may bring on attacks of angina.

Side effects
There are a number of side effects that usually do not require medical attention. These possible side effects may go away during treatment; however, if they continue or are bothersome, check with your doctor, nurse, or pharmacist. More common are: dizziness, lightheadedness, or fainting when standing up; fast pulse; flushing of face and neck; headache; nausea or vomiting.

Side effects that should be reported to your doctor are: blurred vision; dry mouth; severe or prolonged headache; skin rash.

Interactions
This medicine may interact with several other drugs such as tricyclic antidepressants and cough medicines. Before starting to take or apply nitroglycerin, be sure to tell your doctor about any medications you are currently taking.

Storage
Tablets, capsules, and oral spray should be stored as in a tightly capped bottle in a cool, dry place. Ointment and patches should be stored at room temperature in their original containers. Keep out of reach of children. Do not keep outdated medicine or medicine no longer needed.

NITROLIN

Properties
This medicine contains nitroglycerin as active ingredient. Nitrates improve the supply of blood and oxygen to the heart. This medication is for oral use.

Before using this medicine
Before you use this medicine check with your doctor, or pharmacist:
- if you ever had any unusual or allergic reaction to nitrates or nitrites.
- if you are on a low-salt, low-sugar, or any other special diet, or if you are allergic to any substance, such as sulfites or other preservatives or dyes.
- if you are pregnant or intend to become pregnant while using this medicine. Although nitrates have not been shown to cause problems in humans, the chance always exists.
- if you are breast-feeding an infant.
- if you have recently had a heart attack or stroke.
- if you have any of the following medical problems:
  Anemia
  Glaucoma
  Intestinal problems
  Overactive thyroid
- if you are now taking any of the following medicines or types of medicines:
  Antihypertensives
  Asthma or hay fever medicine
  Cold medicine
  Decongestant
  Medicine for appetite control
  Narcotic
  Pain medicine
  Sinus congestion medicine

Treatment
This medication is used to treat and prevent angina (chest pain). Nitroglycerin is a vasodilator, which relaxes the muscles of the blood vessels, causing an increase in the oxygen supply to the heart. The oral tablets, capsules, ointment and patches do not act quickly; they are used to prevent chest pain. The sublingual tablets and oral spray act quickly and can be used to relieve chest pain after it has started.

- Take this medicine exactly as directed by your doctor or pharmacist. It will work only if taken correctly.
- If you are taking this medicine regularly and you miss a dose, take it as soon as possible. However, if your next scheduled dose; is within 2 hours (or within 6 hours for extended-release capsules or tablets), skip the missed dose and go back to your regular dosing schedule.
- If you have been taking this medicine regularly for several weeks or more, do not suddenly stop using it. Stopping suddenly may bring on attacks of angina.

Side effects
There are a number of side effects that usually do not require medical attention. These possible side effects may go away during treatment; however, if they continue or are bothersome, check with your doctor, nurse, or pharmacist. More common are: dizziness, lightheadedness, or fainting when standing up; fast pulse; flushing of face and neck; headache; nausea or vomiting.

Side effects that should be reported to your doctor are: blurred vision; dry mouth; severe or prolonged headache; skin rash.

Interactions
This medicine may interact with several other drugs such as tricyclic antidepressants and cough medicines. Before starting to take or apply nitroglycerin, be sure to tell your doctor about any medications you are currently taking.

Storage
Tablets, capsules, and oral spray should be stored as in a tightly capped bottle in a cool, dry place. Ointment and patches should be stored at room temperature in their original containers. Keep out of reach of children. Do not keep outdated medicine or medicine no longer needed.

NITRO-LONG

Properties
This medicine contains nitroglycerin as active ingredient. Nitrates improve the supply of blood and oxygen to the heart. This medication is for oral use.

Before using this medicine
Before you use this medicine check with your doctor, or pharmacist:
- if you ever had any unusual or allergic reaction to nitrates or nitrites.
- if you are on a low-salt, low-sugar, or any other special diet, or if you are allergic to any substance, such as sulfites or other preservatives or dyes.
- if you are pregnant or intend to become pregnant while using this medicine. Although nitrates have not been shown to cause problems in humans, the chance always exists.
- if you are breast-feeding an infant.
- if you have recently had a heart attack or stroke.
- if you have any of the following medical problems:
  Anemia
  Glaucoma
  Intestinal problems
  Overactive thyroid
- if you are now taking any of the following medicines or types of medicines:
  Antihypertensives
  Asthma or hay fever medicine
  Cold medicine
  Decongestant
  Medicine for appetite control
  Narcotic
  Pain medicine
  Sinus congestion medicine

Treatment
This medication is used to treat and prevent angina (chest pain). Nitroglycerin is a vasodilator, which relaxes the muscles of the blood vessels, causing an increase in the oxygen supply to the heart. The oral tablets, capsules, ointment and patches do not act quickly; they are used to prevent chest pain. The sublingual tablets and oral spray act quickly and can be used to relieve chest pain after it has started.

- Take this medicine exactly as directed by your doctor or pharmacist. It will work only if taken correctly.
- If you are taking this medicine regularly and you miss a dose, take it as soon as possible. However, if your next scheduled dose; is within 2 hours (or within 6 hours for extended-release capsules or tablets), skip the missed dose and go back to your regular dosing schedule.
- If you have been taking this medicine regularly for several weeks or more, do not suddenly stop using it. Stopping suddenly may bring on attacks of angina.

Side effects
There are a number of side effects that usually do not require medical attention. These possible side effects may go away during treatment; however, if they continue or are bothersome, check with your doctor, nurse, or pharmacist. More common are: dizziness, lightheadedness, or fainting when standing up; fast pulse; flushing of face and neck; headache; nausea or vomiting.

Side effects that should be reported to your doctor are: blurred vision; dry mouth; severe or prolonged headache; skin rash.

Interactions
This medicine may interact with several other drugs such as tricyclic antidepressants and cough medicines. Before starting to take or apply nitroglycerin, be sure to tell your doctor about any medications you are currently taking.

Storage
Tablets, capsules, and oral spray should be stored as in a tightly capped bottle in a cool, dry place. Ointment and patches should be stored at room temperature in their original containers. Keep out of reach of children. Do not keep outdated medicine or medicine no longer needed.

NITRONET

Properties
This medicine contains nitroglycerin as active ingredient. Nitrates improve the supply of blood and oxygen to the heart. This medication is for oral use.

Before using this medicine
Before you use this medicine check with your doctor, or pharmacist:
- if you ever had any unusual or allergic reaction to nitrates or nitrites.
- if you are on a low-salt, low-sugar, or any other special diet, or if you are allergic to any substance, such as sulfites or other preservatives or dyes.
- if you are pregnant or intend to become pregnant while using this medicine. Although nitrates have not been shown to cause problems in humans, the chance always exists.
- if you are breast-feeding an infant.
- if you have recently had a heart attack or stroke.
- if you have any of the following medical problems:
  Anemia
  Glaucoma
  Intestinal problems
  Overactive thyroid
- if you are now taking any of the following medicines or types of medicines:
  Antihypertensives
  Asthma or hay fever medicine
  Cold medicine
  Decongestant
  Medicine for appetite control
  Narcotic
  Pain medicine
  Sinus congestion medicine

Treatment
This medication is used to treat and prevent angina (chest pain). Nitroglycerin is a vasodilator, which relaxes the muscles of the blood vessels, causing an increase in the oxygen supply to the heart. The oral tablets, capsules, ointment and patches do not act quickly; they are used to prevent chest pain. The sublingual tablets and oral spray act quickly and can be used to relieve chest pain after it has started.

- Take this medicine exactly as directed by your doctor or pharmacist. It will work only if taken correctly.
- If you are taking this medicine regularly and you miss a dose, take it as soon as possible. However, if your next scheduled dose; is within 2 hours (or within 6 hours for extended-release capsules or tablets), skip the missed dose and go back to your regular dosing schedule.
- If you have been taking this medicine regularly for several weeks or more, do not suddenly stop using it. Stopping suddenly may bring on attacks of angina.

Side effects
There are a number of side effects that usually do not require medical attention. These possible side effects may go away during treatment; however, if they continue or are bothersome, check with your doctor, nurse, or pharmacist. More common are: dizziness, lightheadedness, or fainting when standing up; fast pulse; flushing of face and neck; headache; nausea or vomiting.

Side effects that should be reported to your doctor are: blurred vision; dry mouth; severe or prolonged headache; skin rash.

Interactions
This medicine may interact with several other drugs such as tricyclic antidepressants and cough medicines. Before starting to take or apply nitroglycerin, be sure to tell your doctor about any medications you are currently taking.

Storage
Tablets, capsules, and oral spray should be stored as in a tightly capped bottle in a cool, dry place. Ointment and patches should be stored at room temperature in their original containers. Keep out of reach of children. Do not keep outdated medicine or medicine no longer needed.

NITRONG

Properties
This medicine contains nitroglycerin as active ingredient. Nitrates improve the supply of blood and oxygen to the heart. This medication is for oral use.

Before using this medicine
Before you use this medicine check with your doctor, or pharmacist:
- if you ever had any unusual or allergic reaction to nitrates or nitrites.
- if you are on a low-salt, low-sugar, or any other special diet, or if you are allergic to any substance, such as sulfites or other preservatives or dyes.
- if you are pregnant or intend to become pregnant while using this medicine. Although nitrates have not been shown to cause problems in humans, the chance always exists.
- if you are breast-feeding an infant.
- if you have recently had a heart attack or stroke.
- if you have any of the following medical problems:
  Anemia
  Glaucoma
  Intestinal problems
  Overactive thyroid
- if you are now taking any of the following medicines or types of medicines:
  Antihypertensives
  Asthma or hay fever medicine
  Cold medicine
  Decongestant
  Medicine for appetite control
  Narcotic
  Pain medicine
  Sinus congestion medicine

Treatment
This medication is used to treat and prevent angina (chest pain). Nitroglycerin is a vasodilator, which relaxes the muscles of the blood vessels, causing an increase in the oxygen supply to the heart. The oral tablets, capsules, ointment and patches do not act quickly; they are used to prevent chest pain. The sublingual tablets and oral spray act quickly and can be used to relieve chest pain after it has started.

- Take this medicine exactly as directed by your doctor or pharmacist. It will work only if taken correctly.
- If you are taking this medicine regularly and you miss a dose, take it as soon as possible. However, if your next scheduled dose; is within 2 hours (or within 6 hours for extended-release capsules or tablets), skip the missed dose and go back to your regular dosing schedule.
- If you have been taking this medicine regularly for several weeks or more, do not suddenly stop using it. Stopping suddenly may bring on attacks of angina.

Side effects
There are a number of side effects that usually do not require medical attention. These possible side effects may go away during treatment; however, if they continue or are bothersome, check with your doctor, nurse, or pharmacist. More common are: dizziness, lightheadedness, or fainting when standing up; fast pulse; flushing of face and neck; headache; nausea or vomiting.

Side effects that should be reported to your doctor are: blurred vision; dry mouth; severe or prolonged headache; skin rash.

Interactions
This medicine may interact with several other drugs such as tricyclic antidepressants and cough medicines. Before starting to take or apply nitroglycerin, be sure to tell your doctor about any medications you are currently taking.

Storage
Tablets, capsules, and oral spray should be stored as in a tightly capped bottle in a cool, dry place. Ointment and patches should be stored at room temperature in their original containers. Keep out of reach of children. Do not keep outdated medicine or medicine no longer needed.

NITROSPAN

Properties
This medicine contains nitroglycerin as active ingredient. Nitrates improve the supply of blood and oxygen to the heart. This medication is for oral use.

Before using this medicine
Before you use this medicine check with your doctor, or pharmacist:
- if you ever had any unusual or allergic reaction to nitrates or nitrites.
- if you are on a low-salt, low-sugar, or any other special diet, or if you are allergic to any substance, such as sulfites or other preservatives or dyes.
- if you are pregnant or intend to become pregnant while using this medicine. Although nitrates have not been shown to cause problems in humans, the chance always exists.
- if you are breast-feeding an infant.
- if you have recently had a heart attack or stroke.
- if you have any of the following medical problems:
  Anemia
  Glaucoma
  Intestinal problems
  Overactive thyroid
- if you are now taking any of the following medicines or types of medicines:
  Antihypertensives
  Asthma or hay fever medicine
  Cold medicine
  Decongestant
  Medicine for appetite control
  Narcotic
  Pain medicine
  Sinus congestion medicine

Treatment
This medication is used to treat and prevent angina (chest pain). Nitroglycerin is a vasodilator, which relaxes the muscles of the blood vessels, causing an increase in the oxygen supply to the heart. The oral tablets, capsules, ointment and patches do not act quickly; they are used to prevent chest pain. The sublingual tablets and oral spray act quickly and can be used to relieve chest pain after it has started.

- Take this medicine exactly as directed by your doctor or pharmacist. It will work only if taken correctly.
- If you are taking this medicine regularly and you miss a dose, take it as soon as possible. However, if your next scheduled dose; is within 2 hours (or within 6 hours for extended-release capsules or tablets), skip the missed dose and go back to your regular dosing schedule.
- If you have been taking this medicine regularly for several weeks or more, do not suddenly stop using it. Stopping suddenly may bring on attacks of angina.

Side effects
There are a number of side effects that usually do not require medical attention. These possible side effects may go away during treatment; however, if they continue or are bothersome, check with your doctor, nurse, or pharmacist. More common are: dizziness, lightheadedness, or fainting when standing up; fast pulse; flushing of face and neck; headache; nausea or vomiting.

Side effects that should be reported to your doctor are: blurred vision; dry mouth; severe or prolonged headache; skin rash.

Interactions
This medicine may interact with several other drugs such as tricyclic antidepressants and cough medicines. Before starting to take or apply nitroglycerin, be sure to tell your doctor about any medications you are currently taking.

Storage
Tablets, capsules, and oral spray should be stored as in a tightly capped bottle in a cool, dry place. Ointment and patches should be stored at room temperature in their original containers. Keep out of reach of children. Do not keep outdated medicine or medicine no longer needed.

NITROSTAT SR

Properties
This medicine contains nitroglycerin as active ingredient. Nitrates improve the supply of blood and oxygen to the heart. This medication is for oral use.

Before using this medicine
Before you use this medicine check with your doctor, or pharmacist:
- if you ever had any unusual or allergic reaction to nitrates or nitrites.
- if you are on a low-salt, low-sugar, or any other special diet, or if you are allergic to any substance, such as sulfites or other preservatives or dyes.
- if you are pregnant or intend to become pregnant while using this medicine. Although nitrates have not been shown to cause problems in humans, the chance always exists.
- if you are breast-feeding an infant.
- if you have recently had a heart attack or stroke.
- if you have any of the following medical problems:
  Anemia
  Glaucoma
  Intestinal problems
  Overactive thyroid
- if you are now taking any of the following medicines or types of medicines:
  Antihypertensives
  Asthma or hay fever medicine
  Cold medicine
  Decongestant
  Medicine for appetite control
  Narcotic
  Pain medicine
  Sinus congestion medicine

Treatment
This medication is used to treat and prevent angina (chest pain). Nitroglycerin is a vasodilator, which relaxes the muscles of the blood vessels, causing an increase in the oxygen supply to the heart. The oral tablets, capsules, ointment and patches do not act quickly; they are used to prevent chest pain. The sublingual tablets and oral spray act quickly and can be used to relieve chest pain after it has started.

- Take this medicine exactly as directed by your doctor or pharmacist. It will work only if taken correctly.
- If you are taking this medicine regularly and you miss a dose, take it as soon as possible. However, if your next scheduled dose; is within 2 hours (or within 6 hours for extended-release capsules or tablets), skip the missed dose and go back to your regular dosing schedule.
- If you have been taking this medicine regularly for several weeks or more, do not suddenly stop using it. Stopping suddenly may bring on attacks of angina.

Side effects
There are a number of side effects that usually do not require medical attention. These possible side effects may go away during treatment; however, if they continue or are bothersome, check with your doctor, nurse, or pharmacist. More common are: dizziness, lightheadedness, or fainting when standing up; fast pulse; flushing of face and neck; headache; nausea or vomiting.

Side effects that should be reported to your doctor are: blurred vision; dry mouth; severe or prolonged headache; skin rash.

Interactions
This medicine may interact with several other drugs such as tricyclic antidepressants and cough medicines. Before starting to take or apply nitroglycerin, be sure to tell your doctor about any medications you are currently taking.

Storage
Tablets, capsules, and oral spray should be stored as in a tightly capped bottle in a cool, dry place. Ointment and patches should be stored at room temperature in their original containers. Keep out of reach of children. Do not keep outdated medicine or medicine no longer needed.

NITRO-TIME

Properties
This medicine contains nitroglycerin as active ingredient. Nitrates improve the supply of blood and oxygen to the heart. This medication is for oral use.

Before using this medicine
Before you use this medicine check with your doctor, or pharmacist:
- if you ever had any unusual or allergic reaction to nitrates or nitrites.
- if you are on a low-salt, low-sugar, or any other special diet, or if you are allergic to any substance, such as sulfites or other preservatives or dyes.
- if you are pregnant or intend to become pregnant while using this medicine. Although nitrates have not been shown to cause problems in humans, the chance always exists.
- if you are breast-feeding an infant.
- if you have recently had a heart attack or stroke.
- if you have any of the following medical problems:
  Anemia
  Glaucoma
  Intestinal problems
  Overactive thyroid
- if you are now taking any of the following medicines or types of medicines:
  Antihypertensives
  Asthma or hay fever medicine
  Cold medicine
  Decongestant
  Medicine for appetite control
  Narcotic
  Pain medicine
  Sinus congestion medicine

Treatment
This medication is used to treat and prevent angina (chest pain). Nitroglycerin is a vasodilator, which relaxes the muscles of the blood vessels, causing an increase in the oxygen supply to the heart. The oral tablets, capsules, ointment and patches do not act quickly; they are used to prevent chest pain. The sublingual tablets and oral spray act quickly and can be used to relieve chest pain after it has started.

- Take this medicine exactly as directed by your doctor or pharmacist. It will work only if taken correctly.
- If you are taking this medicine regularly and you miss a dose, take it as soon as possible. However, if your next scheduled dose; is within 2 hours (or within 6 hours for extended-release capsules or tablets), skip the missed dose and go back to your regular dosing schedule.
- If you have been taking this medicine regularly for several weeks or more, do not suddenly stop using it. Stopping suddenly may bring on attacks of angina.

Side effects
There are a number of side effects that usually do not require medical attention. These possible side effects may go away during treatment; however, if they continue or are bothersome, check with your doctor, nurse, or pharmacist. More common are: dizziness, lightheadedness, or fainting when standing up; fast pulse; flushing of face and neck; headache; nausea or vomiting.
Side effects that should be reported to your doctor are: blurred vision; dry mouth; severe or prolonged headache; skin rash.

Interactions
This medicine may interact with several other drugs such as tricyclic antidepressants and cough medicines. Before starting to take or apply nitroglycerin, be sure to tell your doctor about any medications you are currently taking.

Storage
Tablets, capsules, and oral spray should be stored as in a tightly capped bottle in a cool, dry place. Ointment and patches should be stored at room temperature in their original containers. Keep out of reach of children. Do not keep outdated medicine or medicine no longer needed.

NOBESINE-75

Properties
This medicine contains diethylpropion active ingredient; it is prescribed for appetite suppression.

Appetite suppressants are used in the short-term (a few weeks) treatment of obesity. In a few weeks (6 to 12), these medicines in combination with dieting, exercise, and changes in eating habits can help patients lose weight. However, since their appetite reducing effect is only temporary, they are useful only for the first weeks of dieting until new eating habits are established.

Before using this medicine
Before you use this medicine check with your doctor, or pharmacist:
- if you ever had any unusual or allergic reaction to any of the compounds of this medicine.
- if you are on a low-salt, low-sugar, or any other special diet, or if you are allergic to any substance, such as sulfites or other preservatives or dyes.
- if you are pregnant, intend to become pregnant or breast-feeding an infant while using this medicine.
- if you have any of the following medical problems:
  Diabetes mellitus
  Epilepsy
  Glaucoma
  Heart disease
  High blood pressure
  Mental illness (severe)

Treatment
This medication is used to relieve or prevent the symptoms of your medical problem.

Take them as directed. Do not take more of them and do not take them more often than recommended on the label. If too much of the drug is taken, it may become habit-forming.
- The medicine produces central nervous system stimulation, and it should not be taken by people with heart disease or high blood pressure.
- If you think this medicine is not working as well after you have taken it for a few weeks, do not increase the dose. Instead, check with your doctor.

Side effects
The following minor side effects may occur: irritability, nervousness, restlessness, trouble in sleeping.

These side effects should disappear as your body adjusts to the medication. Tell your doctor about any side effects that are persistent or particularly bothersome. It is especially important to tell your doctor about:
  Mental depression
  Nausea or vomiting
  Stomach cramps or pain
  Trembling
  Unusual tiredness
- Discontinue use of the drug; call your doctor right away. Adverse reactions and side effects may be more frequent and severe in people over age 60 than in younger persons.

Interactions
This medicine interacts with several other drugs such as antihypertensives, other appetite suppressants, caffeine, central nervous system depressants, central nervous system stimulants, furazolidone, guanethidine, hydralazine, MAO inhibitors, methyldopa, molindone, phenothiazines, rauwolfia alkaloids, sodium bicarbonate. Interaction with alcoholic beverages may produce drowsiness, sleepiness, and/or inability to concentrate.
- Be sure to tell your doctor about any medications you are currently taking.

Storage
This medicine should be stored at room temperature in tightly closed containers. Store away from heat and direct light. Keep out of reach of children, since overdose may be very dangerous in children.

Do not store this medicine in the bathroom medicine cabinet because the heat and moisture cause the medicine to break down. Do not keep outdated medicine or medicine no longer needed. Flush the contents of the container down the toilet.

NORCEPT-E

Properties
This medicine contains norethindrone and ethinyl estradiol as active ingredients. It is an oral contraceptive prescribed to prevent pregnancy and/or to regulate menstrual periods.

The drug works by altering the mucus at the cervix entrance to prevent the entry of sperm. It also alters the uterus lining to resist implantation of the fertilized egg. Oral contraceptives create the same chemical atmosphere in blood that exists during pregnancy.

Before using this medicine
Before you use this medicine check with your doctor, or pharmacist:
- if you ever had any unusual or allergic reaction to estrogens or progestogen;
- if you are pregnant or want to become pregnant within three months;
- if you are breast-feeding an infant;
- if you have any of the following medical problems:
  Diabetes
  Ailments of the breast
  Disorders of the uterus
  Migraine or epilepsy
  High blood pressure
  Asthma or heart conditions
  Kidney disease
  Gallstones

Treatment
This medication is used to prevent pregnancy or to regulate menstrual periods.

Adverse reactions
Along with the needed effects, a medicine may cause some unwanted effects or adverse reactions.
- *An increased risk of the following adverse reactions has been associated with the use of oral contraceptives:*
  Thrombophlebitis
  Venous thrombosis
  Arterial thromboembolism
  Pulmonary (lung) embolism
  Myocardial infarction
  Cerebral hemorrhage
  Cerebral thrombosis
  Hypertension
  Gallbladder disease
  Hepatic (liver) hepatomas
  Benign lifer tumors
- *The following adverse reactions have been reported in patients receiving oral contraceptives and are believed to be drug-related:*
  Nausea and vomiting
  Abdominal cramps
  Breakthrough bleeding
  Spotting
  Change in menstrual flow
  Amenorrhea
  Temporary infertility
  Edema
  Breast changes
  Weight changes
  Cholestatic jaundice
  Migraine
  Rash (allergic)
  Mental depression
  Vaginal candidiasis

Interactions
This medicine may interact with several other drugs such as antibiotics, anticoagulants, anticonvulsants, antidepressants, oral antidiabetics, antihistamines, barbiturates, oral hypoglycemics, insulin, meperidine.
- Be sure to tell your doctor about any medications you are currently taking.

Storage
Tablets should be stored at room temperature; store away from heat and direct light. Keep out of reach of children, since this medicine may be dangerous in children.

NORDETTE

Properties

This medicine contains levonorgestrel and ethinyl estradiol as active ingredients. It is an oral contraceptive prescribed to prevent pregnancy and/or to regulate menstrual periods.

The drug works by altering the mucus at the cervix entrance to prevent the entry of sperm. It also alters the uterus lining to resist implantation of the fertilized egg. Oral contraceptives create the same chemical atmosphere in blood that exists during pregnancy.

Before using this medicine

Before you use this medicine check with your doctor, or pharmacist:
- if you ever had any unusual or allergic reaction to estrogens or progestogen;
- if you are pregnant or want to become pregnant within three months;
- if you are breast-feeding an infant;
- if you have any of the following medical problems:
  Diabetes
  Ailments of the breast
  Disorders of the uterus
  Migraine or epilepsy
  High blood pressure
  Asthma or heart conditions
  Kidney disease
  Gallstones

Treatment

This medication is used to prevent pregnancy or to regulate menstrual periods.

Adverse reactions

Along with the needed effects, a medicine may cause some unwanted effects or adverse reactions.

- *An increased risk of the following adverse reactions has been associated with the use of oral contraceptives:*
  Thrombophlebitis
  Venous thrombosis
  Arterial thromboembolism
  Pulmonary (lung) embolism
  Myocardial infarction
  Cerebral hemorrhage
  Cerebral thrombosis
  Hypertension
  Gallbladder disease
  Hepatic (liver) hepatomas
  Benign lifer tumors
- *The following adverse reactions have been reported in patients receiving oral contraceptives and are believed to be drug-related:*
  Nausea and vomiting
  Abdominal cramps
  Breakthrough bleeding
  Spotting
  Change in menstrual flow
  Amenorrhea
  Temporary infertility
  Edema
  Breast changes
  Weight changes
  Cholestatic jaundice
  Migraine
  Rash (allergic)
  Mental depression
  Vaginal candidiasis

Interactions

This medicine may interact with several other drugs such as antibiotics, anticoagulants, anticonvulsants, antidepressants, oral antidiabetics, antihistamines, barbiturates, oral hypoglycemics, insulin, meperidine.

- Be sure to tell your doctor about any medications you are currently taking.

Storage

Tablets should be stored at room temperature; store away from heat and direct light. Keep out of reach of children, since this medicine may be dangerous in children.

NORETHIN

Properties

This medicine contains levonorgestrel and ethinyl estradiol as active ingredients. It is an oral contraceptive prescribed to prevent pregnancy and/or to regulate menstrual periods.

The drug works by altering the mucus at the cervix entrance to prevent the entry of sperm. It also alters the uterus lining to resist implantation of the fertilized egg. Oral contraceptives create the same chemical atmosphere in blood that exists during pregnancy.

Before using this medicine

Before you use this medicine check with your doctor, or pharmacist:
- if you ever had any unusual or allergic reaction to estrogens or progestogen;
- if you are pregnant or want to become pregnant within three months;
- if you are breast-feeding an infant;
- if you have any of the following medical problems:
  Diabetes
  Ailments of the breast
  Disorders of the uterus
  Migraine or epilepsy
  High blood pressure
  Asthma or heart conditions
  Kidney disease
  Gallstones

Treatment

This medication is used to prevent pregnancy or to regulate menstrual periods.

Adverse reactions

Along with the needed effects, a medicine may cause some unwanted effects or adverse reactions.
- *An increased risk of the following adverse reactions has been associated with the use of oral contraceptives:*
  Thrombophlebitis
  Venous thrombosis
  Arterial thromboembolism
  Pulmonary (lung) embolism
  Myocardial infarction
  Cerebral hemorrhage
  Cerebral thrombosis
  Hypertension
  Gallbladder disease
  Hepatic (liver) hepatomas
  Benign lifer tumors
- *The following adverse reactions have been reported in patients receiving oral contraceptives and are believed to be drug-related:*
  Nausea and vomiting
  Abdominal cramps
  Breakthrough bleeding
  Spotting
  Change in menstrual flow
  Amenorrhea
  Temporary infertility
  Edema
  Breast changes
  Weight changes
  Cholestatic jaundice
  Migraine
  Rash (allergic)
  Mental depression
  Vaginal candidiasis

Interactions

This medicine may interact with several other drugs such as antibiotics, anticoagulants, anticonvulsants, antidepressants, oral antidiabetics, antihistamines, barbiturates, oral hypoglycemics, insulin, meperidine.
- Be sure to tell your doctor about any medications you are currently taking.

Storage

Tablets should be stored at room temperature; store away from heat and direct light. Keep out of reach of children, since this medicine may be dangerous in children.

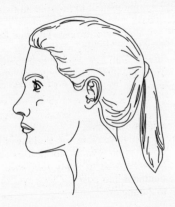

NORFLOXACIN (Ophthalmic)

Properties

This medicine contains an ophthalmic antibacterial as active ingredient. It helps the body to overcome eye infections on surface tissues of the eye. It is most useful when the infecting organism is one known to be sensitive to the antibacterial drug.

The drug penetrates the bacterial cell membrane and prevents cells from multiplying.

Before using this medicine

Before you use this medicine check with your doctor:
- if you ever had any unusual or allergic reaction to any of the compounds of the medicine.
- if you are on a low-salt, low-sugar, or any other special diet, or if you are allergic to any substance, such as sulfites or other preservatives or dyes.
- if you are pregnant or intend to become pregnant while using this medicine. Although ophthalmic antibacterials have been found to be safe for use during pregnancy, you should check with your doctor before taking any drug if you are pregnant.

Treatment

This medication is used to treat an infection caused by bacteria. The medicine may be used in the form of eye drops or as an eye ointment. Use the medication as directed, Do not miss a dose. If you forget a dose, use it as soon as you remember. Notify your doctor if eye symptoms fail to improve in two to four days.

- To apply eye drops: Till the head backward when applying the eye drops. Pull the lower eyelid away from the eye to form a pouch. After applying the drop, keep the eye closed for a minute or so. This allows the medication to come in contact with the infection.
- To apply eye ointment: Pull lower lid down from eye to form a pouch. Squeeze tube to apply thin strip of ointment into pouch. Close eye for 1 to 2 minutes.

Always wash your hands before applying the ointment.

The drug starts to work in about one hour. Treatment may require 7 to 10 days to control infection.

Older adults or seniors may take this medication without special restriction.

Side effects

Along with the needed effects, a medicine may cause some unwanted effects. Side effects that usually do not require medical attention: occasional local irritation after application to the eye. Ointments may cause blurred vision for a few minutes; continue the use of the eye drops or ointment, but tell your doctor at the next visit.

- Discontinue the use of eye drops or eye ointment in the following cases:
  Sore throat
  Aplastic anemia
  Pale skin
  Unusual redness of the eye
  Unusual irritation of the eye
  Fever
  Unusual bleeding
  Unusual bruising
- Tell your doctor about any side effects that are persistent or particularly bothersome. In case of prolonged use sensitivity reactions may develop.

Interactions

Clinically significant interactions with oral or injected medicines are unlikely. Do not use the eye drops or ointment with any other eye drops or ointment without checking with your ophthalmologist.

Storage

Keep bottle (with eye drops) or container (containing ointment) lightly closed. Store in a cool place, but Do not freeze. Wash hands immediately after using. Do not store in the bathroom medicine cabinet because the heat or moisture may cause the medicine to break down.

Do not keep outdated medicine or medicine no longer needed. Flush the contents of the bottle or tube down the toilet, unless otherwise directed.

NORINYL 1

Properties
This medicine contains norethindrone and mestranol as active ingredients. It is an oral contraceptive prescribed to prevent pregnancy and/or to regulate menstrual periods.

The drug works by altering the mucus at the cervix entrance to prevent the entry of sperm. It also alters the uterus lining to resist implantation of the fertilized egg. Oral contraceptives create the same chemical atmosphere in blood that exists during pregnancy.

Before using this medicine
Before you use this medicine check with your doctor, or pharmacist:
- if you ever had any unusual or allergic reaction to estrogens or progestogen;
- if you are pregnant or want to become pregnant within three months;
- if you are breast-feeding an infant;
- if you have any of the following medical problems:
  Diabetes
  Ailments of the breast
  Disorders of the uterus
  Migraine or epilepsy
  High blood pressure
  Asthma or heart conditions
  Kidney disease
  Gallstones

Treatment
This medication is used to prevent pregnancy or to regulate menstrual periods.

Adverse reactions
Along with the needed effects, a medicine may cause some unwanted effects or adverse reactions.
- *An increased risk of the following adverse reactions has been associated with the use of oral contraceptives:*
  Thrombophlebitis
  Venous thrombosis
  Arterial thromboembolism
  Pulmonary (lung) embolism
  Myocardial infarction
  Cerebral hemorrhage
  Cerebral thrombosis
  Hypertension
  Gallbladder disease
  Hepatic (liver) hepatomas
  Benign lifer tumors
- *The following adverse reactions have been reported in patients receiving oral contraceptives and are believed to be drug-related:*
  Nausea and vomiting
  Abdominal cramps
  Breakthrough bleeding
  Spotting
  Change in menstrual flow
  Amenorrhea
  Temporary infertility
  Edema
  Breast changes
  Weight changes
  Cholestatic jaundice
  Migraine
  Rash (allergic)
  Mental depression
  Vaginal candidiasis

Interactions
This medicine may interact with several other drugs such as antibiotics, anticoagulants, anticonvulsants, antidepressants, oral antidiabetics, antihistamines, barbiturates, oral hypoglycemics, insulin, meperidine.
- Be sure to tell your doctor about any medications you are currently taking.

Storage
Tablets should be stored at room temperature; store away from heat and direct light. Keep out of reach of children, since this medicine may be dangerous in children.

NORLESTRIN

Properties

This medicine contains norethindrone and ethinyl acetate as active ingredients. It is an oral contraceptive prescribed to prevent pregnancy and/or to regulate menstrual periods.

The drug works by altering the mucus at the cervix entrance to prevent the entry of sperm. It also alters the uterus lining to resist implantation of the fertilized egg. Oral contraceptives create the same chemical atmosphere in blood that exists during pregnancy.

Before using this medicine

Before you use this medicine check with your doctor, or pharmacist:
- if you ever had any unusual or allergic reaction to estrogens or progestogen;
- if you are pregnant or want to become pregnant within three months;
- if you are breast-feeding an infant;
- if you have any of the following medical problems:
  Diabetes
  Ailments of the breast
  Disorders of the uterus
  Migraine or epilepsy
  High blood pressure
  Asthma or heart conditions
  Kidney disease
  Gallstones

Treatment

This medication is used to prevent pregnancy or to regulate menstrual periods.

Adverse reactions

Along with the needed effects, a medicine may cause some unwanted effects or adverse reactions.
- *An increased risk of the following adverse reactions has been associated with the use of oral contraceptives:*
  Thrombophlebitis
  Venous thrombosis
  Arterial thromboembolism
  Pulmonary (lung) embolism
  Myocardial infarction
  Cerebral hemorrhage
  Cerebral thrombosis
  Hypertension
  Gallbladder disease
  Hepatic (liver) hepatomas
  Benign lifer tumors
- *The following adverse reactions have been reported in patients receiving oral contraceptives and are believed to be drug-related:*
  Nausea and vomiting
  Abdominal cramps
  Breakthrough bleeding
  Spotting
  Change in menstrual flow
  Amenorrhea
  Temporary infertility
  Edema
  Breast changes
  Weight changes
  Cholestatic jaundice
  Migraine
  Rash (allergic)
  Mental depression
  Vaginal candidiasis

Interactions

This medicine may interact with several other drugs such as antibiotics, anticoagulants, anticonvulsants, antidepressants, oral antidiabetics, antihistamines, barbiturates, oral hypoglycemics, insulin, meperidine.
- Be sure to tell your doctor about any medications you are currently taking.

Storage

Tablets should be stored at room temperature; store away from heat and direct light. Keep out of reach of children, since this medicine may be dangerous in children.

NORPRAMIN

Properties
This medicine contains desipramine as active ingredient. It belongs to the group of medicines known as tricyclic antidepressants or 'mood elevators.' It is used to relieve mental depression and depression that sometimes occurs with anxiety. The medication gradually relieves, but doesn't cure, symptoms of depression. The medication may also be used for the treatment of narcolepsy, bulimia, painic attacks, cocaine withdrawal, attention deficit disorder.

Before using this medicine
Before you use this medicine check with your doctor, or pharmacist:
- if you ever had any unusual or allergic reaction to any tricyclic antidepressant, maprotiline or trazodone.
- if you are on a low-salt, low-sugar, or any other special diet, or if you are allergic to any substance, such as sulfites or other preservatives or dyes.
- if you are pregnant or intend to become pregnant while using this medicine. There have been reports of newborns suffering from heart, breathing, and urinary problems when their mothers had taken tricyclic antidepressants before delivery.
- if you are breast-feeding an infant. Some tricyclic antidepressants pass into the breast milk.

Treatment
Take this medicine only as directed by your doctor, to benefit your condition as much as possible. Do not take more of it, do not take it more often, and do not take it for a longer period of time than your doctor ordered.

To lessen stomach upset, take this medicine with food, even for a daily bedtime dose, unless your doctor has told you to take it on an empty stomach. If you forget your once-a-day bedtime dose, Do not take it more than 3 hours late. If more than 3 hours, wait for next scheduled dose;.

Sometimes this medicine must be taken for several weeks before you begin to feel better.

Side effects
Along with the needed effects, a medicine may cause some unwanted effects. Side effects that usually do not require medical attention: difficult or frequent urination; decreased sex drive; muscle aches; abnormal dreams; nasal congestion; weakness and faintness when arising from bed or chair; back pain.
- Other side effects that should be reported to your doctor immediately are:
  Hallucinations
  Shakiness
  Dizziness or fainting
  Blurred vision, eye pain
  Irregular heartbeat or slow pulse
  Inflamed tongue
  Abdominal pain
  Jaundice
  Hair loss, rash
  Fever, chills
  Joint pain
  Palpitations

Interactions
This medicine may interact with several other drugs such as anticoagulants, anticholinergics, cold remedies, oral contraceptives, seizure medicines, sleeping medicines, thyroid medicines, etc.
- Be sure to tell your doctor about any medications you are currently taking.

Storage
Tablets, capsules, etc. should be stored at room temperature in tightly closed, light-resistant containers as directed by your pharmacist. Keep out of reach of children since overdose is especially dangerous in young children. Do not store in the bathroom medicine cabinet because the heat or moisture may cause the medicine to break down. Keep the liquid form of the medicine from freezing.

NORTRIPTYLINE

Properties

This medicine contains nortriptyline as active ingredient. It belongs to the group of medicines known as tricyclic antidepressants or 'mood elevators.' It is used to relieve mental depression and depression that sometimes occurs with anxiety. The medication gradually relieves, but doesn't cure, symptoms of depression. The medication may also be used for the treatment of narcolepsy, bulimia, painic attacks, cocaine withdrawal, attention deficit disorder.

Before using this medicine

Before you use this medicine check with your doctor, or pharmacist:

- if you ever had any unusual or allergic reaction to any tricyclic antidepressant, maprotiline or trazodone.
- if you are on a low-salt, low-sugar, or any other special diet, or if you are allergic to any substance, such as sulfites or other preservatives or dyes.
- if you are pregnant or intend to become pregnant while using this medicine. There have been reports of newborns suffering from heart, breathing, and urinary problems when their mothers had taken tricyclic antidepressants before delivery.
- if you are breast-feeding an infant. Some tricyclic antidepressants pass into the breast milk.

Treatment

Take this medicine only as directed by your doctor, to benefit your condition as much as possible. Do not take more of it, do not take it more often, and do not take it for a longer period of time than your doctor ordered.

To lessen stomach upset, take this medicine with food, even for a daily bedtime dose, unless your doctor has told you to take it on an empty stomach. If you forget your once-a-day bedtime dose, Do not take it more than 3 hours late. If more than 3 hours, wait for next scheduled dose;.

Sometimes this medicine must be taken for several weeks before you begin to feel better.

Side effects

Along with the needed effects, a medicine may cause some unwanted effects. Side effects that usually do not require medical attention: difficult or frequent urination; decreased sex drive; muscle aches; abnormal dreams; nasal congestion; weakness and faintness when arising from bed or chair; back pain.

- Other side effects that should be reported to your doctor immediately are:

Hallucinations
Shakiness
Dizziness or fainting
Blurred vision, eye pain
Irregular heartbeat or slow pulse
Inflamed tongue
Abdominal pain
Jaundice
Hair loss, rash
Fever, chills
Joint pain
Palpitations

Interactions

This medicine may interact with several other drugs such as anticoagulants, anticholinergics, cold remedies, oral contraceptives, seizure medicines, sleeping medicines, thyroid medicines, etc.

- Be sure to tell your doctor about any medications you are currently taking.

Storage

Tablets, capsules, etc. should be stored at room temperature in tightly closed, light-resistant containers as directed by your pharmacist. Keep out of reach of children since overdose is especially dangerous in young children. Do not store in the bathroom medicine cabinet because the heat or moisture may cause the medicine to break down. Keep the liquid form of the medicine from freezing.

NORVASC

Properties

This medicine contains amlodipine as active ingredient. It is a so-called calcium channel blocker, working by blocking the passage of calcium into heart and smooth muscle. Since calcium is an essential factor in muscle contraction, any medicine that affects calcium in this way will interfere with the contraction of these muscles.

The medicine works by:

♦ reducing the work that the heart must perform;
♦ reducing the normal arterial blood pressure;
♦ increasing oxygen to the heart muscle.

The medicine is prescribed for the treatment of attacks of angina pectoris, irregular heartbeat, and high blood pressure. In many cases it can be used for the treatment and prevention of migraine.

Before using this medicine

Before you use this medicine check with your doctor, or pharmacist:

- if you ever had any unusual or allergic reaction to this medicine or any calcium channel blocker;
- if you are pregnant or intend to become pregnant while using this medicine;
- if you have low blood pressure;
- if you have kidney or lifer disease;
- if you are breast-feeding an infant;
- if you easily get a rash or intensity sunburn in areas exposed to sun or ultraviolet light.

Treatment

This medication is used for treatment of heart conditions (for instance, angina pectoris) and high blood pressure. Tablets, capsules or extended-release tablets should be taken with liquid. The usual dose amounts to 30 to 100 milligrams a day.

For safe and effective use of medicine:

♦ Follow your doctor's instructions if this medicine was prescribed.
♦ Follow the manufacturer's package directions if you are treating yourself.

Side effects

Along with the needed effects, a medicine may cause some unwanted effects. Possible side effects include:

Tiredness
Changes in heartbeat
Wheezing
Cough
Shortness of breath
Dizziness
Fainting
Numbness in hands and feet
Tingling in hands and feet
Difficult urination
Constipation

Overdose

The following symptoms may be a sign of overdose:

Unusually fast heartbeat
Unusually slow heartbeat
Loss of consciousness
Cardiac arrest

■ Call a doctor or hospital emergency room for instructions. If necessary start first aid immediately.

Interactions

The effect of this medicine may cause a blood pressure drop if taken together with antihypertensives. Cimetidine may increase the effect of the calcium blocker.

The simultaneous use of diuretics and calcium channel blockers may cause dangerous blood pressure drop.

■ Be sure to tell your doctor about any medications you are currently taking.

Storage

Capsules, tablets, etc. should be stored at room temperature; store away from heat and direct light. Keep out of reach of children, since this medicine may be dangerous in children.

NOVO-NIFEDIN

Properties

This medicine contains nefedipine as active ingredient. It is a so-called calcium channel blocker, working by blocking the passage of calcium into heart and smooth muscle. Since calcium is an essential factor in muscle contraction, any medicine that affects calcium in this way will interfere with the contraction of these muscles.

The medicine works by:
◆ reducing the work that the heart must perform;
◆ reducing the normal arterial blood pressure;
◆ increasing oxygen to the heart muscle.

The medicine is prescribed for the treatment of attacks of angina pectoris, irregular heartbeat, and high blood pressure. In many cases it can be used for the treatment and prevention of migraine.

Before using this medicine

Before you use this medicine check with your doctor, or pharmacist:
– if you ever had any unusual or allergic reaction to this medicine or any calcium channel blocker;
– if you are pregnant or intend to become pregnant while using this medicine;
– if you have low blood pressure;
– if you have kidney or lifer disease;
– if you are breast-feeding an infant;
– if you easily get a rash or intensity sunburn in areas exposed to sun or ultraviolet light.

Treatment

This medication is used for treatment of heart conditions (for instance, angina pectoris) and high blood pressure. Tablets, capsules or extended-release tablets should be taken with liquid. The usual dose amounts to 30 to 100 milligrams a day.

For safe and effective use of medicine:
◆ Follow your doctor's instructions if this medicine was prescribed.
◆ Follow the manufacturer's package directions if you are treating yourself.

Side effects

Along with the needed effects, a medicine may cause some unwanted effects. Possible side effects include:
Tiredness
Changes in heartbeat
Wheezing
Cough
Shortness of breath
Dizziness
Fainting
Numbness in hands and feet
Tingling in hands and feet
Difficult urination
Constipation

Overdose

The following symptoms may be a sign of overdose:
Unusually fast heartbeat
Unusually slow heartbeat
Loss of consciousness
Cardiac arrest
■ Call a doctor or hospital emergency room for instructions. If necessary start first aid immediately.

Interactions

The effect of this medicine may cause a blood pressure drop if taken together with antihypertensives. Cimetidine may increase the effect of the calcium blocker.

The simultaneous use of diuretics and calcium channel blockers may cause dangerous blood pressure drop.
■ Be sure to tell your doctor about any medications you are currently taking.

Storage

Capsules, tablets, etc. should be stored at room temperature; store away from heat and direct light. Keep out of reach of children, since this medicine may be dangerous in children.

NOVOBETAMET

Properties
This medicine contains betamethasone, a corticosteroid, as active ingredient. Corticosteroids are used to help relieve redness, swelling, itching, inflammation, and discomfort of many skin problems. They exert this effect by interfering with natural body mechanisms that produce the rash, itching, or inflammation. They do not cure the underlying cause of the skin problem. This medication is applied to the skin.

Before using this medicine
Before you use this medicine check with your doctor, or pharmacist:
- if you ever had any unusual or allergic reaction to corticosteroids.
- if you are allergic to any substance, such as sulfites or other preservatives or dyes.
- if you are pregnant or intend to become pregnant while using this medicine. Studies have shown that corticosteroids applied to the skin in large amounts or over long periods of time can be the cause of birth defects.
- if you are breast-feeding an infant. Some corticosteroids pass into breast milk and may interfere with the infant's growth.

Treatment
Do not use this medicine more often or for a longer time than ordered. To do so may increase absorption through the skin and the chance of side effects. In addition, too much use, especially on areas with thinner skin (for example, face, armpits, groin), may result in thinning of the skin and stretch marks.

Before applying this medication, wash your hands. than, unless your doctor or pharmacist gives you different instructions, gently wash the area where the medication is to be applied. With a clean towel pat the area dry. Apply a small amount of the medication to the affected area in a thin layer. Do not bandage the area unless your doctor tells you to do so.

If you miss a dose of this medication, apply the dose as soon as possible, unless it is almost time for the next application.

- ◆ Do not use this medicine for other skin problems without first checking with your doctor. You should not use a topical corticosteroid if you have a virus disease (such as herpes), fungal infection of the skin (such as athlete's foot), or tuberculosis of the skin.

Side effects
There are a number of side effects that usually do not require medical attention. Minor side effects are:
Acne
Burning sensations
Itching
Rash
Skin dryness
These possible side effects may go away during treatment; however, if they continue or are bothersome, check with your doctor, nurse, or pharmacist. Tell your doctor about any side effects that are persistent or particularly bothersome, such as:
Blistering
Increased hair growth
Irritation of the affected area
Loss of skin
Secondary infection in the area being treated
Thinning of the skin with easy bruising

Interactions
None known as long as it is used according to the directions given to you by your doctor or pharmacist.

Storage
Cream, ointment, lotion, gel, spray, and aerosol should be stored at room temperature in tightly closed containers. This medication should never be frozen.

NOVOFLUPAM

Properties

This medicine contains as active ingredient flurazepam, a benzodiazepine preparation. Benzodiazepines belong to the group of psychoactive medicines that influence the activity of the brain. Some are used to relieve nervousness or tension. It is effective for this purpose for short periods. Others are used for sleeplessness or to relax muscles or relieve muscle spasm. The benzodiazepines may also be used for other conditions as determined by your doctor.

Before using this medicine

Before you use this medicine check with your doctor:
- if you ever had any unusual or allergic reaction to benzodiazepines.
- if you are on a low-salt, low-sugar, or any other special diet, or if you are allergic to any substance, such as sulfites or other preservatives or dyes.
- if you are pregnant or intend to become pregnant while using this medicine. Some benzodiazepines have been reported to increase the chance of birth defects when used during the first 3 months of pregnancy.
- if you are breast-feeding an infant. Benzodiazepines may pass into the breast milk and cause drowsiness, unusually slow heartbeat, shortness of breath, or troubled breathing in infants of mothers taking this medicine.
- if you have any of the following medical problems: asthma, bronchitis, emphysema, or other chronic lung disease; epilepsy or history of convulsions; hyperactivity (in children); kidney or lifer disease; mental depression or illness; myasthania gravis, porphyria.

Treatment

This medication is used to relieve or prevent the symptoms of your medical problem. Benzodiazepines are mainly used as antianxiety agents, anticonvulsants, or sedatives. Take them as directed. Do not take more of them and do not take them more often than recommended on the label, unless otherwise directed by your doctor. Benzodiazepine tranquilizing drugs can be abused if taken for long periods of time and it is possible to develop withdrawal symptoms if you discontinue the therapy abruptly.

Side effects

Along with the needed effects, a medicine may cause some unwanted effects. Minor side effects are: bitter taste in the mouth, dizziness, drowsiness, depression, constipation, dry mouth, excessive salivation, fatigue, flushing, headache, heartburn, loss of appetite, nausea, nervousness, sweating or vomiting. As your body adjusts to the medicine, these side effects should disappear.

- Tell your doctor about any side effects that are persistent or particularly bothersome. It is especially important to tell your doctor about:
  Blurred or double vision
  Chest pain
  Difficulty in urinating
  Fainting or falling
  Fever or hallucinations
  Joint pain
  Mouth sores
  Nightmares
  Palpitations
  Severe depression
  Shortness of breath
  Slurred speech
  Uncoordinated movements
  Unusual tiredness
  Yellowing of the skin

Interactions

- This medicine may interact with several other drugs. This medicine will add to the effects of alcohol, and CNS depressants.
- Be sure to tell your doctor about any medications you are currently taking.

Storage

Store at room temperature in tightly closed, light-resistent containers. Keep out of the reach of children since overdose may be especially dangerous in children.

NOVOHYDRAZIDE

Properties

This medicine contains as active ingredient hydrochlorothiazide, a thiazide-like diuretic. Thiazide or thiazide-like diuretics are prescribed to treat high blood pressure (hypertension). They are also used to reduce fluid accumulation in the body caused by conditions such as heart failure, cirrhosis, kidney disease, and the long-term use of some medications. Thiazide diuretics may also be used for other conditions as determined by your doctor.

Before using this medicine

Before you use this medicine check with your doctor, or pharmacist:
- if you ever had any unusual or allergic reaction to sulfonamides (sulfa drugs) or any of the thiazide diuretics.
- if you are on a low-salt, low-sugar, or any other special diet, or if you are allergic to any substance, such as sulfites or other preservatives or dyes.
- if you are pregnant or intend to become pregnant while using this medicine. When this medicine is used during pregnancy, it may cause side effects including jaundice, blood problems, and low potassium in the newborn.
- if you are breast-feeding an infant. Although this medicine has not been shown to cause problems in humans, the chance always exists since thiazide diuretics pass into breast milk.
- if you have any of the following medical problems:
  Diabetes
  Gout
  Kidney disease
  Liver disease
  Lupus erythematosus
  Pancreas disease

Treatment

This medication is used to treat high blood pressure (hypertension) and also to help reduce the amount of water in the body by increasing the flow of urine. This medicine will not cure your high blood pressure but it does help control it. You must continue to take it - even if you feel well – if you expect to keep your blood pressure down. You may have to take high blood pressure medicine for the rest of your life.

Thiazide diuretics may cause an unusual feeling of tiredness when you begin to take them. You may also notice an increase in urine or in frequency of urination. To keep this from affecting sleep:
- if you are to take a single dose a day, take it in the morning after breakfast;
- if you are to take more than one dose, take the last one not later than 6 p.m.

Side effects

Along with the needed effects, a medicine may cause some unwanted effects. Side effects that usually do not require medical attention: decreased sexual ability; dizziness or lightheadedness when standing up; increased sensitivity of skin to sunlight; loss of appetite; upset stomach.
- Side effects that should be reported to your doctor: black, tarry stools; blood in urine or stools; cough or hoarseness; fever or chills; joint pain; lower back or side pains; painful or difficult urination; pinpoint red spots on skin; skin rash or hives; stomach pain (severe) with nausea; unusual bleeding or bruising; yellow eyes or skin. This medicine may cause a loss of potassium from your body. Signs of too much potassium loss are: dryness of mouth; increased thirst; mood changes; muscle cramps or pain; nausea or vomiting; unusual tiredness or weakness; weak or irregular heartbeat.

Interactions

This medicine may interact with several other drugs.
- Be sure to tell your doctor about any medications you are currently taking.

Storage

Store at room temperature in a tightly closed container.

NOVOPEN-G

Properties
This medicine contains penicillin G as active ingredient. Penicillins are prescribed to treat infections caused by bacteria. They will not work for colds, flu, or other virus infections. There are several different kinds of penicillins. Each is used to treat different kinds of infections.

Before using this medicine
Before you use this medicine check with your doctor, or pharmacist:
- if you ever had any unusual or allergic reaction to any of the penicillins, cefalosporins, griseofulvin, or penicillamine. Serious reactions may occur in patients who are allergic to penicillins.
- if you are on a low-salt, low-sugar, or any other special diet, or if you are allergic to any substance, such as sulfites or other preservatives or dyes.
- if you are pregnant or intend to become pregnant while using this medicine. Although penicillins have not been shown to cause problems in humans, the chance always exists.
- if you are breast-feeding an infant. Most penicillins (except amdinocillin) pass into the breast milk. Even though only small amounts may pass, allergic reaction, diarrhea, fungal infection, and skin rash may occur in the infant.
- if you have any of the following medical problems:
Allergy
Asthma
Bleeding problems
Eczema
Hay fever, hives
Kidney disease
Liver disease
Mononucleosis
Stomach or intestinal disease

Treatment
This medication is used to treat an infection caused by bacteria. Most penicillins are best taken with a full glass (8 ounces) of water on an empty stomach, some are best taken with a snack or meal. Follow your doctor's or pharmacists's directions on how to take your medicine.
- Keep taking this medicine for the full time of treatment even if you begin to feel better after a few days; do not miss any doses. This is especially important if you have a "strep" infection since serious heart problems could develop later if your infection is not cleared up completely.
- If you do miss a dose of this medicine, take it as soon as possible. However, if it is almost time for your next dose, skip the missed dose and go back to your regular dosing schedule.

Side effects
Along with the needed effects, a medicine may cause some unwanted effects. Side effects that usually do not require medical attention: diarrhea; nausea or vomiting; sore mouth or tongue.
- Stop taking this medicine and get emergency help immediately if you notice: difficulty in breathing; lightheadedness; skin rash, hives, itching; wheezing.

Other side effects that should be reported to your doctor immediately are: abdominal bloating; blood in urine; convulsions (seizures); decreased amount of urine; diarrhea (watery and severe) which may also be bloody; fever; joint pain; sore throat and fever; stomach or abdominal cramps and pain; unusual bleeding or bruising.

Interactions
This medicine may interact with several other drugs such as anticoagulants, diarrhea medicines, heparin, ibuprofen, oral contraceptives, potassium-containing medicines, etc.
- Be sure to tell your doctor about any medications you are currently taking.

Storage
Tablets, capsules, etc. should be stored as directed by your pharmacist or according to instructions on the label.

NOVOPEN-VK

Properties

This medicine contains penicillin V as active ingredient. Penicillins are prescribed to treat infections caused by bacteria. They will not work for colds, flu, or other virus infections. There are several different kinds of penicillins. Each is used to treat different kinds of infections.

Before using this medicine

Before you use this medicine check with your doctor, or pharmacist:
- if you ever had any unusual or allergic reaction to any of the penicillins, cefalosporins, griseofulvin, or penicillamine. Serious reactions may occur in patients who are allergic to penicillins.
- if you are on a low-salt, low-sugar, or any other special diet, or if you are allergic to any substance, such as sulfites or other preservatives or dyes.
- if you are pregnant or intend to become pregnant while using this medicine. Although penicillins have not been shown to cause problems in humans, the chance always exists.
- if you are breast-feeding an infant. Most penicillins (except amdinocillin) pass into the breast milk. Even though only small amounts may pass, allergic reaction, diarrhea, fungal infection, and skin rash may occur in the infant.
- if you have any of the following medical problems:
Allergy
Asthma
Bleeding problems
Eczema
Hay fever, hives
Kidney disease
Liver disease
Mononucleosis
Stomach or intestinal disease

Treatment

This medication is used to treat an infection caused by bacteria. Most penicillins are best taken with a full glass (8 ounces) of water on an empty stomach, some are best taken with a snack or meal. Follow your doctor's or pharmacists's directions on how to take your medicine.
- ◆ Keep taking this medicine for the full time of treatment even if you begin to feel better after a few days; do not miss any doses. This is especially important if you have a "strep" infection since serious heart problems could develop later if your infection is not cleared up completely.
- ◆ If you do miss a dose of this medicine, take it as soon as possible. However, if it is almost time for your next dose, skip the missed dose and go back to your regular dosing schedule.

Side effects

Along with the needed effects, a medicine may cause some unwanted effects. Side effects that usually do not require medical attention: diarrhea; nausea or vomiting; sore mouth or tongue.
- ◆ Stop taking this medicine and get emergency help immediately if you notice: difficulty in breathing; light-headedness; skin rash, hives, itching; wheezing.

Other side effects that should be reported to your doctor immediately are: abdominal bloating; blood in urine; convulsions (seizures); decreased amount of urine; diarrhea (watery and severe) which may also be bloody; fever; joint pain; sore throat and fever; stomach or abdominal cramps and pain; unusual bleeding or bruising.

Interactions

This medicine may interact with several other drugs such as anticoagulants, diarrhea medicines, heparin, ibuprofen, oral contraceptives, potassium-containing medicines, etc.
- ■ Be sure to tell your doctor about any medications you are currently taking.

Storage

Tablets, capsules, etc. should be stored as directed by your pharmacist or according to instructions on the label.

NOVOPENTOBARB

Properties

This medicine contains as active ingredient the barbiturate pentobarbital. Barbiturates belong to the group of medicines called central nervous system depressants (medicines that slow down the nervous system).

Barbiturates may partially block nerve impulses at nerve-cell connections. They may be used to treat insomnia (sleeplessness) by helping patients fall asleep. Also, they may be used to relieve anxiety or tension. Some of the barbiturates are used as anticonvulsants to help control convulsions in certain disorders or diseases, such as epilepsy. If too much of the drug is used, it may become habit-forming (causing mental or physical dependence).

Before using this medicine

Before you use this medicine check with your doctor, or pharmacist:

- if you ever had any unusual or allergic reaction to this medicine or one of its components.
- if you are on a low-salt, low-sugar, or any other special diet, or if you are allergic to preservatives or dyes.
- if you are pregnant or intend to become pregnant while using this medicine, since barbiturates have been shown to increase the chance of birth defects in humans. Taking barbiturates regularly during the last 3 months of pregnancy may cause the baby to become dependent on the medicine. This may lead to withdrawal side effects in the baby after birth.
- if you have any of the following medical problems:
  Anemia (severe)
  Diabetes mellitus (sugar disease)
  Hyperactivity (in children)
  Kidney or lifer disease
  Mental depression
  Overactive thyroid

Treatment

This medication is used to treat the symptoms of your medical condition. Barbiturates act in the central nervous system; some of their side effects are also caused by actions in the central nervous system. Use this medicine as directed by your doctor. Do not use more of it, do not use it more often, and do not use it for a longer period of time than your doctor ordered.

- If you are taking this medication on a regular schedule and you miss a dose, take the missed dose as soon as possible, unless it is almost time for your next dose. In that case do not take the missed dose at all.
- If a barbiturate is used for a long time, it may become habit-forming. Physical dependence may lead to withdrawal side effects when you stop taking this medicine.

Side effects

Along with the needed effects, a medicine may cause some unwanted effects. These side effects may go away during treatment as your body adjusts to the medicine. Such minor side effects are: depression, confusion, diarrhea, nausea, vomiting, joint or muscle pain, slurred speech, hallucinations, headache, decreased sex drive.

- Check with your doctor immediately if any of the following side effects occur:
  Rash or hives
  Face, lip or eyelid swelling
  Sore throat, fever
  Agitation
  Slow heartbeat
  Difficult breathing or chest pain

Interactions

This medicine may interact with several other drugs such as medicines acting on the central nervous system (e.g., antihistamines; beta-adrenergic blockers; MAO inhibitors; mind-altering drugs; nabilone; antidepressants; clozapine; anticonvulsants).

Storage

The medicine should be stored at room temperature in a tightly closed, light-resistant container. Keep out of reach of children since overdose is very dangerous in children.

NOVORIDAZINE

Properties
This medicine contains as active ingredient thioridazine, a phenothiazine derivative. Phenothiazines are a family of medicines used to treat nervous, mental, and emotional conditions. Some are used to control anxiety, restlessness, nausea and vomiting, and severe hiccups. This medicine is available only with your doctor's prescription.

Before using this medicine
Before you use this medicine check with your doctor, or pharmacist:
- if you ever had any unusual or allergic reaction to phenothiazine medicines.
- if you are on a low-salt, low-sugar, or any other special diet, or if you are allergic to any substance, such as sulfites or other preservatives or dyes.
- if you are pregnant or intend to become pregnant while using this medicine. Although phenothiazines have not been shown to cause birth defects, some side effects such as jaundice and muscle tremors have occurred in a few newborns whose mothers received phenothiazines during pregnancy.
- if you are breast-feeding an infant. Although this medicine has not been shown to cause problems in humans but the chance does exist since some phenothiazines are known to pass into the breast milk.
- if you have any of the following medical problems:
  Alcoholism
  Blood disease
  Difficult urination
  Enlarged prostate
  Glaucoma
  Heart or blood vessel disease
  Liver or lung disease
  Parkinson's disease
  Stomach ulcers

Treatment
This medication is prescribed to treat the symptoms of certain types of mental illness or emotional problems. In order to avoid stomach irritation, you can take the tablet or capsule forms of this medication with a meal or with a glass of water or milk (unless your doctor or pharmacist directs you to do otherwise).

Side effects
Along with the needed effects, a medicine may cause some unwanted effects. Minor side effects are: blurred vision, constipation, decreased sweating, diarrhea, dizziness, drooling, drowsiness, dry mouth, fatigue, jitteriness, menstrual irregularities, nasal congestion, restlessness, tremors, vomiting, or weight gain.
- Tell your doctor about any side effects that are persistent or particularly bothersome. It is especially important to tell your doctor about:
  Breast enlargement
  Chest pain or convulsions
  Darkened skin
  Difficulty in swallowing
  Fainting or fever
  Involuntary movements
  Palpitations or sleep disorders
  Rash or sore throat
  Uncoordinated movements
  Unusual bleeding or bruising
  Visual disturbances
  Yellowing of the eyes or skin

Interactions
This medicine may interact with several other drugs such as barbiturates, sleeping pills, narcotics, other tranquilizers, or any other medication that may produce a sedative effect. Avoid alcohol.

Storage
Store this medication as directed on the label. Keep out of the reach of children.

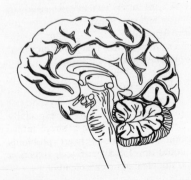

NOVORYTHRO

Properties

This medicine contains erythromycin as active ingredient. This antibiotic is prescribed to treat infections caused by bacteria. They will not work for colds, flu, or other virus infections. Erythromycins are available only with your doctor's prescription.

Before using this medicine

Before you use this medicine check with your doctor, or pharmacist:
- if you ever had any unusual or allergic reaction to any of the erythromycins.
- if you are on a low-salt, low-sugar, or any other special diet, or if you are allergic to any substance, such as sulfites or other preservatives or dyes.
- if you are pregnant or intend to become pregnant while using this medicine. Although erythromycins have not been shown to cause birth defects or other problems in humans, the chance always exists.
- if you are breast-feeding an infant. Most erythromycins pass into the breast milk. Although erythromycins have not been shown to cause problems in humans, the chance always exists.
- if you have lifer disease.

Treatment

This medication belongs to the general family of medicines called antibiotics. It is used to treat a wide variety of bacterial infections. It is also used to treat infections in persons who are allergic to penicillin. Erythromycins are also used to prevent "strep" infections in patients with a history of rheumatic heart disease. They may also be used in Legionnaires' disease and for other problems as determined by your doctor.
- Keep taking this medicine for the full time of treatment even if you begin to feel better after a few days; do not miss any doses. This is especially important if you have a "strep" infection since serious heart problems could develop later if your infection is not cleared up completely.
- If you do miss a dose of this medicine, take it as soon as possible. This will help to keep a constant amount of medicine in the blood. However, if it is almost time for your next dose, skip the missed dose and go back to your regular dosing schedule.
- This medication has been prescribed for your current infection only. Another infection later on, or one that someone else has, may require a different medicine. You should not give your medicine to other people or use it for other infections, unless your doctor specifically directs you to do so.

Side effects

Along with the needed effects, a medicine may cause some unwanted effects. Side effects that usually do not require medical attention: abdominal cramps, black tongue, cough, diarrhea, fatigue, irritation of the mouth, loss of appetite, nausea, or vomiting. These side effects should disappear as your body adjusts to the medication.
- Other side effects that should be reported to your doctor immediately are:
Fever
Hearing loss
Hives or rash
Rectal or vaginal itching
Yellowing of the eyes or skin

Interactions

This medicine may interact with several other drugs such as anticoagulants, theophylline preparations, carbamazepine, etc.
- Be sure to tell your doctor about any medications you are currently taking.

Storage

Tablets, capsules, etc. should be stored at room temperature in tightly closed, light-resistant containers as directed by your pharmacist.

NOVOSECOBARB

Properties
This medicine contains as active ingredient the barbiturate secobarbital. Barbiturates belong to the group of medicines called central nervous system depressants (medicines that slow down the nervous system).

Barbiturates may partially block nerve impulses at nerve-cell connections. They may be used to treat insomnia (sleeplessness) by helping patients fall asleep. Also, they may be used to relieve anxiety or tension. Some of the barbiturates are used as anticonvulsants to help control convulsions in certain disorders or diseases, such as epilepsy. If too much of the drug is used, it may become habit-forming (causing mental or physical dependence).

Before using this medicine
Before you use this medicine check with your doctor, or pharmacist:
- if you ever had any unusual or allergic reaction to this medicine or one of its components.
- if you are on a low-salt, low-sugar, or any other special diet, or if you are allergic to preservatives or dyes.
- if you are pregnant or intend to become pregnant while using this medicine, since barbiturates have been shown to increase the chance of birth defects in humans. Taking barbiturates regularly during the last 3 months of pregnancy may cause the baby to become dependent on the medicine. This may lead to withdrawal side effects in the baby after birth.
- if you have any of the following medical problems:
Anemia (severe)
Diabetes mellitus (sugar disease)
Hyperactivity (in children)
Kidney or lifer disease
Mental depression
Overactive thyroid

Treatment
This medication is used to treat the symptoms of your medical condition. Barbiturates act in the central nervous system; some of their side effects are also caused by actions in the central nervous system. Use this medicine as directed by your doctor. Do not use more of it, do not use it more often, and do not use it for a longer period of time than your doctor ordered.
- If you are taking this medication on a regular schedule and you miss a dose, take the missed dose as soon as possible, unless it is almost time for your next dose. In that case do not take the missed dose at all.
- If a barbiturate is used for a long time, it may become habit-forming. Physical dependence may lead to withdrawal side effects when you stop taking this medicine.

Side effects
Along with the needed effects, a medicine may cause some unwanted effects. These side effects may go away during treatment as your body adjusts to the medicine. Such minor side effects are: depression, confusion, diarrhea, nausea, vomiting, joint or muscle pain, slurred speech, hallucinations, headache, decreased sex drive.
- Check with your doctor immediately if any of the following side effects occur:
Rash or hives
Face, lip or eyelid swelling
Sore throat, fever
Agitation
Slow heartbeat
Difficult breathing or chest pain

Interactions
This medicine may interact with several other drugs such as medicines acting on the central nervous system (e.g., antihistamines; beta-adrenergic blockers; MAO inhibitors; mind-altering drugs; nabilone; antidepressants; clozapine; anticonvulsants).

Storage
The medicine should be stored at room temperature in a tightly closed, light-resistant container. Keep out of reach of children since overdose is very dangerous in children.

NOVOSOXAZOLE

Properties
This medicine contains sulfisoxasole, a sulfonamide, as active ingredient. Sulfonamides are prescribed to treat infections caused by bacteria. They will not work for colds, flu, or other virus infections.

Before using this medicine
Before you use this medicine check with your doctor:
- if you ever had any unusual or allergic reaction to any of the compounds of the medicine.
- if you are on a low-salt, low-sugar, or any other special diet, or if you are allergic to any substance, such as sulfites or other preservatives or dyes.
- if you are pregnant or intend to become pregnant while using this medicine. Although sulfonamides have not been shown to cause defects in humans, the chance may exists.
- if you are breast-feeding an infant. Most sulfonamides pass into the breast milk in small amounts and may cause unwanted effects in infants with some specific conditions.
- if you have any of the following medical problems:
Kidney disease
Liver disease
Porphyria
Deficiency of enzymes such as G6PD

Treatment
This medication is used to treat an infection caused by bacteria. Most sulfonamides are best taken with a full glass (8 ounces) of water on an empty stomach, either one hour before or two hours after a meal. Follow your doctor's or pharmacist's directions on how to take your medicine.
- Keep taking this medicine for the full time of treatment even if you begin to feel better after a few days; do not miss any doses.
- If you do miss a dose of this medicine, take the missed dose immediately.
- This medication works best when the level of medicine in your bloodstream (and urine) is kept constant. It is best, therefore, to take the doses at evenly spaced intervals day and night. if you take two doses a day, the doses should be spaced 12 hours apart.

Side effects
Along with the needed effects, a medicine may cause some unwanted effects. Side effects that usually do not require medical attention: abdominal pain, diarrhea, dizziness, headache, loss of appetite, nausea, sore mouth, or vomiting. These side effects should disappear as your body adjusts to the medication.
Sulfonamides can increase sensitivity to sunlight. It is, therefore, important to avoid prolonged exposure to sunlight and sunlamps.

Tell your doctor about any side effects that are persistent or particularly bothersome. It is especially important to tell your doctor about:
Bloody urine
Difficult urination
Difficulty in breathing
Difficulty in swallowing
Fever or hallucinations
Itching, rash, or pale skin
Joint pain, lower back pain
Ringing in the ears
Sore throat
Swollen or inflamed tongue
Tingling in hands or feet
Unusual bleeding
Yellowing of the eyes or skin

Interactions
This medicine may interact with several other drugs such as anticoagulants, oral antidiabetic agents, aspirin, some antibiotics, or anticancer drugs.
- Be sure to tell your doctor about any medications you are currently taking.

Storage
Tablets, capsules, suspension, etc. should be stored at room temperature as directed by your pharmacist or according to instructions on the label.

NOVOTRIMEL

Properties
This medicine contains sulfamethoxazole, a sulfonamide, and trimethoprim as active ingredients. Sulfonamides are prescribed to treat infections caused by bacteria. They will not work for colds, flu, or other virus infections.

Before using this medicine
Before you use this medicine check with your doctor:
- if you ever had any unusual or allergic reaction to any of the compounds of the medicine.
- if you are on a low-salt, low-sugar, or any other special diet, or if you are allergic to any substance, such as sulfites or other preservatives or dyes.
- if you are pregnant or intend to become pregnant while using this medicine. Although sulfonamides have not been shown to cause defects in humans, the chance may exists.
- if you are breast-feeding an infant. Most sulfonamides pass into the breast milk in small amounts and may cause unwanted effects in infants with some specific conditions.
- if you have any of the following medical problems:
  Kidney disease
  Liver disease
  Porphyria
  Deficiency of enzymes such as G6PD

Treatment
This medication is used to treat an infection caused by bacteria. Most sulfonamides are best taken with a full glass (8 ounces) of water on an empty stomach, either one hour before or two hours after a meal. Follow your doctor's or pharmacist's directions on how to take your medicine.
- Keep taking this medicine for the full time of treatment even if you begin to feel better after a few days; do not miss any doses.
- If you do miss a dose of this medicine, take the missed dose immediately.
- This medication works best when the level of medicine in your bloodstream (and urine) is kept constant. It is best, therefore, to take the doses at evenly spaced intervals day and night. if you take two doses a day, the doses should be spaced 12 hours apart.

Side effects
Along with the needed effects, a medicine may cause some unwanted effects. Side effects that usually do not require medical attention: abdominal pain, diarrhea, dizziness, headache, loss of appetite, nausea, sore mouth, or vomiting. These side effects should disappear as your body adjusts to the medication. Sulfonamides can increase sensitivity to sunlight. It is, therefore, important to avoid prolonged exposure to sunlight and sunlamps.

Tell your doctor about any side effects that are persistent or particularly bothersome. It is especially important to tell your doctor about:
  Bloody urine
  Difficult urination
  Difficulty in breathing
  Difficulty in swallowing
  Fever or hallucinations
  Itching, rash, or pale skin
  Joint pain, lower back pain
  Ringing in the ears
  Sore throat
  Swollen or inflamed tongue
  Tingling in hands or feet
  Unusual bleeding
  Yellowing of the eyes or skin

Interactions
This medicine may interact with several other drugs such as anticoagulants, oral antidiabetic agents, aspirin, some antibiotics, or anticancer drugs.
- Be sure to tell your doctor about any medications you are currently taking.

Storage
Tablets, capsules, suspension, etc. should be stored at room temperature as directed by your pharmacist or according to instructions on the label.

NOVOTRIPTYN

Properties

This medicine contains nortriptyline as active ingredient. It belongs to the group of medicines known as tricyclic antidepressants or 'mood elevators.' It is used to relieve mental depression and depression that sometimes occurs with anxiety. The medication gradually relieves, but doesn't cure, symptoms of depression. The medication may also be used for the treatment of narcolepsy, bulimia, painic attacks, cocaine withdrawal, attention deficit disorder.

Before using this medicine

Before you use this medicine check with your doctor, or pharmacist:
- if you ever had any unusual or allergic reaction to any tricyclic antidepressant, maprotiline or trazodone.
- if you are on a low-salt, low-sugar, or any other special diet, or if you are allergic to any substance, such as sulfites or other preservatives or dyes.
- if you are pregnant or intend to become pregnant while using this medicine. There have been reports of newborns suffering from heart, breathing, and urinary problems when their mothers had taken tricyclic antidepressants before delivery.
- if you are breast-feeding an infant. Some tricyclic antidepressants pass into the breast milk.

Treatment

Take this medicine only as directed by your doctor, to benefit your condition as much as possible. Do not take more of it, do not take it more often, and do not take it for a longer period of time than your doctor ordered.

To lessen stomach upset, take this medicine with food, even for a daily bedtime dose, unless your doctor has told you to take it on an empty stomach. If you forget your once-a-day bedtime dose, Do not take it more than 3 hours late. If more than 3 hours, wait for next scheduled dose;.

Sometimes this medicine must be taken for several weeks before you begin to feel better.

Side effects

Along with the needed effects, a medicine may cause some unwanted effects. Side effects that usually do not require medical attention: difficult or frequent urination; decreased sex drive; muscle aches; abnormal dreams; nasal congestion; weakness and faintness when arising from bed or chair; back pain.
- Other side effects that should be reported to your doctor immediately are:
Hallucinations
Shakiness
Dizziness or fainting
Blurred vision, eye pain
Irregular heartbeat or slow pulse
Inflamed tongue
Abdominal pain
Jaundice
Hair loss, rash
Fever, chills
Joint pain
Palpitations

Interactions

This medicine may interact with several other drugs such as anticoagulants, anticholinergics, cold remedies, oral contraceptives, seizure medicines, sleeping medicines, thyroid medicines, etc.
- Be sure to tell your doctor about any medications you are currently taking.

Storage

Tablets, capsules, etc. should be stored at room temperature in tightly closed, light-resistant containers as directed by your pharmacist. Keep out of reach of children since overdose is especially dangerous in young children. Do not store in the bathroom medicine cabinet because the heat or moisture may cause the medicine to break down. Keep the liquid form of the medicine from freezing.

NU-CEPHALEX

Properties

This medicine contains cephalosporin as active ingredient. Cephalosporins belong to the general family of medicines called antibiotics, used in the treatment of infections caused by bacteria. They work by killing bacteria or preventing their growth. Cephalosporins will not work for colds, flu, or other viral infections.

Before using this medicine

Before you use this medicine check with your doctor:
- if you ever had any unusual or allergic reaction to any of the cephalosporins, penicillins, penicillin-like medicines, or penicillamine.
- if you are on a low-salt, low-sugar, or any other special diet, or if you are allergic to any substance, such as sulfites or other preservatives or dyes.
- if you are pregnant or intend to become pregnant while using this medicine. Although cephalosporins have not been shown to cause birth defects or other problems in humans, the chance always exists.
- if you are breast-feeding an infant. Most cephalosporins pass into the breast milk, usually in small amounts.
- if you have any of the following medical problems:
  Bleeding problem
  Kidney or lifer disease

Treatment

This medication belongs to the general family of medicines called antibiotics. It is used to treat a wide variety of bacterial infections. It is also used to treat infections in persons who are allergic to penicillin.
- Keep taking this medicine for the full time of treatment even if you begin to feel better after a few days; do not miss any doses.
- If you do miss a dose of this medicine, take it as soon as possible. This will help to keep a constant amount of medicine in the blood. However, if it is almost time for your next dose, skip the missed dose and go back to your regular dosing schedule.
- This medication has been prescribed for your current infection only. Another infection later on, or one that someone else has, may require a different medicine. You should not give your medicine to other people or use it for other infections, unless your doctor specifically directs you to do so.
- Take the medicine at the same times each day, 1 hour before or 2 hours after eating.

Side effects

Along with the needed effects, a medicine may cause some unwanted effects. Side effects that usually do not require medical attention: rectal itching, oral or vaginal white spots, mild diarrhea. These side effects should disappear as your body adjusts to the medication.
- Other side effects that should be reported to your doctor immediately are:
  Hives, rash
  Intense itching
  Faintness soon after a dose
  Difficulty in breathing
  Nausea and vomiting
  Severe diarrhea
  Unusual weakness or tiredness
  Bleeding or bruising

Interactions

This medicine may interact with several other drugs such as anticoagulants, theophylline preparations, probenecid, tetracyclines, etc.
- Be sure to tell your doctor about any medications you are currently taking.

Storage

Tablets, capsules, etc. should be stored at room temperature. Store the liquid form in the refrigerator. Keep out of the reach of children. Do not keep outdated medicine or medicine no longer needed.

NU-NIFED

Properties

This medicine contains nefedipine as active ingredient. It is a so-called calcium channel blocker, working by blocking the passage of calcium into heart and smooth muscle. Since calcium is an essential factor in muscle contraction, any medicine that affects calcium in this way will interfere with the contraction of these muscles.

The medicine works by:

* reducing the work that the heart must perform;
* reducing the normal arterial blood pressure;
* increasing oxygen to the heart muscle.

The medicine is prescribed for the treatment of attacks of angina pectoris, irregular heartbeat, and high blood pressure. In many cases it can be used for the treatment and prevention of migraine.

Before using this medicine

Before you use this medicine check with your doctor, or pharmacist:

- if you ever had any unusual or allergic reaction to this medicine or any calcium channel blocker;
- if you are pregnant or intend to become pregnant while using this medicine;
- if you have low blood pressure;
- if you have kidney or lifer disease;
- if you are breast-feeding an infant;
- if you easily get a rash or intensity sunburn in areas exposed to sun or ultraviolet light.

Treatment

This medication is used for treatment of heart conditions (for instance, angina pectoris) and high blood pressure. Tablets, capsules or extended-release tablets should be taken with liquid. The usual dose amounts to 30 to 100 milligrams a day.

For safe and effective use of medicine:

* Follow your doctor's instructions if this medicine was prescribed.
* Follow the manufacturer's package directions if you are treating yourself.

Side effects

Along with the needed effects, a medicine may cause some unwanted effects. Possible side effects include:

Tiredness
Changes in heartbeat
Wheezing
Cough
Shortness of breath
Dizziness
Fainting
Numbness in hands and feet
Tingling in hands and feet
Difficult urination
Constipation

Overdose

The following symptoms may be a sign of overdose:

Unusually fast heartbeat
Unusually slow heartbeat
Loss of consciousness
Cardiac arrest

- Call a doctor or hospital emergency room for instructions. If necessary start first aid immediately.

Interactions

The effect of this medicine may cause a blood pressure drop if taken together with antihypertensives. Cimetidine may increase the effect of the calcium blocker.

The simultaneous use of diuretics and calcium channel blockers may cause dangerous blood pressure drop.

- Be sure to tell your doctor about any medications you are currently taking.

Storage

Capsules, tablets, etc. should be stored at room temperature; store away from heat and direct light. Keep out of reach of children, since this medicine may be dangerous in children.

NUBAIN

Properties
This medicine contains as active ingredient nalbuphine.

It is a narcotic analgesic that acts directly on the central nervous system (brain and spinal cord). It is used to relieve pain or to suppress coughing.

Before using this medicine
Before you use this medicine check with your doctor, or pharmacist:
- if you ever had any unusual or allergic reaction to this medicine or one of its components.
- if you are on a low-salt, low-sugar, or any other special diet, or if you are allergic to any substance, such as sulfites or other preservatives or dyes.
- if you are pregnant or intend to become pregnant while using this medicine. Studies on birth defects have not been done in humans. Too much use of narcotics during pregnancy may cause the baby to become dependent on the medicine.
- if you are breast-feeding an infant. Although this medicine has not been shown to cause problems in humans, it passes into the breast milk in small amounts.
- if you have any of the following medical problems:
  Brain disease or head injury
  Colitis
  Convulsions
  Emphysema, asthma, or chronic lung disease
  Enlarged prostate
  Gallbladder disease or gallstones
  Heart disease
  Kidney or lifer disease
  Underactive thyroid

Treatment
This medication is used to relieve pain or to suppress coughing. Narcotic analgesics act in the central nervous system; some of their side effects are also caused by actions in the central nervous system.
- If you are taking this medication on a regular schedule and you miss a dose, take the missed dose as soon as possible, unless it is almost time for your next dose. In that case do not take the missed dose at all.
- If a narcotic analgesic is used for a long time, it may become habit-forming (causing mental or physical dependence). Physical dependence may lead to withdrawal side effects when you stop taking this medicine.

Unless otherwise directed by your doctor or pharmacist take this as directed. Do not take more of them and do not take them more often than recommended on the label. Children up to 12 years of age should not take this medicine more than 3 times a day or for more than 5 days in a row.

Side effects
Along with the needed effects, a medicine may cause some unwanted effects. These side effects may go away during treatment as your body adjusts to the medicine. Such minor side effects are: constipation, dizziness, drowsiness, dry mouth, false sense of well-being, flushing, light-headedness, loss of appetite, nausea, painful or difficult urination, or sweating.
- Check with your doctor immediately if any of the following side effects occur:
  Anxiety or breathing difficulties
  Excitation or restlessness
  Fatigue, palpitations
  Rash, sore throat and fever
  Tremors or weakness

Interactions
This medicine may interact with several other drugs such as medicines acting on the central nervous system (e.g., antidepressants, tranquilizers), cimetidine, nitrates, quinidine, etc.
- Be sure to tell your doctor about any medications you are currently taking.

Storage
Tablets, elixir, suppository etc. should be stored at room temperature in a tightly closed, light-resistant container.

OBALAN

Properties

This medicine contains phendimetrazine as active ingredient; it is prescribed for appetite suppression.

Appetite suppressants are used in the short-term (a few weeks) treatment of obesity. In a few weeks (6 to 12), these medicines in combination with dieting, exercise, and changes in eating habits can help patients lose weight. However, since their appetite reducing effect is only temporary, they are useful only for the first weeks of dieting until new eating habits are established.

Before using this medicine

Before you use this medicine check with your doctor, or pharmacist:

- if you ever had any unusual or allergic reaction to any of the compounds of this medicine.
- if you are on a low-salt, low-sugar, or any other special diet, or if you are allergic to any substance, such as sulfites or other preservatives or dyes.
- if you are pregnant, intend to become pregnant or breast-feeding an infant while using this medicine.
- if you have any of the following medical problems:
  Diabetes mellitus (sugar diabetes)
  Epilepsy
  Glaucoma
  Heart or blood vessel disease
  High blood pressure
  Mental illness (severe)

Treatment

This medication is used to relieve or prevent the symptoms of your medical problem. Take them as directed. Do not take more of them and do not take them more often than recommended on the label. If too much of the drug is taken, it may become habit-forming.

The medicine produces central nervous system stimulation, and it should not be taken by people with heart disease or high blood pressure.

If you think this medicine is not working as well after you have taken it for a few weeks, do not increase the dose. Instead, check with your doctor.

Side effects

The following minor side effects may occur: irritability, nervousness, restlessness, trouble in sleeping.

These side effects should disappear as your body adjusts to the medication. Tell your doctor about any side effects that are persistent or particularly bothersome. It is especially important to tell your doctor about:

Mental depression
Nausea or vomiting
Stomach cramps or pain
Trembling
Unusual tiredness or weakness

- Discontinue use of the drug; call your doctor right away. Adverse reactions and side effects may be more frequent and severe in people over age 60 than in younger persons.

Interactions

This medicine interacts with several other drugs such as antihypertensives, other appetite suppressants, caffeine, central nervous system depressants, central nervous system stimulants, furazolidone, guanethidine, hydralazine, MAO inhibitors, methyldopa, molindone, phenothiazines, rauwolfia alkaloids, sodium bicarbonate. Interaction with alcoholic beverages may produce drowsiness, sleepiness, and/or inability to concentrate.

- Be sure to tell your doctor about any medications you are currently taking.

Storage

This medicine should be stored at room temperature in tightly closed containers. Store away from heat and direct light. Keep out of reach of children, since overdose may be very dangerous in children.

Do not store this medicine in the bathroom medicine cabinet because the heat and moisture cause the medicine to break down. Do not keep outdated medicine or medicine no longer needed. Flush the contents of the container down the toilet.

OBE-NIX

Properties
This medicine contains phentermine as active ingredient; it is prescribed for appetite suppression. Appetite suppressants are used in the short-term (a few weeks) treatment of obesity. In a few weeks (6 to 12), these medicines in combination with dieting, exercise, and changes in eating habits can help patients lose weight. However, since their appetite reducing effect is only temporary, they are useful only for the first weeks of dieting until new eating habits are established.

Before using this medicine
Before you use this medicine check with your doctor, or pharmacist:
- if you ever had any unusual or allergic reaction to any of the compounds of this medicine.
- if you are on a low-salt, low-sugar, or any other special diet, or if you are allergic to any substance, such as sulfites or other preservatives or dyes.
- if you are pregnant, intend to become pregnant or breast-feeding an infant while using this medicine.
- if you have any of the following medical problems:
Diabetes mellitus
Epilepsy
Glaucoma
Heart disease
High blood pressure
Mental illness (severe)

Treatment
This medication is used to relieve or prevent the symptoms of your medical problem.

Take them as directed. Do not take more of them and do not take them more often than recommended on the label. If too much of the drug is taken, it may become habit-forming.
- The medicine produces central nervous system stimulation, and it should not be taken by people with heart disease or high blood pressure.
- If you think this medicine is not working as well after you have taken it for a few weeks, do not increase the dose. Instead, check with your doctor.

Side effects
The following minor side effects may occur: irritability, nervousness, restlessness, trouble in sleeping.

These side effects should disappear as your body adjusts to the medication. Tell your doctor about any side effects that are persistent or particularly bothersome. It is especially important to tell your doctor about:
Mental depression
Nausea or vomiting
Stomach cramps or pain
Trembling
Unusual tiredness
- Discontinue use of the drug; call your doctor right away. Adverse reactions and side effects may be more frequent and severe in people over age 60 than in younger persons.

Interactions
This medicine interacts with several other drugs such as antihypertensives, other appetite suppressants, caffeine, central nervous system depressants, central nervous system stimulants, furazolidone, guanethidine, hydralazine, MAO inhibitors, methyldopa, molindone, phenothiazines, rauwolfia alkaloids, sodium bicarbonate. Interaction with alcoholic beverages may produce drowsiness, sleepiness, and/or inability to concentrate.
- Be sure to tell your doctor about any medications you are currently taking.

Storage
This medicine should be stored at room temperature in tightly closed containers. Store away from heat and direct light. Keep out of reach of children, since overdose may be very dangerous in children. Do not store this medicine in the bathroom medicine cabinet because the heat and moisture cause the medicine to break down. Do not keep outdated medicine or medicine no longer needed. Flush the contents of the container down the toilet.

OBEPHEN

Properties

This medicine contains phentermine as active ingredient; it is prescribed for appetite suppression.

Appetite suppressants are used in the short-term (a few weeks) treatment of obesity. In a few weeks (6 to 12), these medicines in combination with dieting, exercise, and changes in eating habits can help patients lose weight. However, since their appetite reducing effect is only temporary, they are useful only for the first weeks of dieting until new eating habits are established.

Before using this medicine

Before you use this medicine check with your doctor, or pharmacist:
- if you ever had any unusual or allergic reaction to any of the compounds of this medicine.
- if you are on a low-salt, low-sugar, or any other special diet, or if you are allergic to any substance, such as sulfites or other preservatives or dyes.
- if you are pregnant, intend to become pregnant or breast-feeding an infant while using this medicine.
- if you have any of the following medical problems:
  Diabetes mellitus
  Epilepsy
  Glaucoma
  Heart disease
  High blood pressure
  Mental illness (severe)

Treatment

This medication is used to relieve or prevent the symptoms of your medical problem.

Take them as directed. Do not take more of them and do not take them more often than recommended on the label. If too much of the drug is taken, it may become habit-forming.
- The medicine produces central nervous system stimulation, and it should not be taken by people with heart disease or high blood pressure.
- If you think this medicine is not working as well after you have taken it for a few weeks, do not increase the dose. Instead, check with your doctor.

Side effects

The following minor side effects may occur: irritability, nervousness, restlessness, trouble in sleeping.

These side effects should disappear as your body adjusts to the medication. Tell your doctor about any side effects that are persistent or particularly bothersome. It is especially important to tell your doctor about:
  Mental depression
  Nausea or vomiting
  Stomach cramps or pain
  Trembling
  Unusual tiredness
- Discontinue use of the drug; call your doctor right away. Adverse reactions and side effects may be more frequent and severe in people over age 60 than in younger persons.

Interactions

This medicine interacts with several other drugs such as antihypertensives, other appetite suppressants, caffeine, central nervous system depressants, central nervous system stimulants, furazolidone, guanethidine, hydralazine, MAO inhibitors, methyldopa, molindone, phenothiazines, rauwolfia alkaloids, sodium bicarbonate. Interaction with alcoholic beverages may produce drowsiness, sleepiness, and/or inability to concentrate.

- Be sure to tell your doctor about any medications you are currently taking.

Storage

This medicine should be stored at room temperature in tightly closed containers. Store away from heat and direct light. Keep out of reach of children, since overdose may be very dangerous in children. Do not store this medicine in the bathroom medicine cabinet because the heat and moisture cause the medicine to break down. Do not keep outdated medicine or medicine no longer needed. Flush the contents of the container down the toilet.

OBERMINE

Properties

This medicine contains phentermine as active ingredient; it is prescribed for appetite suppression.

Appetite suppressants are used in the short-term (a few weeks) treatment of obesity. In a few weeks (6 to 12), these medicines in combination with dieting, exercise, and changes in eating habits can help patients lose weight. However, since their appetite reducing effect is only temporary, they are useful only for the first weeks of dieting until new eating habits are established.

Before using this medicine

Before you use this medicine check with your doctor, or pharmacist:
- if you ever had any unusual or allergic reaction to any of the compounds of this medicine.
- if you are on a low-salt, low-sugar, or any other special diet, or if you are allergic to any substance, such as sulfites or other preservatives or dyes.
- if you are pregnant, intend to become pregnant or breast-feeding an infant while using this medicine.
- if you have any of the following medical problems:
Diabetes mellitus
Epilepsy
Glaucoma
Heart disease
High blood pressure
Mental illness (severe)

Treatment

This medication is used to relieve or prevent the symptoms of your medical problem.

Take them as directed. Do not take more of them and do not take them more often than recommended on the label. If too much of the drug is taken, it may become habit-forming.
- The medicine produces central nervous system stimulation, and it should not be taken by people with heart disease or high blood pressure.
- If you think this medicine is not working as well after you have taken it for a few weeks, do not increase the dose. Instead, check with your doctor.

Side effects

The following minor side effects may occur: irritability, nervousness, restlessness, trouble in sleeping.

These side effects should disappear as your body adjusts to the medication. Tell your doctor about any side effects that are persistent or particularly bothersome. It is especially important to tell your doctor about:
Mental depression
Nausea or vomiting
Stomach cramps or pain
Trembling
Unusual tiredness
- Discontinue use of the drug; call your doctor right away. Adverse reactions and side effects may be more frequent and severe in people over age 60 than in younger persons.

Interactions

This medicine interacts with several other drugs such as antihypertensives, other appetite suppressants, caffeine, central nervous system depressants, central nervous system stimulants, furazolidone, guanethidine, hydralazine, MAO inhibitors, methyldopa, molindone, phenothiazines, rauwolfia alkaloids, sodium bicarbonate. Interaction with alcoholic beverages may produce drowsiness, sleepiness, and/or inability to concentrate.
- Be sure to tell your doctor about any medications you are currently taking.

Storage

This medicine should be stored at room temperature in tightly closed containers. Store away from heat and direct light. Keep out of reach of children, since overdose may be very dangerous in children. Do not store this medicine in the bathroom medicine cabinet because the heat and moisture cause the medicine to break down. Do not keep outdated medicine or medicine no longer needed. Flush the contents of the container down the toilet.

OBESTIN-30

Properties

This medicine contains phentermine as active ingredient; it is prescribed for appetite suppression.

Appetite suppressants are used in the short-term (a few weeks) treatment of obesity. In a few weeks (6 to 12), these medicines in combination with dieting, exercise, and changes in eating habits can help patients lose weight. However, since their appetite reducing effect is only temporary, they are useful only for the first weeks of dieting until new eating habits are established.

Before using this medicine

Before you use this medicine check with your doctor, or pharmacist:

- if you ever had any unusual or allergic reaction to any of the compounds of this medicine.
- if you are on a low-salt, low-sugar, or any other special diet, or if you are allergic to any substance, such as sulfites or other preservatives or dyes.
- if you are pregnant, intend to become pregnant or breast-feeding an infant while using this medicine.
- if you have any of the following medical problems:
  Diabetes mellitus
  Epilepsy
  Glaucoma
  Heart disease
  High blood pressure
  Mental illness (severe)

Treatment

This medication is used to relieve or prevent the symptoms of your medical problem.

Take them as directed. Do not take more of them and do not take them more often than recommended on the label. If too much of the drug is taken, it may become habit-forming.

- The medicine produces central nervous system stimulation, and it should not be taken by people with heart disease or high blood pressure.
- If you think this medicine is not working as well after you have taken it for a few weeks, do not increase the dose. Instead, check with your doctor.

Side effects

The following minor side effects may occur: irritability, nervousness, restlessness, trouble in sleeping.

These side effects should disappear as your body adjusts to the medication. Tell your doctor about any side effects that are persistent or particularly bothersome. It is especially important to tell your doctor about:
  Mental depression
  Nausea or vomiting
  Stomach cramps or pain
  Trembling
  Unusual tiredness

- Discontinue use of the drug; call your doctor right away. Adverse reactions and side effects may be more frequent and severe in people over age 60 than in younger persons.

Interactions

This medicine interacts with several other drugs such as antihypertensives, other appetite suppressants, caffeine, central nervous system depressants, central nervous system stimulants, furazolidone, guanethidine, hydralazine, MAO inhibitors, methyldopa, molindone, phenothiazines, rauwolfia alkaloids, sodium bicarbonate. Interaction with alcoholic beverages may produce drowsiness, sleepiness, and/or inability to concentrate.

- Be sure to tell your doctor about any medications you are currently taking.

Storage

This medicine should be stored at room temperature in tightly closed containers. Store away from heat and direct light. Keep out of reach of children, since overdose may be very dangerous in children. Do not store this medicine in the bathroom medicine cabinet because the heat and moisture cause the medicine to break down. Do not keep outdated medicine or medicine no longer needed. Flush the contents of the container down the toilet.

OBEVAL

Properties

This medicine contains phendimetrazine as active ingredient; it is prescribed for appetite suppression.

Appetite suppressants are used in the short-term (a few weeks) treatment of obesity. In a few weeks (6 to 12), these medicines in combination with dieting, exercise, and changes in eating habits can help patients lose weight. However, since their appetite reducing effect is only temporary, they are useful only for the first weeks of dieting until new eating habits are established.

Before using this medicine

Before you use this medicine check with your doctor, or pharmacist:
- if you ever had any unusual or allergic reaction to any of the compounds of this medicine.
- if you are on a low-salt, low-sugar, or any other special diet, or if you are allergic to any substance, such as sulfites or other preservatives or dyes.
- if you are pregnant, intend to become pregnant or breast-feeding an infant while using this medicine.
- if you have any of the following medical problems:
  Diabetes mellitus (sugar diabetes)
  Epilepsy
  Glaucoma
  Heart or blood vessel disease
  High blood pressure
  Mental illness (severe)

Treatment

This medication is used to relieve or prevent the symptoms of your medical problem. Take them as directed. Do not take more of them and do not take them more often than recommended on the label. If too much of the drug is taken, it may become habit-forming.

The medicine produces central nervous system stimulation, and it should not be taken by people with heart disease or high blood pressure.

If you think this medicine is not working as well after you have taken it for a few weeks, do not increase the dose. Instead, check with your doctor.

Side effects

The following minor side effects may occur: irritability, nervousness, restlessness, trouble in sleeping.

These side effects should disappear as your body adjusts to the medication. Tell your doctor about any side effects that are persistent or particularly bothersome. It is especially important to tell your doctor about:
  Mental depression
  Nausea or vomiting
  Stomach cramps or pain
  Trembling
  Unusual tiredness or weakness
- Discontinue use of the drug; call your doctor right away. Adverse reactions and side effects may be more frequent and severe in people over age 60 than in younger persons.

Interactions

This medicine interacts with several other drugs such as antihypertensives, other appetite suppressants, caffeine, central nervous system depressants, central nervous system stimulants, furazolidone, guanethidine, hydralazine, MAO inhibitors, methyldopa, molindone, phenothiazines, rauwolfia alkaloids, sodium bicarbonate. Interaction with alcoholic beverages may produce drowsiness, sleepiness, and/or inability to concentrate.
- Be sure to tell your doctor about any medications you are currently taking.

Storage

This medicine should be stored at room temperature in tightly closed containers. Store away from heat and direct light. Keep out of reach of children, since overdose may be very dangerous in children.

Do not store this medicine in the bathroom medicine cabinet because the heat and moisture cause the medicine to break down. Do not keep outdated medicine or medicine no longer needed. Flush the contents of the container down the toilet.

OBY-TRIM

Properties

This medicine contains phentermine as active ingredient; it is prescribed for appetite suppression.

Appetite suppressants are used in the short-term (a few weeks) treatment of obesity. In a few weeks (6 to 12), these medicines in combination with dieting, exercise, and changes in eating habits can help patients lose weight. However, since their appetite reducing effect is only temporary, they are useful only for the first weeks of dieting until new eating habits are established.

Before using this medicine

Before you use this medicine check with your doctor, or pharmacist:
- if you ever had any unusual or allergic reaction to any of the compounds of this medicine.
- if you are on a low-salt, low-sugar, or any other special diet, or if you are allergic to any substance, such as sulfites or other preservatives or dyes.
- if you are pregnant, intend to become pregnant or breast-feeding an infant while using this medicine.
- if you have any of the following medical problems:
Diabetes mellitus
Epilepsy
Glaucoma
Heart disease
High blood pressure
Mental illness (severe)

Treatment

This medication is used to relieve or prevent the symptoms of your medical problem.

Take them as directed. Do not take more of them and do not take them more often than recommended on the label. If too much of the drug is taken, it may become habit-forming.
- The medicine produces central nervous system stimulation, and it should not be taken by people with heart disease or high blood pressure.
- If you think this medicine is not working as well after you have taken it for a few weeks, do not increase the dose. Instead, check with your doctor.

Side effects

The following minor side effects may occur: irritability, nervousness, restlessness, trouble in sleeping.

These side effects should disappear as your body adjusts to the medication. Tell your doctor about any side effects that are persistent or particularly bothersome. It is especially important to tell your doctor about:
Mental depression
Nausea or vomiting
Stomach cramps or pain
Trembling
Unusual tiredness
- Discontinue use of the drug; call your doctor right away. Adverse reactions and side effects may be more frequent and severe in people over age 60 than in younger persons.

Interactions

This medicine interacts with several other drugs such as antihypertensives, other appetite suppressants, caffeine, central nervous system depressants, central nervous system stimulants, furazolidone, guanethidine, hydralazine, MAO inhibitors, methyldopa, molindone, phenothiazines, rauwolfia alkaloids, sodium bicarbonate. Interaction with alcoholic beverages may produce drowsiness, sleepiness, and/or inability to concentrate.
- Be sure to tell your doctor about any medications you are currently taking.

Storage

This medicine should be stored at room temperature in tightly closed containers. Store away from heat and direct light. Keep out of reach of children, since overdose may be very dangerous in children.

Do not store this medicine in the bathroom medicine cabinet because the heat and moisture cause the medicine to break down. Do not keep outdated medicine or medicine no longer needed. Flush the contents of the container down the toilet.

OCU-CHLOR OPHTHALMIC OINTMENT

Properties
This medicine contains an ophthalmic antibacterial as active ingredient. It helps the body to overcome eye infections on surface tissues of the eye. It is most useful when the infecting organism is one known to be sensitive to the antibacterial drug. The drug penetrates the bacterial cell membrane and prevents cells from multiplying.

Before using this medicine
Before you use this medicine check with your doctor:
- if you ever had any unusual or allergic reaction to any of the compounds of the medicine.
- if you are on a low-salt, low-sugar, or any other special diet, or if you are allergic to any substance, such as sulfites or other preservatives or dyes.
- if you are pregnant or intend to become pregnant while using this medicine. Although ophthalmic antibacterials have been found to be safe for use during pregnancy, you should check with your doctor before taking any drug if you are pregnant.

Treatment
This medication is used to treat an infection caused by bacteria. The medicine may be used in the form of eye drops or as an eye ointment. Use the medication as directed, Do not miss a dose. If you forget a dose, use it as soon as you remember. Notify your doctor if eye symptoms fail to improve in two to four days.
- ◆ To apply eye drops: Till the head backward when applying the eye drops. Pull the lower eyelid away from the eye to form a pouch. After applying the drop, keep the eye closed for a minute or so. This allows the medication to come in contact with the infection.
- ◆ To apply eye ointment: Pull lower lid down from eye to form a pouch. Squeeze tube to apply thin strip of ointment into pouch. Close eye for 1 to 2 minutes.

Always wash your hands before applying the ointment.

The drug starts to work in about one hour. Treatment may require 7 to 10 days to control infection.

Older adults or seniors may take this medication without special restriction.

Side effects
Along with the needed effects, a medicine may cause some unwanted effects. Side effects that usually do not require medical attention: occasional local irritation after application to the eye. Ointments may cause blurred vision for a few minutes; continue the use of the eye drops or ointment, but tell your doctor at the next visit.
- ■ Discontinue the use of eye drops or eye ointment in the following cases:
  Sore throat
  Aplastic anemia
  Pale skin
  Unusual redness of the eye
  Unusual irritation of the eye
  Fever
  Unusual bleeding
  Unusual bruising
- ■ Tell your doctor about any side effects that are persistent or particularly bothersome. In case of prolonged use sensitivity reactions may develop.

Interactions
Clinically significant interactions with oral or injected medicines are unlikely. Do not use the eye drops or ointment with any other eye drops or ointment without checking with your ophthalmologist.

Storage
Keep bottle (with eye drops) or container (containing ointment) lightly closed. Store in a cool place, but Do not freeze. Wash hands immediately after using. Do not store in the bathroom medicine cabinet because the heat or moisture may cause the medicine to break down. Do not keep outdated medicine or medicine no longer needed. Flush the contents of the bottle or tube down the toilet, unless otherwise directed.

OCU-MYCIN (Ophthalmic)

Properties
This medicine contains an ophthalmic antibacterial as active ingredient. It helps the body to overcome eye infections on surface tissues of the eye. It is most useful when the infecting organism is one known to be sensitive to the antibacterial drug.

The drug penetrates the bacterial cell membrane and prevents cells from multiplying.

Before using this medicine
Before you use this medicine check with your doctor:
- if you ever had any unusual or allergic reaction to any of the compounds of the medicine.
- if you are on a low-salt, low-sugar, or any other special diet, or if you are allergic to any substance, such as sulfites or other preservatives or dyes.
- if you are pregnant or intend to become pregnant while using this medicine. Although ophthalmic antibacterials have been found to be safe for use during pregnancy, you should check with your doctor before taking any drug if you are pregnant.

Treatment
This medication is used to treat an infection caused by bacteria. The medicine may be used in the form of eye drops or as an eye ointment. Use the medication as directed, Do not miss a dose. If you forget a dose, use it as soon as you remember. Notify your doctor if eye symptoms fail to improve in two to four days.
- To apply eye drops: Till the head backward when applying the eye drops. Pull the lower eyelid away from the eye to form a pouch. After applying the drop, keep the eye closed for a minute or so. This allows the medication to come in contact with the infection.
- To apply eye ointment: Pull lower lid down from eye to form a pouch. Squeeze tube to apply thin strip of ointment into pouch. Close eye for 1 to 2 minutes.

Always wash your hands before applying the ointment.

The drug starts to work in about one hour. Treatment may require 7 to 10 days to control infection.

Older adults or seniors may take this medication without special restriction.

Side effects
Along with the needed effects, a medicine may cause some unwanted effects. Side effects that usually do not require medical attention: occasional local irritation after application to the eye. Ointments may cause blurred vision for a few minutes; continue the use of the eye drops or ointment, but tell your doctor at the next visit.
- Discontinue the use of eye drops or eye ointment in the following cases:
  Sore throat
  Aplastic anemia
  Pale skin
  Unusual redness of the eye
  Unusual irritation of the eye
  Fever
  Unusual bleeding
  Unusual bruising
- Tell your doctor about any side effects that are persistent or particularly bothersome. In case of prolonged use sensitivity reactions may develop.

Interactions
Clinically significant interactions with oral or injected medicines are unlikely. Do not use the eye drops or ointment with any other eye drops or ointment without checking with your ophthalmologist.

Storage
Keep bottle (with eye drops) or container (containing ointment) lightly closed. Store in a cool place, but Do not freeze. Wash hands immediately after using.

Do not store in the bathroom medicine cabinet because the heat or moisture may cause the medicine to break down.

Do not keep outdated medicine or medicine no longer needed. Flush the contents of the bottle or tube down the toilet, unless otherwise directed.

OCU-SPOR-B (Ophthalmic)

Properties
This medicine contains an ophthalmic antibacterial as active ingredient. It helps the body to overcome eye infections on surface tissues of the eye. It is most useful when the infecting organism is one known to be sensitive to the antibacterial drug.

The drug penetrates the bacterial cell membrane and prevents cells from multiplying.

Before using this medicine
Before you use this medicine check with your doctor:
- if you ever had any unusual or allergic reaction to any of the compounds of the medicine.
- if you are on a low-salt, low-sugar, or any other special diet, or if you are allergic to any substance, such as sulfites or other preservatives or dyes.
- if you are pregnant or intend to become pregnant while using this medicine. Although ophthalmic antibacterials have been found to be safe for use during pregnancy, you should check with your doctor before taking any drug if you are pregnant.

Treatment
This medication is used to treat an infection caused by bacteria. The medicine may be used in the form of eye drops or as an eye ointment. Use the medication as directed, Do not miss a dose. If you forget a dose, use it as soon as you remember. Notify your doctor if eye symptoms fail to improve in two to four days.
- ◆ To apply eye drops: Till the head backward when applying the eye drops. Pull the lower eyelid away from the eye to form a pouch. After applying the drop, keep the eye closed for a minute or so. This allows the medication to come in contact with the infection.
- ◆ To apply eye ointment: Pull lower lid down from eye to form a pouch. Squeeze tube to apply thin strip of ointment into pouch. Close eye for 1 to 2 minutes.

Always wash your hands before applying the ointment.

The drug starts to work in about one hour. Treatment may require 7 to 10 days to control infection.

Older adults or seniors may take this medication without special restriction.

Side effects
Along with the needed effects, a medicine may cause some unwanted effects. Side effects that usually do not require medical attention: occasional local irritation after application to the eye. Ointments may cause blurred vision for a few minutes; continue the use of the eye drops or ointment, but tell your doctor at the next visit.
- ▪ Discontinue the use of eye drops or eye ointment in the following cases:
  Sore throat
  Aplastic anemia
  Pale skin
  Unusual redness of the eye
  Unusual irritation of the eye
  Fever
  Unusual bleeding
  Unusual bruising
- ▪ Tell your doctor about any side effects that are persistent or particularly bothersome. In case of prolonged use sensitivity reactions may develop.

Interactions
Clinically significant interactions with oral or injected medicines are unlikely. Do not use the eye drops or ointment with any other eye drops or ointment without checking with your ophthalmologist.

Storage
Keep bottle (with eye drops) or container (containing ointment) lightly closed. Store in a cool place, but Do not freeze. Wash hands immediately after using. Do not store in the bathroom medicine cabinet because the heat or moisture may cause the medicine to break down.

Do not keep outdated medicine or medicine no longer needed. Flush the contents of the bottle or tube down the toilet, unless otherwise directed.

OCU-SULF-10 Ophthalmic)

Properties

This medicine contains an ophthalmic antibacterial, as active ingredient. It helps the body to overcome eye infections on surface tissues of the eye. It is most useful when the infecting organism is one known to be sensitive to the antibacterial drug.

The drug penetrates the bacterial cell membrane and prevents cells from multiplying.

Before using this medicine

Before you use this medicine check with your doctor:
- if you ever had any unusual or allergic reaction to any of the compounds of the medicine.
- if you are on a low-salt, low-sugar, or any other special diet, or if you are allergic to any substance, such as sulfites or other preservatives or dyes.
- if you are pregnant or intend to become pregnant while using this medicine. Although ophthalmic antibacterials have been found to be safe for use during pregnancy, you should check with your doctor before taking any drug if you are pregnant.

Treatment

This medication is used to treat an infection caused by bacteria. The medicine may be used in the form of eye drops or as an eye ointment. Use the medication as directed, Do not miss a dose. If you forget a dose, use it as soon as you remember. Notify your doctor if eye symptoms fail to improve in two to four days.

◆ To apply eye drops: Till the head backward when applying the eye drops. Pull the lower eyelid away from the eye to form a pouch. After applying the drop, keep the eye closed for a minute or so. This allows the medication to come in contact with the infection.

◆ To apply eye ointment: Pull lower lid down from eye to form a pouch. Squeeze tube to apply thin strip of ointment into pouch. Close eye for 1 to 2 minutes.

Always wash your hands before applying the ointment.

The drug starts to work in about one hour. Treatment may require 7 to 10 days to control infection.

Older adults or seniors may take this medication without special restriction.

Side effects

Along with the needed effects, a medicine may cause some unwanted effects. Side effects that usually do not require medical attention: occasional local irritation after application to the eye. Ointments may cause blurred vision for a few minutes; continue the use of the eye drops or ointment, but tell your doctor at the next visit.

■ Discontinue the use of eye drops or eye ointment in the following cases:
Sore throat
Aplastic anemia
Pale skin
Unusual redness of the eye
Unusual irritation of the eye
Fever
Unusual bleeding
Unusual bruising
■ Tell your doctor about any side effects that are persistent or particularly bothersome. In case of prolonged use sensitivity reactions may develop.

Interactions

Clinically significant interactions with oral or injected medicines are unlikely. Do not use the eye drops or ointment with any other eye drops or ointment without checking with your ophthalmologist.

Storage

Keep bottle (with eye drops) or container (containing ointment) lightly closed. Store in a cool place, but Do not freeze. Wash hands immediately after using. Do not store in the bathroom medicine cabinet because the heat or moisture may cause the medicine to break down. Do not keep outdated medicine or medicine no longer needed. Flush the contents of the bottle or tube down the toilet, unless otherwise directed.

OCUFLOX (Ophthalmic)

Properties
This medicine contains an ophthalmic antibacterial as active ingredient. It helps the body to overcome eye infections on surface tissues of the eye. It is most useful when the infecting organism is one known to be sensitive to the antibacterial drug. The drug penetrates the bacterial cell membrane and prevents cells from multiplying.

Before using this medicine
Before you use this medicine check with your doctor:
- if you ever had any unusual or allergic reaction to any of the compounds of the medicine.
- if you are on a low-salt, low-sugar, or any other special diet, or if you are allergic to any substance, such as sulfites or other preservatives or dyes.
- if you are pregnant or intend to become pregnant while using this medicine. Although ophthalmic antibacterials have been found to be safe for use during pregnancy, you should check with your doctor before taking any drug if you are pregnant.

Treatment
This medication is used to treat an infection caused by bacteria. The medicine may be used in the form of eye drops or as an eye ointment. Use the medication as directed, Do not miss a dose. If you forget a dose, use it as soon as you remember. Notify your doctor if eye symptoms fail to improve in two to four days.
- ◆ To apply eye drops: Till the head backward when applying the eye drops. Pull the lower eyelid away from the eye to form a pouch. After applying the drop, keep the eye closed for a minute or so. This allows the medication to come in contact with the infection.
- ◆ To apply eye ointment: Pull lower lid down from eye to form a pouch. Squeeze tube to apply thin strip of ointment into pouch. Close eye for 1 to 2 minutes.

Always wash your hands before applying the ointment.

The drug starts to work in about one hour. Treatment may require 7 to 10 days to control infection.

Older adults or seniors may take this medication without special restriction.

Side effects
Along with the needed effects, a medicine may cause some unwanted effects. Side effects that usually do not require medical attention: occasional local irritation after application to the eye. Ointments may cause blurred vision for a few minutes; continue the use of the eye drops or ointment, but tell your doctor at the next visit.
- ▪ Discontinue the use of eye drops or eye ointment in the following cases:
  Sore throat
  Aplastic anemia
  Pale skin
  Unusual redness of the eye
  Unusual irritation of the eye
  Fever
  Unusual bleeding
  Unusual bruising
- ▪ Tell your doctor about any side effects that are persistent or particularly bothersome. In case of prolonged use sensitivity reactions may develop.

Interactions
Clinically significant interactions with oral or injected medicines are unlikely. Do not use the eye drops or ointment with any other eye drops or ointment without checking with your ophthalmologist.

Storage
Keep bottle (with eye drops) or container (containing ointment) lightly closed. Store in a cool place, but Do not freeze. Wash hands immediately after using.

Do not store in the bathroom medicine cabinet because the heat or moisture may cause the medicine to break down.

Do not keep outdated medicine or medicine no longer needed. Flush the contents of the bottle or tube down the toilet, unless otherwise directed.

OCUTRICIN (Ophthalmic)

Properties
This medicine contains an ophthalmic antibacterial as active ingredient. It helps the body to overcome eye infections on surface tissues of the eye. It is most useful when the infecting organism is one known to be sensitive to the antibacterial drug.

The drug penetrates the bacterial cell membrane and prevents cells from multiplying.

Before using this medicine
Before you use this medicine check with your doctor:
- if you ever had any unusual or allergic reaction to any of the compounds of the medicine.
- if you are on a low-salt, low-sugar, or any other special diet, or if you are allergic to any substance, such as sulfites or other preservatives or dyes.
- if you are pregnant or intend to become pregnant while using this medicine. Although ophthalmic antibacterials have been found to be safe for use during pregnancy, you should check with your doctor before taking any drug if you are pregnant.

Treatment
This medication is used to treat an infection caused by bacteria. The medicine may be used in the form of eye drops or as an eye ointment. Use the medication as directed, Do not miss a dose. If you forget a dose, use it as soon as you remember. Notify your doctor if eye symptoms fail to improve in two to four days.
- ♦ To apply eye drops: Till the head backward when applying the eye drops. Pull the lower eyelid away from the eye to form a pouch. After applying the drop, keep the eye closed for a minute or so. This allows the medication to come in contact with the infection.
- ♦ To apply eye ointment: Pull lower lid down from eye to form a pouch. Squeeze tube to apply thin strip of ointment into pouch. Close eye for 1 to 2 minutes.

Always wash your hands before applying the ointment.

The drug starts to work in about one hour. Treatment may require 7 to 10 days to control infection.

Older adults or seniors may take this medication without special restriction.

Side effects
Along with the needed effects, a medicine may cause some unwanted effects. Side effects that usually do not require medical attention: occasional local irritation after application to the eye. Ointments may cause blurred vision for a few minutes; continue the use of the eye drops or ointment, but tell your doctor at the next visit.
- Discontinue the use of eye drops or eye ointment in the following cases:
  Sore throat
  Aplastic anemia
  Pale skin
  Unusual redness of the eye
  Unusual irritation of the eye
  Fever
  Unusual bleeding
  Unusual bruising
- Tell your doctor about any side effects that are persistent or particularly bothersome. In case of prolonged use sensitivity reactions may develop.

Interactions
Clinically significant interactions with oral or injected medicines are unlikely. Do not use the eye drops or ointment with any other eye drops or ointment without checking with your ophthalmologist.

Storage
Keep bottle (with eye drops) or container (containing ointment) lightly closed. Store in a cool place, but Do not freeze. Wash hands immediately after using.

Do not store in the bathroom medicine cabinet because the heat or moisture may cause the medicine to break down. Do not keep outdated medicine or medicine no longer needed. Flush the contents of the bottle or tube down the toilet, unless otherwise directed.

OFLOXACIN (Ophthalmic)

Properties
This medicine contains an ophthalmic antibacterial as active ingredient. It helps the body to overcome eye infections on surface tissues of the eye. It is most useful when the infecting organism is one known to be sensitive to the antibacterial drug.

The drug penetrates the bacterial cell membrane and prevents cells from multiplying.

Before using this medicine
Before you use this medicine check with your doctor:
– if you ever had any unusual or allergic reaction to any of the compounds of the medicine.
– if you are on a low-salt, low-sugar, or any other special diet, or if you are allergic to any substance, such as sulfites or other preservatives or dyes.
– if you are pregnant or intend to become pregnant while using this medicine. Although ophthalmic antibacterials have been found to be safe for use during pregnancy, you should check with your doctor before taking any drug if you are pregnant.

Treatment
This medication is used to treat an infection caused by bacteria. The medicine may be used in the form of eye drops or as an eye ointment. Use the medication as directed, Do not miss a dose. If you forget a dose, use it as soon as you remember. Notify your doctor if eye symptoms fail to improve in two to four days.
◆ To apply eye drops: Till the head backward when applying the eye drops. Pull the lower eyelid away from the eye to form a pouch. After applying the drop, keep the eye closed for a minute or so. This allows the medication to come in contact with the infection.
◆ To apply eye ointment: Pull lower lid down from eye to form a pouch. Squeeze tube to apply thin strip of ointment into pouch. Close eye for 1 to 2 minutes.

Always wash your hands before applying the ointment.

The drug starts to work in about one hour. Treatment may require 7 to 10 days to control infection.

Older adults or seniors may take this medication without special restriction.

Side effects
Along with the needed effects, a medicine may cause some unwanted effects. Side effects that usually do not require medical attention: occasional local irritation after application to the eye. Ointments may cause blurred vision for a few minutes; continue the use of the eye drops or ointment, but tell your doctor at the next visit.
■ Discontinue the use of eye drops or eye ointment in the following cases:
Sore throat
Aplastic anemia
Pale skin
Unusual redness of the eye
Unusual irritation of the eye
Fever
Unusual bleeding
Unusual bruising
■ Tell your doctor about any side effects that are persistent or particularly bothersome. In case of prolonged use sensitivity reactions may develop.

Interactions
Clinically significant interactions with oral or injected medicines are unlikely. Do not use the eye drops or ointment with any other eye drops or ointment without checking with your ophthalmologist.

Storage
Keep bottle (with eye drops) or container (containing ointment) lightly closed. Store in a cool place, but Do not freeze. Wash hands immediately after using. Do not store in the bathroom medicine cabinet because the heat or moisture may cause the medicine to break down. Do not keep outdated medicine or medicine no longer needed. Flush the contents of the bottle or tube down the toilet, unless otherwise directed.

OGEN

Properties
This medicine contains estradiol as active ingredient. The medicine is prescribed for treatment of estrogen deficiency; it restores normal estrogen levels in tissues. There is no evidence that this drug is effective for nervous symptoms or depression occurring during menopause. They should not be used to treat this condition; they should be used only to replace the estrogen that is naturally absent after menopause.

Before using this medicine
Before you use this medicine check with your doctor, or pharmacist:
- if you ever had any unusual or allergic reaction to estrogens;
- if you are pregnant or intend to become pregnant within three months;
- if you are breast-feeding an infant;
- if you have any of the following medical problems:
  Diabetes
  Breast cancer
  Fibrocystic breast disease
  Fibroid uterine tumors
  Endometriosis
  Migraine headaches
  Epilepsy
  Porphyria
  High blood pressure
  Asthma
  Congestive heart failure
  Kidney disease
  Gallstones

Treatment
This medication is used to treat estrogen deficiency, specific symptoms of menopause, estrogen-deficiency osteoporosis, atrophic vaginitis, prostate cancer.
For safe and effective use of this medicine:
- Follow your doctor's instructions if this medicine was prescribed.
- Follow the manufacturer's package directions if you are treating yourself.
- Estrogens have been reported to increase the risk of endometrial carcinoma.

Side effects
Along with the needed effects, a medicine may cause some unwanted effects. Possible side effects include:
  Stomach cramps
  Profuse bleeding
  Appetite loss
  Nausea and vomiting
  Swollen breasts
  Change in menstruation
  Rash, skin blisters
  Depression
  Dizziness

Overdose
The following symptoms may indicate an overdose:
  Nausea and vomiting
  Fluid retention
  Breast enlargement
  Abnormal vaginal bleeding
- Call a doctor or hospital emergency room for instructions.

Interactions
This medicine may interact with several other drugs such as adrenocorticosteroids, antidepressants, oral antidiabetics, insulin, phenobarbital, primidone.
- Be sure to tell your doctor about any medications you are currently taking.

Storage
Capsules, tablets, vaginal cream, transdermal patches, etc. should be stored at room temperature; store away from heat and direct light. Keep out of reach of children, since this medicine may be dangerous in children.

OMEPRAZOLE

Properties
This medicine contains omeprazole as active ingredient. It is a so-called proton pump inhibitor, a medicine that inhibits the production and secretion of hydrochloric acid from the cells in the mucosal lining of the stomach.

The medicine is prescribed for the short-term treatment of duodenal (intestinal) and gastric (stomach) ulcers. It is also prescribed for gastroesophageal reflex, that is the splashing of stomach acid from the stomach up onto the lower end of the esophagus.

Before using this medicine
Before you use this medicine check with your doctor, or pharmacist:
- if you ever had any unusual or allergic reaction to this medicine or any proton pump inhibitor;
- if you are allergic to any medicines, foods or other substances;
- if you are pregnant or intend to become pregnant while using this medicine (animal studies have shown toxic effects to developing fetuses);
- if you are breast-feeding an infant.

Treatment
This medication is used for treatment of peptic ulcers (duodenal or gastric ulcers), and certain ailments of the esophagus. The usual dose amounts to 20 to 80 milligrams a day. If you forget to take a dose of this medicine, take it as soon as you remember.

The medicine should be taken immediately before a meal or with an antacid if it upsets the stomach.

For safe and effective use of medicine:
♦ Follow your doctor's instructions if this medicine was prescribed.
♦ Follow the manufacturer's package directions if you are treating yourself.

Side effects
Along with the needed effects, a medicine may cause some unwanted effects. Possible side effects include:
  Abdominal pain
  Headache
  Diarrhea
  Nausea
  Sore throat
  Vomiting
  Dizziness
  Constipation
  Back pain
  Urinary infections
  Skin rash
  Heartburn
  Drowsiness
  Unusual bleeding
  Unusual bruising
  Muscle cramps
  Appetite loss

Overdose
The following symptoms may be a sign of overdose:
  Seizures
  Breathing difficulty
  Severe drowsiness
■ Call a doctor or hospital emergency room for instructions. If necessary, give first aid immediately.

Interactions
The effect of this medicine may be reduced if it is taken together with sucralfate. Taken together with anticoagulants it may increase the effect of the latter.
■ Be sure to tell your doctor about any medications you are currently taking.

Storage
Delayed-release and extended-release capsules should be stored at room temperature; store away from heat and direct light. Keep out of reach of children, since overdose may be dangerous in children.

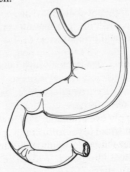

OPHTHACET (Ophthalmic)

Properties

This medicine contains an ophthalmic antibacterial as active ingredient. It helps the body to overcome eye infections on surface tissues of the eye. It is most useful when the infecting organism is one known to be sensitive to the antibacterial drug.

The drug penetrates the bacterial cell membrane and prevents cells from multiplying.

Before using this medicine

Before you use this medicine check with your doctor:

- if you ever had any unusual or allergic reaction to any of the compounds of the medicine.
- if you are on a low-salt, low-sugar, or any other special diet, or if you are allergic to any substance, such as sulfites or other preservatives or dyes.
- if you are pregnant or intend to become pregnant while using this medicine. Although ophthalmic antibacterials have been found to be safe for use during pregnancy, you should check with your doctor before taking any drug if you are pregnant.

Treatment

This medication is used to treat an infection caused by bacteria. The medicine may be used in the form of eye drops or as an eye ointment. Use the medication as directed, Do not miss a dose. If you forget a dose, use it as soon as you remember. Notify your doctor if eye symptoms fail to improve in two to four days.

♦ To apply eye drops: Till the head backward when applying the eye drops. Pull the lower eyelid away from the eye to form a pouch. After applying the drop, keep the eye closed for a minute or so. This allows the medication to come in contact with the infection.

♦ To apply eye ointment: Pull lower lid down from eye to form a pouch. Squeeze tube to apply thin strip of ointment into pouch. Close eye for 1 to 2 minutes.

Always wash your hands before applying the ointment.

The drug starts to work in about one hour. Treatment may require 7 to 10 days to control infection.

Older adults or seniors may take this medication without special restriction.

Side effects

Along with the needed effects, a medicine may cause some unwanted effects. Side effects that usually do not require medical attention: occasional local irritation after application to the eye. Ointments may cause blurred vision for a few minutes; continue the use of the eye drops or ointment, but tell your doctor at the next visit.

- Discontinue the use of eye drops or eye ointment in the following cases:
  Sore throat
  Aplastic anemia
  Pale skin
  Unusual redness of the eye
  Unusual irritation of the eye
  Fever
  Unusual bleeding
  Unusual bruising
- Tell your doctor about any side effects that are persistent or particularly bothersome. In case of prolonged use sensitivity reactions may develop.

Interactions

Clinically significant interactions with oral or injected medicines are unlikely. Do not use the eye drops or ointment with any other eye drops or ointment without checking with your ophthalmologist.

Storage

Keep bottle (with eye drops) or container (containing ointment) lightly closed. Store in a cool place, but Do not freeze. Wash hands immediately after using. Do not store in the bathroom medicine cabinet because the heat or moisture may cause the medicine to break down. Do not keep outdated medicine or medicine no longer needed. Flush the contents of the bottle or tube down the toilet, unless otherwise directed.

ORETIC

Properties
This medicine contains as active ingredient hydrochlorothiazide, a thiazide-like diuretic. Thiazide or thiazide-like diuretics are prescribed to treat high blood pressure (hypertension). They are also used to reduce fluid accumulation in the body caused by conditions such as heart failure, cirrhosis, kidney disease, and the long-term use of some medications. Thiazide diuretics may also be used for other conditions as determined by your doctor.

Before using this medicine
Before you use this medicine check with your doctor, or pharmacist:
- if you ever had any unusual or allergic reaction to sulfonamides (sulfa drugs) or any of the thiazide diuretics.
- if you are on a low-salt, low-sugar, or any other special diet, or if you are allergic to any substance, such as sulfites or other preservatives or dyes.
- if you are pregnant or intend to become pregnant while using this medicine. When this medicine is used during pregnancy, it may cause side effects including jaundice, blood problems, and low potassium in the newborn.
- if you are breast-feeding an infant. Although this medicine has not been shown to cause problems in humans, the chance always exists since thiazide diuretics pass into breast milk.
- if you have any of the following medical problems:
Diabetes
Gout
Kidney disease
Liver disease
Lupus erythematosus
Pancreas disease

Treatment
This medication is used to treat high blood pressure (hypertension) and also to help reduce the amount of water in the body by increasing the flow of urine. This medicine will not cure your high blood pressure but it does help control it. You must continue to take it - even if you feel well -if you expect to keep your blood pressure down. You may have to take high blood pressure medicine for the rest of your life.

Thiazide diuretics may cause an unusual feeling of tiredness when you begin to take them. You may also notice an increase in urine or in frequency of urination. To keep this from affecting sleep:
- if you are to take a single dose a day, take it in the morning after breakfast;
- if you are to take more than one dose, take the last one not later than 6 p.m.

Side effects
Along with the needed effects, a medicine may cause some unwanted effects. Side effects that usually do not require medical attention: decreased sexual ability; dizziness or lightheadedness when standing up; increased sensitivity of skin to sunlight; loss of appetite; upset stomach.
- Side effects that should be reported to your doctor: black, tarry stools; blood in urine or stools; cough or hoarseness; fever or chills; joint pain; lower back or side pains; painful or difficult urination; pinpoint red spots on skin; skin rash or hives; stomach pain (severe) with nausea; unusual bleeding or bruising; yellow eyes or skin. This medicine may cause a loss of potassium from your body. Signs of too much potassium loss are: dryness of mouth; increased thirst; mood changes; muscle cramps or pain; nausea or vomiting; unusual tiredness or weakness; weak or irregular heartbeat.

Interactions
This medicine may interact with several other drugs.
- Be sure to tell your doctor about any medications you are currently taking.

Storage
Store at room temperature in a tightly closed container.

ORMAZINE

Properties

This medicine contains as active ingredient chlorpromazine, a phenothiazine derivative. Phenothiazines are a family of medicines used to treat nervous, mental, and emotional conditions. Some are used to control anxiety, restlessness, nausea and vomiting, and severe hiccups. This medicine is available only with your doctor's prescription.

Before using this medicine

Before you use this medicine check with your doctor, or pharmacist:
- if you ever had any unusual or allergic reaction to phenothiazine medicines.
- if you are on a low-salt, low-sugar, or any other special diet, or if you are allergic to any substance, such as sulfites or other preservatives or dyes.
- if you are pregnant or intend to become pregnant while using this medicine. Although phenothiazines have not been shown to cause birth defects, some side effects such as jaundice and muscle tremors have occurred in a few newborns whose mothers received phenothiazines during pregnancy.
- if you are breast-feeding an infant. Although this medicine has not been shown to cause problems in humans but the chance does exist since some phenothiazines are known to pass into the breast milk.
- if you have any of the following medical problems:
Alcoholism
Blood disease
Difficult urination
Enlarged prostate
Glaucoma
Heart or blood vessel disease
Liver or lung disease
Parkinson's disease
Stomach ulcers

Treatment

This medication is prescribed to treat the symptoms of certain types of mental illness or emotional problems. In order to avoid stomach irritation, you can take the tablet or capsule forms of this medication with a meal or with a glass of water or milk (unless your doctor or pharmacist directs you to do otherwise).

Side effects

Along with the needed effects, a medicine may cause some unwanted effects. Minor side effects are: blurred vision, constipation, decreased sweating, diarrhea, dizziness, drooling, drowsiness, dry mouth, fatigue, jitteriness, menstrual irregularities, nasal congestion, restlessness, tremors, vomiting, or weight gain.
- Tell your doctor about any side effects that are persistent or particularly bothersome. It is especially important to tell your doctor about:
Breast enlargement
Chest pain or convulsions
Darkened skin
Difficulty in swallowing
Fainting or fever
Involuntary movements
Palpitations or sleep disorders
Rash or sore throat
Uncoordinated movements
Unusual bleeding or bruising
Visual disturbances
Yellowing of the eyes or skin

Interactions

This medicine may interact with several other drugs such as barbiturates, sleeping pills, narcotics, other tranquilizers, or any other medication that may produce a sedative effect. Avoid alcohol.

Storage

Store this medication as directed on the label. Keep out of the reach of children.

ORTHO

Properties
This medicine contains norethindrone and ethinyl estradiol as active ingredients. It is an oral contraceptive prescribed to prevent pregnancy and/or to regulate menstrual periods.

The drug works by altering the mucus at the cervix entrance to prevent the entry of sperm. It also alters the uterus lining to resist implantation of the fertilized egg. Oral contraceptives create the same chemical atmosphere in blood that exists during pregnancy.

Before using this medicine
Before you use this medicine check with your doctor, or pharmacist:
- if you ever had any unusual or allergic reaction to estrogens or progestogen;
- if you are pregnant or want to become pregnant within three months;
- if you are breast-feeding an infant;
- if you have any of the following medical problems:
Diabetes
Ailments of the breast
Disorders of the uterus
Migraine or epilepsy
High blood pressure
Asthma or heart conditions
Kidney disease
Gallstones

Treatment
This medication is used to prevent pregnancy or to regulate menstrual periods.

Adverse reactions
Along with the needed effects, a medicine may cause some unwanted effects or adverse reactions.
■ *An increased risk of the following adverse reactions has been associated with the use of oral contraceptives:*
Thrombophlebitis
Venous thrombosis
Arterial thromboembolism
Pulmonary (lung) embolism
Myocardial infarction
Cerebral hemorrhage
Cerebral thrombosis
Hypertension
Gallbladder disease
Hepatic (liver) hepatomas
Benign lifer tumors
■ *The following adverse reactions have been reported in patients receiving oral contraceptives and are believed to be drug-related:*
Nausea and vomiting
Abdominal cramps
Breakthrough bleeding
Spotting
Change in menstrual flow
Amenorrhea
Temporary infertility
Edema
Breast changes
Weight changes
Cholestatic jaundice
Migraine
Rash (allergic)
Mental depression
Vaginal candidiasis

Interactions
This medicine may interact with several other drugs such as antibiotics, anticoagulants, anticonvulsants, antidepressants, oral antidiabetics, antihistamines, barbiturates, oral hypoglycemics, insulin, meperidine.
■ Be sure to tell your doctor about any medications you are currently taking.

Storage
Tablets should be stored at room temperature; store away from heat and direct light. Keep out of reach of children, since this medicine may be dangerous in children.

ORTHO-CEPT

Properties
This medicine contains desogestrel and ethinyl estradiol as active ingredients. It is an oral contraceptive prescribed to prevent pregnancy and/or to regulate menstrual periods.

The drug works by altering the mucus at the cervix entrance to prevent the entry of sperm. It also alters the uterus lining to resist implantation of the fertilized egg. Oral contraceptives create the same chemical atmosphere in blood that exists during pregnancy.

Before using this medicine
Before you use this medicine check with your doctor, or pharmacist:
- if you ever had any unusual or allergic reaction to estrogens or progestogen;
- if you are pregnant or want to become pregnant within three months;
- if you are breast-feeding an infant;
- if you have any of the following medical problems:
  Diabetes
  Ailments of the breast
  Disorders of the uterus
  Migraine or epilepsy
  High blood pressure
  Asthma or heart conditions
  Kidney disease
  Gallstones

Treatment
This medication is used to prevent pregnancy or to regulate menstrual periods.

Adverse reactions
Along with the needed effects, a medicine may cause some unwanted effects or adverse reactions.
- *An increased risk of the following adverse reactions has been associated with the use of oral contraceptives:*
  Thrombophlebitis
  Venous thrombosis
  Arterial thromboembolism
  Pulmonary (lung) embolism
  Myocardial infarction
  Cerebral hemorrhage
  Cerebral thrombosis
  Hypertension
  Gallbladder disease
  Hepatic (liver) hepatomas
  Benign lifer tumors
- *The following adverse reactions have been reported in patients receiving oral contraceptives and are believed to be drug-related:*
  Nausea and vomiting
  Abdominal cramps
  Breakthrough bleeding
  Spotting
  Change in menstrual flow
  Amenorrhea
  Temporary infertility
  Edema
  Breast changes
  Weight changes
  Cholestatic jaundice
  Migraine
  Rash (allergic)
  Mental depression
  Vaginal candidiasis

Interactions
This medicine may interact with several other drugs such as antibiotics, anticoagulants, anticonvulsants, antidepressants, oral antidiabetics, antihistamines, barbiturates, oral hypoglycemics, insulin, meperidine.
- Be sure to tell your doctor about any medications you are currently taking.

Storage
Tablets should be stored at room temperature; store away from heat and direct light. Keep out of reach of children, since this medicine may be dangerous in children.

ORTHO-CYCLEN

Properties
This medicine contains norgestimate and ethinyl estradiol as active ingredients. It is an oral contraceptive prescribed to prevent pregnancy and/or to regulate menstrual periods.

The drug works by altering the mucus at the cervix entrance to prevent the entry of sperm. It also alters the uterus lining to resist implantation of the fertilized egg. Oral contraceptives create the same chemical atmosphere in blood that exists during pregnancy.

Before using this medicine
Before you use this medicine check with your doctor, or pharmacist:
- if you ever had any unusual or allergic reaction to estrogens or progestogen;
- if you are pregnant or want to become pregnant within three months;
- if you are breast-feeding an infant;
- if you have any of the following medical problems:
  Diabetes
  Ailments of the breast
  Disorders of the uterus
  Migraine or epilepsy
  High blood pressure
  Asthma or heart conditions
  Kidney disease
  Gallstones

Treatment
This medication is used to prevent pregnancy or to regulate menstrual periods.

Adverse reactions
Along with the needed effects, a medicine may cause some unwanted effects or adverse reactions.
- *An increased risk of the following adverse reactions has been associated with the use of oral contraceptives:*
  Thrombophlebitis
  Venous thrombosis
  Arterial thromboembolism
  Pulmonary (lung) embolism
  Myocardial infarction
  Cerebral hemorrhage
  Cerebral thrombosis
  Hypertension
  Gallbladder disease
  Hepatic (liver) hepatomas
  Benign lifer tumors
- *The following adverse reactions have been reported in patients receiving oral contraceptives and are believed to be drug-related:*
  Nausea and vomiting
  Abdominal cramps
  Breakthrough bleeding
  Spotting
  Change in menstrual flow
  Amenorrhea
  Temporary infertility
  Edema
  Breast changes
  Weight changes
  Cholestatic jaundice
  Migraine
  Rash (allergic)
  Mental depression
  Vaginal candidiasis

Interactions
This medicine may interact with several other drugs such as antibiotics, anticoagulants, anticonvulsants, antidepressants, oral antidiabetics, antihistamines, barbiturates, oral hypoglycemics, insulin, meperidine.
- Be sure to tell your doctor about any medications you are currently taking.

Storage
Tablets should be stored at room temperature; store away from heat and direct light. Keep out of reach of children, since this medicine may be dangerous in children.

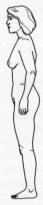

ORTHO-EST

Properties
This medicine contains estropipate as active ingredient. The medicine is prescribed for treatment of estrogen deficiency; it restores normal estrogen levels in tissues. There is no evidence that this drug is effective for nervous symptoms or depression occurring during menopause. They should not be used to treat this condition; they should be used only to replace the estrogen that is naturally absent after menopause.

Before using this medicine
Before you use this medicine check with your doctor, or pharmacist:
- if you ever had any unusual or allergic reaction to estrogens;
- if you are pregnant or intend to become pregnant within three months;
- if you are breast-feeding an infant;
- if you have any of the following medical problems:
  Diabetes
  Breast cancer
  Fibrocystic breast disease
  Fibroid uterine tumors
  Endometriosis
  Migraine headaches
  Epilepsy
  Porphyria
  High blood pressure
  Asthma
  Congestive heart failure
  Kidney disease
  Gallstones

Treatment
This medication is used to treat estrogen deficiency, specific symptoms of menopause, estrogen-deficiency osteoporosis, atrophic vaginitis, prostate cancer.

For safe and effective use of this medicine:
- ◆ Follow your doctor's instructions if this medicine was prescribed.
- ◆ Follow the manufacturer's package directions if you are treating yourself.
- ◆ Estrogens have been reported to increase the risk of endometrial carcinoma.

Side effects
Along with the needed effects, a medicine may cause some unwanted effects. Possible side effects include:
  Stomach cramps
  Profuse bleeding
  Appetite loss
  Nausea and vomiting
  Swollen breasts
  Change in menstruation
  Rash, skin blisters
  Depression
  Dizziness

Overdose
The following symptoms may indicate an overdose:
  Nausea and vomiting
  Fluid retention
  Breast enlargement
  Abnormal vaginal bleeding
- ▪ Call a doctor or hospital emergency room for instructions.

Interactions
This medicine may interact with several other drugs such as adrenocorticosteroids, antidepressants, oral antidiabetics, insulin, phenobarbital, primidone.
- ▪ Be sure to tell your doctor about any medications you are currently taking.

Storage
Capsules, tablets, vaginal cream, transdermal patches, etc. should be stored at room temperature; store away from heat and direct light. Keep out of reach of children, since this medicine may be dangerous in children.

ORTHO-NOVUM

Properties

This medicine contains norethindrone and ethinyl estradiol as active ingredients. It is an oral contraceptive prescribed to prevent pregnancy and/or to regulate menstrual periods.

The drug works by altering the mucus at the cervix entrance to prevent the entry of sperm. It also alters the uterus lining to resist implantation of the fertilized egg. Oral contraceptives create the same chemical atmosphere in blood that exists during pregnancy.

Before using this medicine

Before you use this medicine check with your doctor, or pharmacist:
- if you ever had any unusual or allergic reaction to estrogens or progestogen;
- if you are pregnant or want to become pregnant within three months;
- if you are breast-feeding an infant;
- if you have any of the following medical problems:
  Diabetes
  Ailments of the breast
  Disorders of the uterus
  Migraine or epilepsy
  High blood pressure
  Asthma or heart conditions
  Kidney disease
  Gallstones

Treatment

This medication is used to prevent pregnancy or to regulate menstrual periods.

Adverse reactions

Along with the needed effects, a medicine may cause some unwanted effects or adverse reactions.
- *An increased risk of the following adverse reactions has been associated with the use of oral contraceptives:*
  Thrombophlebitis
  Venous thrombosis
  Arterial thromboembolism
  Pulmonary (lung) embolism
  Myocardial infarction
  Cerebral hemorrhage
  Cerebral thrombosis
  Hypertension
  Gallbladder disease
  Hepatic (liver) hepatomas
  Benign lifer tumors
- *The following adverse reactions have been reported in patients receiving oral contraceptives and are believed to be drug-related:*
  Nausea and vomiting
  Abdominal cramps
  Breakthrough bleeding
  Spotting
  Change in menstrual flow
  Amenorrhea
  Temporary infertility
  Edema
  Breast changes
  Weight changes
  Cholestatic jaundice
  Migraine
  Rash (allergic)
  Mental depression
  Vaginal candidiasis

Interactions

This medicine may interact with several other drugs such as antibiotics, anticoagulants, anticonvulsants, antidepressants, oral antidiabetics, antihistamines, barbiturates, oral hypoglycemics, insulin, meperidine.
- Be sure to tell your doctor about any medications you are currently taking.

Storage

Tablets should be stored at room temperature; store away from heat and direct light. Keep out of reach of children, since this medicine may be dangerous in children.

ORTHO-TRI-CYCLEN

Properties
This medicine contains norethindrone and mestranol as active ingredients. It is an oral contraceptive prescribed to prevent pregnancy and/or to regulate menstrual periods.

The drug works by altering the mucus at the cervix entrance to prevent the entry of sperm. It also alters the uterus lining to resist implantation of the fertilized egg. Oral contraceptives create the same chemical atmosphere in blood that exists during pregnancy.

Before using this medicine
Before you use this medicine check with your doctor, or pharmacist:
- if you ever had any unusual or allergic reaction to estrogens or progestogen;
- if you are pregnant or want to become pregnant within three months;
- if you are breast-feeding an infant;
- if you have any of the following medical problems:
  Diabetes
  Ailments of the breast
  Disorders of the uterus
  Migraine or epilepsy
  High blood pressure
  Asthma or heart conditions
  Kidney disease
  Gallstones

Treatment
This medication is used to prevent pregnancy or to regulate menstrual periods.

Adverse reactions
Along with the needed effects, a medicine may cause some unwanted effects or adverse reactions.
- *An increased risk of the following adverse reactions has been associated with the use of oral contraceptives:*
  Thrombophlebitis
  Venous thrombosis
  Arterial thromboembolism
  Pulmonary (lung) embolism
  Myocardial infarction
  Cerebral hemorrhage
  Cerebral thrombosis
  Hypertension
  Gallbladder disease
  Hepatic (liver) hepatomas
  Benign lifer tumors
- *The following adverse reactions have been reported in patients receiving oral contraceptives and are believed to be drug-related:*
  Nausea and vomiting
  Abdominal cramps
  Breakthrough bleeding
  Spotting
  Change in menstrual flow
  Amenorrhea
  Temporary infertility
  Edema
  Breast changes
  Weight changes
  Cholestatic jaundice
  Migraine
  Rash (allergic)
  Mental depression
  Vaginal candidiasis

Interactions
This medicine may interact with several other drugs such as antibiotics, anticoagulants, anticonvulsants, antidepressants, oral antidiabetics, antihistamines, barbiturates, oral hypoglycemics, insulin, meperidine.
- Be sure to tell your doctor about any medications you are currently taking.

Storage
Tablets should be stored at room temperature; store away from heat and direct light. Keep out of reach of children, since this medicine may be dangerous in children.

OVCON

Properties

This medicine contains norethindrone and ethinyl estradiol as active ingredients. It is an oral contraceptive prescribed to prevent pregnancy and/or to regulate menstrual periods.

The drug works by altering the mucus at the cervix entrance to prevent the entry of sperm. It also alters the uterus lining to resist implantation of the fertilized egg. Oral contraceptives create the same chemical atmosphere in blood that exists during pregnancy.

Before using this medicine

Before you use this medicine check with your doctor, or pharmacist:
- if you ever had any unusual or allergic reaction to estrogens or progestogen;
- if you are pregnant or want to become pregnant within three months;
- if you are breast-feeding an infant;
- if you have any of the following medical problems:
  Diabetes
  Ailments of the breast
  Disorders of the uterus
  Migraine or epilepsy
  High blood pressure
  Asthma or heart conditions
  Kidney disease
  Gallstones

Treatment

This medication is used to prevent pregnancy or to regulate menstrual periods.

Adverse reactions

Along with the needed effects, a medicine may cause some unwanted effects or adverse reactions.
- *An increased risk of the following adverse reactions has been associated with the use of oral contraceptives:*
  Thrombophlebitis
  Venous thrombosis
  Arterial thromboembolism
  Pulmonary (lung) embolism
  Myocardial infarction
  Cerebral hemorrhage
  Cerebral thrombosis
  Hypertension
  Gallbladder disease
  Hepatic (liver) hepatomas
  Benign lifer tumors
- *The following adverse reactions have been reported in patients receiving oral contraceptives and are believed to be drug-related:*
  Nausea and vomiting
  Abdominal cramps
  Breakthrough bleeding
  Spotting
  Change in menstrual flow
  Amenorrhea
  Temporary infertility
  Edema
  Breast changes
  Weight changes
  Cholestatic jaundice
  Migraine
  Rash (allergic)
  Mental depression
  Vaginal candidiasis

Interactions

This medicine may interact with several other drugs such as antibiotics, anticoagulants, anticonvulsants, antidepressants, oral antidiabetics, antihistamines, barbiturates, oral hypoglycemics, insulin, meperidine.
- Be sure to tell your doctor about any medications you are currently taking.

Storage

Tablets should be stored at room temperature; store away from heat and direct light. Keep out of reach of children, since this medicine may be dangerous in children.

OVRAL

Properties

This medicine contains norgestrel and ethinyl estradiol as active ingredients. It is an oral contraceptive prescribed to prevent pregnancy and/or to regulate menstrual periods.

The drug works by altering the mucus at the cervix entrance to prevent the entry of sperm. It also alters the uterus lining to resist implantation of the fertilized egg. Oral contraceptives create the same chemical atmosphere in blood that exists during pregnancy.

Before using this medicine

Before you use this medicine check with your doctor, or pharmacist:
- if you ever had any unusual or allergic reaction to estrogens or progestogen;
- if you are pregnant or want to become pregnant within three months;
- if you are breast-feeding an infant;
- if you have any of the following medical problems:
  Diabetes
  Ailments of the breast
  Disorders of the uterus
  Migraine or epilepsy
  High blood pressure
  Asthma or heart conditions
  Kidney disease
  Gallstones

Treatment

This medication is used to prevent pregnancy or to regulate menstrual periods.

Adverse reactions

Along with the needed effects, a medicine may cause some unwanted effects or adverse reactions.
- *An increased risk of the following adverse reactions has been associated with the use of oral contraceptives:*
Thrombophlebitis
Venous thrombosis
Arterial thromboembolism
Pulmonary (lung) embolism
Myocardial infarction
Cerebral hemorrhage
Cerebral thrombosis
Hypertension
Gallbladder disease
Hepatic (liver) hepatomas
Benign lifer tumors
- *The following adverse reactions have been reported in patients receiving oral contraceptives and are believed to be drug-related:*
Nausea and vomiting
Abdominal cramps
Breakthrough bleeding
Spotting
Change in menstrual flow
Amenorrhea
Temporary infertility
Edema
Breast changes
Weight changes
Cholestatic jaundice
Migraine
Rash (allergic)
Mental depression
Vaginal candidiasis

Interactions

This medicine may interact with several other drugs such as antibiotics, anticoagulants, anticonvulsants, antidepressants, oral antidiabetics, antihistamines, barbiturates, oral hypoglycemics, insulin, meperidine.
- Be sure to tell your doctor about any medications you are currently taking.

Storage

Tablets should be stored at room temperature; store away from heat and direct light. Keep out of reach of children, since this medicine may be dangerous in children.

OX-PAM

Properties

This medicine contains as active ingredient oxazepam, a benzodiazepine preparation. Benzodiazepines belong to the group of psychoactive medicines that influence the activity of the brain. Some are used to relieve nervousness or tension. It is effective for this purpose for short periods. Others are used for sleeplessness or to relax muscles or relieve muscle spasm. The benzodiazepines may also be used for other conditions as determined by your doctor.

Before using this medicine

Before you use this medicine check with your doctor:
- if you ever had any unusual or allergic reaction to benzodiazepines.
- if you are on a low-salt, low-sugar, or any other special diet, or if you are allergic to any substance, such as sulfites or other preservatives or dyes.
- if you are pregnant or intend to become pregnant while using this medicine. Some benzodiazepines have been reported to increase the chance of birth defects when used during the first 3 months of pregnancy.
- if you are breast-feeding an infant. Benzodiazepines may pass into the breast milk and cause drowsiness, unusually slow heartbeat, shortness of breath, or troubled breathing in infants of mothers taking this medicine.
- if you have any of the following medical problems: asthma, bronchitis, emphysema, or other chronic lung disease; epilepsy or history of convulsions; hyperactivity (in children); kidney or lifer disease; mental depression or illness; myasthania gravis, porphyria.

Treatment

This medication is used to relieve or prevent the symptoms of your medical problem. Benzodiazepines are mainly used as antianxiety agents, anticonvulsants, or sedatives. Take them as directed. Do not take more of them and do not take them more often than recommended on the label, unless otherwise directed by your doctor. Benzodiazepine tranquilizing drugs can be abused if taken for long periods of time and it is possible to develop withdrawal symptoms if you discontinue the therapy abruptly.

Side effects

Along with the needed effects, a medicine may cause some unwanted effects. Minor side effects are: bitter taste in the mouth, dizziness, drowsiness, depression, constipation, dry mouth, excessive salivation, fatigue, flushing, headache, heartburn, loss of appetite, nausea, nervousness, sweating or vomiting. As your body adjusts to the medicine, these side effects should disappear.

- Tell your doctor about any side effects that are persistent or particularly bothersome. It is especially important to tell your doctor about:
  Blurred or double vision
  Chest pain
  Difficulty in urinating
  Fainting or falling
  Fever or hallucinations
  Joint pain
  Mouth sores
  Nightmares
  Palpitations
  Severe depression
  Shortness of breath
  Slurred speech
  Uncoordinated movements
  Unusual tiredness
  Yellowing of the skin

Interactions

- This medicine may interact with several other drugs. This medicine will add to the effects of alcohol, and CNS depressants.
- Be sure to tell your doctor about any medications you are currently taking.

Storage

Store at room temperature in tightly closed, light-resistent containers. Keep out of the reach of children since overdose may be especially dangerous in children.

OXAZEPAM

Properties

This medicine contains as active ingredient oxazepam, a benzodiazepine preparation. Benzodiazepines belong to the group of psychoactive medicines that influence the activity of the brain. Some are used to relieve nervousness or tension. It is effective for this purpose for short periods. Others are used for sleeplessness or to relax muscles or relieve muscle spasm. The benzodiazepines may also be used for other conditions as determined by your doctor.

Before using this medicine

Before you use this medicine check with your doctor:

- if you ever had any unusual or allergic reaction to benzodiazepines.
- if you are on a low-salt, low-sugar, or any other special diet, or if you are allergic to any substance, such as sulfites or other preservatives or dyes.
- if you are pregnant or intend to become pregnant while using this medicine. Some benzodiazepines have been reported to increase the chance of birth defects when used during the first 3 months of pregnancy.
- if you are breast-feeding an infant. Benzodiazepines may pass into the breast milk and cause drowsiness, unusually slow heartbeat, shortness of breath, or troubled breathing in infants of mothers taking this medicine.
- if you have any of the following medical problems: asthma, bronchitis, emphysema, or other chronic lung disease; epilepsy or history of convulsions; hyperactivity (in children); kidney or lifer disease; mental depression or illness; myasthania gravis, porphyria.

Treatment

This medication is used to relieve or prevent the symptoms of your medical problem. Benzodiazepines are mainly used as antianxiety agents, anticonvulsants, or sedatives. Take them as directed. Do not take more of them and do not take them more often than recommended on the label, unless otherwise directed by your doctor. Benzodiazepine tranquilizing drugs can be abused if taken for long periods of time and it is possible to develop withdrawal symptoms if you discontinue the therapy abruptly.

Side effects

Along with the needed effects, a medicine may cause some unwanted effects. Minor side effects are: bitter taste in the mouth, dizziness, drowsiness, depression, constipation, dry mouth, excessive salivation, fatigue, flushing, headache, heartburn, loss of appetite, nausea, nervousness, sweating or vomiting. As your body adjusts to the medicine, these side effects should disappear.

- Tell your doctor about any side effects that are persistent or particularly bothersome. It is especially important to tell your doctor about:
  Blurred or double vision
  Chest pain
  Difficulty in urinating
  Fainting or falling
  Fever or hallucinations
  Joint pain
  Mouth sores
  Nightmares
  Palpitations
  Severe depression
  Shortness of breath
  Slurred speech
  Uncoordinated movements
  Unusual tiredness
  Yellowing of the skin

Interactions

- This medicine may interact with several other drugs. This medicine will add to the effects of alcohol, and CNS depressants.
- Be sure to tell your doctor about any medications you are currently taking.

Storage

Store at room temperature in tightly closed, light-resistent containers. Keep out of the reach of children since overdose may be especially dangerous in children.

PAMELOR

Properties

This medicine contains nortriptyline as active ingredient. It belongs to the group of medicines known as tricyclic antidepressants or 'mood elevators.' It is used to relieve mental depression and depression that sometimes occurs with anxiety. The medication gradually relieves, but doesn't cure, symptoms of depression. The medication may also be used for the treatment of narcolepsy, bulimia, painic attacks, cocaine withdrawal, attention deficit disorder.

Before using this medicine

Before you use this medicine check with your doctor, or pharmacist:
- if you ever had any unusual or allergic reaction to any tricyclic antidepressant, maprotiline or trazodone.
- if you are on a low-salt, low-sugar, or any other special diet, or if you are allergic to any substance, such as sulfites or other preservatives or dyes.
- if you are pregnant or intend to become pregnant while using this medicine. There have been reports of newborns suffering from heart, breathing, and urinary problems when their mothers had taken tricyclic antidepressants before delivery.
- if you are breast-feeding an infant. Some tricyclic antidepressants pass into the breast milk.

Treatment

Take this medicine only as directed by your doctor, to benefit your condition as much as possible. Do not take more of it, do not take it more often, and do not take it for a longer period of time than your doctor ordered.

To lessen stomach upset, take this medicine with food, even for a daily bedtime dose, unless your doctor has told you to take it on an empty stomach. If you forget your once-a-day bedtime dose, Do not take it more than 3 hours late. If more than 3 hours, wait for next scheduled dose;.

Sometimes this medicine must be taken for several weeks before you begin to feel better.

Side effects

Along with the needed effects, a medicine may cause some unwanted effects. Side effects that usually do not require medical attention: difficult or frequent urination; decreased sex drive; muscle aches; abnormal dreams; nasal congestion; weakness and faintness when arising from bed or chair; back pain.
- Other side effects that should be reported to your doctor immediately are:
  Hallucinations
  Shakiness
  Dizziness or fainting
  Blurred vision, eye pain
  Irregular heartbeat or slow pulse
  Inflamed tongue
  Abdominal pain
  Jaundice
  Hair loss, rash
  Fever, chills
  Joint pain
  Palpitations

Interactions

This medicine may interact with several other drugs such as anticoagulants, anticholinergics, cold remedies, oral contraceptives, seizure medicines, sleeping medicines, thyroid medicines, etc.
- Be sure to tell your doctor about any medications you are currently taking.

Storage

Tablets, capsules, etc. should be stored at room temperature in tightly closed, light-resistant containers as directed by your pharmacist. Keep out of reach of children since overdose is especially dangerous in young children. Do not store in the bathroom medicine cabinet because the heat or moisture may cause the medicine to break down. Keep the liquid form of the medicine from freezing.

PANTOPON

Properties

This medicine contains as active ingredient opium.

It is a narcotic analgesic that acts directly on the central nervous system (brain and spinal cord). It is used to relieve pain or to suppress coughing.

Before using this medicine

Before you use this medicine check with your doctor, or pharmacist:
- if you ever had any unusual or allergic reaction to this medicine or one of its components.
- if you are on a low-salt, low-sugar, or any other special diet, or if you are allergic to any substance, such as sulfites or other preservatives or dyes.
- if you are pregnant or intend to become pregnant while using this medicine. Studies on birth defects have not been done in humans. Too much use of narcotics during pregnancy may cause the baby to become dependent on the medicine.
- if you are breast-feeding an infant. Although this medicine has not been shown to cause problems in humans, it passes into the breast milk in small amounts.
- if you have any of the following medical problems:
  Brain disease or head injury
  Colitis
  Convulsions
  Emphysema, asthma, or chronic lung disease
  Enlarged prostate
  Gallbladder disease or gallstones
  Heart disease
  Kidney or lifer disease
  Underactive thyroid

Treatment

This medication is used to relieve pain or to suppress coughing. Narcotic analgesics act in the central nervous system; some of their side effects are also caused by actions in the central nervous system.
- If you are taking this medication on a regular schedule and you miss a dose, take the missed dose as soon as possible, unless it is almost time for your next dose. In that case do not take the missed dose at all.
- If a narcotic analgesic is used for a long time, it may become habit-forming (causing mental or physical dependence). Physical dependence may lead to withdrawal side effects when you stop taking this medicine.

Unless otherwise directed by your doctor or pharmacist take this as directed. Do not take more of them and do not take them more often than recommended on the label. Children up to 12 years of age should not take this medicine more than 3 times a day or for more than 5 days in a row.

Side effects

Along with the needed effects, a medicine may cause some unwanted effects. These side effects may go away during treatment as your body adjusts to the medicine. Such minor side effects are: constipation, dizziness, drowsiness, dry mouth, false sense of well-being, flushing, light-headedness, loss of appetite, nausea, painful or difficult urination, or sweating.
- Check with your doctor immediately if any of the following side effects occur:
  Anxiety or breathing difficulties
  Excitation or restlessness
  Fatigue, palpitations
  Rash, sore throat and fever
  Tremors or weakness

Interactions

This medicine may interact with several other drugs such as medicines acting on the central nervous system (e.g., antidepressants, tranquilizers), cimetidine, nitrates, quinidine, etc.
- Be sure to tell your doctor about any medications you are currently taking.

Storage

Tablets, elixir, suppository etc. should be stored at room temperature in a tightly closed, light-resistant container.

PARMINE

Properties

This medicine contains phentermine as active ingredient; it is prescribed for appetite suppression.

Appetite suppressants are used in the short-term (a few weeks) treatment of obesity. In a few weeks (6 to 12), these medicines in combination with dieting, exercise, and changes in eating habits can help patients lose weight. However, since their appetite reducing effect is only temporary, they are useful only for the first weeks of dieting until new eating habits are established.

Before using this medicine

Before you use this medicine check with your doctor, or pharmacist:
- if you ever had any unusual or allergic reaction to any of the compounds of this medicine.
- if you are on a low-salt, low-sugar, or any other special diet, or if you are allergic to any substance, such as sulfites or other preservatives or dyes.
- if you are pregnant, intend to become pregnant or breast-feeding an infant while using this medicine.
- if you have any of the following medical problems:
  Diabetes mellitus
  Epilepsy
  Glaucoma
  Heart disease
  High blood pressure
  Mental illness (severe)

Treatment

This medication is used to relieve or prevent the symptoms of your medical problem.

Take them as directed. Do not take more of them and do not take them more often than recommended on the label. If too much of the drug is taken, it may become habit-forming.
- The medicine produces central nervous system stimulation, and it should not be taken by people with heart disease or high blood pressure.
- If you think this medicine is not working as well after you have taken it for a few weeks, do not increase the dose. Instead, check with your doctor.

Side effects

The following minor side effects may occur: irritability, nervousness, restlessness, trouble in sleeping.

These side effects should disappear as your body adjusts to the medication. Tell your doctor about any side effects that are persistent or particularly bothersome. It is especially important to tell your doctor about:
  Mental depression
  Nausea or vomiting
  Stomach cramps or pain
  Trembling
  Unusual tiredness
- Discontinue use of the drug; call your doctor right away. Adverse reactions and side effects may be more frequent and severe in people over age 60 than in younger persons.

Interactions

This medicine interacts with several other drugs such as antihypertensives, other appetite suppressants, caffeine, central nervous system depressants, central nervous system stimulants, furazolidone, guanethidine, hydralazine, MAO inhibitors, methyldopa, molindone, phenothiazines, rauwolfia alkaloids, sodium bicarbonate. Interaction with alcoholic beverages may produce drowsiness, sleepiness, and/or inability to concentrate.
- Be sure to tell your doctor about any medications you are currently taking.

Storage

This medicine should be stored at room temperature in tightly closed containers. Store away from heat and direct light. Keep out of reach of children, since overdose may be very dangerous in children.

Do not store this medicine in the bathroom medicine cabinet because the heat and moisture cause the medicine to break down. Do not keep outdated medicine or medicine no longer needed. Flush the contents of the container down the toilet.

PAVERAL

Properties
This medicine contains as active ingredient codeine.

It is a narcotic analgesic that acts directly on the central nervous system (brain and spinal cord). It is used to relieve pain or to suppress coughing.

Before using this medicine
Before you use this medicine check with your doctor, or pharmacist:
- if you ever had any unusual or allergic reaction to this medicine or one of its components.
- if you are on a low-salt, low-sugar, or any other special diet, or if you are allergic to any substance, such as sulfites or other preservatives or dyes.
- if you are pregnant or intend to become pregnant while using this medicine. Studies on birth defects have not been done in humans. Too much use of narcotics during pregnancy may cause the baby to become dependent on the medicine.
- if you are breast-feeding an infant. Although this medicine has not been shown to cause problems in humans, it passes into the breast milk in small amounts.
- if you have any of the following medical problems:
Brain disease or head injury
Colitis
Convulsions
Emphysema, asthma, or chronic lung disease
Enlarged prostate
Gallbladder disease or gallstones
Heart disease
Kidney or lifer disease
Underactive thyroid

Treatment
This medication is used to relieve pain or to suppress coughing. Narcotic analgesics act in the central nervous system; some of their side effects are also caused by actions in the central nervous system.
- If you are taking this medication on a regular schedule and you miss a dose, take the missed dose as soon as possible, unless it is almost time for your next dose. In that case do not take the missed dose at all.
- If a narcotic analgesic is used for a long time, it may become habit-forming (causing mental or physical dependence). Physical dependence may lead to withdrawal side effects when you stop taking this medicine.

Unless otherwise directed by your doctor or pharmacist take this as directed. Do not take more of them and do not take them more often than recommended on the label. Children up to 12 years of age should not take this medicine more than 3 times a day or for more than 5 days in a row.

Side effects
Along with the needed effects, a medicine may cause some unwanted effects. These side effects may go away during treatment as your body adjusts to the medicine. Such minor side effects are: constipation, dizziness, drowsiness, dry mouth, false sense of well-being, flushing, light-headedness, loss of appetite, nausea, painful or difficult urination, or sweating.
- Check with your doctor immediately if any of the following side effects occur:
Anxiety or breathing difficulties
Excitation or restlessness
Fatigue, palpitations
Rash, sore throat and fever
Tremors or weakness

Interactions
This medicine may interact with several other drugs such as medicines acting on the central nervous system (e.g., antidepressants, tranquilizers), cimetidine, nitrates, quinidine, etc.
- Be sure to tell your doctor about any medications you are currently taking.

Storage
Tablets, elixir, suppository etc. should be stored at room temperature in a tightly closed, light-resistant container.

PAXIL

Properties
This medicine contains paroxetine as active ingredient. It is an antidepressant drug that has a specific effect on certain areas of the brain. The medicine is known to affect serotonin, one of the chemicals in the brain called neuro-transmitters or chemical messengers, that play a role in the steering of psy-choactive behavior. It is prescribed for the treatment of depressive disorders.

Before using this medicine
Before you use this medicine check with your doctor, or pharmacist:
- if you ever had any unusual or aller-gic reaction to this medicine or any psychoactive drug;
- if you are allergic to any medicines, foods or other substances;
- if you are pregnant or intend to be-come pregnant while using this medicine (animal studies have shown toxic effects to developing fetuses);
- if you are breast-feeding an infant;
- if you have thought of suicide;
- if you have kidney or lifer disease.

Treatment
This medication is used for treatment of certain types of mental depression and obsessive-compulsive disorders. Tablets should be swallowed with liquid. If you forget to take a dose of this medicine, take it as soon as you remember up to two hours late. If more than two hours, wait for the next scheduled dose;. In pa-tients over 60 years of age, adverse re-actions may be more frequent and se-vere than in younger persons.

For safe and effective use of medi-cine:
- ◆ Follow your doctor's instructions if this medicine was prescribed.
- ◆ Follow the manufacturer's package directions if you are treating your-self.

Side effects
Along with the needed effects, a medi-cine may cause some unwanted effects. Possible side effects include:
Headache
Nervousness
Increased sweating
Nausea
Insomnia
Anxiety
Joint pain
Muscle pain
Blurred vision
Problems urinating
Nightmares
Sensory changes
Decreased sex drive
Dry mouth

Overdose
The following symptoms may be a sign of overdose:
Vomiting
Severe drowsiness
Heart rhythm disturbances
Dilated pupils
Severe mouth dryness
- ■ Call a doctor or hospital emergency room for instructions. If necessary, give first aid immediately.

Interactions
The effect of this medicine may be in-creased by other antidepressants. Lith-ium, may increase the occurrence of side effects. Anticoagulants may cause an increase in anticoagulation. Alcohol will sometimes augment the depression.
- ■ Be sure to tell your doctor about any medications you are currently taking.

Storage
The tablets should be stored at room temperature; store away from heat and direct light. Keep out of reach of chil-dren, since this medicine may be dan-gerous to children.

PAXIPAM

Properties
This medicine contains as active ingredient halazepam, a benzodiazepine preparation. Benzodiazepines belong to the group of psychoactive medicines that influence the activity of the brain. Some are used to relieve nervousness or tension. It is effective for this purpose for short periods. Others are used for sleeplessness or to relax muscles or relieve muscle spasm. The benzodiazepines may also be used for other conditions as determined by your doctor.

Before using this medicine
Before you use this medicine check with your doctor:
- if you ever had any unusual or allergic reaction to benzodiazepines.
- if you are on a low-salt, low-sugar, or any other special diet, or if you are allergic to any substance, such as sulfites or other preservatives or dyes.
- if you are pregnant or intend to become pregnant while using this medicine. Some benzodiazepines have been reported to increase the chance of birth defects when used during the first 3 months of pregnancy.
- if you are breast-feeding an infant. Benzodiazepines may pass into the breast milk and cause drowsiness, unusually slow heartbeat, shortness of breath, or troubled breathing in infants of mothers taking this medicine.
- if you have any of the following medical problems: asthma, bronchitis, emphysema, or other chronic lung disease; epilepsy or history of convulsions; hyperactivity (in children); kidney or lifer disease; mental depression or illness; myasthania gravis, porphyria.

Treatment
This medication is used to relieve or prevent the symptoms of your medical problem. Benzodiazepines are mainly used as antianxiety agents, anticonvulsants, or sedatives. Take them as directed. Do not take more of them and do not take them more often than recommended on the label, unless otherwise directed by your doctor. Benzodiazepine tranquilizing drugs can be abused if taken for long periods of time and it is possible to develop withdrawal symptoms if you discontinue the therapy abruptly.

Side effects
Along with the needed effects, a medicine may cause some unwanted effects. Minor side effects are: bitter taste in the mouth, dizziness, drowsiness, depression, constipation, dry mouth, excessive salivation, fatigue, flushing, headache, heartburn, loss of appetite, nausea, nervousness, sweating or vomiting. As your body adjusts to the medicine, these side effects should disappear.
- Tell your doctor about any side effects that are persistent or particularly bothersome. It is especially important to tell your doctor about:
  Blurred or double vision
  Chest pain
  Difficulty in urinating
  Fainting or falling
  Fever or hallucinations
  Joint pain
  Mouth sores
  Nightmares
  Palpitations
  Severe depression
  Shortness of breath
  Slurred speech
  Uncoordinated movements
  Unusual tiredness
  Yellowing of the skin

Interactions
This medicine may interact with several other drugs. Be sure to tell your doctor about any medications you are currently taking. This medicine will add to the effects of alcohol, and CNS depressants.

Storage
Store at room temperature in tightly closed, light-resistant-resistant containers. Keep out of the reach of children since overdose may be especially dangerous in children.

PBR/12

Properties
This medicine contains as active ingredient the barbiturate phenobarbital. Barbiturates belong to the group of medicines called central nervous system depressants (medicines that slow down the nervous system).

Barbiturates may partially block nerve impulses at nerve-cell connections. They may be used to treat insomnia (sleeplessness) by helping patients fall asleep. Also, they may be used to relieve anxiety or tension. Some of the barbiturates are used as anticonvulsants to help control convulsions in certain disorders or diseases, such as epilepsy. If too much of the drug is used, it may become habit-forming (causing mental or physical dependence).

Before using this medicine
Before you use this medicine check with your doctor, or pharmacist:
- if you ever had any unusual or allergic reaction to this medicine or one of its components.
- if you are on a low-salt, low-sugar, or any other special diet, or if you are allergic to preservatives or dyes.
- if you are pregnant or intend to become pregnant while using this medicine, since barbiturates have been shown to increase the chance of birth defects in humans. Taking barbiturates regularly during the last 3 months of pregnancy may cause the baby to become dependent on the medicine. This may lead to withdrawal side effects in the baby after birth.
- if you have any of the following medical problems:
  Anemia (severe)
  Diabetes mellitus (sugar disease)
  Hyperactivity (in children)
  Kidney or lifer disease
  Mental depression
  Overactive thyroid

Treatment
This medication is used to treat the symptoms of your medical condition. Barbiturates act in the central nervous system; some of their side effects are also caused by actions in the central nervous system. Use this medicine as directed by your doctor. Do not use more of it, do not use it more often, and do not use it for a longer period of time than your doctor ordered.
- If you are taking this medication on a regular schedule and you miss a dose, take the missed dose as soon as possible, unless it is almost time for your next dose. In that case do not take the missed dose at all.
- If a barbiturate is used for a long time, it may become habit-forming. Physical dependence may lead to withdrawal side effects when you stop taking this medicine.

Side effects
Along with the needed effects, a medicine may cause some unwanted effects. These side effects may go away during treatment as your body adjusts to the medicine. Such minor side effects are: depression, confusion, diarrhea, nausea, vomiting, joint or muscle pain, slurred speech, hallucinations, headache, decreased sex drive.
- Check with your doctor immediately if any of the following side effects occur:
  Rash or hives
  Face, lip or eyelid swelling
  Sore throat, fever
  Agitation
  Slow heartbeat
  Difficult breathing or chest pain

Interactions
This medicine may interact with several other drugs such as medicines acting on the central nervous system (e.g., antihistamines; beta-adrenergic blockers; MAO inhibitors; mind-altering drugs; nabilone; antidepressants; clozapine; anticonvulsants).

Storage
The medicine should be stored at room temperature in a tightly closed, light-resistant container. Keep out of reach of children since overdose is very dangerous in children.

PCE DISPERTAB

Properties

This medicine contains erythromycin as active ingredient. This antibiotic is prescribed to treat infections caused by bacteria. They will not work for colds, flu, or other virus infections. Erythromycins are available only with your doctor's prescription.

Before using this medicine

Before you use this medicine check with your doctor, or pharmacist:

– if you ever had any unusual or allergic reaction to any of the erythromycins.
– if you are on a low-salt, low-sugar, or any other special diet, or if you are allergic to any substance, such as sulfites or other preservatives or dyes.
– if you are pregnant or intend to become pregnant while using this medicine. Although erythromycins have not been shown to cause birth defects or other problems in humans, the chance always exists.
– if you are breast-feeding an infant. Most erythromycins pass into the breast milk. Although erythromycins have not been shown to cause problems in humans, the chance always exists.
– if you have lifer disease.

Treatment

This medication belongs to the general family of medicines called antibiotics. It is used to treat a wide variety of bacterial infections. It is also used to treat infections in persons who are allergic to penicillin. Erythromycins are also used to prevent "strep" infections in patients with a history of rheumatic heart disease. They may also be used in Legionnaires' disease and for other problems as determined by your doctor.

■ Keep taking this medicine for the full time of treatment even if you begin to feel better after a few days; do not miss any doses. This is especially important if you have a "strep" infection since serious heart problems could develop later if your infection is not cleared up completely.

■ If you do miss a dose of this medicine, take it as soon as possible. This will help to keep a constant amount of medicine in the blood. However, if it is almost time for your next dose, skip the missed dose and go back to your regular dosing schedule.

■ This medication has been prescribed for your current infection only. Another infection later on, or one that someone else has, may require a different medicine. You should not give your medicine to other people or use it for other infections, unless your doctor specifically directs you to do so.

Side effects

Along with the needed effects, a medicine may cause some unwanted effects. Side effects that usually do not require medical attention: abdominal cramps, black tongue, cough, diarrhea, fatigue, irritation of the mouth, loss of appetite, nausea, or vomiting. These side effects should disappear as your body adjusts to the medication.

■ Other side effects that should be reported to your doctor immediately are:
Fever
Hearing loss
Hives or rash
Rectal or vaginal itching
Yellowing of the eyes or skin

Interactions

This medicine may interact with several other drugs such as anticoagulants, theophylline preparations, carbamazepine, etc.

■ Be sure to tell your doctor about any medications you are currently taking.

Storage

Tablets, capsules, etc. should be stored at room temperature in tightly closed, light-resistant containers as directed by your pharmacist.

PEDIAMYCIN

Properties
This medicine contains erythromycin as active ingredient. This antibiotic is prescribed to treat infections caused by bacteria. They will not work for colds, flu, or other virus infections. Erythromycins are available only with your doctor's prescription.

Before using this medicine
Before you use this medicine check with your doctor, or pharmacist:
- if you ever had any unusual or allergic reaction to any of the erythromycins.
- if you are on a low-salt, low-sugar, or any other special diet, or if you are allergic to any substance, such as sulfites or other preservatives or dyes.
- if you are pregnant or intend to become pregnant while using this medicine. Although erythromycins have not been shown to cause birth defects or other problems in humans, the chance always exists.
- if you are breast-feeding an infant. Most erythromycins pass into the breast milk. Although erythromycins have not been shown to cause problems in humans, the chance always exists.
- if you have lifer disease.

Treatment
This medication belongs to the general family of medicines called antibiotics. It is used to treat a wide variety of bacterial infections. It is also used to treat infections in persons who are allergic to penicillin. Erythromycins are also used to prevent "strep" infections in patients with a history of rheumatic heart disease. They may also be used in Legionnaires' disease and for other problems as determined by your doctor.
- Keep taking this medicine for the full time of treatment even if you begin to feel better after a few days; do not miss any doses. This is especially important if you have a "strep" infection since serious heart problems could develop later if your infection is not cleared up completely.
- If you do miss a dose of this medicine, take it as soon as possible. This will help to keep a constant amount of medicine in the blood. However, if it is almost time for your next dose, skip the missed dose and go back to your regular dosing schedule.
- This medication has been prescribed for your current infection only. Another infection later on, or one that someone else has, may require a different medicine. You should not give your medicine to other people or use it for other infections, unless your doctor specifically directs you to do so.

Side effects
Along with the needed effects, a medicine may cause some unwanted effects. Side effects that usually do not require medical attention: abdominal cramps, black tongue, cough, diarrhea, fatigue, irritation of the mouth, loss of appetite, nausea, or vomiting. These side effects should disappear as your body adjusts to the medication.
- Other side effects that should be reported to your doctor immediately are:
Fever
Hearing loss
Hives or rash
Rectal or vaginal itching
Yellowing of the eyes or skin

Interactions
This medicine may interact with several other drugs such as anticoagulants, theophylline preparations, carbamazepine, etc.
- Be sure to tell your doctor about any medications you are currently taking.

Storage
Tablets, capsules, etc. should be stored at room temperature in tightly closed, light-resistant containers as directed by your pharmacist.

PEN VEE K

Properties

This medicine contains penicillin V as active ingredient. Penicillins are prescribed to treat infections caused by bacteria. They will not work for colds, flu, or other virus infections. There are several different kinds of penicillins. Each is used to treat different kinds of infections.

Before using this medicine

Before you use this medicine check with your doctor, or pharmacist:

- if you ever had any unusual or allergic reaction to any of the penicillins, cefalosporins, griseofulvin, or penicillamine. Serious reactions may occur in patients who are allergic to penicillins.
- if you are on a low-salt, low-sugar, or any other special diet, or if you are allergic to any substance, such as sulfites or other preservatives or dyes.
- if you are pregnant or intend to become pregnant while using this medicine. Although penicillins have not been shown to cause problems in humans, the chance always exists.
- if you are breast-feeding an infant. Most penicillins (except amdinocillin) pass into the breast milk. Even though only small amounts may pass, allergic reaction, diarrhea, fungal infection, and skin rash may occur in the infant.
- if you have any of the following medical problems:
  Allergy
  Asthma
  Bleeding problems
  Eczema
  Hay fever, hives
  Kidney disease
  Liver disease
  Mononucleosis
  Stomach or intestinal disease

Treatment

This medication is used to treat an infection caused by bacteria. Most penicillins are best taken with a full glass (8 ounces) of water on an empty stomach, some are best taken with a snack or meal. Follow your doctor's or pharmacist's directions on how to take your medicine.

- Keep taking this medicine for the full time of treatment even if you begin to feel better after a few days; do not miss any doses. This is especially important if you have a "strep" infection since serious heart problems could develop later if your infection is not cleared up completely.
- If you do miss a dose of this medicine, take it as soon as possible. However, if it is almost time for your next dose, skip the missed dose and go back to your regular dosing schedule.

Side effects

Along with the needed effects, a medicine may cause some unwanted effects. Side effects that usually do not require medical attention: diarrhea; nausea or vomiting; sore mouth or tongue.

- Stop taking this medicine and get emergency help immediately if you notice: difficulty in breathing; lightheadedness; skin rash, hives, itching; wheezing.

  Other side effects that should be reported to your doctor immediately are: abdominal bloating; blood in urine; convulsions (seizures); decreased amount of urine; diarrhea (watery and severe) which may also be bloody; fever; joint pain; sore throat and fever; stomach or abdominal cramps and pain; unusual bleeding or bruising.

Interactions

This medicine may interact with several other drugs such as anticoagulants, diarrhea medicines, heparin, ibuprofen, oral contraceptives, potassium-containing medicines, etc.

- Be sure to tell your doctor about any medications you are currently taking.

Storage

Tablets, capsules, etc. should be stored as directed by your pharmacist or according to instructions on the label.

PENAPAR VK

Properties
This medicine contains penicillin V as active ingredient. Penicillins are prescribed to treat infections caused by bacteria. They will not work for colds, flu, or other virus infections. There are several different kinds of penicillins. Each is used to treat different kinds of infections.

Before using this medicine
Before you use this medicine check with your doctor, or pharmacist:
- if you ever had any unusual or allergic reaction to any of the penicillins, cefalosporins, griseofulvin, or penicillamine. Serious reactions may occur in patients who are allergic to penicillins.
- if you are on a low-salt, low-sugar, or any other special diet, or if you are allergic to any substance, such as sulfites or other preservatives or dyes.
- if you are pregnant or intend to become pregnant while using this medicine. Although penicillins have not been shown to cause problems in humans, the chance always exists.
- if you are breast-feeding an infant. Most penicillins (except amdinocillin) pass into the breast milk. Even though only small amounts may pass, allergic reaction, diarrhea, fungal infection, and skin rash may occur in the infant.
- if you have any of the following medical problems:
  Allergy
  Asthma
  Bleeding problems
  Eczema
  Hay fever, hives
  Kidney disease
  Liver disease
  Mononucleosis
  Stomach or intestinal disease

Treatment
This medication is used to treat an infection caused by bacteria. Most penicillins are best taken with a full glass (8 ounces) of water on an empty stomach, some are best taken with a snack or meal. Follow your doctor's or pharmacist's directions on how to take your medicine.
- Keep taking this medicine for the full time of treatment even if you begin to feel better after a few days; do not miss any doses. This is especially important if you have a "strep" infection since serious heart problems could develop later if your infection is not cleared up completely.
- If you do miss a dose of this medicine, take it as soon as possible. However, if it is almost time for your next dose, skip the missed dose and go back to your regular dosing schedule.

Side effects
Along with the needed effects, a medicine may cause some unwanted effects. Side effects that usually do not require medical attention: diarrhea; nausea or vomiting; sore mouth or tongue.
- Stop taking this medicine and get emergency help immediately if you notice: difficulty in breathing; light-headedness; skin rash, hives, itching; wheezing.

Other side effects that should be reported to your doctor immediately are: abdominal bloating; blood in urine; convulsions (seizures); decreased amount of urine; diarrhea (watery and severe) which may also be bloody; fever; joint pain; sore throat and fever; stomach or abdominal cramps and pain; unusual bleeding or bruising.

Interactions
This medicine may interact with several other drugs such as anticoagulants, diarrhea medicines, heparin, ibuprofen, oral contraceptives, potassium-containing medicines, etc.
- Be sure to tell your doctor about any medications you are currently taking.

Storage
Tablets, capsules, etc. should be stored as directed by your pharmacist or according to instructions on the label.

PENICILLIN V

Properties

This medicine contains penicillin V as active ingredient. Penicillins are prescribed to treat infections caused by bacteria. They will not work for colds, flu, or other virus infections. There are several different kinds of penicillins. Each is used to treat different kinds of infections.

Before using this medicine

Before you use this medicine check with your doctor, or pharmacist:

- if you ever had any unusual or allergic reaction to any of the penicillins, cefalosporins, griseofulvin, or penicillamine. Serious reactions may occur in patients who are allergic to penicillins.
- if you are on a low-salt, low-sugar, or any other special diet, or if you are allergic to any substance, such as sulfites or other preservatives or dyes.
- if you are pregnant or intend to become pregnant while using this medicine. Although penicillins have not been shown to cause problems in humans, the chance always exists.
- if you are breast-feeding an infant. Most penicillins (except amdinocillin) pass into the breast milk. Even though only small amounts may pass, allergic reaction, diarrhea, fungal infection, and skin rash may occur in the infant.
- if you have any of the following medical problems:
Allergy
Asthma
Bleeding problems
Eczema
Hay fever, hives
Kidney disease
Liver disease
Mononucleosis
Stomach or intestinal disease

Treatment

This medication is used to treat an infection caused by bacteria. Most penicillins are best taken with a full glass (8 ounces) of water on an empty stomach, some are best taken with a snack or meal. Follow your doctor's or pharmacist's directions on how to take your medicine.

- Keep taking this medicine for the full time of treatment even if you begin to feel better after a few days; do not miss any doses. This is especially important if you have a "strep" infection since serious heart problems could develop later if your infection is not cleared up completely.
- If you do miss a dose of this medicine, take it as soon as possible. However, if it is almost time for your next dose, skip the missed dose and go back to your regular dosing schedule.

Side effects

Along with the needed effects, a medicine may cause some unwanted effects. Side effects that usually do not require medical attention: diarrhea; nausea or vomiting; sore mouth or tongue.

- Stop taking this medicine and get emergency help immediately if you notice: difficulty in breathing; light-headedness; skin rash, hives, itching; wheezing.

Other side effects that should be reported to your doctor immediately are: abdominal bloating; blood in urine; convulsions (seizures); decreased amount of urine; diarrhea (watery and severe) which may also be bloody; fever; joint pain; sore throat and fever; stomach or abdominal cramps and pain; unusual bleeding or bruising.

Interactions

This medicine may interact with several other drugs such as anticoagulants, diarrhea medicines, heparin, ibuprofen, oral contraceptives, potassium-containing medicines, etc.

- Be sure to tell your doctor about any medications you are currently taking.

Storage

Tablets, capsules, etc. should be stored as directed by your pharmacist or according to instructions on the label.

PENTAMYCETIN (Ophthalmic)

Properties

This medicine contains an ophthalmic antibacterial, as active ingredient. It helps the body to overcome eye infections on surface tissues of the eye. It is most useful when the infecting organism is one known to be sensitive to the antibacterial drug.

The drug penetrates the bacterial cell membrane and prevents cells from multiplying.

Before using this medicine

Before you use this medicine check with your doctor:

– if you ever had any unusual or allergic reaction to any of the compounds of the medicine.
– if you are on a low-salt, low-sugar, or any other special diet, or if you are allergic to any substance, such as sulfites or other preservatives or dyes.
– if you are pregnant or intend to become pregnant while using this medicine. Although ophthalmic antibacterials have been found to be safe for use during pregnancy, you should check with your doctor before taking any drug if you are pregnant.

Treatment

This medication is used to treat an infection caused by bacteria. The medicine may be used in the form of eye drops or as an eye ointment. Use the medication as directed, Do not miss a dose. If you forget a dose, use it as soon as you remember. Notify your doctor if eye symptoms fail to improve in two to four days.

♦ To apply eye drops: Till the head backward when applying the eye drops. Pull the lower eyelid away from the eye to form a pouch. After applying the drop, keep the eye closed for a minute or so. This allows the medication to come in contact with the infection.
♦ To apply eye ointment: Pull lower lid down from eye to form a pouch. Squeeze tube to apply thin strip of ointment into pouch. Close eye for 1 to 2 minutes.

Always wash your hands before applying the ointment.

The drug starts to work in about one hour. Treatment may require 7 to 10 days to control infection.

Older adults or seniors may take this medication without special restriction.

Side effects

Along with the needed effects, a medicine may cause some unwanted effects. Side effects that usually do not require medical attention: occasional local irritation after application to the eye. Ointments may cause blurred vision for a few minutes; continue the use of the eye drops or ointment, but tell your doctor at the next visit.

■ Discontinue the use of eye drops or eye ointment in the following cases:
Sore throat
Aplastic anemia
Pale skin
Unusual redness of the eye
Unusual irritation of the eye
Fever
Unusual bleeding
Unusual bruising
■ Tell your doctor about any side effects that are persistent or particularly bothersome. In case of prolonged use sensitivity reactions may develop.

Interactions

Clinically significant interactions with oral or injected medicines are unlikely. Do not use the eye drops or ointment with any other eye drops or ointment without checking with your ophthalmologist.

Storage

Keep bottle (with eye drops) or container (containing ointment) lightly closed. Store in a cool place, but Do not freeze. Wash handss immediately after using.

Do not store in the bathroom medicine cabinet because the heat or moisture may cause the medicine to break down.

Do not keep outdated medicine or medicine no longer needed. Flush the contents of the bottle or tube down the toilet, unless otherwise directed.

PENTIDS

Properties
This medicine contains penicillin G as active ingredient. Penicillins are prescribed to treat infections caused by bacteria. They will not work for colds, flu, or other virus infections. There are several different kinds of penicillins. Each is used to treat different kinds of infections.

Before using this medicine
Before you use this medicine check with your doctor, or pharmacist:
- if you ever had any unusual or allergic reaction to any of the penicillins, cefalosporins, griseofulvin, or penicillamine. Serious reactions may occur in patients who are allergic to penicillins.
- if you are on a low-salt, low-sugar, or any other special diet, or if you are allergic to any substance, such as sulfites or other preservatives or dyes.
- if you are pregnant or intend to become pregnant while using this medicine. Although penicillins have not been shown to cause problems in humans, the chance always exists.
- if you are breast-feeding an infant. Most penicillins (except amdinocillin) pass into the breast milk. Even though only small amounts may pass, allergic reaction, diarrhea, fungal infection, and skin rash may occur in the infant.
- if you have any of the following medical problems:
  Allergy
  Asthma
  Bleeding problems
  Eczema
  Hay fever, hives
  Kidney disease
  Liver disease
  Mononucleosis
  Stomach or intestinal disease

Treatment
This medication is used to treat an infection caused by bacteria. Most penicillins are best taken with a full glass (8 ounces) of water on an empty stomach, some are best taken with a snack or meal. Follow your doctor's or pharmacist's directions on how to take your medicine.
- ◆ Keep taking this medicine for the full time of treatment even if you begin to feel better after a few days; do not miss any doses. This is especially important if you have a "strep" infection since serious heart problems could develop later if your infection is not cleared up completely.
- ◆ If you do miss a dose of this medicine, take it as soon as possible. However, if it is almost time for your next dose, skip the missed dose and go back to your regular dosing schedule.

Side effects
Along with the needed effects, a medicine may cause some unwanted effects. Side effects that usually do not require medical attention: diarrhea; nausea or vomiting; sore mouth or tongue.
- ◆ Stop taking this medicine and get emergency help immediately if you notice: difficulty in breathing; lightheadedness; skin rash, hives, itching; wheezing.
Other side effects that should be reported to your doctor immediately are: abdominal bloating; blood in urine; convulsions (seizures); decreased amount of urine; diarrhea (watery and severe) which may also be bloody; fever; joint pain; sore throat and fever; stomach or abdominal cramps and pain; unusual bleeding or bruising.

Interactions
This medicine may interact with several other drugs such as anticoagulants, diarrhea medicines, heparin, ibuprofen, oral contraceptives, potassium-containing medicines, etc.
- ■ Be sure to tell your doctor about any medications you are currently taking.

Storage
Tablets, capsules, etc. should be stored as directed by your pharmacist or according to instructions on the label.

PENTOBARBITAL

Properties
This medicine contains as active ingredient the barbiturate pentobarbital. Barbiturates belong to the group of medicines called central nervous system depressants (medicines that slow down the nervous system).

Barbiturates may partially block nerve impulses at nerve-cell connections. They may be used to treat insomnia (sleeplessness) by helping patients fall asleep. Also, they may be used to relieve anxiety or tension. Some of the barbiturates are used as anticonvulsants to help control convulsions in certain disorders or diseases, such as epilepsy. If too much of the drug is used, it may become habit-forming (causing mental or physical dependence).

Before using this medicine
Before you use this medicine check with your doctor, or pharmacist:
- if you ever had any unusual or allergic reaction to this medicine or one of its components.
- if you are on a low-salt, low-sugar, or any other special diet, or if you are allergic to preservatives or dyes.
- if you are pregnant or intend to become pregnant while using this medicine, since barbiturates have been shown to increase the chance of birth defects in humans. Taking barbiturates regularly during the last 3 months of pregnancy may cause the baby to become dependent on the medicine. This may lead to withdrawal side effects in the baby after birth.
- if you have any of the following medical problems:
  Anemia (severe)
  Diabetes mellitus (sugar disease)
  Hyperactivity (in children)
  Kidney or lifer disease
  Mental depression
  Overactive thyroid

Treatment
This medication is used to treat the symptoms of your medical condition. Barbiturates act in the central nervous system; some of their side effects are also caused by actions in the central nervous system. Use this medicine as directed by your doctor. Do not use more of it, do not use it more often, and do not use it for a longer period of time than your doctor ordered.
- If you are taking this medication on a regular schedule and you miss a dose, take the missed dose as soon as possible, unless it is almost time for your next dose. In that case do not take the missed dose at all.
- If a barbiturate is used for a long time, it may become habit-forming. Physical dependence may lead to withdrawal side effects when you stop taking this medicine.

Side effects
Along with the needed effects, a medicine may cause some unwanted effects. These side effects may go away during treatment as your body adjusts to the medicine. Such minor side effects are: depression, confusion, diarrhea, nausea, vomiting, joint or muscle pain, slurred speech, hallucinations, headache, decreased sex drive.
- Check with your doctor immediately if any of the following side effects occur:
  Rash or hives
  Face, lip or eyelid swelling
  Sore throat, fever
  Agitation
  Slow heartbeat
  Difficult breathing or chest pain

Interactions
This medicine may interact with several other drugs such as medicines acting on the central nervous system (e.g., antihistamines; beta-adrenergic blockers; MAO inhibitors; mind-altering drugs; nabilone; antidepressants; clozapine; anticonvulsants).

Storage
The medicine should be stored at room temperature in a tightly closed, light-resistant container. Keep out of reach of children since overdose is very dangerous in children.

PERMAPEN

Properties
This medicine contains penicillin G as active ingredient. Penicillins are prescribed to treat infections caused by bacteria. They will not work for colds, flu, or other virus infections. There are several different kinds of penicillins. Each is used to treat different kinds of infections.

Before using this medicine
Before you use this medicine check with your doctor, or pharmacist:
- if you ever had any unusual or allergic reaction to any of the penicillins, cefalosporins, griseofulvin, or penicillamine. Serious reactions may occur in patients who are allergic to penicillins.
- if you are on a low-salt, low-sugar, or any other special diet, or if you are allergic to any substance, such as sulfites or other preservatives or dyes.
- if you are pregnant or intend to become pregnant while using this medicine. Although penicillins have not been shown to cause problems in humans, the chance always exists.
- if you are breast-feeding an infant. Most penicillins (except amdinocillin) pass into the breast milk. Even though only small amounts may pass, allergic reaction, diarrhea, fungal infection, and skin rash may occur in the infant.
- if you have any of the following medical problems:
  Allergy
  Asthma
  Bleeding problems
  Eczema
  Hay fever, hives
  Kidney disease
  Liver disease
  Mononucleosis
  Stomach or intestinal disease

Treatment
This medication is used to treat an infection caused by bacteria. Most penicillins are best taken with a full glass (8 ounces) of water on an empty stomach, some are best taken with a snack or meal. Follow your doctor's or pharmacist's directions on how to take your medicine.
- Keep taking this medicine for the full time of treatment even if you begin to feel better after a few days; do not miss any doses. This is especially important if you have a "strep" infection since serious heart problems could develop later if your infection is not cleared up completely.
- If you do miss a dose of this medicine, take it as soon as possible. However, if it is almost time for your next dose, skip the missed dose and go back to your regular dosing schedule.

Side effects
Along with the needed effects, a medicine may cause some unwanted effects. Side effects that usually do not require medical attention: diarrhea; nausea or vomiting; sore mouth or tongue.
- Stop taking this medicine and get emergency help immediately if you notice: difficulty in breathing; light-headedness; skin rash, hives, itching; wheezing.
  Other side effects that should be reported to your doctor immediately are: abdominal bloating; blood in urine; convulsions (seizures); decreased amount of urine; diarrhea (watery and severe) which may also be bloody; fever; joint pain; sore throat and fever; stomach or abdominal cramps and pain; unusual bleeding or bruising.

Interactions
This medicine may interact with several other drugs such as anticoagulants, diarrhea medicines, heparin, ibuprofen, oral contraceptives, potassium-containing medicines, etc.
- Be sure to tell your doctor about any medications you are currently taking.

Storage
Tablets, capsules, etc. should be stored as directed by your pharmacist or according to instructions on the label.

PERMITIL

Properties

This medicine contains as active ingredient fluphenazine, a phenothiazine derivative. Phenothiazines are a family of medicines used to treat nervous, mental, and emotional conditions. Some are used to control anxiety, restlessness, nausea and vomiting, and severe hiccups. This medicine is available only with your doctor's prescription.

Before using this medicine

Before you use this medicine check with your doctor, or pharmacist:
- if you ever had any unusual or allergic reaction to phenothiazine medicines.
- if you are on a low-salt, low-sugar, or any other special diet, or if you are allergic to any substance, such as sulfites or other preservatives or dyes.
- if you are pregnant or intend to become pregnant while using this medicine. Although phenothiazines have not been shown to cause birth defects, some side effects such as jaundice and muscle tremors have occurred in a few newborns whose mothers received phenothiazines during pregnancy.
- if you are breast-feeding an infant. Although this medicine has not been shown to cause problems in humans but the chance does exist since some phenothiazines are known to pass into the breast milk.
- if you have any of the following medical problems:
  Alcoholism
  Blood disease
  Difficult urination
  Enlarged prostate
  Glaucoma
  Heart or blood vessel disease
  Liver or lung disease
  Parkinson's disease
  Stomach ulcers

Treatment

This medication is prescribed to treat the symptoms of certain types of mental illness or emotional problems. In order to avoid stomach irritation, you can take the tablet or capsule forms of this medication with a meal or with a glass of water or milk (unless your doctor or pharmacist directs you to do otherwise).

Side effects

Along with the needed effects, a medicine may cause some unwanted effects. Minor side effects are: blurred vision, constipation, decreased sweating, diarrhea, dizziness, drooling, drowsiness, dry mouth, fatigue, jitteriness, menstrual irregularities, nasal congestion, restlessness, tremors, vomiting, or weight gain.
- Tell your doctor about any side effects that are persistent or particularly bothersome. It is especially important to tell your doctor about:
  Breast enlargement
  Chest pain or convulsions
  Darkened skin
  Difficulty in swallowing
  Fainting or fever
  Involuntary movements
  Palpitations or sleep disorders
  Rash or sore throat
  Uncoordinated movements
  Unusual bleeding or bruising
  Visual disturbances
  Yellowing of the eyes or skin

Interactions

This medicine may interact with several other drugs such as barbiturates, sleeping pills, narcotics, other tranquilizers, or any other medication that may produce a sedative effect. Avoid alcohol.

Storage

Store this medication as directed on the label. Keep out of the reach of children.

PERPHENAZINE

Properties

This medicine contains as active ingredient perphenazine, a phenothiazine derivative. Phenothiazines are a family of medicines used to treat nervous, mental, and emotional conditions. Some are used to control anxiety, restlessness, nausea and vomiting, and severe hiccups. This medicine is available only with your doctor's prescription.

Before using this medicine

Before you use this medicine check with your doctor, or pharmacist:
- if you ever had any unusual or allergic reaction to phenothiazine medicines.
- if you are on a low-salt, low-sugar, or any other special diet, or if you are allergic to any substance, such as sulfites or other preservatives or dyes.
- if you are pregnant or intend to become pregnant while using this medicine. Although phenothiazines have not been shown to cause birth defects, some side effects such as jaundice and muscle tremors have occurred in a few newborns whose mothers received phenothiazines during pregnancy.
- if you are breast-feeding an infant. Although this medicine has not been shown to cause problems in humans but the chance does exist since some phenothiazines are known to pass into the breast milk.
- if you have any of the following medical problems:
Alcoholism
Blood disease
Difficult urination
Enlarged prostate
Glaucoma
Heart or blood vessel disease
Liver or lung disease
Parkinson's disease
Stomach ulcers

Treatment

This medication is prescribed to treat the symptoms of certain types of mental illness or emotional problems. In order to avoid stomach irritation, you can take the tablet or capsule forms of this medication with a meal or with a glass of water or milk (unless your doctor or pharmacist directs you to do otherwise).

Side effects

Along with the needed effects, a medicine may cause some unwanted effects. Minor side effects are: blurred vision, constipation, decreased sweating, diarrhea, dizziness, drooling, drowsiness, dry mouth, fatigue, jitteriness, menstrual irregularities, nasal congestion, restlessness, tremors, vomiting, or weight gain.
- Tell your doctor about any side effects that are persistent or particularly bothersome. It is especially important to tell your doctor about:
Breast enlargement
Chest pain or convulsions
Darkened skin
Difficulty in swallowing
Fainting or fever
Involuntary movements
Palpitations or sleep disorders
Rash or sore throat
Uncoordinated movements
Unusual bleeding or bruising
Visual disturbances
Yellowing of the eyes or skin

Interactions

This medicine may interact with several other drugs such as barbiturates, sleeping pills, narcotics, other tranquilizers, or any other medication that may produce a sedative effect. Avoid alcohol.

Storage

Store this medication as directed on the label. Keep out of the reach of children.

PERTOFRANE

Properties
This medicine contains desipramine as active ingredient. It belongs to the group of medicines known as tricyclic antidepressants or 'mood elevators.' It is used to relieve mental depression and depression that sometimes occurs with anxiety. The medication gradually relieves, but doesn't cure, symptoms of depression. The medication may also be used for the treatment of narcolepsy, bulimia, painic attacks, cocaine withdrawal, attention deficit disorder.

Before using this medicine
Before you use this medicine check with your doctor, or pharmacist:
- if you ever had any unusual or allergic reaction to any tricyclic antidepressant, maprotiline or trazodone.
- if you are on a low-salt, low-sugar, or any other special diet, or if you are allergic to any substance, such as sulfites or other preservatives or dyes.
- if you are pregnant or intend to become pregnant while using this medicine. There have been reports of newborns suffering from heart, breathing, and urinary problems when their mothers had taken tricyclic antidepressants before delivery.
- if you are breast-feeding an infant. Some tricyclic antidepressants pass into the breast milk.

Treatment
Take this medicine only as directed by your doctor, to benefit your condition as much as possible. Do not take more of it, do not take it more often, and do not take it for a longer period of time than your doctor ordered.

To lessen stomach upset, take this medicine with food, even for a daily bedtime dose, unless your doctor has told you to take it on an empty stomach. If you forget your once-a-day bedtime dose, Do not take it more than 3 hours late. If more than 3 hours, wait for next scheduled dose;.

Sometimes this medicine must be taken for several weeks before you begin to feel better.

Side effects
Along with the needed effects, a medicine may cause some unwanted effects. Side effects that usually do not require medical attention: difficult or frequent urination; decreased sex drive; muscle aches; abnormal dreams; nasal congestion; weakness and faintness when arising from bed or chair; back pain.
- Other side effects that should be reported to your doctor immediately are:
  Hallucinations
  Shakiness
  Dizziness or fainting
  Blurred vision, eye pain
  Irregular heartbeat or slow pulse
  Inflamed tongue
  Abdominal pain
  Jaundice
  Hair loss, rash
  Fever, chills
  Joint pain
  Palpitations

Interactions
This medicine may interact with several other drugs such as anticoagulants, anticholinergics, cold remedies, oral contraceptives, seizure medicines, sleeping medicines, thyroid medicines, etc.
- Be sure to tell your doctor about any medications you are currently taking.

Storage
Tablets, capsules, etc. should be stored at room temperature in tightly closed, light-resistant containers as directed by your pharmacist. Keep out of reach of children since overdose is especially dangerous in young children. Do not store in the bathroom medicine cabinet because the heat or moisture may cause the medicine to break down. Keep the liquid form of the medicine from freezing.

PETHADOL

Properties
This medicine contains as active ingredient meperidine.

It is a narcotic analgesic that acts directly on the central nervous system (brain and spinal cord). It is used to relieve pain or to suppress coughing.

Before using this medicine
Before you use this medicine check with your doctor, or pharmacist:
– if you ever had any unusual or allergic reaction to this medicine or one of its components.
– if you are on a low-salt, low-sugar, or any other special diet, or if you are allergic to any substance, such as sulfites or other preservatives or dyes.
– if you are pregnant or intend to become pregnant while using this medicine. Studies on birth defects have not been done in humans. Too much use of narcotics during pregnancy may cause the baby to become dependent on the medicine.
– if you are breast-feeding an infant. Although this medicine has not been shown to cause problems in humans, it passes into the breast milk in small amounts.
– if you have any of the following medical problems:
Brain disease or head injury
Colitis
Convulsions
Emphysema, asthma, or chronic lung disease
Enlarged prostate
Gallbladder disease or gallstones
Heart disease
Kidney or lifer disease
Underactive thyroid

Treatment
This medication is used to relieve pain or to suppress coughing. Narcotic analgesics act in the central nervous system; some of their side effects are also caused by actions in the central nervous system.
■ If you are taking this medication on a regular schedule and you miss a dose, take the missed dose as soon as possible, unless it is almost time for your next dose. In that case do not take the missed dose at all.
■ If a narcotic analgesic is used for a long time, it may become habit-forming (causing mental or physical dependence). Physical dependence may lead to withdrawal side effects when you stop taking this medicine.
Unless otherwise directed by your doctor or pharmacist take this as directed. Do not take more of them and do not take them more often than recommended on the label. Children up to 12 years of age should not take this medicine more than 3 times a day or for more than 5 days in a row.

Side effects
Along with the needed effects, a medicine may cause some unwanted effects. These side effects may go away during treatment as your body adjusts to the medicine. Such minor side effects are: constipation, dizziness, drowsiness, dry mouth, false sense of well-being, flushing, light-headedness, loss of appetite, nausea, painful or difficult urination, or sweating.
■ Check with your doctor immediately if any of the following side effects occur:
Anxiety or breathing difficulties
Excitation or restlessness
Fatigue, palpitations
Rash, sore throat and fever
Tremors or weakness

Interactions
This medicine may interact with several other drugs such as medicines acting on the central nervous system (e.g., antidepressants, tranquilizers), cimetidine, nitrates, quinidine, etc.
■ Be sure to tell your doctor about any medications you are currently taking.

Storage
Tablets, elixir, suppository etc. should be stored at room temperature in a tightly closed, light-resistant container.

PETHIDINE

Properties

This medicine contains as active ingredient meperidine.

It is a narcotic analgesic that acts directly on the central nervous system (brain and spinal cord). It is used to relieve pain or to suppress coughing.

Before using this medicine

Before you use this medicine check with your doctor, or pharmacist:

- if you ever had any unusual or allergic reaction to this medicine or one of its components.
- if you are on a low-salt, low-sugar, or any other special diet, or if you are allergic to any substance, such as sulfites or other preservatives or dyes.
- if you are pregnant or intend to become pregnant while using this medicine. Studies on birth defects have not been done in humans. Too much use of narcotics during pregnancy may cause the baby to become dependent on the medicine.
- if you are breast-feeding an infant. Although this medicine has not been shown to cause problems in humans, it passes into the breast milk in small amounts.
- if you have any of the following medical problems:
  Brain disease or head injury
  Colitis
  Convulsions
  Emphysema, asthma, or chronic lung disease
  Enlarged prostate
  Gallbladder disease or gallstones
  Heart disease
  Kidney or lifer disease
  Underactive thyroid

Treatment

This medication is used to relieve pain or to suppress coughing. Narcotic analgesics act in the central nervous system; some of their side effects are also caused by actions in the central nervous system.

- If you are taking this medication on a regular schedule and you miss a dose, take the missed dose as soon as possible, unless it is almost time for your next dose. In that case do not take the missed dose at all.
- If a narcotic analgesic is used for a long time, it may become habit-forming (causing mental or physical dependence). Physical dependence may lead to withdrawal side effects when you stop taking this medicine.

Unless otherwise directed by your doctor or pharmacist take this as directed. Do not take more of them and do not take them more often than recommended on the label. Children up to 12 years of age should not take this medicine more than 3 times a day or for more than 5 days in a row.

Side effects

Along with the needed effects, a medicine may cause some unwanted effects. These side effects may go away during treatment as your body adjusts to the medicine. Such minor side effects are: constipation, dizziness, drowsiness, dry mouth, false sense of well-being, flushing, light-headedness, loss of appetite, nausea, painful or difficult urination, or sweating.

- Check with your doctor immediately if any of the following side effects occur:
  Anxiety or breathing difficulties
  Excitation or restlessness
  Fatigue, palpitations
  Rash, sore throat and fever
  Tremors or weakness

Interactions

This medicine may interact with several other drugs such as medicines acting on the central nervous system (e.g., antidepressants, tranquilizers), cimetidine, nitrates, quinidine, etc.

- Be sure to tell your doctor about any medications you are currently taking.

Storage

Tablets, elixir, suppository etc. should be stored at room temperature in a tightly closed, light-resistant container.

PFIZERPEN

Properties
This medicine contains penicillin G as active ingredient. Penicillins are prescribed to treat infections caused by bacteria. They will not work for colds, flu, or other virus infections. There are several different kinds of penicillins. Each is used to treat different kinds of infections.

Before using this medicine
Before you use this medicine check with your doctor, or pharmacist:
- if you ever had any unusual or allergic reaction to any of the penicillins, cefalosporins, griseofulvin, or penicillamine. Serious reactions may occur in patients who are allergic to penicillins.
- if you are on a low-salt, low-sugar, or any other special diet, or if you are allergic to any substance, such as sulfites or other preservatives or dyes.
- if you are pregnant or intend to become pregnant while using this medicine. Although penicillins have not been shown to cause problems in humans, the chance always exists.
- if you are breast-feeding an infant. Most penicillins (except amdinocillin) pass into the breast milk. Even though only small amounts may pass, allergic reaction, diarrhea, fungal infection, and skin rash may occur in the infant.
- if you have any of the following medical problems:
Allergy
Asthma
Bleeding problems
Eczema
Hay fever, hives
Kidney disease
Liver disease
Mononucleosis
Stomach or intestinal disease

Treatment
This medication is used to treat an infection caused by bacteria. Most penicillins are best taken with a full glass (8 ounces) of water on an empty stomach, some are best taken with a snack or meal. Follow your doctor's or pharmacist's directions on how to take your medicine.

- Keep taking this medicine for the full time of treatment even if you begin to feel better after a few days; do not miss any doses. This is especially important if you have a "strep" infection since serious heart problems could develop later if your infection is not cleared up completely.
- If you do miss a dose of this medicine, take it as soon as possible. However, if it is almost time for your next dose, skip the missed dose and go back to your regular dosing schedule.

Side effects
Along with the needed effects, a medicine may cause some unwanted effects. Side effects that usually do not require medical attention: diarrhea; nausea or vomiting; sore mouth or tongue.

- Stop taking this medicine and get emergency help immediately if you notice: difficulty in breathing; light-headedness; skin rash, hives, itching; wheezing.

Other side effects that should be reported to your doctor immediately are: abdominal bloating; blood in urine; convulsions (seizures); decreased amount of urine; diarrhea (watery and severe) which may also be bloody; fever; joint pain; sore throat and fever; stomach or abdominal cramps and pain; unusual bleeding or bruising.

Interactions
This medicine may interact with several other drugs such as anticoagulants, diarrhea medicines, heparin, ibuprofen, oral contraceptives, potassium-containing medicines, etc.

- Be sure to tell your doctor about any medications you are currently taking.

Storage
Tablets, capsules, etc. should be stored as directed by your pharmacist or according to instructions on the label.

PHENAZINE

Properties

This medicine contains as active ingredient perphenazine, a phenothiazine derivative. Phenothiazines are a family of medicines used to treat nervous, mental, and emotional conditions. Some are used to control anxiety, restlessness, nausea and vomiting, and severe hiccups. This medicine is available only with your doctor's prescription.

Before using this medicine

Before you use this medicine check with your doctor, or pharmacist:

- if you ever had any unusual or allergic reaction to phenothiazine medicines.
- if you are on a low-salt, low-sugar, or any other special diet, or if you are allergic to any substance, such as sulfites or other preservatives or dyes.
- if you are pregnant or intend to become pregnant while using this medicine. Although phenothiazines have not been shown to cause birth defects, some side effects such as jaundice and muscle tremors have occurred in a few newborns whose mothers received phenothiazines during pregnancy.
- if you are breast-feeding an infant. Although this medicine has not been shown to cause problems in humans but the chance does exist since some phenothiazines are known to pass into the breast milk.
- if you have any of the following medical problems:
  Alcoholism
  Blood disease
  Difficult urination
  Enlarged prostate
  Glaucoma
  Heart or blood vessel disease
  Liver or lung disease
  Parkinson's disease
  Stomach ulcers

Treatment

This medication is prescribed to treat the symptoms of certain types of mental illness or emotional problems. In order to avoid stomach irritation, you can take the tablet or capsule forms of this medication with a meal or with a glass of water or milk (unless your doctor or pharmacist directs you to do otherwise).

Side effects

Along with the needed effects, a medicine may cause some unwanted effects.

Minor side effects are: blurred vision, constipation, decreased sweating, diarrhea, dizziness, drooling, drowsiness, dry mouth, fatigue, jitteriness, menstrual irregularities, nasal congestion, restlessness, tremors, vomiting, or weight gain.

- Tell your doctor about any side effects that are persistent or particularly bothersome. It is especially important to tell your doctor about:
  Breast enlargement
  Chest pain or convulsions
  Darkened skin
  Difficulty in swallowing
  Fainting or fever
  Involuntary movements
  Palpitations or sleep disorders
  Rash or sore throat
  Uncoordinated movements
  Unusual bleeding or bruising
  Visual disturbances
  Yellowing of the eyes or skin

Interactions

This medicine may interact with several other drugs such as barbiturates, sleeping pills, narcotics, other tranquilizers, or any other medication that may produce a sedative effect. Avoid alcohol.

Storage

Store this medication as directed on the label. Keep out of the reach of children.

PHENDIMETRAZINE

Properties
This medicine contains phendimetrazine as active ingredient; it is prescribed for appetite suppression.

Appetite suppressants are used in the short-term (a few weeks) treatment of obesity. In a few weeks (6 to 12), these medicines in combination with dieting, exercise, and changes in eating habits can help patients lose weight. However, since their appetite reducing effect is only temporary, they are useful only for the first weeks of dieting until new eating habits are established.

Before using this medicine
Before you use this medicine check with your doctor, or pharmacist:
- if you ever had any unusual or allergic reaction to any of the compounds of this medicine.
- if you are on a low-salt, low-sugar, or any other special diet, or if you are allergic to any substance, such as sulfites or other preservatives or dyes.
- if you are pregnant, intend to become pregnant or breast-feeding an infant while using this medicine.
- if you have any of the following medical problems:
  Diabetes mellitus (sugar diabetes)
  Epilepsy
  Glaucoma
  Heart or blood vessel disease
  High blood pressure
  Mental illness (severe)

Treatment
This medication is used to relieve or prevent the symptoms of your medical problem. Take them as directed. Do not take more of them and do not take them more often than recommended on the label. If too much of the drug is taken, it may become habit-forming.

The medicine produces central nervous system stimulation, and it should not be taken by people with heart disease or high blood pressure.

If you think this medicine is not working as well after you have taken it for a few weeks, do not increase the dose. Instead, check with your doctor.

Side effects
The following minor side effects may occur: irritability, nervousness, restlessness, trouble in sleeping.

These side effects should disappear as your body adjusts to the medication. Tell your doctor about any side effects that are persistent or particularly bothersome. It is especially important to tell your doctor about:
  Mental depression
  Nausea or vomiting
  Stomach cramps or pain
  Trembling
  Unusual tiredness or weakness
- Discontinue use of the drug; call your doctor right away. Adverse reactions and side effects may be more frequent and severe in people over age 60 than in younger persons.

Interactions
This medicine interacts with several other drugs such as antihypertensives, other appetite suppressants, caffeine, central nervous system depressants, central nervous system stimulants, furazolidone, guanethidine, hydralazine, MAO inhibitors, methyldopa, molindone, phenothiazines, rauwolfia alkaloids, sodium bicarbonate. Interaction with alcoholic beverages may produce drowsiness, sleepiness, and/or inability to concentrate.
- Be sure to tell your doctor about any medications you are currently taking.

Storage
This medicine should be stored at room temperature in tightly closed containers. Store away from heat and direct light. Keep out of reach of children, since overdose may be very dangerous in children.

Do not store this medicine in the bathroom medicine cabinet because the heat and moisture cause the medicine to break down. Do not keep outdated medicine or medicine no longer needed. Flush the contents of the container down the toilet.

PHENOBARB

Properties

This medicine contains as active ingredient the barbiturate   phenobarbital. Barbiturates belong to the group of medicines called central nervous system depressants (medicines that slow down the nervous system).

Barbiturates may partially block nerve impulses at nerve-cell connections. They may be used to treat insomnia (sleeplessness) by helping patients fall asleep. Also, they may be used to relieve anxiety or tension. Some of the barbiturates are used as anticonvulsants to help control convulsions in certain disorders or diseases, such as epilepsy. If too much of the drug is used, it may become habit-forming (causing mental or physical dependence).

Before using this medicine

Before you use this medicine check with your doctor, or pharmacist:
- if you ever had any unusual or allergic reaction to this medicine or one of its components.
- if you are on a low-salt, low-sugar, or any other special diet, or if you are allergic to preservatives or dyes.
- if you are pregnant or intend to become pregnant while using this medicine, since barbiturates have been shown to increase the chance of birth defects in humans. Taking barbiturates regularly during the last 3 months of pregnancy may cause the baby to become dependent on the medicine. This may lead to withdrawal side effects in the baby after birth.
- if you have any of the following medical problems:
  Anemia (severe)
  Diabetes mellitus (sugar disease)
  Hyperactivity (in children)
  Kidney or lifer disease
  Mental depression
  Overactive thyroid

Treatment

This medication is used to treat the symptoms of your medical condition. Barbiturates act in the central nervous system; some of their side effects are also caused by actions in the central nervous system. Use this medicine as directed by your doctor. Do not use more of it, do not use it more often, and do not use it for a longer period of time than your doctor ordered.

- If you are taking this medication on a regular schedule and you miss a dose, take the missed dose as soon as possible, unless it is almost time for your next dose. In that case do not take the missed dose at all.
- If a barbiturate is used for a long time, it may become habit-forming. Physical dependence may lead to withdrawal side effects when you stop taking this medicine.

Side effects

Along with the needed effects, a medicine may cause some unwanted effects. These side effects may go away during treatment as your body adjusts to the medicine. Such minor side effects are: depression, confusion, diarrhea, nausea, vomiting, joint or muscle pain, slurred speech, hallucinations, headache, decreased sex drive.

- Check with your doctor immediately if any of the following side effects occur:
  Rash or hives
  Face, lip or eyelid swelling
  Sore throat, fever
  Agitation
  Slow heartbeat
  Difficult breathing or chest pain

Interactions

This medicine may interact with several other drugs such as medicines acting on the central nervous system (e.g., antihistamines; beta-adrenergic blockers; MAO inhibitors; mind-altering drugs; nabilone; antidepressants; clozapine; anticonvulsants).

Storage

The medicine should be stored at room temperature in a tightly closed, light-resistant container. Keep out of reach of children since overdose is very dangerous in children.

PHENOBARBITAL

Properties
This medicine contains as active ingredient the barbiturate phenobarbital. Barbiturates belong to the group of medicines called central nervous system depressants (medicines that slow down the nervous system).

Barbiturates may partially block nerve impulses at nerve-cell connections. They may be used to treat insomnia (sleeplessness) by helping patients fall asleep. Also, they may be used to relieve anxiety or tension. Some of the barbiturates are used as anticonvulsants to help control convulsions in certain disorders or diseases, such as epilepsy. If too much of the drug is used, it may become habit-forming (causing mental or physical dependence).

Before using this medicine
Before you use this medicine check with your doctor, or pharmacist:
- if you ever had any unusual or allergic reaction to this medicine or one of its components.
- if you are on a low-salt, low-sugar, or any other special diet, or if you are allergic to preservatives or dyes.
- if you are pregnant or intend to become pregnant while using this medicine, since barbiturates have been shown to increase the chance of birth defects in humans. Taking barbiturates regularly during the last 3 months of pregnancy may cause the baby to become dependent on the medicine. This may lead to withdrawal side effects in the baby after birth.
- if you have any of the following medical problems:
Anemia (severe)
Diabetes mellitus (sugar disease)
Hyperactivity (in children)
Kidney or lifer disease
Mental depression
Overactive thyroid

Treatment
This medication is used to treat the symptoms of your medical condition. Barbiturates act in the central nervous system; some of their side effects are also caused by actions in the central nervous system. Use this medicine as directed by your doctor. Do not use more of it, do not use it more often, and do not use it for a longer period of time than your doctor ordered.
- If you are taking this medication on a regular schedule and you miss a dose, take the missed dose as soon as possible, unless it is almost time for your next dose. In that case do not take the missed dose at all.
- If a barbiturate is used for a long time, it may become habit-forming. Physical dependence may lead to withdrawal side effects when you stop taking this medicine.

Side effects
Along with the needed effects, a medicine may cause some unwanted effects. These side effects may go away during treatment as your body adjusts to the medicine. Such minor side effects are: depression, confusion, diarrhea, nausea, vomiting, joint or muscle pain, slurred speech, hallucinations, headache, decreased sex drive.
- Check with your doctor immediately if any of the following side effects occur:
Rash or hives
Face, lip or eyelid swelling
Sore throat, fever
Agitation
Slow heartbeat
Difficult breathing or chest pain

Interactions
This medicine may interact with several other drugs such as medicines acting on the central nervous system (e.g., antihistamines; beta-adrenergic blockers; MAO inhibitors; mind-altering drugs; nabilone; antidepressants; clozapine; anticonvulsants).

Storage
The medicine should be stored at room temperature in a tightly closed, light-resistant container. Keep out of reach of children since overdose is very dangerous in children.

PHENTAMINE

Properties
This medicine contains phentermine as active ingredient; it is prescribed for appetite suppression.

Appetite suppressants are used in the short-term (a few weeks) treatment of obesity. In a few weeks (6 to 12), these medicines in combination with dieting, exercise, and changes in eating habits can help patients lose weight. However, since their appetite reducing effect is only temporary, they are useful only for the first weeks of dieting until new eating habits are established.

Before using this medicine
Before you use this medicine check with your doctor, or pharmacist:
- if you ever had any unusual or allergic reaction to any of the compounds of this medicine.
- if you are on a low-salt, low-sugar, or any other special diet, or if you are allergic to any substance, such as sulfites or other preservatives or dyes.
- if you are pregnant, intend to become pregnant or breast-feeding an infant while using this medicine.
- if you have any of the following medical problems:
  Diabetes mellitus
  Epilepsy
  Glaucoma
  Heart disease
  High blood pressure
  Mental illness (severe)

Treatment
This medication is used to relieve or prevent the symptoms of your medical problem. Take them as directed.

Do not take more of them and do not take them more often than recommended on the label. If too much of the drug is taken, it may become habit-forming.
- The medicine produces central nervous system stimulation, and it should not be taken by people with heart disease or high blood pressure.
- If you think this medicine is not working as well after you have taken it for a few weeks, do not increase the dose. Instead, check with your doctor.

Side effects
The following minor side effects may occur: irritability, nervousness, restlessness, trouble in sleeping.

These side effects should disappear as your body adjusts to the medication. Tell your doctor about any side effects that are persistent or particularly bothersome. It is especially important to tell your doctor about:
  Mental depression
  Nausea or vomiting
  Stomach cramps or pain
  Trembling
  Unusual tiredness
- Discontinue use of the drug; call your doctor right away. Adverse reactions and side effects may be more frequent and severe in people over age 60 than in younger persons.

Interactions
This medicine interacts with several other drugs such as antihypertensives, other appetite suppressants, caffeine, central nervous system depressants, central nervous system stimulants, furazolidone, guanethidine, hydralazine, MAO inhibitors, methyldopa, molindone, phenothiazines, rauwolfia alkaloids, sodium bicarbonate. Interaction with alcoholic beverages may produce drowsiness, sleepiness, and/or inability to concentrate.
- Be sure to tell your doctor about any medications you are currently taking.

Storage
This medicine should be stored at room temperature in tightly closed containers. Store away from heat and direct light. Keep out of reach of children, since overdose may be very dangerous in children.

Do not store this medicine in the bathroom medicine cabinet because the heat and moisture cause the medicine to break down. Do not keep outdated medicine or medicine no longer needed. Flush the contents of the container down the toilet.

PHENTERMINE

Properties

This medicine contains phentermine as active ingredient; it is prescribed for appetite suppression.

Appetite suppressants are used in the short-term (a few weeks) treatment of obesity. In a few weeks (6 to 12), these medicines in combination with dieting, exercise, and changes in eating habits can help patients lose weight. However, since their appetite reducing effect is only temporary, they are useful only for the first weeks of dieting until new eating habits are established.

Before using this medicine

Before you use this medicine check with your doctor, or pharmacist:
- if you ever had any unusual or allergic reaction to any of the compounds of this medicine.
- if you are on a low-salt, low-sugar, or any other special diet, or if you are allergic to any substance, such as sulfites or other preservatives or dyes.
- if you are pregnant, intend to become pregnant or breast-feeding an infant while using this medicine.
- if you have any of the following medical problems:
  Diabetes mellitus
  Epilepsy
  Glaucoma
  Heart disease
  High blood pressure
  Mental illness (severe)

Treatment

This medication is used to relieve or prevent the symptoms of your medical problem.

Take them as directed. Do not take more of them and do not take them more often than recommended on the label. If too much of the drug is taken, it may become habit-forming.
- The medicine produces central nervous system stimulation, and it should not be taken by people with heart disease or high blood pressure.
- If you think this medicine is not working as well after you have taken it for a few weeks, do not increase the dose. Instead, check with your doctor.

Side effects

The following minor side effects may occur: irritability, nervousness, restlessness, trouble in sleeping.

These side effects should disappear as your body adjusts to the medication. Tell your doctor about any side effects that are persistent or particularly bothersome. It is especially important to tell your doctor about:
  Mental depression
  Nausea or vomiting
  Stomach cramps or pain
  Trembling
  Unusual tiredness
- Discontinue use of the drug; call your doctor right away. Adverse reactions and side effects may be more frequent and severe in people over age 60 than in younger persons.

Interactions

This medicine interacts with several other drugs such as antihypertensives, other appetite suppressants, caffeine, central nervous system depressants, central nervous system stimulants, furazolidone, guanethidine, hydralazine, MAO inhibitors, methyldopa, molindone, phenothiazines, rauwolfia alkaloids, sodium bicarbonate. Interaction with alcoholic beverages may produce drowsiness, sleepiness, and/or inability to concentrate.
- Be sure to tell your doctor about any medications you are currently taking.

Storage

This medicine should be stored at room temperature in tightly closed containers. Store away from heat and direct light. Keep out of reach of children, since overdose may be very dangerous in children. Do not store this medicine in the bathroom medicine cabinet because the heat and moisture cause the medicine to break down. Do not keep outdated medicine or medicine no longer needed. Flush the contents of the container down the toilet.

PHENTROL

Properties
This medicine contains phentermine as active ingredient; it is prescribed for appetite suppression.

Appetite suppressants are used in the short-term (a few weeks) treatment of obesity. In a few weeks (6 to 12), these medicines in combination with dieting, exercise, and changes in eating habits can help patients lose weight. However, since their appetite reducing effect is only temporary, they are useful only for the first weeks of dieting until new eating habits are established.

Before using this medicine
Before you use this medicine check with your doctor, or pharmacist:
- if you ever had any unusual or allergic reaction to any of the compounds of this medicine.
- if you are on a low-salt, low-sugar, or any other special diet, or if you are allergic to any substance, such as sulfites or other preservatives or dyes.
- if you are pregnant, intend to become pregnant or breast-feeding an infant while using this medicine.
- if you have any of the following medical problems:
Diabetes mellitus
Epilepsy
Glaucoma
Heart disease
High blood pressure
Mental illness (severe)

Treatment
This medication is used to relieve or prevent the symptoms of your medical problem.

Take them as directed. Do not take more of them and do not take them more often than recommended on the label. If too much of the drug is taken, it may become habit-forming.
- The medicine produces central nervous system stimulation, and it should not be taken by people with heart disease or high blood pressure.
- If you think this medicine is not working as well after you have taken it for a few weeks, do not increase the dose. Instead, check with your doctor.

Side effects
The following minor side effects may occur: irritability, nervousness, restlessness, trouble in sleeping.

These side effects should disappear as your body adjusts to the medication. Tell your doctor about any side effects that are persistent or particularly bothersome. It is especially important to tell your doctor about:
Mental depression
Nausea or vomiting
Stomach cramps or pain
Trembling
Unusual tiredness
- Discontinue use of the drug; call your doctor right away. Adverse reactions and side effects may be more frequent and severe in people over age 60 than in younger persons.

Interactions
This medicine interacts with several other drugs such as antihypertensives, other appetite suppressants, caffeine, central nervous system depressants, central nervous system stimulants, furazolidone, guanethidine, hydralazine, MAO inhibitors, methyldopa, molindone, phenothiazines, rauwolfia alkaloids, sodium bicarbonate. Interaction with alcoholic beverages may produce drowsiness, sleepiness, and/or inability to concentrate.
- Be sure to tell your doctor about any medications you are currently taking.

Storage
This medicine should be stored at room temperature in tightly closed containers. Store away from heat and direct light. Keep out of reach of children, since overdose may be very dangerous in children.

Do not store this medicine in the bathroom medicine cabinet because the heat and moisture cause the medicine to break down. Do not keep outdated medicine or medicine no longer needed. Flush the contents of the container down the toilet.

PHENZINE

Properties

This medicine contains phendimetrazine as active ingredient; it is prescribed for appetite suppression.

Appetite suppressants are used in the short-term (a few weeks) treatment of obesity. In a few weeks (6 to 12), these medicines in combination with dieting, exercise, and changes in eating habits can help patients lose weight. However, since their appetite reducing effect is only temporary, they are useful only for the first weeks of dieting until new eating habits are established.

Before using this medicine

Before you use this medicine check with your doctor, or pharmacist:
- if you ever had any unusual or allergic reaction to any of the compounds of this medicine.
- if you are on a low-salt, low-sugar, or any other special diet, or if you are allergic to any substance, such as sulfites or other preservatives or dyes.
- if you are pregnant, intend to become pregnant or breast-feeding an infant while using this medicine.
- if you have any of the following medical problems:
  Diabetes mellitus (sugar diabetes)
  Epilepsy
  Glaucoma
  Heart or blood vessel disease
  High blood pressure
  Mental illness (severe)

Treatment

This medication is used to relieve or prevent the symptoms of your medical problem. Take them as directed. Do not take more of them and do not take them more often than recommended on the label. If too much of the drug is taken, it may become habit-forming.

The medicine produces central nervous system stimulation, and it should not be taken by people with heart disease or high blood pressure.

If you think this medicine is not working as well after you have taken it for a few weeks, do not increase the dose. Instead, check with your doctor.

Side effects

The following minor side effects may occur: irritability, nervousness, restlessness, trouble in sleeping.

These side effects should disappear as your body adjusts to the medication. Tell your doctor about any side effects that are persistent or particularly bothersome. It is especially important to tell your doctor about:
  Mental depression
  Nausea or vomiting
  Stomach cramps or pain
  Trembling
  Unusual tiredness or weakness
- Discontinue use of the drug; call your doctor right away. Adverse reactions and side effects may be more frequent and severe in people over age 60 than in younger persons.

Interactions

This medicine interacts with several other drugs such as antihypertensives, other appetite suppressants, caffeine, central nervous system depressants, central nervous system stimulants, furazolidone, guanethidine, hydralazine, MAO inhibitors, methyldopa, molindone, phenothiazines, rauwolfia alkaloids, sodium bicarbonate. Interaction with alcoholic beverages may produce drowsiness, sleepiness, and/or inability to concentrate.
- Be sure to tell your doctor about any medications you are currently taking.

Storage

This medicine should be stored at room temperature in tightly closed containers. Store away from heat and direct light. Keep out of reach of children, since overdose may be very dangerous in children.

Do not store this medicine in the bathroom medicine cabinet because the heat and moisture cause the medicine to break down. Do not keep outdated medicine or medicine no longer needed. Flush the contents of the container down the toilet.

PIPERACILLIN

Properties
This medicine contains piperacillin (penicillin) as active ingredient. Penicillins are prescribed to treat infections caused by bacteria. They will not work for colds, flu, or other virus infections. There are several different kinds of penicillins. Each is used to treat different kinds of infections.

Before using this medicine
Before you use this medicine check with your doctor, or pharmacist:
- if you ever had any unusual or allergic reaction to any of the penicillins, cefalosporins, griseofulvin, or penicillamine. Serious reactions may occur in patients who are allergic to penicillins.
- if you are on a low-salt, low-sugar, or any other special diet, or if you are allergic to any substance, such as sulfites or other preservatives or dyes.
- if you are pregnant or intend to become pregnant while using this medicine. Although penicillins have not been shown to cause problems in humans, the chance always exists.
- if you are breast-feeding an infant. Most penicillins (except amdinocillin) pass into the breast milk. Even though only small amounts may pass, allergic reaction, diarrhea, fungal infection, and skin rash may occur in the infant.
- if you have any of the following medical problems:
Allergy
Asthma
Bleeding problems
Eczema
Hay fever, hives
Kidney disease
Liver disease
Mononucleosis
Stomach or intestinal disease

Treatment
This medication is used to treat an infection caused by bacteria. Most penicillins are best taken with a full glass (8 ounces) of water on an empty stomach, some are best taken with a snack or meal. Follow your doctor's or pharmacist's directions on how to take your medicine.
◆ Keep taking this medicine for the full time of treatment even if you begin to feel better after a few days; do not miss any doses. This is especially important if you have a "strep" infection since serious heart problems could develop later if your infection is not cleared up completely.
◆ If you do miss a dose of this medicine, take it as soon as possible. However, if it is almost time for your next dose, skip the missed dose and go back to your regular dosing schedule.

Side effects
Along with the needed effects, a medicine may cause some unwanted effects. Side effects that usually do not require medical attention: diarrhea; nausea or vomiting; sore mouth or tongue.
◆ Stop taking this medicine and get emergency help immediately if you notice: difficulty in breathing; light-headedness; skin rash, hives, itching; wheezing.

Other side effects that should be reported to your doctor immediately are: abdominal bloating; blood in urine; convulsions (seizures); decreased amount of urine; diarrhea (watery and severe) which may also be bloody; fever; joint pain; sore throat and fever; stomach or abdominal cramps and pain; unusual bleeding or bruising.

Interactions
This medicine may interact with several other drugs such as anticoagulants, diarrhea medicines, heparin, ibuprofen, oral contraceptives, potassium-containing medicines, etc.
■ Be sure to tell your doctor about any medications you are currently taking.

Storage
Tablets, capsules, etc. should be stored as directed by your pharmacist or according to instructions on the label.

PIPERAZINE

Properties

This medicine contains estropipate as active ingredient. The medicine is prescribed for treatment of estrogen deficiency; it restores normal estrogen levels in tissues. There is no evidence that this drug is effective for nervous symptoms or depression occurring during menopause. They should not be used to treat this condition; they should be used only to replace the estrogen that is naturally absent after menopause.

Before using this medicine

Before you use this medicine check with your doctor, or pharmacist:
- if you ever had any unusual or allergic reaction to estrogens;
- if you are pregnant or intend to become pregnant within three months;
- if you are breast-feeding an infant;
- if you have any of the following medical problems:
  Diabetes
  Breast cancer
  Fibrocystic breast disease
  Fibroid uterine tumors
  Endometriosis
  Migraine headaches
  Epilepsy
  Porphyria
  High blood pressure
  Asthma
  Congestive heart failure
  Kidney disease
  Gallstones

Treatment

This medication is used to treat estrogen deficiency, specific symptoms of menopause, estrogen-deficiency osteoporosis, atrophic vaginitis, prostate cancer.

For safe and effective use of this medicine:
- ◆ Follow your doctor's instructions if this medicine was prescribed.
- ◆ Follow the manufacturer's package directions if you are treating yourself.
- ◆ Estrogens have been reported to increase the risk of endometrial carcinoma.

Side effects

Along with the needed effects, a medicine may cause some unwanted effects. Possible side effects include:
  Stomach cramps
  Profuse bleeding
  Appetite loss
  Nausea and vomiting
  Swollen breasts
  Change in menstruation
  Rash, skin blisters
  Depression
  Dizziness

Overdose

The following symptoms may indicate an overdose:
  Nausea and vomiting
  Fluid retention
  Breast enlargement
  Abnormal vaginal bleeding
- ▪ Call a doctor or hospital emergency room for instructions.

Interactions

This medicine may interact with several other drugs such as adrenocorticosteroids, antidepressants, oral antidiabetics, insulin, phenobarbital, primidone.
- ▪ Be sure to tell your doctor about any medications you are currently taking.

Storage

Capsules, tablets, vaginal cream, transdermal patches, etc. should be stored at room temperature; store away from heat and direct light. Keep out of reach of children, since this medicine may be dangerous in children.

PIPRACIL

Properties
This medicine contains piperacillin (penicillin) as active ingredient. Penicillins are prescribed to treat infections caused by bacteria. They will not work for colds, flu, or other virus infections. There are several different kinds of penicillins. Each is used to treat different kinds of infections.

Before using this medicine
Before you use this medicine check with your doctor, or pharmacist:
- if you ever had any unusual or allergic reaction to any of the penicillins, cefalosporins, griseofulvin, or penicillamine. Serious reactions may occur in patients who are allergic to penicillins.
- if you are on a low-salt, low-sugar, or any other special diet, or if you are allergic to any substance, such as sulfites or other preservatives or dyes.
- if you are pregnant or intend to become pregnant while using this medicine. Although penicillins have not been shown to cause problems in humans, the chance always exists.
- if you are breast-feeding an infant. Most penicillins (except amdinocillin) pass into the breast milk. Even though only small amounts may pass, allergic reaction, diarrhea, fungal infection, and skin rash may occur in the infant.
- if you have any of the following medical problems:
  Allergy
  Asthma
  Bleeding problems
  Eczema
  Hay fever, hives
  Kidney disease
  Liver disease
  Mononucleosis
  Stomach or intestinal disease

Treatment
This medication is used to treat an infection caused by bacteria. Most penicillins are best taken with a full glass (8 ounces) of water on an empty stomach, some are best taken with a snack or meal. Follow your doctor's or pharmacist's directions on how to take your medicine.
- Keep taking this medicine for the full time of treatment even if you begin to feel better after a few days; do not miss any doses. This is especially important if you have a "strep" infection since serious heart problems could develop later if your infection is not cleared up completely.
- If you do miss a dose of this medicine, take it as soon as possible. However, if it is almost time for your next dose, skip the missed dose and go back to your regular dosing schedule.

Side effects
Along with the needed effects, a medicine may cause some unwanted effects. Side effects that usually do not require medical attention: diarrhea; nausea or vomiting; sore mouth or tongue.
- Stop taking this medicine and get emergency help immediately if you notice: difficulty in breathing; light-headedness; skin rash, hives, itching; wheezing.

  Other side effects that should be reported to your doctor immediately are: abdominal bloating; blood in urine; convulsions (seizures); decreased amount of urine; diarrhea (watery and severe) which may also be bloody; fever; joint pain; sore throat and fever; stomach or abdominal cramps and pain; unusual bleeding or bruising.

Interactions
This medicine may interact with several other drugs such as anticoagulants, diarrhea medicines, heparin, ibuprofen, oral contraceptives, potassium-containing medicines, etc.
- Be sure to tell your doctor about any medications you are currently taking.

Storage
Tablets, capsules, etc. should be stored as directed by your pharmacist or according to instructions on the label.

PLEGINE

Properties
This medicine contains phendimetrazine as active ingredient; it is prescribed for appetite suppression.

Appetite suppressants are used in the short-term (a few weeks) treatment of obesity. In a few weeks (6 to 12), these medicines in combination with dieting, exercise, and changes in eating habits can help patients lose weight. However, since their appetite reducing effect is only temporary, they are useful only for the first weeks of dieting until new eating habits are established.

Before using this medicine
Before you use this medicine check with your doctor, or pharmacist:
- if you ever had any unusual or allergic reaction to any of the compounds of this medicine.
- if you are on a low-salt, low-sugar, or any other special diet, or if you are allergic to any substance, such as sulfites or other preservatives or dyes.
- if you are pregnant, intend to become pregnant or breast-feeding an infant while using this medicine.
- if you have any of the following medical problems:
Diabetes mellitus (sugar diabetes)
Epilepsy
Glaucoma
Heart or blood vessel disease
High blood pressure
Mental illness (severe)

Treatment
This medication is used to relieve or prevent the symptoms of your medical problem. Take them as directed. Do not take more of them and do not take them more often than recommended on the label. If too much of the drug is taken, it may become habit-forming.

The medicine produces central nervous system stimulation, and it should not be taken by people with heart disease or high blood pressure.

If you think this medicine is not working as well after you have taken it for a few weeks, do not increase the dose. Instead, check with your doctor.

Side effects
The following minor side effects may occur: irritability, nervousness, restlessness, trouble in sleeping.

These side effects should disappear as your body adjusts to the medication. Tell your doctor about any side effects that are persistent or particularly bothersome. It is especially important to tell your doctor about:
Mental depression
Nausea or vomiting
Stomach cramps or pain
Trembling
Unusual tiredness or weakness
- Discontinue use of the drug; call your doctor right away. Adverse reactions and side effects may be more frequent and severe in people over age 60 than in younger persons.

Interactions
This medicine interacts with several other drugs such as antihypertensives, other appetite suppressants, caffeine, central nervous system depressants, central nervous system stimulants, furazolidone, guanethidine, hydralazine, MAO inhibitors, methyldopa, molindone, phenothiazines, rauwolfia alkaloids, sodium bicarbonate. Interaction with alcoholic beverages may produce drowsiness, sleepiness, and/or inability to concentrate.
- Be sure to tell your doctor about any medications you are currently taking.

Storage
This medicine should be stored at room temperature in tightly closed containers. Store away from heat and direct light. Keep out of reach of children, since overdose may be very dangerous in children.

Do not store this medicine in the bathroom medicine cabinet because the heat and moisture cause the medicine to break down. Do not keep outdated medicine or medicine no longer needed. Flush the contents of the container down the toilet.

PLENDIL

Properties
This medicine contains felodipine as active ingredient. It is a so-called calcium channel blocker, working by blocking the passage of calcium into heart and smooth muscle. Since calcium is an essential factor in muscle contraction, any medicine that affects calcium in this way will interfere with the contraction of these muscles.

The medicine works by:
◆ reducing the work that the heart must perform;
◆ reducing the normal arterial blood pressure;
◆ increasing oxygen to the heart muscle.

The medicine is prescribed for the treatment of attacks of angina pectoris, irregular heartbeat, and high blood pressure. In many cases it can be used for the treatment and prevention of migraine.

Before using this medicine
Before you use this medicine check with your doctor, or pharmacist:
– if you ever had any unusual or allergic reaction to this medicine or any calcium channel blocker;
– if you are pregnant or intend to become pregnant while using this medicine;
– if you have low blood pressure;
– if you have kidney or lifer disease;
– if you are breast-feeding an infant;
– if you easily get a rash or intensity sunburn in areas exposed to sun or ultraviolet light.

Treatment
This medication is used for treatment of heart conditions (for instance, angina pectoris) and high blood pressure. Tablets, capsules or extended-release tablets should be taken with liquid. The usual dose amounts to 30 to 100 milligrams a day.

For safe and effective use of medicine:
◆ Follow your doctor's instructions if this medicine was prescribed.
◆ Follow the manufacturer's package directions if you are treating yourself.

Side effects
Along with the needed effects, a medicine may cause some unwanted effects. Possible side effects include:
Tiredness
Changes in heartbeat
Wheezing
Cough
Shortness of breath
Dizziness
Fainting
Numbness in hands and feet
Tingling in hands and feet
Difficult urination
Constipation

Overdose
The following symptoms may be a sign of overdose:
Unusually fast heartbeat
Unusually slow heartbeat
Loss of consciousness
Cardiac arrest
■ Call a doctor or hospital emergency room for instructions. If necessary start first aid immediately.

Interactions
The effect of this medicine may cause a blood pressure drop if taken together with antihypertensives. Cimetidine may increase the effect of the calcium blocker.

The simultaneous use of diuretics and calcium channel blockers may cause dangerous blood pressure drop.
■ Be sure to tell your doctor about any medications you are currently taking.

Storage
Capsules, tablets, etc. should be stored at room temperature; store away from heat and direct light. Keep out of reach of children, since this medicine may be dangerous in children.

PMS AMITRIPTYLINE

Properties
This medicine contains amitriptyline as active ingredient. It belongs to the group of medicines known as tricyclic antidepressants or 'mood elevators.' It is used to relieve mental depression and depression that sometimes occurs with anxiety. The medication gradually relieves, but doesn't cure, symptoms of depression. The medication may also be used for the treatment of narcolepsy, bulimia, painic attacks, cocaine withdrawal, attention deficit disorder.

Before using this medicine
Before you use this medicine check with your doctor, or pharmacist:
- if you ever had any unusual or allergic reaction to any tricyclic antidepressant, maprotiline or trazodone.
- if you are on a low-salt, low-sugar, or any other special diet, or if you are allergic to any substance, such as sulfites or other preservatives or dyes.
- if you are pregnant or intend to become pregnant while using this medicine. There have been reports of newborns suffering from heart, breathing, and urinary problems when their mothers had taken tricyclic antidepressants before delivery.
- if you are breast-feeding an infant. Some tricyclic antidepressants pass into the breast milk.

Treatment
Take this medicine only as directed by your doctor, to benefit your condition as much as possible. Do not take more of it, do not take it more often, and do not take it for a longer period of time than your doctor ordered.

To lessen stomach upset, take this medicine with food, even for a daily bedtime dose, unless your doctor has told you to take it on an empty stomach. If you forget your once-a-day bedtime dose, Do not take it more than 3 hours late. If more than 3 hours, wait for next scheduled dose;.

Sometimes this medicine must be taken for several weeks before you begin to feel better.

Side effects
Along with the needed effects, a medicine may cause some unwanted effects. Side effects that usually do not require medical attention: difficult or frequent urination; decreased sex drive; muscle aches; abnormal dreams; nasal congestion; weakness and faintness when arising from bed or chair; back pain.
- Other side effects that should be reported to your doctor immediately are:
  Hallucinations
  Shakiness
  Dizziness or fainting
  Blurred vision, eye pain
  Irregular heartbeat or slow pulse
  Inflamed tongue
  Abdominal pain
  Jaundice
  Hair loss, rash
  Fever, chills
  Joint pain
  Palpitations

Interactions
This medicine may interact with several other drugs such as anticoagulants, anticholinergics, cold remedies, oral contraceptives, seizure medicines, sleeping medicines, thyroid medicines, etc. Be sure to tell your doctor about any medications you are currently taking.

Storage
Tablets, capsules, etc. should be stored at room temperature in tightly closed, light-resistant containers as directed by your pharmacist. Keep out of reach of children since overdose is especially dangerous in young children. Do not store in the bathroom medicine cabinet because the heat or moisture may cause the medicine to break down. Keep the liquid form of the medicine from freezing.

PMS IMIPRAMINE

Properties
This medicine contains imipramine as active ingredient. It belongs to the group of medicines known as tricyclic antidepressants or 'mood elevators.' It is used to relieve mental depression and depression that sometimes occurs with anxiety. The medication gradually relieves, but doesn't cure, symptoms of depression. The medication may also be used for the treatment of narcolepsy, bulimia, painic attacks, cocaine withdrawal, attention deficit disorder.

Before using this medicine
Before you use this medicine check with your doctor, or pharmacist:
- if you ever had any unusual or allergic reaction to any tricyclic antidepressant, maprotiline or trazodone.
- if you are on a low-salt, low-sugar, or any other special diet, or if you are allergic to any substance, such as sulfites or other preservatives or dyes.
- if you are pregnant or intend to become pregnant while using this medicine. There have been reports of newborns suffering from heart, breathing, and urinary problems when their mothers had taken tricyclic antidepressants before delivery.
- if you are breast-feeding an infant. Some tricyclic antidepressants pass into the breast milk.

Treatment
Take this medicine only as directed by your doctor, to benefit your condition as much as possible. Do not take more of it, do not take it more often, and do not take it for a longer period of time than your doctor ordered.

To lessen stomach upset, take this medicine with food, even for a daily bedtime dose, unless your doctor has told you to take it on an empty stomach. If you forget your once-a-day bedtime dose, Do not take it more than 3 hours late. If more than 3 hours, wait for next scheduled dose;.

Sometimes this medicine must be taken for several weeks before you begin to feel better.

Side effects
Along with the needed effects, a medicine may cause some unwanted effects. Side effects that usually do not require medical attention: difficult or frequent urination; decreased sex drive; muscle aches; abnormal dreams; nasal congestion; weakness and faintness when arising from bed or chair; back pain.
- Other side effects that should be reported to your doctor immediately are:
  Hallucinations
  Shakiness
  Dizziness or fainting
  Blurred vision, eye pain
  Irregular heartbeat or slow pulse
  Inflamed tongue
  Abdominal pain
  Jaundice
  Hair loss, rash
  Fever, chills
  Joint pain
  Palpitations

Interactions
This medicine may interact with several other drugs such as anticoagulants, anticholinergics, cold remedies, oral contraceptives, seizure medicines, sleeping medicines, thyroid medicines, etc.
- Be sure to tell your doctor about any medications you are currently taking.

Storage
Tablets, capsules, etc. should be stored at room temperature in tightly closed, light-resistant containers as directed by your pharmacist. Keep out of reach of children since overdose is especially dangerous in young children. Do not store in the bathroom medicine cabinet because the heat or moisture may cause the medicine to break down. Keep the liquid form of the medicine from freezing.

PMS THEOPHYLLINE

Properties
This medicine contains theophylline as active ingredient; it is used to treat or prevent breathing problems (wheezing and shortness of breath) caused by asthma, bronchitis, or emphysema. This medication belongs to a group known as xanthine-derivative bronchodilators. They work by opening up the bronchial tubes or air passages of the lungs and increasing the flow of air through them. These medicines are available only with your doctor's prescription.

Before using this medicine
Before you use this medicine check with your doctor, or pharmacist:
- if you ever had any unusual or allergic reaction to xanthine-derivative bronchodilators.
- if you are on a low-salt, low-sugar, or any other special diet, or if you are allergic to any substance, such as sulfites or other preservatives or dyes.
- if you are pregnant or intend to become pregnant while using this medicine.
- if you are breast-feeding an infant. Theophylline passes into the breast milk and may cause irritability, fretfulness, or trouble in sleeping in infants of mothers taking this medicine.
- if you have any of the following medical problems:
Diarrhea
Enlarged prostate
Fibrocystic breast disease
Heart disease
Stomach ulcer

Treatment
This medication is used to relieve or prevent the symptoms of your medical problem. Take them as directed. Do not take more of them and do not take them more often than recommended on the label, unless otherwise directed by your doctor. To do so may increase the chance of side effects. The medicine should be taken on an empty stomach 30 to 60 minutes before a meal or two hours after a meal. Try not to miss any doses of this medication. If you do miss a dose, take the missed dose as soon as possible, unless it is almost time for the next dose. Do not double the next dose. It works best when taken with a glass of water.

Side effects
The following minor side effects may occur:
Dizziness Or Flushing
Headache
Diarrhea
Heartburn
Increased Urination
Insomnia
Nervousness Or Irritability
Loss Of Appetite
Nausea Or Stomach Upset
Stomach Pain.
These side effects should disappear as your body adjusts to the medication. Tell your doctor about any side effects that are persistent or particularly bothersome. It is especially important to tell your doctor about black, tarry stools; confusion; convulsions; difficulty in breathing; fainting; muscle twitching; palpitations; rash; severe abdominal pain; or unusual weakness.

Interactions
This medicine interacts with several other drugs such as diuretics, reserpine, beta blockers, phenytoin, lithium, phenobarbital, birth control pills, and other medications.
- Be sure to tell your doctor about any medications you are currently taking.

Storage
Tablets, capsules, liquid and suspension should be stored at room temperature in tightly closed containers. Store away from heat and direct light. Keep out of reach of children, since overdose may be very dangerous in children. Discard any outdated medication.

P.N. OPHTHALMIC (Ophthalmic)

Properties
This medicine contains an ophthalmic antibacterial, as active ingredient. It helps the body to overcome eye infections on surface tissues of the eye. It is most useful when the infecting organism is one known to be sensitive to the antibacterial drug.

The drug penetrates the bacterial cell membrane and prevents cells from multiplying.

Before using this medicine
Before you use this medicine check with your doctor:
– if you ever had any unusual or allergic reaction to any of the compounds of the medicine.
– if you are on a low-salt, low-sugar, or any other special diet, or if you are allergic to any substance, such as sulfites or other preservatives or dyes.
– if you are pregnant or intend to become pregnant while using this medicine. Although ophthalmic antibacterials have been found to be safe for use during pregnancy, you should check with your doctor before taking any drug if you are pregnant.

Treatment
This medication is used to treat an infection caused by bacteria. The medicine may be used in the form of eye drops or as an eye ointment. Use the medication as directed, Do not miss a dose. If you forget a dose, use it as soon as you remember. Notify your doctor if eye symptoms fail to improve in two to four days.
◆ To apply eye drops: Till the head backward when applying the eye drops. Pull the lower eyelid away from the eye to form a pouch. After applying the drop, keep the eye closed for a minute or so. This allows the medication to come in contact with the infection.
◆ To apply eye ointment: Pull lower lid down from eye to form a pouch. Squeeze tube to apply thin strip of ointment into pouch. Close eye for 1 to 2 minutes.

Always wash your hands before applying the ointment.
The drug starts to work in about one hour. Treatment may require 7 to 10 days to control infection.
Older adults or seniors may take this medication without special restriction.

Side effects
Along with the needed effects, a medicine may cause some unwanted effects. Side effects that usually do not require medical attention: occasional local irritation after application to the eye. Ointments may cause blurred vision for a few minutes; continue the use of the eye drops or ointment, but tell your doctor at the next visit.
■ Discontinue the use of eye drops or eye ointment in the following cases:
Sore throat
Aplastic anemia
Pale skin
Unusual redness of the eye
Unusual irritation of the eye
Fever
Unusual bleeding
Unusual bruising
■ Tell your doctor about any side effects that are persistent or particularly bothersome. In case of prolonged use sensitivity reactions may develop.

Interactions
Clinically significant interactions with oral or injected medicines are unlikely. Do not use the eye drops or ointment with any other eye drops or ointment without checking with your ophthalmologist.

Storage
Keep bottle (with eye drops) or container (containing ointment) lightly closed. Store in a cool place, but Do not freeze. Wash handss immediately after using.
Do not store in the bathroom medicine cabinet because the heat or moisture may cause the medicine to break down.
Do not keep outdated medicine or medicine no longer needed. Flush the contents of the bottle or tube down the toilet, unless otherwise directed.

POLYMYXIN B Ophthalmic)

Properties
This medicine contains an ophthalmic antibacterial, as active ingredient. It helps the body to overcome eye infections on surface tissues of the eye. It is most useful when the infecting organism is one known to be sensitive to the antibacterial drug.

The drug penetrates the bacterial cell membrane and prevents cells from multiplying.

Before using this medicine
Before you use this medicine check with your doctor:
- if you ever had any unusual or allergic reaction to any of the compounds of the medicine.
- if you are on a low-salt, low-sugar, or any other special diet, or if you are allergic to any substance, such as sulfites or other preservatives or dyes.
- if you are pregnant or intend to become pregnant while using this medicine. Although ophthalmic antibacterials have been found to be safe for use during pregnancy, you should check with your doctor before taking any drug if you are pregnant.

Treatment
This medication is used to treat an infection caused by bacteria. The medicine may be used in the form of eye drops or as an eye ointment. Use the medication as directed, Do not miss a dose. If you forget a dose, use it as soon as you remember. Notify your doctor if eye symptoms fail to improve in two to four days.
- ♦ To apply eye drops: Till the head backward when applying the eye drops. Pull the lower eyelid away from the eye to form a pouch. After applying the drop, keep the eye closed for a minute or so. This allows the medication to come in contact with the infection.
- ♦ To apply eye ointment: Pull lower lid down from eye to form a pouch. Squeeze tube to apply thin strip of ointment into pouch. Close eye for 1 to 2 minutes.

Always wash your hands before applying the ointment.

The drug starts to work in about one hour. Treatment may require 7 to 10 days to control infection.

Older adults or seniors may take this medication without special restriction.

Side effects
Along with the needed effects, a medicine may cause some unwanted effects. Side effects that usually do not require medical attention: occasional local irritation after application to the eye. Ointments may cause blurred vision for a few minutes; continue the use of the eye drops or ointment, but tell your doctor at the next visit.
- ■ Discontinue the use of eye drops or eye ointment in the following cases:
  Sore throat
  Aplastic anemia
  Pale skin
  Unusual redness of the eye
  Unusual irritation of the eye
  Fever
  Unusual bleeding
  Unusual bruising
- ■ Tell your doctor about any side effects that are persistent or particularly bothersome. In case of prolonged use sensitivity reactions may develop.

Interactions
Clinically significant interactions with oral or injected medicines are unlikely. Do not use the eye drops or ointment with any other eye drops or ointment without checking with your ophthalmologist.

Storage
Keep bottle (with eye drops) or container (containing ointment) lightly closed. Store in a cool place, but Do not freeze. Wash handss immediately after using. Do not store in the bathroom medicine cabinet because the heat or moisture may cause the medicine to break down. Do not keep outdated medicine or medicine no longer needed. Flush the contents of the bottle or tube down the toilet, unless otherwise directed.

POTACHLOR

Properties
This medicine contains potassium chloride as active ingredient; it is used to treat or prevent potassium deficiency, especially potassium deficiency that is caused by the use of diuretics (water pills).

Potassium is needed to maintain good health. Potassium supplements may be needed by patients who do not have enough potassium in their regular diet and by those who have lost too much potassium because of illness or treatment with certain medicines.

Since too much potassium may also cause health problems, most potassium supplements are available only with your doctor's prescription.

Before using this medicine
Before you use this medicine check with your doctor, or pharmacist:
- if you ever had any unusual or allergic reaction to potassium preparations;
- if you are on a low-salt, low-sugar, or any other special diet, or if you are allergic to any substance, such as sulfites or other preservatives or dyes.
- if you are pregnant or intend to become pregnant while using this medicine. Although potassium supplements have not been shown to cause problems in humans, the chance always exists.
- if you are breast-feeding an infant. Although this medicine has not been shown to cause problems in humans, the chance always exists since small amounts of potassium pass into the breast milk.
- if you have any of the following medical problems:
Addison's disease
Heart disease
Diarrhea
Kidney disease
Stomach ulcer

Treatment
This medication is used to relieve or prevent the symptoms of your medical problem. Take them as directed. Do not take more of them and do not take them more often than recommended on the label, unless otherwise directed by your doctor. To do so may increase the chance of side effects.

In order to avoid stomach irritation, you should take potassium supplements with food or immediately after a meal. If you miss a dose of this medication, take the missed dose as soon as possible, unless it is within two hours of the next scheduled dose;.

Side effects
The following minor side effects may occur:
Diarrhea
Nausea
Stomach Pains
Vomiting.
These side effects should disappear as your body adjusts to the medication. Tell your doctor about any side effects that are persistent or particularly bothersome. It is especially important to tell your doctor about anxiety; bloody or black, tarry stools; confusion; difficulty in breathing; numbness or tingling in the arms, legs, or feet; palpitations; severe abdominal pain; or unusual weakness.

Interactions
This medicine interacts with several other drugs such as adrenocorticosteroids, antimuscarinics, calcium-containing medicines; heart medicines such as digitalis or digoxin; laxatives; other potassium-containing medicines.
- Be sure to tell your doctor about any medications you are currently taking.

Storage
Tablets, elixir, etc. should be stored at room temperature in tightly closed containers. Store away from heat and direct light. Keep out of reach of children, since overdose may be very dangerous in children. Do not keep outdated medicine or medicine no longer needed. Flush the contents of the container down the toilet, unless otherwise directed.

POTAGE

Properties
This medicine contains potassium chloride as active ingredient; it is used to treat or prevent potassium deficiency, especially potassium deficiency that is caused by the use of diuretics (water pills).

Potassium is needed to maintain good health. Potassium supplements may be needed by patients who do not have enough potassium in their regular diet and by those who have lost too much potassium because of illness or treatment with certain medicines.

Since too much potassium may also cause health problems, most potassium supplements are available only with your doctor's prescription.

Before using this medicine
Before you use this medicine check with your doctor, or pharmacist:
- if you ever had any unusual or allergic reaction to potassium preparations;
- if you are on a low-salt, low-sugar, or any other special diet, or if you are allergic to any substance, such as sulfites or other preservatives or dyes.
- if you are pregnant or intend to become pregnant while using this medicine. Although potassium supplements have not been shown to cause problems in humans, the chance always exists.
- if you are breast-feeding an infant. Although this medicine has not been shown to cause problems in humans, the chance always exists since small amounts of potassium pass into the breast milk.
- if you have any of the following medical problems:
Addison's disease
Heart disease
Diarrhea
Kidney disease
Stomach ulcer

Treatment
This medication is used to relieve or prevent the symptoms of your medical problem. Take them as directed. Do not take more of them and do not take them more often than recommended on the label, unless otherwise directed by your doctor. To do so may increase the chance of side effects.

In order to avoid stomach irritation, you should take potassium supplements with food or immediately after a meal. If you miss a dose of this medication, take the missed dose as soon as possible, unless it is within two hours of the next scheduled dose;.

Side effects
The following minor side effects may occur:
Diarrhea
Nausea
Stomach pains
Vomiting.
These side effects should disappear as your body adjusts to the medication. Tell your doctor about any side effects that are persistent or particularly bothersome. It is especially important to tell your doctor about anxiety; bloody or black, tarry stools; confusion; difficulty in breathing; numbness or tingling in the arms, legs, or feet; palpitations; severe abdominal pain; or unusual weakness.

Interactions
This medicine interacts with several other drugs such as adrenocorticosteroids, antimuscarinics, calcium-containing medicines; heart medicines such as digitalis or digoxin; laxatives; other potassium-containing medicines.
- Be sure to tell your doctor about any medications you are currently taking.

Storage
Tablets, elixir, etc. should be stored at room temperature in tightly closed containers. Store away from heat and direct light. Keep out of reach of children, since overdose may be very dangerous in children. Do not keep outdated medicine or medicine no longer needed. Flush the contents of the container down the toilet, unless otherwise directed.

POTASALAN

Properties
This medicine contains potassium chloride as active ingredient; it is used to treat or prevent potassium deficiency, especially potassium deficiency that is caused by the use of diuretics (water pills).

Potassium is needed to maintain good health. Potassium supplements may be needed by patients who do not have enough potassium in their regular diet and by those who have lost too much potassium because of illness or treatment with certain medicines.

Since too much potassium may also cause health problems, most potassium supplements are available only with your doctor's prescription.

Before using this medicine
Before you use this medicine check with your doctor, or pharmacist:
- if you ever had any unusual or allergic reaction to potassium preparations;
- if you are on a low-salt, low-sugar, or any other special diet, or if you are allergic to any substance, such as sulfites or other preservatives or dyes.
- if you are pregnant or intend to become pregnant while using this medicine. Although potassium supplements have not been shown to cause problems in humans, the chance always exists.
- if you are breast-feeding an infant. Although this medicine has not been shown to cause problems in humans, the chance always exists since small amounts of potassium pass into the breast milk.
- if you have any of the following medical problems:
Addison's disease
Heart disease
Diarrhea
Kidney disease
Stomach ulcer

Treatment
This medication is used to relieve or prevent the symptoms of your medical problem. Take them as directed. Do not take more of them and do not take them more often than recommended on the label, unless otherwise directed by your doctor. To do so may increase the chance of side effects.

In order to avoid stomach irritation, you should take potassium supplements with food or immediately after a meal. If you miss a dose of this medication, take the missed dose as soon as possible, unless it is within two hours of the next scheduled dose;.

Side effects
The following minor side effects may occur:
Diarrhea
Nausea
Stomach pains
Vomiting.
These side effects should disappear as your body adjusts to the medication. Tell your doctor about any side effects that are persistent or particularly bothersome. It is especially important to tell your doctor about anxiety; bloody or black, tarry stools; confusion; difficulty in breathing; numbness or tingling in the arms, legs, or feet; palpitations; severe abdominal pain; or unusual weakness.

Interactions
This medicine interacts with several other drugs such as adrenocorticosteroids, antimuscarinics, calcium-containing medicines; heart medicines such as digitalis or digoxin; laxatives; other potassium-containing medicines.
- Be sure to tell your doctor about any medications you are currently taking.

Storage
Tablets, elixir, etc. should be stored at room temperature in tightly closed containers. Store away from heat and direct light. Keep out of reach of children, since overdose may be very dangerous in children. Do not keep outdated medicine or medicine no longer needed. Flush the contents of the container down the toilet, unless otherwise directed.

POTASSINE

Properties

This medicine contains potassium chloride as active ingredient; it is used to treat or prevent potassium deficiency, especially potassium deficiency that is caused by the use of diuretics (water pills).

Potassium is needed to maintain good health. Potassium supplements may be needed by patients who do not have enough potassium in their regular diet and by those who have lost too much potassium because of illness or treatment with certain medicines.

Since too much potassium may also cause health problems, most potassium supplements are available only with your doctor's prescription.

Before using this medicine

Before you use this medicine check with your doctor, or pharmacist:
- if you ever had any unusual or allergic reaction to potassium preparations;
- if you are on a low-salt, low-sugar, or any other special diet, or if you are allergic to any substance, such as sulfites or other preservatives or dyes.
- if you are pregnant or intend to become pregnant while using this medicine. Although potassium supplements have not been shown to cause problems in humans, the chance always exists.
- if you are breast-feeding an infant. Although this medicine has not been shown to cause problems in humans, the chance always exists since small amounts of potassium pass into the breast milk.
- if you have any of the following medical problems:
Addison's disease
Heart disease
Diarrhea
Kidney disease
Stomach ulcer

Treatment

This medication is used to relieve or prevent the symptoms of your medical problem. Take them as directed. Do not take more of them and do not take them more often than recommended on the label, unless otherwise directed by your doctor. To do so may increase the chance of side effects.

In order to avoid stomach irritation, you should take potassium supplements with food or immediately after a meal. If you miss a dose of this medication, take the missed dose as soon as possible, unless it is within two hours of the next scheduled dose;.

Side effects

The following minor side effects may occur:
Diarrhea
Nausea
Stomach pains
Vomiting.

These side effects should disappear as your body adjusts to the medication. Tell your doctor about any side effects that are persistent or particularly bothersome. It is especially important to tell your doctor about anxiety; bloody or black, tarry stools; confusion; difficulty in breathing; numbness or tingling in the arms, legs, or feet; palpitations; severe abdominal pain; or unusual weakness.

Interactions

This medicine interacts with several other drugs such as adrenocorticosteroids, antimuscarinics, calcium-containing medicines; heart medicines such as digitalis or digoxin; laxatives; other potassium-containing medicines.
- Be sure to tell your doctor about any medications you are currently taking.

Storage

Tablets, elixir, etc. should be stored at room temperature in tightly closed containers. Store away from heat and direct light. Keep out of reach of children, since overdose may be very dangerous in children. Do not keep outdated medicine or medicine no longer needed. Flush the contents of the container down the toilet, unless otherwise directed.

POTASSIUM ACETATE

Properties
This medicine contains potassium acetate as active ingredient; it is used to treat or prevent potassium deficiency, especially potassium deficiency that is caused by the use of diuretics (water pills).

Potassium is needed to maintain good health. Potassium supplements may be needed by patients who do not have enough potassium in their regular diet and by those who have lost too much potassium because of illness or treatment with certain medicines.

Since too much potassium may also cause health problems, most potassium supplements are available only with your doctor's prescription.

Before using this medicine
Before you use this medicine check with your doctor, or pharmacist:
- if you ever had any unusual or allergic reaction to potassium preparations;
- if you are on a low-salt, low-sugar, or any other special diet, or if you are allergic to any substance, such as sulfites or other preservatives or dyes.
- if you are pregnant or intend to become pregnant while using this medicine. Although potassium supplements have not been shown to cause problems in humans, the chance always exists.
- if you are breast-feeding an infant. Although this medicine has not been shown to cause problems in humans, the chance always exists since small amounts of potassium pass into the breast milk.
- if you have any of the following medical problems:
Addison's disease
Heart disease
Diarrhea
Kidney disease
Stomach ulcer

Treatment
This medication is used to relieve or prevent the symptoms of your medical problem. Take them as directed. Do not take more of them and do not take them more often than recommended on the label, unless otherwise directed by your doctor. To do so may increase the chance of side effects.

In order to avoid stomach irritation, you should take potassium supplements with food or immediately after a meal. If you miss a dose of this medication, take the missed dose as soon as possible, unless it is within two hours of the next scheduled dose;.

Side effects
The following minor side effects may occur:
Diarrhea
Nausea
Stomach pains
Vomiting.

These side effects should disappear as your body adjusts to the medication. Tell your doctor about any side effects that are persistent or particularly bothersome. It is especially important to tell your doctor about anxiety; bloody or black, tarry stools; confusion; difficulty in breathing; numbness or tingling in the arms, legs, or feet; palpitations; severe abdominal pain; or unusual weakness.

Interactions
This medicine interacts with several other drugs such as adrenocorticosteroids, antimuscarinics, calcium-containing medicines; heart medicines such as digitalis or digoxin; laxatives; other potassium-containing medicines.
- Be sure to tell your doctor about any medications you are currently taking.

Storage
Tablets, elixir, etc. should be stored at room temperature in tightly closed containers. Store away from heat and direct light. Keep out of reach of children, since overdose may be very dangerous in children. Do not keep outdated medicine or medicine no longer needed. Flush the contents of the container down the toilet, unless otherwise directed.

POTASSIUM TRIPLEX

Properties
This medicine contains trikates as active ingredient; it is used to treat or prevent potassium deficiency, especially potassium deficiency that is caused by the use of diuretics (water pills).

Potassium is needed to maintain good health. Potassium supplements may be needed by patients who do not have enough potassium in their regular diet and by those who have lost too much potassium because of illness or treatment with certain medicines.

Since too much potassium may also cause health problems, most potassium supplements are available only with your doctor's prescription.

Before using this medicine
Before you use this medicine check with your doctor, or pharmacist:
- if you ever had any unusual or allergic reaction to potassium preparations;
- if you are on a low-salt, low-sugar, or any other special diet, or if you are allergic to any substance, such as sulfites or other preservatives or dyes.
- if you are pregnant or intend to become pregnant while using this medicine. Although potassium supplements have not been shown to cause problems in humans, the chance always exists.
- if you are breast-feeding an infant. Although this medicine has not been shown to cause problems in humans, the chance always exists since small amounts of potassium pass into the breast milk.
- if you have any of the following medical problems:
Addison's disease
Heart disease
Diarrhea
Kidney disease
Stomach ulcer

Treatment
This medication is used to relieve or prevent the symptoms of your medical problem. Take them as directed. Do not take more of them and do not take them more often than recommended on the label, unless otherwise directed by your doctor. To do so may increase the chance of side effects.

In order to avoid stomach irritation, you should take potassium supplements with food or immediately after a meal. If you miss a dose of this medication, take the missed dose as soon as possible, unless it is within two hours of the next scheduled dose;.

Side effects
The following minor side effects may occur:
Diarrhea
Nausea
Stomach pains
Vomiting.
These side effects should disappear as your body adjusts to the medication. Tell your doctor about any side effects that are persistent or particularly bothersome. It is especially important to tell your doctor about anxiety; bloody or black, tarry stools; confusion; difficulty in breathing; numbness or tingling in the arms, legs, or feet; palpitations; severe abdominal pain; or unusual weakness.

Interactions
This medicine interacts with several other drugs such as adrenocorticosteroids, antimuscarinics, calcium-containing medicines; heart medicines such as digitalis or digoxin; laxatives; other potassium-containing medicines.
- Be sure to tell your doctor about any medications you are currently taking.

Storage
Tablets, elixir, etc. should be stored at room temperature in tightly closed containers. Store away from heat and direct light. Keep out of reach of children, since overdose may be very dangerous in children. Do not keep outdated medicine or medicine no longer needed. Flush the contents of the container down the toilet, unless otherwise directed.

POTASSIUM CHLORIDE

Properties
This medicine contains potassium chloride as active ingredient; it is used to treat or prevent potassium deficiency, especially potassium deficiency that is caused by the use of diuretics (water pills).

Potassium is needed to maintain good health. Potassium supplements may be needed by patients who do not have enough potassium in their regular diet and by those who have lost too much potassium because of illness or treatment with certain medicines.

Since too much potassium may also cause health problems, most potassium supplements are available only with your doctor's prescription.

Before using this medicine
Before you use this medicine check with your doctor, or pharmacist:
- if you ever had any unusual or allergic reaction to potassium preparations;
- if you are on a low-salt, low-sugar, or any other special diet, or if you are allergic to any substance, such as sulfites or other preservatives or dyes.
- if you are pregnant or intend to become pregnant while using this medicine. Although potassium supplements have not been shown to cause problems in humans, the chance always exists.
- if you are breast-feeding an infant. Although this medicine has not been shown to cause problems in humans, the chance always exists since small amounts of potassium pass into the breast milk.
- if you have any of the following medical problems:
  Addison's disease
  Heart disease
  Diarrhea
  Kidney disease
  Stomach ulcer

Treatment
This medication is used to relieve or prevent the symptoms of your medical problem. Take them as directed. Do not take more of them and do not take them more often than recommended on the label, unless otherwise directed by your doctor. To do so may increase the chance of side effects.

In order to avoid stomach irritation, you should take potassium supplements with food or immediately after a meal. If you miss a dose of this medication, take the missed dose as soon as possible, unless it is within two hours of the next scheduled dose;.

Side effects
The following minor side effects may occur:
  Diarrhea
  Nausea
  Stomach pains
  Vomiting.
These side effects should disappear as your body adjusts to the medication. Tell your doctor about any side effects that are persistent or particularly bothersome. It is especially important to tell your doctor about anxiety; bloody or black, tarry stools; confusion; difficulty in breathing; numbness or tingling in the arms, legs, or feet; palpitations; severe abdominal pain; or unusual weakness.

Interactions
This medicine interacts with several other drugs such as adrenocorticosteroids, antimuscarinics, calcium-containing medicines; heart medicines such as digitalis or digoxin; laxatives; other potassium-containing medicines.
- Be sure to tell your doctor about any medications you are currently taking.

Storage
Tablets, elixir, etc. should be stored at room temperature in tightly closed containers. Store away from heat and direct light. Keep out of reach of children, since overdose may be very dangerous in children. Do not keep outdated medicine or medicine no longer needed. Flush the contents of the container down the toilet, unless otherwise directed.

POTASSIUM BICARBONATE

Properties

This medicine contains potassium bicarbonate as active ingredient; it is used to treat or prevent potassium deficiency, especially potassium deficiency that is caused by the use of diuretics (water pills).

Potassium is needed to maintain good health. Potassium supplements may be needed by patients who do not have enough potassium in their regular diet and by those who have lost too much potassium because of illness or treatment with certain medicines.

Since too much potassium may also cause health problems, most potassium supplements are available only with your doctor's prescription.

Before using this medicine

Before you use this medicine check with your doctor, or pharmacist:
- if you ever had any unusual or allergic reaction to potassium preparations;
- if you are on a low-salt, low-sugar, or any other special diet, or if you are allergic to any substance, such as sulfites or other preservatives or dyes.
- if you are pregnant or intend to become pregnant while using this medicine. Although potassium supplements have not been shown to cause problems in humans, the chance always exists.
- if you are breast-feeding an infant. Although this medicine has not been shown to cause problems in humans, the chance always exists since small amounts of potassium pass into the breast milk.
- if you have any of the following medical problems:
Addison's disease
Heart disease
Diarrhea
Kidney disease
Stomach ulcer

Treatment

This medication is used to relieve or prevent the symptoms of your medical problem. Take them as directed. Do not take more of them and do not take them more often than recommended on the label, unless otherwise directed by your doctor. To do so may increase the chance of side effects.

In order to avoid stomach irritation, you should take potassium supplements with food or immediately after a meal. If you miss a dose of this medication, take the missed dose as soon as possible, unless it is within two hours of the next scheduled dose;.

Side effects

The following minor side effects may occur:
Diarrhea
Nausea
Stomach pains
Vomiting.
These side effects should disappear as your body adjusts to the medication. Tell your doctor about any side effects that are persistent or particularly bothersome. It is especially important to tell your doctor about anxiety; bloody or black, tarry stools; confusion; difficulty in breathing; numbness or tingling in the arms, legs, or feet; palpitations; severe abdominal pain; or unusual weakness.

Interactions

This medicine interacts with several other drugs such as adrenocorticosteroids, antimuscarinics, calcium-containing medicines; heart medicines such as digitalis or digoxin; laxatives; other potassium-containing medicines.
- Be sure to tell your doctor about any medications you are currently taking.

Storage

Tablets, elixir, etc. should be stored at room temperature in tightly closed containers. Store away from heat and direct light. Keep out of reach of children, since overdose may be very dangerous in children. Do not keep outdated medicine or medicine no longer needed. Flush the contents of the container down the toilet, unless otherwise directed.

POTASSIUM GLUCONATE

Properties
This medicine contains potassium gluconate as active ingredient; it is used to
treat or prevent potassium deficiency,
especially potassium deficiency that is
caused by the use of diuretics (water
pills).

Potassium is needed to maintain
good health. Potassium supplements
may be needed by patients who do not
have enough potassium in their regular
diet and by those who have lost too
much potassium because of illness or
treatment with certain medicines.

Since too much potassium may also
cause health problems, most potassium
supplements are available only with
your doctor's prescription.

Before using this medicine
Before you use this medicine check
with your doctor, or pharmacist:
- if you ever had any unusual or allergic reaction to potassium preparations;
- if you are on a low-salt, low-sugar,
  or any other special diet, or if you are
  allergic to any substance, such as sulfites or other preservatives or dyes.
- if you are pregnant or intend to become pregnant while using this
  medicine. Although potassium supplements have not been shown to
  cause problems in humans, the
  chance always exists.
- if you are breast-feeding an infant.
  Although this medicine has not been
  shown to cause problems in humans,
  the chance always exists since small
  amounts of potassium pass into the
  breast milk.
- if you have any of the following
  medical problems:
  Addison's disease
  Heart disease
  Diarrhea
  Kidney disease
  Stomach ulcer

Treatment
This medication is used to relieve or
prevent the symptoms of your medical
problem. Take them as directed. Do not
take more of them and do not take them
more often than recommended on the
label, unless otherwise directed by your
doctor. To do so may increase the
chance of side effects.

In order to avoid stomach irritation,
you should take potassium supplements
with food or immediately after a meal.
If you miss a dose of this medication,
take the missed dose as soon as possible, unless it is within two hours of the
next scheduled dose;.

Side effects
The following minor side effects may
occur:
  Diarrhea
  Nausea
  Stomach pains
  Vomiting.
These side effects should disappear as
your body adjusts to the medication.
Tell your doctor about any side effects
that are persistent or particularly bothersome. It is especially important to tell
your doctor about anxiety; bloody or
black, tarry stools; confusion; difficulty
in breathing; numbness or tingling in
the arms, legs, or feet; palpitations; severe abdominal pain; or unusual weakness.

Interactions
This medicine interacts with several
other drugs such as adrenocorticosteroids, antimuscarinics, calcium-containing medicines; heart medicines such
as digitalis or digoxin; laxatives; other
potassium-containing medicines.
- Be sure to tell your doctor about any
  medications you are currently taking.

Storage
Tablets, elixir, etc. should be stored at
room temperature in tightly closed containers. Store away from heat and direct
light. Keep out of reach of children,
since overdose may be very dangerous
in children. Do not keep outdated
medicine or medicine no longer needed.
Flush the contents of the container
down the toilet, unless otherwise directed.

PRAZEPAM

Properties

This medicine contains as active ingredient prazepam, a benzodiazepine preparation. Benzodiazepines belong to the group of psychoactive medicines that influence the activity of the brain. Some are used to relieve nervousness or tension. It is effective for this purpose for short periods. Others are used for sleeplessness or to relax muscles or relieve muscle spasm. The benzodiazepines may also be used for other conditions as determined by your doctor.

Before using this medicine

Before you use this medicine check with your doctor:
- if you ever had any unusual or allergic reaction to benzodiazepines.
- if you are on a low-salt, low-sugar, or any other special diet, or if you are allergic to any substance, such as sulfites or other preservatives or dyes.
- if you are pregnant or intend to become pregnant while using this medicine. Some benzodiazepines have been reported to increase the chance of birth defects when used during the first 3 months of pregnancy.
- if you are breast-feeding an infant. Benzodiazepines may pass into the breast milk and cause drowsiness, unusually slow heartbeat, shortness of breath, or troubled breathing in infants of mothers taking this medicine.
- if you have any of the following medical problems: asthma, bronchitis, emphysema, or other chronic lung disease; epilepsy or history of convulsions; hyperactivity (in children); kidney or lifer disease; mental depression or illness; myasthania gravis, porphyria.

Treatment

This medication is used to relieve or prevent the symptoms of your medical problem. Benzodiazepines are mainly used as antianxiety agents, anticonvulsants, or sedatives. Take them as directed. Do not take more of them and do not take them more often than recommended on the label, unless otherwise directed by your doctor. Benzodiazepine tranquilizing drugs can be abused if taken for long periods of time and it is possible to develop withdrawal symptoms if you discontinue the therapy abruptly.

Side effects

Along with the needed effects, a medicine may cause some unwanted effects. Minor side effects are: bitter taste in the mouth, dizziness, drowsiness, depression, constipation, dry mouth, excessive salivation, fatigue, flushing, headache, heartburn, loss of appetite, nausea, nervousness, sweating or vomiting. As your body adjusts to the medicine, these side effects should disappear.
- Tell your doctor about any side effects that are persistent or particularly bothersome. It is especially important to tell your doctor about:
  Blurred or double vision
  Chest pain
  Difficulty in urinating
  Fainting or falling
  Fever or hallucinations
  Joint pain
  Mouth sores
  Nightmares
  Palpitations
  Severe depression
  Shortness of breath
  Slurred speech
  Uncoordinated movements
  Unusual tiredness
  Yellowing of the skin

Interactions
- This medicine may interact with several other drugs. This medicine will add to the effects of alcohol, and CNS depressants.
- Be sure to tell your doctor about any medications you are currently taking.

Storage

Store at room temperature in tightly closed, light-resistant-resistant containers. Keep out of the reach of children since overdose may be especially dangerous in children.

PRECEF

Properties
This medicine contains cephalosporin as active ingredient. Cephalosporins belong to the general family of medicines called antibiotics, used in the treatment of infections caused by bacteria. They work by killing bacteria or preventing their growth. Cephalosporins will not work for colds, flu, or other viral infections.

Before using this medicine
Before you use this medicine check with your doctor:
- if you ever had any unusual or allergic reaction to any of the cephalosporins, penicillins, penicillin-like medicines, or penicillamine.
- if you are on a low-salt, low-sugar, or any other special diet, or if you are allergic to any substance, such as sulfites or other preservatives or dyes.
- if you are pregnant or intend to become pregnant while using this medicine. Although cephalosporins have not been shown to cause birth defects or other problems in humans, the chance always exists.
- if you are breast-feeding an infant. Most cephalosporins pass into the breast milk, usually in small amounts.
- if you have any of the following medical problems:
  Bleeding problem
  Kidney or lifer disease

Treatment
This medication belongs to the general family of medicines called antibiotics. It is used to treat a wide variety of bacterial infections. It is also used to treat infections in persons who are allergic to penicillin.
- Keep taking this medicine for the full time of treatment even if you begin to feel better after a few days; do not miss any doses.
- If you do miss a dose of this medicine, take it as soon as possible. This will help to keep a constant amount of medicine in the blood. However, if it is almost time for your next dose, skip the missed dose and go back to your regular dosing schedule.
- This medication has been prescribed for your current infection only. Another infection later on, or one that someone else has, may require a different medicine. You should not give your medicine to other people or use it for other infections, unless your doctor specifically directs you to do so.
- Take the medicine at the same times each day, 1 hour before or 2 hours after eating.

Side effects
Along with the needed effects, a medicine may cause some unwanted effects. Side effects that usually do not require medical attention: rectal itching, oral or vaginal white spots, mild diarrhea. These side effects should disappear as your body adjusts to the medication.
- Other side effects that should be reported to your doctor immediately are:
  Hives, rash
  Intense itching
  Faintness soon after a dose
  Difficulty in breathing
  Nausea and vomiting
  Severe diarrhea
  Unusual weakness or tiredness
  Bleeding or bruising

Interactions
This medicine may interact with several other drugs such as anticoagulants, theophylline preparations, probenecid, tetracyclines, etc.
- Be sure to tell your doctor about any medications you are currently taking.

Storage
Tablets, capsules, etc. should be stored at room temperature. Store the liquid form in the refrigerator. Keep out of the reach of children. Do not keep outdated medicine or medicine no longer needed.

PRELU-2

Properties

This medicine contains phendimetrazine as active ingredient; it is prescribed for appetite suppression.

Appetite suppressants are used in the short-term (a few weeks) treatment of obesity. In a few weeks (6 to 12), these medicines in combination with dieting, exercise, and changes in eating habits can help patients lose weight. However, since their appetite reducing effect is only temporary, they are useful only for the first weeks of dieting until new eating habits are established.

Before using this medicine

Before you use this medicine check with your doctor, or pharmacist:
- if you ever had any unusual or allergic reaction to any of the compounds of this medicine.
- if you are on a low-salt, low-sugar, or any other special diet, or if you are allergic to any substance, such as sulfites or other preservatives or dyes.
- if you are pregnant, intend to become pregnant or breast-feeding an infant while using this medicine.
- if you have any of the following medical problems:
  Diabetes mellitus (sugar diabetes)
  Epilepsy
  Glaucoma
  Heart or blood vessel disease
  High blood pressure
  Mental illness (severe)

Treatment

This medication is used to relieve or prevent the symptoms of your medical problem. Take them as directed. Do not take more of them and do not take them more often than recommended on the label. If too much of the drug is taken, it may become habit-forming.

The medicine produces central nervous system stimulation, and it should not be taken by people with heart disease or high blood pressure.

If you think this medicine is not working as well after you have taken it for a few weeks, do not increase the dose. Instead, check with your doctor.

Side effects

The following minor side effects may occur: irritability, nervousness, restlessness, trouble in sleeping.

These side effects should disappear as your body adjusts to the medication. Tell your doctor about any side effects that are persistent or particularly bothersome. It is especially important to tell your doctor about:
  Mental depression
  Nausea or vomiting
  Stomach cramps or pain
  Trembling
  Unusual tiredness or weakness
- Discontinue use of the drug; call your doctor right away. Adverse reactions and side effects may be more frequent and severe in people over age 60 than in younger persons.

Interactions

This medicine interacts with several other drugs such as antihypertensives, other appetite suppressants, caffeine, central nervous system depressants, central nervous system stimulants, furazolidone, guanethidine, hydralazine, MAO inhibitors, methyldopa, molindone, phenothiazines, rauwolfia alkaloids, sodium bicarbonate.
- Be sure to tell your doctor about any medications you are currently taking.

Interaction with alcoholic beverages may produce drowsiness, sleepiness, and/or inability to concentrate.

Storage

This medicine should be stored at room temperature in tightly closed containers. Store away from heat and direct light. Keep out of reach of children, since overdose may be very dangerous in children.

Do not store this medicine in the bathroom medicine cabinet because the heat and moisture cause the medicine to break down. Do not keep outdated medicine or medicine no longer needed. Flush the contents of the container down the toilet.

PREMARIN

Properties
This medicine contains conjugated estrogens as active ingredients. The medicine is prescribed for treatment of estrogen deficiency; it restores normal estrogen levels in tissues. There is no evidence that this drug is effective for nervous symptoms or depression occurring during menopause. They should not be used to treat this condition; they should be used only to replace the estrogen that is naturally absent after menopause.

Before using this medicine
Before you use this medicine check with your doctor, or pharmacist:
- if you ever had any unusual or allergic reaction to estrogens;
- if you are pregnant or intend to become pregnant within three months;
- if you are breast-feeding an infant;
- if you have any of the following medical problems:
  Diabetes
  Breast cancer
  Fibrocystic breast disease
  Fibroid uterine tumors
  Endometriosis
  Migraine headaches
  Epilepsy
  Porphyria
  High blood pressure
  Asthma
  Congestive heart failure
  Kidney disease
  Gallstones

Treatment
This medication is used to treat estrogen deficiency, specific symptoms of menopause, estrogen-deficiency osteoporosis, atrophic vaginitis, prostate cancer. For safe and effective use of this medicine:
- ◆ Follow your doctor's instructions if this medicine was prescribed.
- ◆ Follow the manufacturer's package directions if you are treating yourself.
- ◆ Estrogens have been reported to increase the risk of endometrial carcinoma.

Side effects
Along with the needed effects, a medicine may cause some unwanted effects. Possible side effects include:
  Stomach cramps
  Profuse bleeding
  Appetite loss
  Nausea and vomiting
  Swollen breasts
  Change in menstruation
  Rash, skin blisters
  Depression
  Dizziness

Overdose
The following symptoms may indicate an overdose:
  Nausea and vomiting
  Fluid retention
  Breast enlargement
  Abnormal vaginal bleeding
- ■ Call a doctor or hospital emergency room for instructions.

Interactions
This medicine may interact with several other drugs such as adrenocorticosteroids, antidepressants, oral antidiabetics, insulin, phenobarbital, primidone.
- ■ Be sure to tell your doctor about any medications you are currently taking.

Storage
Capsules, tablets, vaginal cream, transdermal patches, etc. should be stored at room temperature; store away from heat and direct light. Keep out of reach of children, since this medicine may be dangerous in children.

PREMPHASE

Properties
This medicine contains conjugated estrogens as active ingredients. The medicine is prescribed for treatment of estrogen deficiency; it restores normal estrogen levels in tissues. There is no evidence that this drug is effective for nervous symptoms or depression occurring during menopause. They should not be used to treat this condition; they should be used only to replace the estrogen that is naturally absent after menopause.

Before using this medicine
Before you use this medicine check with your doctor, or pharmacist:
- if you ever had any unusual or allergic reaction to estrogens;
- if you are pregnant or intend to become pregnant within three months;
- if you are breast-feeding an infant;
- if you have any of the following medical problems:
  Diabetes
  Breast cancer
  Fibrocystic breast disease
  Fibroid uterine tumors
  Endometriosis
  Migraine headaches
  Epilepsy
  Porphyria
  High blood pressure
  Asthma
  Congestive heart failure
  Kidney disease
  Gallstones

Treatment
This medication is used to treat estrogen deficiency, specific symptoms of menopause, estrogen-deficiency osteoporosis, atrophic vaginitis, prostate cancer. For safe and effective use of this medicine:
- ◆ Follow your doctor's instructions if this medicine was prescribed.
- ◆ Follow the manufacturer's package directions if you are treating yourself.
- ◆ Estrogens have been reported to increase the risk of endometrial carcinoma.

Side effects
Along with the needed effects, a medicine may cause some unwanted effects. Possible side effects include:
  Stomach cramps
  Profuse bleeding
  Appetite loss
  Nausea and vomiting
  Swollen breasts
  Change in menstruation
  Rash, skin blisters
  Depression
  Dizziness

Overdose
The following symptoms may indicate an overdose:
  Nausea and vomiting
  Fluid retention
  Breast enlargement
  Abnormal vaginal bleeding
- ▪ Call a doctor or hospital emergency room for instructions.

Interactions
This medicine may interact with several other drugs such as adrenocorticosteroids, antidepressants, oral antidiabetics, insulin, phenobarbital, primidone.
- ▪ Be sure to tell your doctor about any medications you are currently taking.

Storage
Capsules, tablets, vaginal cream, transdermal patches, etc. should be stored at room temperature; store away from heat and direct light. Keep out of reach of children, since this medicine may be dangerous in children.

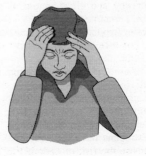

PREVACID

Properties
This medicine contains lansperazole as active ingredient. It is a so-called proton pump inhibitor, a medicine that inhibits the production and secretion of hydrochloric acid from the cells in the mucosal lining of the stomach.

The medicine is prescribed for the short-term treatment of duodenal (intestinal) and gastric (stomach) ulcers. It is also prescribed for gastroesophageal reflex, that is the splashing of stomach acid from the stomach up onto the lower end of the esophagus.

Before using this medicine
Before you use this medicine check with your doctor, or pharmacist:
– if you ever had any unusual or allergic reaction to this medicine or any proton pump inhibitor;
– if you are allergic to any medicines, foods or other substances;
– if you are pregnant or intend to become pregnant while using this medicine (animal studies have shown toxic effects to developing fetuses);
– if you are breast-feeding an infant.

Treatment
This medication is used for treatment of peptic ulcers (duodenal or gastric ulcers), and certain ailments of the esophagus. The usual dose amounts to 20 to 80 milligrams a day. If you forget to take a dose of this medicine, take it as soon as you remember.

The medicine should be taken immediately before a meal or with an antacid if it upsets the stomach.

For safe and effective use of medicine:
♦ Follow your doctor's instructions if this medicine was prescribed.
♦ Follow the manufacturer's package directions if you are treating yourself.

Side effects
Along with the needed effects, a medicine may cause some unwanted effects. Possible side effects include:
  Abdominal pain
  Headache
  Diarrhea
  Nausea
  Sore throat
  Vomiting
  Dizziness
  Constipation
  Back pain
  Urinary infections
  Skin rash
  Heartburn
  Drowsiness
  Unusual bleeding
  Unusual bruising
  Muscle cramps
  Appetite loss

Overdose
The following symptoms may be a sign of overdose:
  Seizures
  Breathing difficulty
  Severe drowsiness
▪ Call a doctor or hospital emergency room for instructions. If necessary, give first aid immediately.

Interactions
The effect of this medicine may be reduced if it is taken together with sucralfate. Taken together with anticoagulants it may increase the effect of the latter.
▪ Be sure to tell your doctor about any medications you are currently taking.

Storage
Delayed-release and extended-release capsules should be stored at room temperature; store away from heat and direct light. Keep out of reach of children, since overdose may be dangerous in children.

PRILOSEC

Properties

This medicine contains omeprazole as active ingredient. It is a so-called proton pump inhibitor, a medicine that inhibits the production and secretion of hydrochloric acid from the cells in the mucosal lining of the stomach.

The medicine is prescribed for the short-term treatment of duodenal (intestinal) and gastric (stomach) ulcers. It is also prescribed for gastroesophageal reflex, that is the splashing of stomach acid from the stomach up onto the lower end of the esophagus.

Before using this medicine

Before you use this medicine check with your doctor, or pharmacist:
- if you ever had any unusual or allergic reaction to this medicine or any proton pump inhibitor;
- if you are allergic to any medicines, foods or other substances;
- if you are pregnant or intend to become pregnant while using this medicine (animal studies have shown toxic effects to developing fetuses);
- if you are breast-feeding an infant.

Treatment

This medication is used for treatment of peptic ulcers (duodenal or gastric ulcers), and certain ailments of the esophagus. The usual dose amounts to 20 to 80 milligrams a day. If you forget to take a dose of this medicine, take it as soon as you remember.

The medicine should be taken immediately before a meal or with an antacid if it upsets the stomach.

For safe and effective use of medicine:
- ◆ Follow your doctor's instructions if this medicine was prescribed.
- ◆ Follow the manufacturer's package directions if you are treating yourself.

Side effects

Along with the needed effects, a medicine may cause some unwanted effects. Possible side effects include:
Abdominal pain
Headache
Diarrhea
Nausea
Sore throat
Vomiting
Dizziness
Constipation
Back pain
Urinary infections
Skin rash
Heartburn
Drowsiness
Unusual bleeding
Unusual bruising
Muscle cramps
Appetite loss

Overdose

The following symptoms may be a sign of overdose:
Seizures
Breathing difficulty
Severe drowsiness
- ■ Call a doctor or hospital emergency room for instructions. If necessary, give first aid immediately.

Interactions

The effect of this medicine may be reduced if it is taken together with sucralfate. Taken together with anticoagulants it may increase the effect of the latter.
- ■ Be sure to tell your doctor about any medications you are currently taking.

Storage

Delayed-release and extended-release capsules should be stored at room temperature; store away from heat and direct light. Keep out of reach of children, since overdose may be dangerous in children.

PROCARDIA

Properties
This medicine contains nefedipine as active ingredient. It is a so-called calcium channel blocker, working by blocking the passage of calcium into heart and smooth muscle. Since calcium is an essential factor in muscle contraction, any medicine that affects calcium in this way will interfere with the contraction of these muscles.

The medicine works by:
◆ reducing the work that the heart must perform;
◆ reducing the normal arterial blood pressure;
◆ increasing oxygen to the heart muscle.

The medicine is prescribed for the treatment of attacks of angina pectoris, irregular heartbeat, and high blood pressure. In many cases it can be used for the treatment and prevention of migraine.

Before using this medicine
Before you use this medicine check with your doctor, or pharmacist:
- if you ever had any unusual or allergic reaction to this medicine or any calcium channel blocker;
- if you are pregnant or intend to become pregnant while using this medicine;
- if you have low blood pressure;
- if you have kidney or lifer disease;
- if you are breast-feeding an infant;
- if you easily get a rash or intensity sunburn in areas exposed to sun or ultraviolet light.

Treatment
This medication is used for treatment of heart conditions (for instance, angina pectoris) and high blood pressure. Tablets, capsules or extended-release tablets should be taken with liquid. The usual dose amounts to 30 to 100 milligrams a day.

For safe and effective use of medicine:
◆ Follow your doctor's instructions if this medicine was prescribed.
◆ Follow the manufacturer's package directions if you are treating yourself.

Side effects
Along with the needed effects, a medicine may cause some unwanted effects. Possible side effects include:
Tiredness
Changes in heartbeat
Wheezing
Cough
Shortness of breath
Dizziness
Fainting
Numbness in hands and feet
Tingling in hands and feet
Difficult urination
Constipation

Overdose
The following symptoms may be a sign of overdose:
Unusually fast heartbeat
Unusually slow heartbeat
Loss of consciousness
Cardiac arrest
■ Call a doctor or hospital emergency room for instructions. If necessary start first aid immediately.

Interactions
The effect of this medicine may cause a blood pressure drop if taken together with antihypertensives. Cimetidine may increase the effect of the calcium blocker.

The simultaneous use of diuretics and calcium channel blockers may cause dangerous blood pressure drop.
■ Be sure to tell your doctor about any medications you are currently taking.

Storage
Capsules, tablets, etc. should be stored at room temperature; store away from heat and direct light. Keep out of reach of children, since this medicine may be dangerous in children.

PROCHLORPERAZINE

Properties

This medicine contains as active ingredient prochlorperazine, a phenothiazine derivative. Phenothiazines are a family of medicines used to treat nervous, mental, and emotional conditions. Some are used to control anxiety, restlessness, nausea and vomiting, and severe hiccups. This medicine is available only with your doctor's prescription.

Before using this medicine

Before you use this medicine check with your doctor, or pharmacist:
- if you ever had any unusual or allergic reaction to phenothiazine medicines.
- if you are on a low-salt, low-sugar, or any other special diet, or if you are allergic to any substance, such as sulfites or other preservatives or dyes.
- if you are pregnant or intend to become pregnant while using this medicine. Although phenothiazines have not been shown to cause birth defects, some side effects such as jaundice and muscle tremors have occurred in a few newborns whose mothers received phenothiazines during pregnancy.
- if you are breast-feeding an infant. Although this medicine has not been shown to cause problems in humans the chance does exist since some phenothiazines are known to pass into the breast milk.
- if you have any of the following medical problems:
Alcoholism
Blood disease
Difficult urination
Enlarged prostate
Glaucoma
Heart or blood vessel disease
Liver or lung disease
Parkinson's disease
Stomach ulcers

Treatment

This medication is prescribed to treat the symptoms of certain types of mental illness or emotional problems. In order to avoid stomach irritation, you can take the tablet or capsule forms of this medication with a meal or with a glass of water or milk (unless your doctor or pharmacist directs you to do otherwise).

Side effects

Along with the needed effects, a medicine may cause some unwanted effects. Minor side effects are: blurred vision, constipation, decreased sweating, diarrhea, dizziness, drooling, drowsiness, dry mouth, fatigue, jitteriness, menstrual irregularities, nasal congestion, restlessness, tremors, vomiting, or weight gain.
- Tell your doctor about any side effects that are persistent or particularly bothersome. It is especially important to tell your doctor about:
Breast enlargement
Chest pain or convulsions
Darkened skin
Difficulty in swallowing
Fainting or fever
Involuntary movements
Palpitations or sleep disorders
Rash or sore throat
Uncoordinated movements
Unusual bleeding or bruising
Visual disturbances
Yellowing of the eyes or skin

Interactions

This medicine may interact with several other drugs such as barbiturates, sleeping pills, narcotics, other tranquilizers, or any other medication that may produce a sedative effect. Avoid alcohol.

Storage

Store this medication as directed on the label. Keep out of the reach of children.

PROKLAR

Properties
This medicine contains sulfamethiazole, a sulfonamide, as active ingredient. Sulfonamides are prescribed to treat infections caused by bacteria. They will not work for colds, flu, or other virus infections.

Before using this medicine
Before you use this medicine check with your doctor:
- if you ever had any unusual or allergic reaction to any of the compounds of the medicine.
- if you are on a low-salt, low-sugar, or any other special diet, or if you are allergic to any substance, such as sulfites or other preservatives or dyes.
- if you are pregnant or intend to become pregnant while using this medicine. Although sulfonamides have not been shown to cause defects in humans, the chance may exists.
- if you are breast-feeding an infant. Most sulfonamides pass into the breast milk in small amounts and may cause unwanted effects in infants with some specific conditions.
- if you have any of the following medical problems:
Kidney disease
Liver disease
Porphyria
Deficiency of enzymes such as G6PD

Treatment
This medication is used to treat an infection caused by bacteria. Most sulfonamides are best taken with a full glass (8 ounces) of water on an empty stomach, either one hour before or two hours after a meal. Follow your doctor's or pharmacist's directions on how to take your medicine.
- Keep taking this medicine for the full time of treatment even if you begin to feel better after a few days; do not miss any doses.
- If you do miss a dose of this medicine, take the missed dose immediately.
- This medication works best when the level of medicine in your bloodstream (and urine) is kept constant. It is best, therefore, to take the doses at evenly spaced intervals day and night. if you take two doses a day, the doses should be spaced 12 hours apart.

Side effects
Along with the needed effects, a medicine may cause some unwanted effects. Side effects that usually do not require medical attention: abdominal pain, diarrhea, dizziness, headache, loss of appetite, nausea, sore mouth, or vomiting. These side effects should disappear as your body adjusts to the medication.

Sulfonamides can increase sensitivity to sunlight. It is, therefore, important to avoid prolonged exposure to sunlight and sunlamps.

Tell your doctor about any side effects that are persistent or particularly bothersome. It is especially important to tell your doctor about:
Bloody urine
Difficult urination
Difficulty in breathing
Difficulty in swallowing
Fever or hallucinations
Itching, rash, or pale skin
Joint pain, lower back pain
Ringing in the ears
Sore throat
Swollen or inflamed tongue
Tingling in hands or feet
Unusual bleeding
Yellowing of the eyes or skin

Interactions
This medicine may interact with several other drugs such as anticoagulants, oral antidiabetic agents, aspirin, some antibiotics, or anticancer drugs.
- Be sure to tell your doctor about any medications you are currently taking.

Storage
Tablets, capsules, suspension, etc. should be stored at room temperature as directed by your pharmacist or according to instructions on the label.

PROLIXIN

Properties
This medicine contains as active ingredient fluphenazine, a phenothiazine derivative. Phenothiazines are a family of medicines used to treat nervous, mental, and emotional conditions. Some are used to control anxiety, restlessness, nausea and vomiting, and severe hiccups. This medicine is available only with your doctor's prescription.

Before using this medicine
Before you use this medicine check with your doctor, or pharmacist:
- if you ever had any unusual or allergic reaction to phenothiazine medicines.
- if you are on a low-salt, low-sugar, or any other special diet, or if you are allergic to any substance, such as sulfites or other preservatives or dyes.
- if you are pregnant or intend to become pregnant while using this medicine. Although phenothiazines have not been shown to cause birth defects, some side effects such as jaundice and muscle tremors have occurred in a few newborns whose mothers received phenothiazines during pregnancy.
- if you are breast-feeding an infant. Although this medicine has not been shown to cause problems in humans the chance does exist since some phenothiazines are known to pass into the breast milk.
- if you have any of the following medical problems:
Alcoholism
Blood disease
Difficult urination
Enlarged prostate
Glaucoma
Heart or blood vessel disease
Liver or lung disease
Parkinson's disease
Stomach ulcers

Treatment
This medication is prescribed to treat the symptoms of certain types of mental illness or emotional problems. In order to avoid stomach irritation, you can take the tablet or capsule forms of this medication with a meal or with a glass of water or milk (unless your doctor or pharmacist directs you to do otherwise).

Side effects
Along with the needed effects, a medicine may cause some unwanted effects. Minor side effects are: blurred vision, constipation, decreased sweating, diarrhea, dizziness, drooling, drowsiness, dry mouth, fatigue, jitteriness, menstrual irregularities, nasal congestion, restlessness, tremors, vomiting, or weight gain.
- Tell your doctor about any side effects that are persistent or particularly bothersome. It is especially important to tell your doctor about:
Breast enlargement
Chest pain or convulsions
Darkened skin
Difficulty in swallowing
Fainting or fever
Involuntary movements
Palpitations or sleep disorders
Rash or sore throat
Uncoordinated movements
Unusual bleeding or bruising
Visual disturbances
Yellowing of the eyes or skin

Interactions
This medicine may interact with several other drugs such as barbiturates, sleeping pills, narcotics, other tranquilizers, or any other medication that may produce a sedative effect. Avoid alcohol.

Storage
Store this medication as directed on the label. Keep out of the reach of children.

PROLIXIN DECANOATE

Properties

This medicine contains as active ingredient fluphenazine, a phenothiazine derivative. Phenothiazines are a family of medicines used to treat nervous, mental, and emotional conditions. Some are used to control anxiety, restlessness, nausea and vomiting, and severe hiccups. This medicine is available only with your doctor's prescription.

Before using this medicine

Before you use this medicine check with your doctor, or pharmacist:
- if you ever had any unusual or allergic reaction to phenothiazine medicines.
- if you are on a low-salt, low-sugar, or any other special diet, or if you are allergic to any substance, such as sulfites or other preservatives or dyes.
- if you are pregnant or intend to become pregnant while using this medicine. Although phenothiazines have not been shown to cause birth defects, some side effects such as jaundice and muscle tremors have occurred in a few newborns whose mothers received phenothiazines during pregnancy.
- if you are breast-feeding an infant. Although this medicine has not been shown to cause problems in humans the chance does exist since some phenothiazines are known to pass into the breast milk.
- if you have any of the following medical problems:
Alcoholism
Blood disease
Difficult urination
Enlarged prostate
Glaucoma
Heart or blood vessel disease
Liver or lung disease
Parkinson's disease
Stomach ulcers

Treatment

This medication is prescribed to treat the symptoms of certain types of mental illness or emotional problems. In order to avoid stomach irritation, you can take the tablet or capsule forms of this medication with a meal or with a glass of water or milk (unless your doctor or pharmacist directs you to do otherwise).

Side effects

Along with the needed effects, a medicine may cause some unwanted effects.

Minor side effects are: blurred vision, constipation, decreased sweating, diarrhea, dizziness, drooling, drowsiness, dry mouth, fatigue, jitteriness, menstrual irregularities, nasal congestion, restlessness, tremors, vomiting, or weight gain.
- Tell your doctor about any side effects that are persistent or particularly bothersome. It is especially important to tell your doctor about:
Breast enlargement
Chest pain or convulsions
Darkened skin
Difficulty in swallowing
Fainting or fever
Involuntary movements
Palpitations or sleep disorders
Rash or sore throat
Uncoordinated movements
Unusual bleeding or bruising
Visual disturbances
Yellowing of the eyes or skin

Interactions

This medicine may interact with several other drugs such as barbiturates, sleeping pills, narcotics, other tranquilizers, or any other medication that may produce a sedative effect. Avoid alcohol.

Storage

Store this medication as directed on the label. Keep out of the reach of children.

PROMAPAR

Properties

This medicine contains as active ingredient chlorpromazine, a phenothiazine derivative. Phenothiazines are a family of medicines used to treat nervous, mental, and emotional conditions. Some are used to control anxiety, restlessness, nausea and vomiting, and severe hiccups. This medicine is available only with your doctor's prescription.

Before using this medicine

Before you use this medicine check with your doctor, or pharmacist:
- if you ever had any unusual or allergic reaction to phenothiazine medicines.
- if you are on a low-salt, low-sugar, or any other special diet, or if you are allergic to any substance, such as sulfites or other preservatives or dyes.
- if you are pregnant or intend to become pregnant while using this medicine. Although phenothiazines have not been shown to cause birth defects, some side effects such as jaundice and muscle tremors have occurred in a few newborns whose mothers received phenothiazines during pregnancy.
- if you are breast-feeding an infant. Although this medicine has not been shown to cause problems in humans the chance does exist since some phenothiazines are known to pass into the breast milk.
- if you have any of the following medical problems:
Alcoholism
Blood disease
Difficult urination
Enlarged prostate
Glaucoma
Heart or blood vessel disease
Liver or lung disease
Parkinson's disease
Stomach ulcers

Treatment

This medication is prescribed to treat the symptoms of certain types of mental illness or emotional problems. In order to avoid stomach irritation, you can take the tablet or capsule forms of this medication with a meal or with a glass of water or milk (unless your doctor or pharmacist directs you to do otherwise).

Side effects

Along with the needed effects, a medicine may cause some unwanted effects.
Minor side effects are: blurred vision, constipation, decreased sweating, diarrhea, dizziness, drooling, drowsiness, dry mouth, fatigue, jitteriness, menstrual irregularities, nasal congestion, restlessness, tremors, vomiting, or weight gain.
- Tell your doctor about any side effects that are persistent or particularly bothersome. It is especially important to tell your doctor about:
Breast enlargement
Chest pain or convulsions
Darkened skin
Difficulty in swallowing
Fainting or fever
Involuntary movements
Palpitations or sleep disorders
Rash or sore throat
Uncoordinated movements
Unusual bleeding or bruising
Visual disturbances
Yellowing of the eyes or skin

Interactions

This medicine may interact with several other drugs such as barbiturates, sleeping pills, narcotics, other tranquilizers, or any other medication that may produce a sedative effect. Avoid alcohol.

Storage

Store this medication as directed on the label. Keep out of the reach of children.

PROMAZ

Properties

This medicine contains as active ingredient chlorpromazine, a phenothiazine derivative. Phenothiazines are a family of medicines used to treat nervous, mental, and emotional conditions. Some are used to control anxiety, restlessness, nausea and vomiting, and severe hiccups. This medicine is available only with your doctor's prescription.

Before using this medicine

Before you use this medicine check with your doctor, or pharmacist:

- if you ever had any unusual or allergic reaction to phenothiazine medicines.
- if you are on a low-salt, low-sugar, or any other special diet, or if you are allergic to any substance, such as sulfites or other preservatives or dyes.
- if you are pregnant or intend to become pregnant while using this medicine. Although phenothiazines have not been shown to cause birth defects, some side effects such as jaundice and muscle tremors have occurred in a few newborns whose mothers received phenothiazines during pregnancy.
- if you are breast-feeding an infant. Although this medicine has not been shown to cause problems in humans the chance does exist since some phenothiazines are known to pass into the breast milk.
- if you have any of the following medical problems:
Alcoholism
Blood disease
Difficult urination
Enlarged prostate
Glaucoma
Heart or blood vessel disease
Liver or lung disease
Parkinson's disease
Stomach ulcers

Treatment

This medication is prescribed to treat the symptoms of certain types of mental illness or emotional problems. In order to avoid stomach irritation, you can take the tablet or capsule forms of this medication with a meal or with a glass of water or milk (unless your doctor or pharmacist directs you to do otherwise).

Side effects

Along with the needed effects, a medicine may cause some unwanted effects. Minor side effects are: blurred vision, constipation, decreased sweating, diarrhea, dizziness, drooling, drowsiness, dry mouth, fatigue, jitteriness, menstrual irregularities, nasal congestion, restlessness, tremors, vomiting, or weight gain.

- Tell your doctor about any side effects that are persistent or particularly bothersome. It is especially important to tell your doctor about:
Breast enlargement
Chest pain or convulsions
Darkened skin
Difficulty in swallowing
Fainting or fever
Involuntary movements
Palpitations or sleep disorders
Rash or sore throat
Uncoordinated movements
Unusual bleeding or bruising
Visual disturbances
Yellowing of the eyes or skin

Interactions

This medicine may interact with several other drugs such as barbiturates, sleeping pills, narcotics, other tranquilizers, or any other medication that may produce a sedative effect. Avoid alcohol.

Storage

Store this medication as directed on the label. Keep out of the reach of children.

PROMAZINE

Properties
This medicine contains as active ingredient promazine, a phenothiazine derivative. Phenothiazines are a family of medicines used to treat nervous, mental, and emotional conditions. Some are used to control anxiety, restlessness, nausea and vomiting, and severe hiccups. This medicine is available only with your doctor's prescription.

Before using this medicine
Before you use this medicine check with your doctor, or pharmacist:
- if you ever had any unusual or allergic reaction to phenothiazine medicines.
- if you are on a low-salt, low-sugar, or any other special diet, or if you are allergic to any substance, such as sulfites or other preservatives or dyes.
- if you are pregnant or intend to become pregnant while using this medicine. Although phenothiazines have not been shown to cause birth defects, some side effects such as jaundice and muscle tremors have occurred in a few newborns whose mothers received phenothiazines during pregnancy.
- if you are breast-feeding an infant. Although this medicine has not been shown to cause problems in humans the chance does exist since some phenothiazines are known to pass into the breast milk.
- if you have any of the following medical problems:
  Alcoholism
  Blood disease
  Difficult urination
  Enlarged prostate
  Glaucoma
  Heart or blood vessel disease
  Liver or lung disease
  Parkinson's disease
  Stomach ulcers

Treatment
This medication is prescribed to treat the symptoms of certain types of mental illness or emotional problems. In order to avoid stomach irritation, you can take the tablet or capsule forms of this medication with a meal or with a glass of water or milk (unless your doctor or pharmacist directs you to do otherwise).

Side effects
Along with the needed effects, a medicine may cause some unwanted effects. Minor side effects are: blurred vision, constipation, decreased sweating, diarrhea, dizziness, drooling, drowsiness, dry mouth, fatigue, jitteriness, menstrual irregularities, nasal congestion, restlessness, tremors, vomiting, or weight gain.
- Tell your doctor about any side effects that are persistent or particularly bothersome. It is especially important to tell your doctor about:
  Breast enlargement
  Chest pain or convulsions
  Darkened skin
  Difficulty in swallowing
  Fainting or fever
  Involuntary movements
  Palpitations or sleep disorders
  Rash or sore throat
  Uncoordinated movements
  Unusual bleeding or bruising
  Visual disturbances
  Yellowing of the eyes or skin

Interactions
This medicine may interact with several other drugs such as barbiturates, sleeping pills, narcotics, other tranquilizers, or any other medication that may produce a sedative effect. Avoid alcohol.

Storage
Store this medication as directed on the label. Keep out of the reach of children.

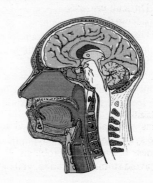

PROTRIN

Properties

This medicine contains sulfamethoxazole, a sulfonamide, and trimethoprim as active ingredients. Sulfonamides are prescribed to treat infections caused by bacteria. They will not work for colds, flu, or other virus infections.

Before using this medicine

Before you use this medicine check with your doctor:
- if you ever had any unusual or allergic reaction to any of the compounds of the medicine.
- if you are on a low-salt, low-sugar, or any other special diet, or if you are allergic to any substance, such as sulfites or other preservatives or dyes.
- if you are pregnant or intend to become pregnant while using this medicine. Although sulfonamides have not been shown to cause defects in humans, the chance may exists.
- if you are breast-feeding an infant. Most sulfonamides pass into the breast milk in small amounts and may cause unwanted effects in infants with some specific conditions.
- if you have any of the following medical problems:
Kidney disease
Liver disease
Porphyria
Deficiency of enzymes such as G6PD

Treatment

This medication is used to treat an infection caused by bacteria. Most sulfonamides are best taken with a full glass (8 ounces) of water on an empty stomach, either one hour before or two hours after a meal. Follow your doctor's or pharmacist's directions on how to take your medicine.
- Keep taking this medicine for the full time of treatment even if you begin to feel better after a few days; do not miss any doses.
- If you do miss a dose of this medicine, take the missed dose immediately.
- This medication works best when the level of medicine in your bloodstream (and urine) is kept constant. It is best, therefore, to take the doses at evenly spaced intervals day and night. if you take two doses a day, the doses should be spaced 12 hours apart.

Side effects

Along with the needed effects, a medicine may cause some unwanted effects. Side effects that usually do not require medical attention: abdominal pain, diarrhea, dizziness, headache, loss of appetite, nausea, sore mouth, or vomiting. These side effects should disappear as your body adjusts to the medication.

Sulfonamides can increase sensitivity to sunlight. It is, therefore, important to avoid prolonged exposure to sunlight and sunlamps.

Tell your doctor about any side effects that are persistent or particularly bothersome. It is especially important to tell your doctor about:
Bloody urine
Difficult urination
Difficulty in breathing
Difficulty in swallowing
Fever or hallucinations
Itching, rash, or pale skin
Joint pain, lower back pain
Ringing in the ears
Sore throat
Swollen or inflamed tongue
Tingling in hands or feet
Unusual bleeding
Yellowing of the eyes or skin

Interactions

This medicine may interact with several other drugs such as anticoagulants, oral antidiabetic agents, aspirin, some antibiotics, or anticancer drugs.
- Be sure to tell your doctor about any medications you are currently taking.

Storage

Tablets, capsules, suspension, etc. should be stored at room temperature as directed by your pharmacist or according to instructions on the label.

PROTRIPTYINE

Properties

This medicine contains protriptyline as active ingredient. It belongs to the group of medicines known as tricyclic antidepressants or 'mood elevators.' It is used to relieve mental depression and depression that sometimes occurs with anxiety. The medication gradually relieves, but doesn't cure, symptoms of depression. The medication may also be used for the treatment of narcolepsy, bulimia, painic attacks, cocaine withdrawal, attention deficit disorder.

Before using this medicine

Before you use this medicine check with your doctor, or pharmacist:
- if you ever had any unusual or allergic reaction to any tricyclic antidepressant, maprotiline or trazodone.
- if you are on a low-salt, low-sugar, or any other special diet, or if you are allergic to any substance, such as sulfites or other preservatives or dyes.
- if you are pregnant or intend to become pregnant while using this medicine. There have been reports of newborns suffering from heart, breathing, and urinary problems when their mothers had taken tricyclic antidepressants before delivery.
- if you are breast-feeding an infant. Some tricyclic antidepressants pass into the breast milk.

Treatment

Take this medicine only as directed by your doctor, to benefit your condition as much as possible. Do not take more of it, do not take it more often, and do not take it for a longer period of time than your doctor ordered.

To lessen stomach upset, take this medicine with food, even for a daily bedtime dose, unless your doctor has told you to take it on an empty stomach. If you forget your once-a-day bedtime dose, Do not take it more than 3 hours late. If more than 3 hours, wait for next scheduled dose;.

Sometimes this medicine must be taken for several weeks before you begin to feel better.

Side effects

Along with the needed effects, a medicine may cause some unwanted effects. Side effects that usually do not require medical attention: difficult or frequent urination; decreased sex drive; muscle aches; abnormal dreams; nasal congestion; weakness and faintness when arising from bed or chair; back pain.
- Other side effects that should be reported to your doctor immediately are:
Hallucinations
Shakiness
Dizziness or fainting
Blurred vision, eye pain
Irregular heartbeat or slow pulse
Inflamed tongue
Abdominal pain
Jaundice
Hair loss, rash
Fever, chills
Joint pain
Palpitations

Interactions

This medicine may interact with several other drugs such as anticoagulants, anticholinergics, cold remedies, oral contraceptives, seizure medicines, sleeping medicines, thyroid medicines, etc.
- Be sure to tell your doctor about any medications you are currently taking.

Storage

Tablets, capsules, etc. should be stored at room temperature in tightly closed, light-resistant containers as directed by your pharmacist. Keep out of reach of children since overdose is especially dangerous in young children. Do not store in the bathroom medicine cabinet because the heat or moisture may cause the medicine to break down. Keep the liquid form of the medicine from freezing.

PROZAC

Properties
This medicine contains fluoxethine as active ingredient. It is an antidepressant drug that has a specific effect on certain areas of the brain. The medicine is known to affect serotonin, one of the chemicals in the brain called neuro-transmitters or chemical messengers, that play a role in the steering of psychoactive behavior. The medicine is effective in treating common symptoms of depression. It can also help to improve mood and mental alertness.

Before using this medicine
Before you use this medicine check with your doctor, or pharmacist:
- if you ever had any unusual or allergic reaction to this medicine or any psychoactive drug;
- if you are allergic to any medicines, foods or other substances;
- if you are pregnant or intend to become pregnant while using this medicine (animal studies have shown toxic effects to developing fetuses);
- if you are breast-feeding an infant.

Treatment
This medication is used for treatment of certain types of mental depression, mood changes, obsessive-compulsive disorders, bulimia and obesity.

Capsules should be swallowed with liquid or food to lessen stomach irritation. If you forget to take a dose of this medicine, take it as soon as you remember up to two hours late. If more than two hours, wait for the next scheduled dose;.

For safe and effective use of medicine:
◆ Follow your doctor's instructions if this medicine was prescribed.
◆ Follow the manufacturer's package directions if you are treating yourself.

Side effects
Along with the needed effects, a medicine may cause some unwanted effects. Possible side effects include:
Rash, itchy skin
Headache
Nervousness
Increased sweating
Nausea
Insomnia
Anxiety
Joint pain
Muscle pain
Blurred vision
Nightmares
Sensory changes
Decreased sex drive
Dry mouth
Changes in heartbeat
Flushing
Tremors

Overdose
The following symptoms may be a sign of overdose:
Seizures
Agitation
Violent vomiting
■ Call a doctor or hospital emergency room for instructions. If necessary, give first aid immediately.

Interactions
The effect of this medicine may be increased by other antidepressants. Lithium, may increase the occurrence of side effects. Anticoagulants may cause an increase in anticoagulation. Alcohol will sometimes augment the depression.
■ Be sure to tell your doctor about any medications you are currently taking.

Storage
Liquid and tablets should be stored at room temperature; store away from heat and direct light. Keep out of reach of children, since this medicine may be dangerous in children.

PROZINE

Properties

This medicine contains as active ingredient promazine, a phenothiazine derivative. Phenothiazines are a family of medicines used to treat nervous, mental, and emotional conditions. Some are used to control anxiety, restlessness, nausea and vomiting, and severe hiccups. This medicine is available only with your doctor's prescription.

Before using this medicine

Before you use this medicine check with your doctor, or pharmacist:
- if you ever had any unusual or allergic reaction to phenothiazine medicines.
- if you are on a low-salt, low-sugar, or any other special diet, or if you are allergic to any substance, such as sulfites or other preservatives or dyes.
- if you are pregnant or intend to become pregnant while using this medicine. Although phenothiazines have not been shown to cause birth defects, some side effects such as jaundice and muscle tremors have occurred in a few newborns whose mothers received phenothiazines during pregnancy.
- if you are breast-feeding an infant. Although this medicine has not been shown to cause problems in humans the chance does exist since some phenothiazines are known to pass into the breast milk.
- if you have any of the following medical problems:
  Alcoholism
  Blood disease
  Difficult urination
  Enlarged prostate
  Glaucoma
  Heart or blood vessel disease
  Liver or lung disease
  Parkinson's disease
  Stomach ulcers

Treatment

This medication is prescribed to treat the symptoms of certain types of mental illness or emotional problems. In order to avoid stomach irritation, you can take the tablet or capsule forms of this medication with a meal or with a glass of water or milk (unless your doctor or pharmacist directs you to do otherwise).

Side effects

Along with the needed effects, a medicine may cause some unwanted effects. Minor side effects are: blurred vision, constipation, decreased sweating, diarrhea, dizziness, drooling, drowsiness, dry mouth, fatigue, jitteriness, menstrual irregularities, nasal congestion, restlessness, tremors, vomiting, or weight gain.
- Tell your doctor about any side effects that are persistent or particularly bothersome. It is especially important to tell your doctor about:
  Breast enlargement
  Chest pain or convulsions
  Darkened skin
  Difficulty in swallowing
  Fainting or fever
  Involuntary movements
  Palpitations or sleep disorders
  Rash or sore throat
  Uncoordinated movements
  Unusual bleeding or bruising
  Visual disturbances
  Yellowing of the eyes or skin

Interactions

This medicine may interact with several other drugs such as barbiturates, sleeping pills, narcotics, other tranquilizers, or any other medication that may produce a sedative effect. Avoid alcohol.

Storage

Store this medication as directed on the label. Keep out of the reach of children.

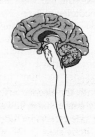

PULMOPHYLLINE

Properties

This medicine contains theophylline as active ingredient; it is used to treat or prevent breathing problems (wheezing and shortness of breath) caused by asthma, bronchitis, or emphysema. This medication belongs to a group known as xanthine-derivative bronchodilators. They work by opening up the bronchial tubes or air passages of the lungs and increasing the flow of air through them. These medicines are available only with your doctor's prescription.

Before using this medicine

Before you use this medicine check with your doctor, or pharmacist:
- if you ever had any unusual or allergic reaction to xanthine-derivative bronchodilators.
- if you are on a low-salt, low-sugar, or any other special diet, or if you are allergic to any substance, such as sulfites or other preservatives or dyes.
- if you are pregnant or intend to become pregnant while using this medicine.
- if you are breast-feeding an infant. Theophylline passes into the breast milk and may cause irritability, fretfulness, or trouble in sleeping in infants of mothers taking this medicine.
- if you have any of the following medical problems:
Diarrhea
Enlarged prostate
Fibrocystic breast disease
Heart disease
Stomach ulcer

Treatment

This medication is used to relieve or prevent the symptoms of your medical problem. Take them as directed. Do not take more of them and do not take them more often than recommended on the label, unless otherwise directed by your doctor. To do so may increase the chance of side effects. The medicine should be taken on an empty stomach 30 to 60 minutes before a meal or two hours after a meal. Try not to miss any doses of this medication. If you do miss a dose, take the missed dose as soon as possible, unless it is almost time for the next dose. Do not double the next dose. It works best when taken with a glass of water.

Side effects

The following minor side effects may occur:
    Dizziness Or Flushing
    Headache
    Diarrhea
    Heartburn
    Increased Urination
    Insomnia
    Nervousness Or Irritability
    Loss Of Appetite
    Nausea Or Stomach Upset
    Stomach Pain.
These side effects should disappear as your body adjusts to the medication. Tell your doctor about any side effects that are persistent or particularly bothersome. It is especially important to tell your doctor about black, tarry stools; confusion; convulsions; difficulty in breathing; fainting; muscle twitching; palpitations; rash; severe abdominal pain; or unusual weakness.

Interactions

This medicine interacts with several other drugs such as diuretics, reserpine, beta blockers, phenytoin, lithium, phenobarbital, birth control pills, and other medications.
- Be sure to tell your doctor about any medications you are currently taking.

Storage

Tablets, capsules, liquid and suspension should be stored at room temperature in tightly closed containers. Store away from heat and direct light. Keep out of reach of children, since overdose may be very dangerous in children. Discard any outdated medication.

QUIBRON-T

Properties
This medicine contains theophylline as active ingredient; it is used to treat or prevent breathing problems (wheezing and shortness of breath) caused by asthma, bronchitis, or emphysema. This medication belongs to a group known as xanthine-derivative bronchodilators. They work by opening up the bronchial tubes or air passages of the lungs and increasing the flow of air through them. These medicines are available only with your doctor's prescription.

Before using this medicine
Before you use this medicine check with your doctor, or pharmacist:
- if you ever had any unusual or allergic reaction to xanthine-derivative bronchodilators.
- if you are on a low-salt, low-sugar, or any other special diet, or if you are allergic to any substance, such as sulfites or other preservatives or dyes.
- if you are pregnant or intend to become pregnant while using this medicine.
- if you are breast-feeding an infant. Theophylline passes into the breast milk and may cause irritability, fretfulness, or trouble in sleeping in infants of mothers taking this medicine.
- if you have any of the following medical problems:
Diarrhea
Enlarged prostate
Fibrocystic breast disease
Heart disease
Stomach ulcer

Treatment
This medication is used to relieve or prevent the symptoms of your medical problem. Take them as directed. Do not take more of them and do not take them more often than recommended on the label, unless otherwise directed by your doctor. To do so may increase the chance of side effects. The medicine should be taken on an empty stomach 30 to 60 minutes before a meal or two hours after a meal. Try not to miss any doses of this medication. If you do miss a dose, take the missed dose as soon as possible, unless it is almost time for the next dose. Do not double the next dose. It works best when taken with a glass of water.

Side effects
The following minor side effects may occur:
Dizziness Or Flushing
Headache
Diarrhea
Heartburn
Increased Urination
Insomnia
Nervousness Or Irritability
Loss Of Appetite
Nausea Or Stomach Upset
Stomach Pain.
These side effects should disappear as your body adjusts to the medication. Tell your doctor about any side effects that are persistent or particularly bothersome. It is especially important to tell your doctor about black, tarry stools; confusion; convulsions; difficulty in breathing; fainting; muscle twitching; palpitations; rash; severe abdominal pain; or unusual weakness.

Interactions
This medicine interacts with several other drugs such as diuretics, reserpine, beta blockers, phenytoin, lithium, phenobarbital, birth control pills, and other medications.
- Be sure to tell your doctor about any medications you are currently taking.

Storage
Tablets, capsules, liquid and suspension should be stored at room temperature in tightly closed containers. Store away from heat and direct light. Keep out of reach of children, since overdose may be very dangerous in children. Discard any outdated medication.

QUINESTROL

Properties
This medicine contains quinestrol as active ingredient. The medicine is prescribed for treatment of estrogen deficiency; it restores normal estrogen levels in tissues. There is no evidence that this drug is effective for nervous symptoms or depression occurring during menopause. They should not be used to treat this condition; they should be used only to replace the estrogen that is naturally absent after menopause.

Before using this medicine
Before you use this medicine check with your doctor, or pharmacist:
- if you ever had any unusual or allergic reaction to estrogens;
- if you are pregnant or intend to become pregnant within three months;
- if you are breast-feeding an infant;
- if you have any of the following medical problems:
  Diabetes
  Breast cancer
  Fibrocystic breast disease
  Fibroid uterine tumors
  Endometriosis
  Migraine headaches
  Epilepsy
  Porphyria
  High blood pressure
  Asthma
  Congestive heart failure
  Kidney disease
  Gallstones

Treatment
This medication is used to treat estrogen deficiency, specific symptoms of menopause, estrogen-deficiency osteoporosis, atrophic vaginitis, prostate cancer.

For safe and effective use of this medicine:
- ◆ Follow your doctor's instructions if this medicine was prescribed.
- ◆ Follow the manufacturer's package directions if you are treating yourself.
- ◆ Estrogens have been reported to increase the risk of endometrial carcinoma.

Side effects
Along with the needed effects, a medicine may cause some unwanted effects. Possible side effects include:
  Stomach cramps
  Profuse bleeding
  Appetite loss
  Nausea and vomiting
  Swollen breasts
  Change in menstruation
  Rash, skin blisters
  Depression
  Dizziness

Overdose
The following symptoms may indicate an overdose:
  Nausea and vomiting
  Fluid retention
  Breast enlargement
  Abnormal vaginal bleeding
- ■ Call a doctor or hospital emergency room for instructions.

Interactions
This medicine may interact with several other drugs such as adrenocorticosteroids, antidepressants, oral antidiabetics, insulin, phenobarbital, primidone.
- ■ Be sure to tell your doctor about any medications you are currently taking.

Storage
Capsules, tablets, vaginal cream, transdermal patches, etc. should be stored at room temperature; store away from heat and direct light. Keep out of reach of children, since this medicine may be dangerous in children.

REGIBON

Properties
This medicine contains diethylpropion active ingredient; it is prescribed for appetite suppression.

Appetite suppressants are used in the short-term (a few weeks) treatment of obesity. In a few weeks (6 to 12), these medicines in combination with dieting, exercise, and changes in eating habits can help patients lose weight. However, since their appetite reducing effect is only temporary, they are useful only for the first weeks of dieting until new eating habits are established.

Before using this medicine
Before you use this medicine check with your doctor, or pharmacist:
- if you ever had any unusual or allergic reaction to any of the compounds of this medicine.
- if you are on a low-salt, low-sugar, or any other special diet, or if you are allergic to any substance, such as sulfites or other preservatives or dyes.
- if you are pregnant, intend to become pregnant or breast-feeding an infant while using this medicine.
- if you have any of the following medical problems:
  Diabetes mellitus
  Epilepsy
  Glaucoma
  Heart disease
  High blood pressure
  Mental illness (severe)

Treatment
This medication is used to relieve or prevent the symptoms of your medical problem.

Take them as directed. Do not take more of them and do not take them more often than recommended on the label. If too much of the drug is taken, it may become habit-forming.
- The medicine produces central nervous system stimulation, and it should not be taken by people with heart disease or high blood pressure.
- If you think this medicine is not working as well after you have taken it for a few weeks, do not increase the dose. Instead, check with your doctor.

Side effects
The following minor side effects may occur: irritability, nervousness, restlessness, trouble in sleeping.

These side effects should disappear as your body adjusts to the medication. Tell your doctor about any side effects that are persistent or particularly bothersome. It is especially important to tell your doctor about:
  Mental depression
  Nausea or vomiting
  Stomach cramps or pain
  Trembling
  Unusual tiredness
- Discontinue use of the drug; call your doctor right away. Adverse reactions and side effects may be more frequent and severe in people over age 60 than in younger persons.

Interactions
This medicine interacts with several other drugs such as antihypertensives, other appetite suppressants, caffeine, central nervous system depressants, central nervous system stimulants, furazolidone, guanethidine, hydralazine, MAO inhibitors, methyldopa, molindone, phenothiazines, rauwolfia alkaloids, sodium bicarbonate. Interaction with alcoholic beverages may produce drowsiness, sleepiness, and/or inability to concentrate.
- Be sure to tell your doctor about any medications you are currently taking.

Storage
This medicine should be stored at room temperature in tightly closed containers. Store away from heat and direct light. Keep out of reach of children, since overdose may be very dangerous in children.

Do not store this medicine in the bathroom medicine cabinet because the heat and moisture cause the medicine to break down. Do not keep outdated medicine or medicine no longer needed. Flush the contents of the container down the toilet.

RENEDIL

Properties
This medicine contains felodipine as active ingredient. It is a so-called calcium channel blocker, working by blocking the passage of calcium into heart and smooth muscle. Since calcium is an essential factor in muscle contraction, any medicine that affects calcium in this way will interfere with the contraction of these muscles.

The medicine works by:
- reducing the work that the heart must perform;
- reducing the normal arterial blood pressure;
- increasing oxygen to the heart muscle.

The medicine is prescribed for the treatment of attacks of angina pectoris, irregular heartbeat, and high blood pressure. In many cases it can be used for the treatment and prevention of migraine.

Before using this medicine
Before you use this medicine check with your doctor, or pharmacist:
- if you ever had any unusual or allergic reaction to this medicine or any calcium channel blocker;
- if you are pregnant or intend to become pregnant while using this medicine;
- if you have low blood pressure;
- if you have kidney or lifer disease;
- if you are breast-feeding an infant;
- if you easily get a rash or intensity sunburn in areas exposed to sun or ultraviolet light.

Treatment
This medication is used for treatment of heart conditions (for instance, angina pectoris) and high blood pressure. Tablets, capsules or extended-release tablets should be taken with liquid. The usual dose amounts to 30 to 100 milligrams a day.

For safe and effective use of medicine:
- Follow your doctor's instructions if this medicine was prescribed.
- Follow the manufacturer's package directions if you are treating yourself.

Side effects
Along with the needed effects, a medicine may cause some unwanted effects. Possible side effects include:
Tiredness
Changes in heartbeat
Wheezing
Cough
Shortness of breath
Dizziness
Fainting
Numbness in hands and feet
Tingling in hands and feet
Difficult urination
Constipation

Overdose
The following symptoms may be a sign of overdose:
Unusually fast heartbeat
Unusually slow heartbeat
Loss of consciousness
Cardiac arrest
- Call a doctor or hospital emergency room for instructions. If necessary start first aid immediately.

Interactions
The effect of this medicine may cause a blood pressure drop if taken together with antihypertensives. Cimetidine may increase the effect of the calcium blocker.

The simultaneous use of diuretics and calcium channel blockers may cause dangerous blood pressure drop.
- Be sure to tell your doctor about any medications you are currently taking.

Storage
Capsules, tablets, etc. should be stored at room temperature; store away from heat and direct light. Keep out of reach of children, since this medicine may be dangerous in children.

RENOQUID

Properties
This medicine contains sulfacytine, a sulfonamide, as active ingredient. Sulfonamides are prescribed to treat infections caused by bacteria. They will not work for colds, flu, or other virus infections.

Before using this medicine
Before you use this medicine check with your doctor:
- if you ever had any unusual or allergic reaction to any of the compounds of the medicine.
- if you are on a low-salt, low-sugar, or any other special diet, or if you are allergic to any substance, such as sulfites or other preservatives or dyes.
- if you are pregnant or intend to become pregnant while using this medicine. Although sulfonamides have not been shown to cause defects in humans, the chance may exists.
- if you are breast-feeding an infant. Most sulfonamides pass into the breast milk in small amounts and may cause unwanted effects in infants with some specific conditions.
- if you have any of the following medical problems:
Kidney disease
Liver disease
Porphyria
Deficiency of enzymes such as G6PD

Treatment
This medication is used to treat an infection caused by bacteria. Most sulfonamides are best taken with a full glass (8 ounces) of water on an empty stomach, either one hour before or two hours after a meal. Follow your doctor's or pharmacist's directions on how to take your medicine.
- Keep taking this medicine for the full time of treatment even if you begin to feel better after a few days; do not miss any doses.
- If you do miss a dose of this medicine, take the missed dose immediately.
- This medication works best when the level of medicine in your bloodstream (and urine) is kept constant. It is best, therefore, to take the doses at evenly spaced intervals day and night. if you take two doses a day, the doses should be spaced 12 hours apart.

Side effects
Along with the needed effects, a medicine may cause some unwanted effects. Side effects that usually do not require medical attention: abdominal pain, diarrhea, dizziness, headache, loss of appetite, nausea, sore mouth, or vomiting. These side effects should disappear as your body adjusts to the medication.

Sulfonamides can increase sensitivity to sunlight. It is, therefore, important to avoid prolonged exposure to sunlight and sunlamps.

Tell your doctor about any side effects that are persistent or particularly bothersome. It is especially important to tell your doctor about:
Bloody urine
Difficult or painful urination
Difficulty in breathing
Difficulty in swallowing
Fever or hallucinations
Itching, rash, or pale skin
Joint pain, lower back pain
Ringing in the ears
Sore throat
Swollen or inflamed tongue
Tingling in hands or feet
Unusual bleeding, bruising
Yellowing of the eyes or skin

Interactions
This medicine may interact with several other drugs such as anticoagulants, oral antidiabetic agents, aspirin, some antibiotics, or anticancer drugs.
- Be sure to tell your doctor about any medications you are currently taking.

Storage
Tablets, capsules, suspension, etc. should be stored at room temperature as directed by your pharmacist or according to instructions on the label.

RESPBID

Properties

This medicine contains theophylline as active ingredient; it is used to treat or prevent breathing problems (wheezing and shortness of breath) caused by asthma, bronchitis, or emphysema. This medication belongs to a group known as xanthine-derivative bronchodilators. They work by opening up the bronchial tubes or air passages of the lungs and increasing the flow of air through them. These medicines are available only with your doctor's prescription.

Before using this medicine

Before you use this medicine check with your doctor, or pharmacist:
- if you ever had any unusual or allergic reaction to xanthine-derivative bronchodilators.
- if you are on a low-salt, low-sugar, or any other special diet, or if you are allergic to any substance, such as sulfites or other preservatives or dyes.
- if you are pregnant or intend to become pregnant while using this medicine.
- if you are breast-feeding an infant. Theophylline passes into the breast milk and may cause irritability, fretfulness, or trouble in sleeping in infants of mothers taking this medicine.
- if you have any of the following medical problems:
  Diarrhea
  Enlarged prostate
  Fibrocystic breast disease
  Heart disease
  Stomach ulcer

Treatment

This medication is used to relieve or prevent the symptoms of your medical problem. Take them as directed. Do not take more of them and do not take them more often than recommended on the label, unless otherwise directed by your doctor. To do so may increase the chance of side effects. The medicine should be taken on an empty stomach 30 to 60 minutes before a meal or two hours after a meal. Try not to miss any doses of this medication. If you do miss a dose, take the missed dose as soon as possible, unless it is almost time for the next dose. Do not double the next dose. It works best when taken with a glass of water.

Side effects

The following minor side effects may occur:
  Dizziness Or Flushing
  Headache
  Diarrhea
  Heartburn
  Increased Urination
  Insomnia
  Nervousness Or Irritability
  Loss Of Appetite
  Nausea Or Stomach Upset
  Stomach Pain.

These side effects should disappear as your body adjusts to the medication. Tell your doctor about any side effects that are persistent or particularly bothersome. It is especially important to tell your doctor about black, tarry stools; confusion; convulsions; difficulty in breathing; fainting; muscle twitching; palpitations; rash; severe abdominal pain; or unusual weakness.

Interactions

This medicine interacts with several other drugs such as diuretics, reserpine, beta blockers, phenytoin, lithium, phenobarbital, birth control pills, and other medications.
- Be sure to tell your doctor about any medications you are currently taking.

Storage

Tablets, capsules, liquid and suspension should be stored at room temperature in tightly closed containers. Store away from heat and direct light. Keep out of reach of children, since overdose may be very dangerous in children. Discard any outdated medication.

RESTORIL

Properties

This medicine contains as active ingredient temazepam, a benzodiazepine preparation. Benzodiazepines belong to the group of psychoactive medicines that influence the activity of the brain. Some are used to relieve nervousness or tension. It is effective for this purpose for short periods. Others are used for sleeplessness or to relax muscles or relieve muscle spasm. The benzodiazepines may also be used for other conditions as determined by your doctor.

Before using this medicine

Before you use this medicine check with your doctor:
- if you ever had any unusual or allergic reaction to benzodiazepines.
- if you are on a low-salt, low-sugar, or any other special diet, or if you are allergic to any substance, such as sulfites or other preservatives or dyes.
- if you are pregnant or intend to become pregnant while using this medicine. Some benzodiazepines have been reported to increase the chance of birth defects when used during the first 3 months of pregnancy.
- if you are breast-feeding an infant. Benzodiazepines may pass into the breast milk and cause drowsiness, unusually slow heartbeat, shortness of breath, or troubled breathing in infants of mothers taking this medicine.
- if you have any of the following medical problems: asthma, bronchitis, emphysema, or other chronic lung disease; epilepsy or history of convulsions; hyperactivity (in children); kidney or lifer disease; mental depression or illness; myasthania gravis, porphyria.

Treatment

This medication is used to relieve or prevent the symptoms of your medical problem. Benzodiazepines are mainly used as antianxiety agents, anticonvulsants, or sedatives. Take them as directed. Do not take more of them and do not take them more often than recommended on the label, unless otherwise directed by your doctor. Benzodiazepine tranquilizing drugs can be abused if taken for long periods of time and it is possible to develop withdrawal symptoms if you discontinue the therapy abruptly.

Side effects

Along with the needed effects, a medicine may cause some unwanted effects. Minor side effects are: bitter taste in the mouth, dizziness, drowsiness, depression, constipation, dry mouth, excessive salivation, fatigue, flushing, headache, heartburn, loss of appetite, nausea, nervousness, sweating or vomiting. As your body adjusts to the medicine, these side effects should disappear.
- Tell your doctor about any side effects that are persistent or particularly bothersome. It is especially important to tell your doctor about:
  Blurred or double vision
  Chest pain
  Difficulty in urinating
  Fainting or falling
  Fever or hallucinations
  Joint pain
  Mouth sores
  Nightmares
  Palpitations
  Severe depression
  Shortness of breath
  Slurred speech
  Uncoordinated movements
  Unusual tiredness
  Yellowing of the skin

Interactions

This medicine may interact with several other drugs. This medicine will add to the effects of alcohol, and CNS depressants.
- Be sure to tell your doctor about any medications you are currently taking.

Storage

Store at room temperature in tightly closed, light-resistant-resistant containers. Keep out of the reach of children since overdose may be especially dangerous in children.

RISPERAL

Properties
This medicine contains risperidone as active ingredient. It is an antipsychotic drug, belonging to the class of psychoactive medicines, that has a specific effect on certain neurotransmitters, the chemical messengers in the brain.

Before using this medicine
Before you use this medicine check with your doctor, or pharmacist:
- if you ever had any unusual or allergic reaction to this medicine or any psychoactive drug;
- if you are pregnant or intend to become pregnant while using this medicine;
- if you are breast-feeding an infant;
- if you have lifer or kidney disease;
- if you have a heart problem;
- if you have a history of seizures (convulsions, epilepsy).

Treatment
This medication is used for treatment of severe mental, nervous and emotional conditions. The drug is known to help the management of signs and symptoms of schizophrenia and schizoid-like mental disorders.

If you forget to take a dose of this medicine, take it as soon as you remember. The tablets should be swallowed with liquid. The oral solution should be diluted in 3 to 4 ounces of liquid (water or orange juice).

Do not discontinue the use of this drug without consulting your doctor. Dosage may require a gradual reduction before stopping.

For safe and effective use of medicine:
◆ Follow your doctor's instructions if this medicine was prescribed.
◆ Follow the manufacturer's package directions if you are treating yourself.

Side effects
Along with the needed effects, a medicine may cause some unwanted effects. Possible side effects include:
Drowsiness
Anxiety
High fever
Rapid heartbeat
Tremor
Profuse sweating
Confusion
Irritability
Dizziness
Constipation
Difficulty urinating
Involuntary movements
Digestive problems
Rash
Sexual dysfunction

Overdose
The following symptoms may be a sign of overdose:
Extreme drowsiness
Rapid heartbeat
Faintness
Convulsions
Difficulty in breathing
Excessive sweating
Call a doctor or hospital emergency room for instructions. If necessary start first aid immediately.

Interactions
The effect of this medicine may be reduced if it is taken together with carbamazepine. It may increase the effect of antihypertensives. Taken together with central nervous system depressants it may increase the sedative effect.
■ Be sure to tell your doctor about any medications you are currently taking.

Storage
Tablets and oral solution should be stored at room temperature; store away from heat and direct light. Keep out of reach of children, since this medicine may be dangerous in children.

RMS UNISERTS

Properties
This medicine contains as active ingredient morphine.

It is a narcotic analgesic that acts directly on the central nervous system (brain and spinal cord). It is used to relieve pain or to suppress coughing.

Before using this medicine
Before you use this medicine check with your doctor, or pharmacist:
- if you ever had any unusual or allergic reaction to this medicine or one of its components.
- if you are on a low-salt, low-sugar, or any other special diet, or if you are allergic to any substance, such as sulfites or other preservatives or dyes.
- if you are pregnant or intend to become pregnant while using this medicine. Studies on birth defects have not been done in humans. Too much use of narcotics during pregnancy may cause the baby to become dependent on the medicine.
- if you are breast-feeding an infant. Although this medicine has not been shown to cause problems in humans, it passes into the breast milk in small amounts.
- if you have any of the following medical problems:
  Brain disease or head injury
  Colitis
  Convulsions
  Emphysema, asthma, or chronic lung disease
  Enlarged prostate
  Gallbladder disease or gallstones
  Heart disease
  Kidney or lifer disease
  Underactive thyroid

Treatment
This medication is used to relieve pain or to suppress coughing. Narcotic analgesics act in the central nervous system; some of their side effects are also caused by actions in the central nervous system.
- If you are taking this medication on a regular schedule and you miss a dose, take the missed dose as soon as possible, unless it is almost time for your next dose. In that case do not take the missed dose at all.
- If a narcotic analgesic is used for a long time, it may become habit-forming (causing mental or physical dependence). Physical dependence may lead to withdrawal side effects when you stop taking this medicine.

Unless otherwise directed by your doctor or pharmacist take this as directed. Do not take more of them and do not take them more often than recommended on the label. Children up to 12 years of age should not take this medicine more than 3 times a day or for more than 5 days in a row.

Side effects
Along with the needed effects, a medicine may cause some unwanted effects. These side effects may go away during treatment as your body adjusts to the medicine. Such minor side effects are: constipation, dizziness, drowsiness, dry mouth, false sense of well-being, flushing, light-headedness, loss of appetite, nausea, painful or difficult urination, or sweating.
- Check with your doctor immediately if any of the following side effects occur:
  Anxiety or breathing difficulties
  Excitation or restlessness
  Fatigue, palpitations
  Rash, sore throat and fever
  Tremors or weakness

Interactions
This medicine may interact with several other drugs such as medicines acting on the central nervous system (e.g., antidepressants, tranquilizers), cimetidine, nitrates, quinidine, etc.
- Be sure to tell your doctor about any medications you are currently taking.

Storage
Tablets, elixir, suppository etc. should be stored at room temperature in a tightly closed, light-resistant container.

RO-CEF

Properties

This medicine contains cephalosporin as active ingredient. Cephalosporins belong to the general family of medicines called antibiotics, used in the treatment of infections caused by bacteria. They work by killing bacteria or preventing their growth. Cephalosporins will not work for colds, flu, or other viral infections.

Before using this medicine

Before you use this medicine check with your doctor:
- if you ever had any unusual or allergic reaction to any of the cephalosporins, penicillins, penicillin-like medicines, or penicillamine.
- if you are on a low-salt, low-sugar, or any other special diet, or if you are allergic to any substance, such as sulfites or other preservatives or dyes.
- if you are pregnant or intend to become pregnant while using this medicine. Although cephalosporins have not been shown to cause birth defects or other problems in humans, the chance always exists.
- if you are breast-feeding an infant. Most cephalosporins pass into the breast milk, usually in small amounts.
- if you have any of the following medical problems:
  Bleeding problem
  Kidney or lifer disease

Treatment

This medication belongs to the general family of medicines called antibiotics. It is used to treat a wide variety of bacterial infections. It is also used to treat infections in persons who are allergic to penicillin.
- Keep taking this medicine for the full time of treatment even if you begin to feel better after a few days; do not miss any doses.
- If you do miss a dose of this medicine, take it as soon as possible. This will help to keep a constant amount of medicine in the blood. However, if it is almost time for your next dose,

skip the missed dose and go back to your regular dosing schedule.
- This medication has been prescribed for your current infection only. Another infection later on, or one that someone else has, may require a different medicine. You should not give your medicine to other people or use it for other infections, unless your doctor specifically directs you to do so.
- Take the medicine at the same times each day, 1 hour before or 2 hours after eating.

Side effects

Along with the needed effects, a medicine may cause some unwanted effects. Side effects that usually do not require medical attention: rectal itching, oral or vaginal white spots, mild diarrhea. These side effects should disappear as your body adjusts to the medication.
- Other side effects that should be reported to your doctor immediately are:
  Hives, rash
  Intense itching
  Faintness soon after a dose
  Difficulty in breathing
  Nausea and vomiting
  Severe diarrhea
  Unusual weakness or tiredness
  Bleeding or bruising

Interactions

This medicine may interact with several other drugs such as anticoagulants, theophylline preparations, probenecid, tetracyclines, etc.
- Be sure to tell your doctor about any medications you are currently taking.

Storage

Tablets, capsules, etc. should be stored at room temperature. Store the liquid form in the refrigerator. Keep out of the reach of children. Do not keep outdated medicine or medicine no longer needed.

ROBICILLIN VK

Properties

This medicine contains penicillin V as active ingredient. Penicillins are prescribed to treat infections caused by bacteria. They will not work for colds, flu, or other virus infections. There are several different kinds of penicillins. Each is used to treat different kinds of infections.

Before using this medicine

Before you use this medicine check with your doctor, or pharmacist:

- if you ever had any unusual or allergic reaction to any of the penicillins, cefalosporins, griseofulvin, or penicillamine. Serious reactions may occur in patients who are allergic to penicillins.
- if you are on a low-salt, low-sugar, or any other special diet, or if you are allergic to any substance, such as sulfites or other preservatives or dyes.
- if you are pregnant or intend to become pregnant while using this medicine. Although penicillins have not been shown to cause problems in humans, the chance always exists.
- if you are breast-feeding an infant. Most penicillins (except amdinocillin) pass into the breast milk. Even though only small amounts may pass, allergic reaction, diarrhea, fungal infection, and skin rash may occur in the infant.
- if you have any of the following medical problems:
  Allergy
  Asthma
  Bleeding problems
  Eczema
  Hay fever, hives
  Kidney disease
  Liver disease
  Mononucleosis
  Stomach or intestinal disease

Treatment

This medication is used to treat an infection caused by bacteria. Most penicillins are best taken with a full glass (8 ounces) of water on an empty stomach, some are best taken with a snack or meal. Follow your doctor's or pharmacist's directions on how to take your medicine.

- ◆ Keep taking this medicine for the full time of treatment even if you begin to feel better after a few days; do not miss any doses. This is especially important if you have a "strep" infection since serious heart problems could develop later if your infection is not cleared up completely.
- ◆ If you do miss a dose of this medicine, take it as soon as possible. However, if it is almost time for your next dose, skip the missed dose and go back to your regular dosing schedule.

Side effects

Along with the needed effects, a medicine may cause some unwanted effects. Side effects that usually do not require medical attention: diarrhea; nausea or vomiting; sore mouth or tongue.

- ◆ Stop taking this medicine and get emergency help immediately if you notice: difficulty in breathing; lightheadedness; skin rash, hives, itching; wheezing.

Other side effects that should be reported to your doctor immediately are: abdominal bloating; blood in urine; convulsions (seizures); decreased amount of urine; diarrhea (watery and severe) which may also be bloody; fever; joint pain; sore throat and fever; stomach or abdominal cramps and pain; unusual bleeding or bruising.

Interactions

This medicine may interact with several other drugs such as anticoagulants, diarrhea medicines, heparin, ibuprofen, oral contraceptives, potassium-containing medicines, etc.

- ■ Be sure to tell your doctor about any medications you are currently taking.

Storage

Tablets, capsules, etc. should be stored as directed by your pharmacist or according to instructions on the label.

ROBIDONE

Properties

This medicine contains as active ingredient hydrocodone.

It is a narcotic analgesic that acts directly on the central nervous system (brain and spinal cord). It is used to relieve pain or to suppress coughing.

Before using this medicine

Before you use this medicine check with your doctor, or pharmacist:

- if you ever had any unusual or allergic reaction to this medicine or one of its components.
- if you are on a low-salt, low-sugar, or any other special diet, or if you are allergic to any substance, such as sulfites or other preservatives or dyes.
- if you are pregnant or intend to become pregnant while using this medicine. Studies on birth defects have not been done in humans. Too much use of narcotics during pregnancy may cause the baby to become dependent on the medicine.
- if you are breast-feeding an infant. Although this medicine has not been shown to cause problems in humans, it passes into the breast milk in small amounts.
- if you have any of the following medical problems:
  Brain disease or head injury
  Colitis
  Convulsions
  Emphysema, asthma, or chronic lung disease
  Enlarged prostate
  Gallbladder disease or gallstones
  Heart disease
  Kidney or lifer disease
  Underactive thyroid

Treatment

This medication is used to relieve pain or to suppress coughing. Narcotic analgesics act in the central nervous system; some of their side effects are also caused by actions in the central nervous system.

- If you are taking this medication on a regular schedule and you miss a dose, take the missed dose as soon as possible, unless it is almost time for your next dose. In that case do not take the missed dose at all.
- If a narcotic analgesic is used for a long time, it may become habit-forming (causing mental or physical dependence). Physical dependence may lead to withdrawal side effects when you stop taking this medicine.

Unless otherwise directed by your doctor or pharmacist take this as directed. Do not take more of them and do not take them more often than recommended on the label. Children up to 12 years of age should not take this medicine more than 3 times a day or for more than 5 days in a row.

Side effects

Along with the needed effects, a medicine may cause some unwanted effects. These side effects may go away during treatment as your body adjusts to the medicine. Such minor side effects are: constipation, dizziness, drowsiness, dry mouth, false sense of well-being, flushing, light-headedness, loss of appetite, nausea, painful or difficult urination, or sweating.

- Check with your doctor immediately if any of the following side effects occur:
  Anxiety or breathing difficulties
  Excitation or restlessness
  Fatigue, palpitations
  Rash, sore throat and fever
  Tremors or weakness

Interactions

This medicine may interact with several other drugs such as medicines acting on the central nervous system (e.g., antidepressants, tranquilizers), cimetidine, nitrates, quinidine, etc.

- Be sure to tell your doctor about any medications you are currently taking.

Storage

Tablets, elixir, suppository etc. should be stored at room temperature in a tightly closed, light-resistant container.

ROBIMYCIN

Properties
This medicine contains erythromycin as active ingredient. This antibiotic is prescribed to treat infections caused by bacteria. They will not work for colds, flu, or other virus infections. Erythromycins are available only with your doctor's prescription.

Before using this medicine
Before you use this medicine check with your doctor, or pharmacist:
– if you ever had any unusual or allergic reaction to any of the erythromycins.
– if you are on a low-salt, low-sugar, or any other special diet, or if you are allergic to any substance, such as sulfites or other preservatives or dyes.
– if you are pregnant or intend to become pregnant while using this medicine. Although erythromycins have not been shown to cause birth defects or other problems in humans, the chance always exists.
– if you are breast-feeding an infant. Most erythromycins pass into the breast milk. Although erythromycins have not been shown to cause problems in humans, the chance always exists.
– if you have lifer disease.

Treatment
This medication belongs to the general family of medicines called antibiotics. It is used to treat a wide variety of bacterial infections. It is also used to treat infections in persons who are allergic to penicillin. Erythromycins are also used to prevent "strep" infections in patients with a history of rheumatic heart disease. They may also be used in Legionnaires' disease and for other problems as determined by your doctor.
■ Keep taking this medicine for the full time of treatment even if you begin to feel better after a few days; do not miss any doses. This is especially important if you have a "strep" infection since serious heart problems could develop later if your infection is not cleared up completely.

■ If you do miss a dose of this medicine, take it as soon as possible. This will help to keep a constant amount of medicine in the blood. However, if it is almost time for your next dose, skip the missed dose and go back to your regular dosing schedule.
■ This medication has been prescribed for your current infection only. Another infection later on, or one that someone else has, may require a different medicine. You should not give your medicine to other people or use it for other infections, unless your doctor specifically directs you to do so.

Side effects
Along with the needed effects, a medicine may cause some unwanted effects. Side effects that usually do not require medical attention: abdominal cramps, black tongue, cough, diarrhea, fatigue, irritation of the mouth, loss of appetite, nausea, or vomiting. These side effects should disappear as your body adjusts to the medication.
■ Other side effects that should be reported to your doctor immediately are:
Fever
Hearing loss
Hives or rash
Rectal or vaginal itching
Yellowing of the eyes or skin

Interactions
This medicine may interact with several other drugs such as anticoagulants, theophylline preparations, carbamazepine, etc.
■ Be sure to tell your doctor about any medications you are currently taking.

Storage
Tablets, capsules, etc. should be stored at room temperature in tightly closed, light-resistant containers as directed by your pharmacist.

ROCEPHIN

Properties

This medicine contains cephalosporin as active ingredient. Cephalosporins belong to the general family of medicines called antibiotics, used in the treatment of infections caused by bacteria. They work by killing bacteria or preventing their growth. Cephalosporins will not work for colds, flu, or other viral infections.

Before using this medicine

Before you use this medicine check with your doctor:
- if you ever had any unusual or allergic reaction to any of the cephalosporins, penicillins, penicillin-like medicines, or penicillamine.
- if you are on a low-salt, low-sugar, or any other special diet, or if you are allergic to any substance, such as sulfites or other preservatives or dyes.
- if you are pregnant or intend to become pregnant while using this medicine. Although cephalosporins have not been shown to cause birth defects or other problems in humans, the chance always exists.
- if you are breast-feeding an infant. Most cephalosporins pass into the breast milk, usually in small amounts.
- if you have any of the following medical problems:
  Bleeding problem
  Kidney or lifer disease

Treatment

This medication belongs to the general family of medicines called antibiotics. It is used to treat a wide variety of bacterial infections. It is also used to treat infections in persons who are allergic to penicillin.
- Keep taking this medicine for the full time of treatment even if you begin to feel better after a few days; do not miss any doses.
- If you do miss a dose of this medicine, take it as soon as possible. This will help to keep a constant amount of medicine in the blood. However, if it is almost time for your next dose, skip the missed dose and go back to your regular dosing schedule.
- This medication has been prescribed for your current infection only. Another infection later on, or one that someone else has, may require a different medicine. You should not give your medicine to other people or use it for other infections, unless your doctor specifically directs you to do so.
- Take the medicine at the same times each day, 1 hour before or 2 hours after eating.

Side effects

Along with the needed effects, a medicine may cause some unwanted effects. Side effects that usually do not require medical attention: rectal itching, oral or vaginal white spots, mild diarrhea. These side effects should disappear as your body adjusts to the medication.
- Other side effects that should be reported to your doctor immediately are:
  Hives, rash
  Intense itching
  Faintness soon after a dose
  Difficulty in breathing
  Nausea and vomiting
  Severe diarrhea
  Unusual weakness or tiredness
  Bleeding or bruising

Interactions

This medicine may interact with several other drugs such as anticoagulants, theophylline preparations, probenecid, tetracyclines, etc.
- Be sure to tell your doctor about any medications you are currently taking.

Storage

Tablets, capsules, etc. should be stored at room temperature. Store the liquid form in the refrigerator. Keep out of the reach of children. Do not keep outdated medicine or medicine no longer needed.

ROUBAC

Properties

This medicine contains sulfamethoxazole, a sulfonamide, and trimethoprim as active ingredients. Sulfonamides are prescribed to treat infections caused by bacteria. They will not work for colds, flu, or other virus infections.

Before using this medicine

Before you use this medicine check with your doctor:
- if you ever had any unusual or allergic reaction to any of the compounds of the medicine.
- if you are on a low-salt, low-sugar, or any other special diet, or if you are allergic to any substance, such as sulfites or other preservatives or dyes.
- if you are pregnant or intend to become pregnant while using this medicine. Although sulfonamides have not been shown to cause defects in humans, the chance may exists.
- if you are breast-feeding an infant. Most sulfonamides pass into the breast milk in small amounts and may cause unwanted effects in infants with some specific conditions.
- if you have any of the following medical problems:
Kidney disease
Liver disease
Porphyria
Deficiency of enzymes such as G6PD

Treatment

This medication is used to treat an infection caused by bacteria. Most sulfonamides are best taken with a full glass (8 ounces) of water on an empty stomach, either one hour before or two hours after a meal. Follow your doctor's or pharmacist's directions on how to take your medicine.
- Keep taking this medicine for the full time of treatment even if you begin to feel better after a few days; do not miss any doses.
- If you do miss a dose of this medicine, take the missed dose immediately.
- This medication works best when the level of medicine in your bloodstream (and urine) is kept constant. It is best, therefore, to take the doses at evenly spaced intervals day and night. if you take two doses a day, the doses should be spaced 12 hours apart.

Side effects

Along with the needed effects, a medicine may cause some unwanted effects. Side effects that usually do not require medical attention: abdominal pain, diarrhea, dizziness, headache, loss of appetite, nausea, sore mouth, or vomiting. These side effects should disappear as your body adjusts to the medication.
Sulfonamides can increase sensitivity to sunlight. It is, therefore, important to avoid prolonged exposure to sunlight and sunlamps.

Tell your doctor about any side effects that are persistent or particularly bothersome. It is especially important to tell your doctor about:
Bloody urine
Difficult urination
Difficulty in breathing
Difficulty in swallowing
Fever or hallucinations
Itching, rash, or pale skin
Joint pain, lower back pain
Ringing in the ears
Sore throat
Swollen or inflamed tongue
Tingling in hands or feet
Unusual bleeding
Yellowing of the eyes or skin

Interactions

This medicine may interact with several other drugs such as anticoagulants, oral antidiabetic agents, aspirin, some antibiotics, or anticancer drugs.
- Be sure to tell your doctor about any medications you are currently taking.

Storage

Tablets, capsules, suspension, etc. should be stored at room temperature as directed by your pharmacist or according to instructions on the label.

ROXANOL

Properties
This medicine contains as active ingredient morphine.
It is a narcotic analgesic that acts directly on the central nervous system (brain and spinal cord). It is used to relieve pain or to suppress coughing.

Before using this medicine
Before you use this medicine check with your doctor, or pharmacist:
- if you ever had any unusual or allergic reaction to this medicine or one of its components.
- if you are on a low-salt, low-sugar, or any other special diet, or if you are allergic to any substance, such as sulfites or other preservatives or dyes.
- if you are pregnant or intend to become pregnant while using this medicine. Studies on birth defects have not been done in humans. Too much use of narcotics during pregnancy may cause the baby to become dependent on the medicine.
- if you are breast-feeding an infant. Although this medicine has not been shown to cause problems in humans, it passes into the breast milk in small amounts.
- if you have any of the following medical problems:
Brain disease or head injury
Colitis
Convulsions
Emphysema, asthma, or chronic lung disease
Enlarged prostate
Gallbladder disease or gallstones
Heart disease
Kidney or lifer disease
Underactive thyroid

Treatment
This medication is used to relieve pain or to suppress coughing. Narcotic analgesics act in the central nervous system; some of their side effects are also caused by actions in the central nervous system.
- If you are taking this medication on a regular schedule and you miss a dose, take the missed dose as soon as possible, unless it is almost time for your next dose. In that case do not take the missed dose at all.
- If a narcotic analgesic is used for a long time, it may become habit-forming (causing mental or physical dependence). Physical dependence may lead to withdrawal side effects when you stop taking this medicine.

Unless otherwise directed by your doctor or pharmacist take this as directed. Do not take more of them and do not take them more often than recommended on the label. Children up to 12 years of age should not take this medicine more than 3 times a day or for more than 5 days in a row.

Side effects
Along with the needed effects, a medicine may cause some unwanted effects. These side effects may go away during treatment as your body adjusts to the medicine. Such minor side effects are: constipation, dizziness, drowsiness, dry mouth, false sense of well-being, flushing, light-headedness, loss of appetite, nausea, painful or difficult urination, or sweating.
- Check with your doctor immediately if any of the following side effects occur:
Anxiety or breathing difficulties
Excitation or restlessness
Fatigue, palpitations
Rash, sore throat and fever
Tremors or weakness

Interactions
This medicine may interact with several other drugs such as medicines acting on the central nervous system (e.g., antidepressants, tranquilizers), cimetidine, nitrates, quinidine, etc.
- Be sure to tell your doctor about any medications you are currently taking.

Storage
Tablets, elixir, suppository etc. should be stored at room temperature in a tightly closed, light-resistant container.

RP-MYCIN

Properties
This medicine contains erythromycin as active ingredient. This antibiotic is prescribed to treat infections caused by bacteria. They will not work for colds, flu, or other virus infections. Erythromycins are available only with your doctor's prescription.

Before using this medicine
Before you use this medicine check with your doctor, or pharmacist:
- if you ever had any unusual or allergic reaction to any of the erythromycins.
- if you are on a low-salt, low-sugar, or any other special diet, or if you are allergic to any substance, such as sulfites or other preservatives or dyes.
- if you are pregnant or intend to become pregnant while using this medicine. Although erythromycins have not been shown to cause birth defects or other problems in humans, the chance always exists.
- if you are breast-feeding an infant. Most erythromycins pass into the breast milk. Although erythromycins have not been shown to cause problems in humans, the chance always exists.
- if you have lifer disease.

Treatment
This medication belongs to the general family of medicines called antibiotics. It is used to treat a wide variety of bacterial infections. It is also used to treat infections in persons who are allergic to penicillin. Erythromycins are also used to prevent "strep" infections in patients with a history of rheumatic heart disease. They may also be used in Legionnaires' disease and for other problems as determined by your doctor.
- Keep taking this medicine for the full time of treatment even if you begin to feel better after a few days; do not miss any doses. This is especially important if you have a "strep" infection since serious heart problems could develop later if your infection is not cleared up completely.
- If you do miss a dose of this medicine, take it as soon as possible. This will help to keep a constant amount of medicine in the blood. However, if it is almost time for your next dose, skip the missed dose and go back to your regular dosing schedule.
- This medication has been prescribed for your current infection only. Another infection later on, or one that someone else has, may require a different medicine. You should not give your medicine to other people or use it for other infections, unless your doctor specifically directs you to do so.

Side effects
Along with the needed effects, a medicine may cause some unwanted effects. Side effects that usually do not require medical attention: abdominal cramps, black tongue, cough, diarrhea, fatigue, irritation of the mouth, loss of appetite, nausea, or vomiting. These side effects should disappear as your body adjusts to the medication.
- Other side effects that should be reported to your doctor immediately are:
Fever
Hearing loss
Hives or rash
Rectal or vaginal itching
Yellowing of the eyes or skin

Interactions
This medicine may interact with several other drugs such as anticoagulants, theophylline preparations, carbamazepine, etc.
- Be sure to tell your doctor about any medications you are currently taking.

Storage
Tablets, capsules, etc. should be stored at room temperature in tightly closed, light-resistant containers as directed by your pharmacist.

RUM-K

Properties

This medicine contains potassium chloride as active ingredient; it is used to treat or prevent potassium deficiency, especially potassium deficiency that is caused by the use of diuretics (water pills).

Potassium is needed to maintain good health. Potassium supplements may be needed by patients who do not have enough potassium in their regular diet and by those who have lost too much potassium because of illness or treatment with certain medicines.

Since too much potassium may also cause health problems, most potassium supplements are available only with your doctor's prescription.

Before using this medicine

Before you use this medicine check with your doctor, or pharmacist:

- if you ever had any unusual or allergic reaction to potassium preparations;
- if you are on a low-salt, low-sugar, or any other special diet, or if you are allergic to any substance, such as sulfites or other preservatives or dyes.
- if you are pregnant or intend to become pregnant while using this medicine. Although potassium supplements have not been shown to cause problems in humans, the chance always exists.
- if you are breast-feeding an infant. Although this medicine has not been shown to cause problems in humans, the chance always exists since small amounts of potassium pass into the breast milk.
- if you have any of the following medical problems:
  Addison's disease
  Heart disease
  Diarrhea
  Kidney disease
  Stomach ulcer

Treatment

This medication is used to relieve or prevent the symptoms of your medical problem. Take them as directed. Do not take more of them and do not take them more often than recommended on the label, unless otherwise directed by your doctor. To do so may increase the chance of side effects.

In order to avoid stomach irritation, you should take potassium supplements with food or immediately after a meal. If you miss a dose of this medication, take the missed dose as soon as possible, unless it is within two hours of the next scheduled dose;.

Side effects

The following minor side effects may occur:
  Diarrhea
  Nausea
  Stomach pains
  Vomiting.

These side effects should disappear as your body adjusts to the medication. Tell your doctor about any side effects that are persistent or particularly bothersome. It is especially important to tell your doctor about anxiety; bloody or black, tarry stools; confusion; difficulty in breathing; numbness or tingling in the arms, legs, or feet; palpitations; severe abdominal pain; or unusual weakness.

Interactions

This medicine interacts with several other drugs such as adrenocorticosteroids, antimuscarinics, calcium-containing medicines; heart medicines such as digitalis or digoxin; laxatives; other potassium-containing medicines.

- Be sure to tell your doctor about any medications you are currently taking.

Storage

Tablets, elixir, etc. should be stored at room temperature in tightly closed containers. Store away from heat and direct light. Keep out of reach of children, since overdose may be very dangerous in children. Do not keep outdated medicine or medicine no longer needed. Flush the contents of the container down the toilet, unless otherwise directed.

SANOREX

Properties

This medicine contains mazindol as active ingredient; it is prescribed for appetite suppression.

Appetite suppressants are used in the short-term (a few weeks) treatment of obesity. In a few weeks (6 to 12), these medicines in combination with dieting, exercise, and changes in eating habits can help patients lose weight. However, since their appetite reducing effect is only temporary, they are useful only for the first weeks of dieting until new eating habits are established.

Before using this medicine

Before you use this medicine check with your doctor, or pharmacist:
- if you ever had any unusual or allergic reaction to any of the compounds of this medicine.
- if you are on a low-salt, low-sugar, or any other special diet, or if you are allergic to any substance, such as sulfites or other preservatives or dyes.
- if you are pregnant, intend to become pregnant or breast-feeding an infant while using this medicine.
- if you have any of the following medical problems:
  Diabetes mellitus
  Epilepsy
  Glaucoma
  Heart disease
  High blood pressure
  Mental illness (severe)

Treatment

This medication is used to relieve or prevent the symptoms of your medical problem.

Take them as directed. Do not take more of them and do not take them more often than recommended on the label. If too much of the drug is taken, it may become habit-forming.
- The medicine produces central nervous system stimulation, and it should not be taken by people with heart disease or high blood pressure.
- If you think this medicine is not working as well after you have taken it for a few weeks, do not increase the dose. Instead, check with your doctor.

Side effects

The following minor side effects may occur: irritability, nervousness, restlessness, trouble in sleeping.

These side effects should disappear as your body adjusts to the medication. Tell your doctor about any side effects that are persistent or particularly bothersome. It is especially important to tell your doctor about:
  Mental depression
  Nausea or vomiting
  Stomach cramps or pain
  Trembling
  Unusual tiredness
- Discontinue use of the drug; call your doctor right away. Adverse reactions and side effects may be more frequent and severe in people over age 60 than in younger persons.

Interactions

This medicine interacts with several other drugs such as antihypertensives, other appetite suppressants, caffeine, central nervous system depressants, central nervous system stimulants, furazolidone, guanethidine, hydralazine, MAO inhibitors, methyldopa, molindone, phenothiazines, rauwolfia alkaloids, sodium bicarbonate. Interaction with alcoholic beverages may produce drowsiness, sleepiness, and/or inability to concentrate.
- Be sure to tell your doctor about any medications you are currently taking.

Storage

This medicine should be stored at room temperature in tightly closed containers. Store away from heat and direct light. Keep out of reach of children, since overdose may be very dangerous in children. Do not store this medicine in the bathroom medicine cabinet because the heat and moisture cause the medicine to break down. Do not keep outdated medicine or medicine no longer needed. Flush the contents of the container down the toilet.

SARISOL NO.2

Properties
This medicine contains as active ingredient the barbiturate butabarbital. Barbiturates belong to the group of medicines called central nervous system depressants (medicines that slow down the nervous system).

Barbiturates may partially block nerve impulses at nerve-cell connections. They may be used to treat insomnia (sleeplessness) by helping patients fall asleep. Also, they may be used to relieve anxiety or tension. Some of the barbiturates are used as anticonvulsants to help control convulsions in certain disorders or diseases, such as epilepsy. If too much of the drug is used, it may become habit-forming (causing mental or physical dependence).

Before using this medicine
Before you use this medicine check with your doctor, or pharmacist:
- if you ever had any unusual or allergic reaction to this medicine or one of its components.
- if you are on a low-salt, low-sugar, or any other special diet, or if you are allergic to preservatives or dyes.
- if you are pregnant or intend to become pregnant while using this medicine, since barbiturates have been shown to increase the chance of birth defects in humans. Taking barbiturates regularly during the last 3 months of pregnancy may cause the baby to become dependent on the medicine. This may lead to withdrawal side effects in the baby after birth.
- if you have any of the following medical problems:
Anemia (severe)
Diabetes mellitus (sugar disease)
Hyperactivity (in children)
Kidney or lifer disease
Mental depression
Overactive thyroid

Treatment
This medication is used to treat the symptoms of your medical condition. Barbiturates act in the central nervous system; some of their side effects are also caused by actions in the central nervous system. Use this medicine as directed by your doctor. Do not use more of it, do not use it more often, and do not use it for a longer period of time than your doctor ordered.
- If you are taking this medication on a regular schedule and you miss a dose, take the missed dose as soon as possible, unless it is almost time for your next dose. In that case do not take the missed dose at all.
- If a barbiturate is used for a long time, it may become habit-forming. Physical dependence may lead to withdrawal side effects when you stop taking this medicine.

Side effects
Along with the needed effects, a medicine may cause some unwanted effects. These side effects may go away during treatment as your body adjusts to the medicine. Such minor side effects are: depression, confusion, diarrhea, nausea, vomiting, joint or muscle pain, slurred speech, hallucinations, headache, decreased sex drive.
- Check with your doctor immediately if any of the following side effects occur:
Rash or hives
Face, lip or eyelid swelling
Sore throat, fever
Agitation
Slow heartbeat
Difficult breathing or chest pain

Interactions
This medicine may interact with several other drugs such as medicines acting on the central nervous system (e.g., antihistamines; beta-adrenergic blockers; MAO inhibitors; mind-altering drugs; nabilone; antidepressants; clozapine; anticonvulsants).

Storage
The medicine should be stored at room temperature in a tightly closed, light-resistant container. Keep out of reach of children since overdose is very dangerous in children.

SECOBARBITAL

Properties
This medicine contains as active ingredient the barbiturate secobarbital. Barbiturates belong to the group of medicines called central nervous system depressants (medicines that slow down the nervous system).

Barbiturates may partially block nerve impulses at nerve-cell connections. They may be used to treat insomnia (sleeplessness) by helping patients fall asleep. Also, they may be used to relieve anxiety or tension. Some of the barbiturates are used as anticonvulsants to help control convulsions in certain disorders or diseases, such as epilepsy. If too much of the drug is used, it may become habit-forming (causing mental or physical dependence).

Before using this medicine
Before you use this medicine check with your doctor, or pharmacist:
- if you ever had any unusual or allergic reaction to this medicine or one of its components.
- if you are on a low-salt, low-sugar, or any other special diet, or if you are allergic to preservatives or dyes.
- if you are pregnant or intend to become pregnant while using this medicine, since barbiturates have been shown to increase the chance of birth defects in humans. Taking barbiturates regularly during the last 3 months of pregnancy may cause the baby to become dependent on the medicine. This may lead to withdrawal side effects in the baby after birth.
- if you have any of the following medical problems:
Anemia (severe)
Diabetes mellitus (sugar disease)
Hyperactivity (in children)
Kidney or lifer disease
Mental depression
Overactive thyroid

Treatment
This medication is used to treat the symptoms of your medical condition. Barbiturates act in the central nervous system; some of their side effects are also caused by actions in the central nervous system. Use this medicine as directed by your doctor. Do not use more of it, do not use it more often, and do not use it for a longer period of time than your doctor ordered.
- If you are taking this medication on a regular schedule and you miss a dose, take the missed dose as soon as possible, unless it is almost time for your next dose. In that case do not take the missed dose at all.
- If a barbiturate is used for a long time, it may become habit-forming. Physical dependence may lead to withdrawal side effects when you stop taking this medicine.

Side effects
Along with the needed effects, a medicine may cause some unwanted effects. These side effects may go away during treatment as your body adjusts to the medicine. Such minor side effects are: depression, confusion, diarrhea, nausea, vomiting, joint or muscle pain, slurred speech, hallucinations, headache, decreased sex drive.
- Check with your doctor immediately if any of the following side effects occur:
Rash or hives
Face, lip or eyelid swelling
Sore throat, fever
Agitation
Slow heartbeat
Difficult breathing or chest pain

Interactions
This medicine may interact with several other drugs such as medicines acting on the central nervous system (e.g., antihistamines; beta-adrenergic blockers; MAO inhibitors; mind-altering drugs; nabilone; antidepressants; clozapine; anticonvulsants).

Storage
The medicine should be stored at room temperature in a tightly closed, light-resistant container. Keep out of reach of children since overdose is very dangerous in children.

SECONAL

Properties

This medicine contains as active ingredient the barbiturate secobarbital. Barbiturates belong to the group of medicines called central nervous system depressants (medicines that slow down the nervous system).

Barbiturates may partially block nerve impulses at nerve-cell connections. They may be used to treat insomnia (sleeplessness) by helping patients fall asleep. Also, they may be used to relieve anxiety or tension. Some of the barbiturates are used as anticonvulsants to help control convulsions in certain disorders or diseases, such as epilepsy. If too much of the drug is used, it may become habit-forming (causing mental or physical dependence).

Before using this medicine

Before you use this medicine check with your doctor, or pharmacist:
- if you ever had any unusual or allergic reaction to this medicine or one of its components.
- if you are on a low-salt, low-sugar, or any other special diet, or if you are allergic to preservatives or dyes.
- if you are pregnant or intend to become pregnant while using this medicine, since barbiturates have been shown to increase the chance of birth defects in humans. Taking barbiturates regularly during the last 3 months of pregnancy may cause the baby to become dependent on the medicine. This may lead to withdrawal side effects in the baby after birth.
- if you have any of the following medical problems:
  Anemia (severe)
  Diabetes mellitus (sugar disease)
  Hyperactivity (in children)
  Kidney or lifer disease
  Mental depression
  Overactive thyroid

Treatment

This medication is used to treat the symptoms of your medical condition. Barbiturates act in the central nervous system; some of their side effects are also caused by actions in the central nervous system. Use this medicine as directed by your doctor. Do not use more of it, do not use it more often, and do not use it for a longer period of time than your doctor ordered.
- If you are taking this medication on a regular schedule and you miss a dose, take the missed dose as soon as possible, unless it is almost time for your next dose. In that case do not take the missed dose at all.
- If a barbiturate is used for a long time, it may become habit-forming. Physical dependence may lead to withdrawal side effects when you stop taking this medicine.

Side effects

Along with the needed effects, a medicine may cause some unwanted effects. These side effects may go away during treatment as your body adjusts to the medicine. Such minor side effects are: depression, confusion, diarrhea, nausea, vomiting, joint or muscle pain, slurred speech, hallucinations, headache, decreased sex drive.
- Check with your doctor immediately if any of the following side effects occur:
  Rash or hives
  Face, lip or eyelid swelling
  Sore throat, fever
  Agitation
  Slow heartbeat
  Difficult breathing or chest pain

Interactions

This medicine may interact with several other drugs such as medicines acting on the central nervous system (e.g., antihistamines; beta-adrenergic blockers; MAO inhibitors; mind-altering drugs; nabilone; antidepressants; clozapine; anticonvulsants).

Storage

The medicine should be stored at room temperature in a tightly closed, light-resistant container. Keep out of reach of children since overdose is very dangerous in children.

SEDAPAP

Properties

This medicine contains as active ingredient the barbiturate secobarbital. Barbiturates belong to the group of medicines called central nervous system depressants (medicines that slow down the nervous system).

Barbiturates may partially block nerve impulses at nerve-cell connections. They may be used to treat insomnia (sleeplessness) by helping patients fall asleep. Also, they may be used to relieve anxiety or tension. Some of the barbiturates are used as anticonvulsants to help control convulsions in certain disorders or diseases, such as epilepsy. If too much of the drug is used, it may become habit-forming (causing mental or physical dependence).

Before using this medicine

Before you use this medicine check with your doctor, or pharmacist:
- if you ever had any unusual or allergic reaction to this medicine or one of its components.
- if you are on a low-salt, low-sugar, or any other special diet, or if you are allergic to preservatives or dyes.
- if you are pregnant or intend to become pregnant while using this medicine, since barbiturates have been shown to increase the chance of birth defects in humans. Taking barbiturates regularly during the last 3 months of pregnancy may cause the baby to become dependent on the medicine. This may lead to withdrawal side effects in the baby after birth.
- if you have any of the following medical problems:
Anemia (severe)
Diabetes mellitus (sugar disease)
Hyperactivity (in children)
Kidney or lifer disease
Mental depression
Overactive thyroid

Treatment

This medication is used to treat the symptoms of your medical condition. Barbiturates act in the central nervous system; some of their side effects are also caused by actions in the central nervous system. Use this medicine as directed by your doctor. Do not use more of it, do not use it more often, and do not use it for a longer period of time than your doctor ordered.

- If you are taking this medication on a regular schedule and you miss a dose, take the missed dose as soon as possible, unless it is almost time for your next dose. In that case do not take the missed dose at all.
- If a barbiturate is used for a long time, it may become habit-forming. Physical dependence may lead to withdrawal side effects when you stop taking this medicine.

Side effects

Along with the needed effects, a medicine may cause some unwanted effects. These side effects may go away during treatment as your body adjusts to the medicine. Such minor side effects are: depression, confusion, diarrhea, nausea, vomiting, joint or muscle pain, slurred speech, hallucinations, headache, decreased sex drive.

- Check with your doctor immediately if any of the following side effects occur:
Rash or hives
Face, lip or eyelid swelling
Sore throat, fever
Agitation
Slow heartbeat
Difficult breathing or chest pain

Interactions

This medicine may interact with several other drugs such as medicines acting on the central nervous system (e.g., antihistamines; beta-adrenergic blockers; MAO inhibitors; mind-altering drugs; nabilone; antidepressants; clozapine; anticonvulsants).

Storage

The medicine should be stored at room temperature in a tightly closed, light-resistant container. Keep out of reach of children since overdose is very dangerous in children.

SEPTRA

Properties

This medicine contains sulfamethoxazole, a sulfonamide, and trimethoprim as active ingredients. Sulfonamides are prescribed to treat infections caused by bacteria. They will not work for colds, flu, or other virus infections.

Before using this medicine

Before you use this medicine check with your doctor:

- if you ever had any unusual or allergic reaction to any of the compounds of the medicine.
- if you are on a low-salt, low-sugar, or any other special diet, or if you are allergic to any substance, such as sulfites or other preservatives or dyes.
- if you are pregnant or intend to become pregnant while using this medicine. Although sulfonamides have not been shown to cause defects in humans, the chance may exists.
- if you are breast-feeding an infant. Most sulfonamides pass into the breast milk in small amounts and may cause unwanted effects in infants with some specific conditions.
- if you have any of the following medical problems:
Kidney disease
Liver disease
Porphyria
Deficiency of enzymes such as G6PD

Treatment

This medication is used to treat an infection caused by bacteria. Most sulfonamides are best taken with a full glass (8 ounces) of water on an empty stomach, either one hour before or two hours after a meal. Follow your doctor's or pharmacist's directions on how to take your medicine.

- Keep taking this medicine for the full time of treatment even if you begin to feel better after a few days; do not miss any doses.
- If you do miss a dose of this medicine, take the missed dose immediately.
- This medication works best when the level of medicine in your bloodstream (and urine) is kept constant. It is best, therefore, to take the doses at evenly spaced intervals day and night. if you take two doses a day, the doses should be spaced 12 hours apart.

Side effects

Along with the needed effects, a medicine may cause some unwanted effects. Side effects that usually do not require medical attention: abdominal pain, diarrhea, dizziness, headache, loss of appetite, nausea, sore mouth, or vomiting. These side effects should disappear as your body adjusts to the medication.
Sulfonamides can increase sensitivity to sunlight. It is, therefore, important to avoid prolonged exposure to sunlight and sunlamps.

Tell your doctor about any side effects that are persistent or particularly bothersome. It is especially important to tell your doctor about:
Bloody urine
Difficult urination
Difficulty in breathing
Difficulty in swallowing
Fever or hallucinations
Itching, rash, or pale skin
Joint pain, lower back pain
Ringing in the ears
Sore throat
Swollen or inflamed tongue
Tingling in hands or feet
Unusual bleeding
Yellowing of the eyes or skin

Interactions

This medicine may interact with several other drugs such as anticoagulants, oral antidiabetic agents, aspirin, some antibiotics, or anticancer drugs.

- Be sure to tell your doctor about any medications you are currently taking.

Storage

Tablets, capsules, suspension, etc. should be stored at room temperature as directed by your pharmacist or according to instructions on the label.

SERAL

Properties

This medicine contains as active ingredient the barbiturate secobarbital. Barbiturates belong to the group of medicines called central nervous system depressants (medicines that slow down the nervous system).

Barbiturates may partially block nerve impulses at nerve-cell connections. They may be used to treat insomnia (sleeplessness) by helping patients fall asleep. Also, they may be used to relieve anxiety or tension. Some of the barbiturates are used as anticonvulsants to help control convulsions in certain disorders or diseases, such as epilepsy. If too much of the drug is used, it may become habit-forming (causing mental or physical dependence).

Before using this medicine

Before you use this medicine check with your doctor, or pharmacist:
- if you ever had any unusual or allergic reaction to this medicine or one of its components.
- if you are on a low-salt, low-sugar, or any other special diet, or if you are allergic to preservatives or dyes.
- if you are pregnant or intend to become pregnant while using this medicine, since barbiturates have been shown to increase the chance of birth defects in humans. Taking barbiturates regularly during the last 3 months of pregnancy may cause the baby to become dependent on the medicine. This may lead to withdrawal side effects in the baby after birth.
- if you have any of the following medical problems:
Anemia (severe)
Diabetes mellitus (sugar disease)
Hyperactivity (in children)
Kidney or lifer disease
Mental depression
Overactive thyroid

Treatment

This medication is used to treat the symptoms of your medical condition. Barbiturates act in the central nervous system; some of their side effects are also caused by actions in the central nervous system. Use this medicine as directed by your doctor. Do not use more of it, do not use it more often, and do not use it for a longer period of time than your doctor ordered.
- If you are taking this medication on a regular schedule and you miss a dose, take the missed dose as soon as possible, unless it is almost time for your next dose. In that case do not take the missed dose at all.
- If a barbiturate is used for a long time, it may become habit-forming. Physical dependence may lead to withdrawal side effects when you stop taking this medicine.

Side effects

Along with the needed effects, a medicine may cause some unwanted effects. These side effects may go away during treatment as your body adjusts to the medicine. Such minor side effects are: depression, confusion, diarrhea, nausea, vomiting, joint or muscle pain, slurred speech, hallucinations, headache, decreased sex drive.
- Check with your doctor immediately if any of the following side effects occur:
Rash or hives
Face, lip or eyelid swelling
Sore throat, fever
Agitation
Slow heartbeat
Difficult breathing or chest pain

Interactions

This medicine may interact with several other drugs such as medicines acting on the central nervous system (e.g., antihistamines; beta-adrenergic blockers; MAO inhibitors; mind-altering drugs; nabilone; antidepressants; clozapine; anticonvulsants).

Storage

The medicine should be stored at room temperature in a tightly closed, light-resistant container. Keep out of reach of children since overdose is very dangerous in children.

SERAX

Properties

This medicine contains as active ingredient oxazepam, a benzodiazepine preparation. Benzodiazepines belong to the group of psychoactive medicines that influence the activity of the brain. Some are used to relieve nervousness or tension. It is effective for this purpose for short periods. Others are used for sleeplessness or to relax muscles or relieve muscle spasm. The benzodiazepines may also be used for other conditions as determined by your doctor.

Before using this medicine

Before you use this medicine check with your doctor:
- if you ever had any unusual or allergic reaction to benzodiazepines.
- if you are on a low-salt, low-sugar, or any other special diet, or if you are allergic to any substance, such as sulfites or other preservatives or dyes.
- if you are pregnant or intend to become pregnant while using this medicine. Some benzodiazepines have been reported to increase the chance of birth defects when used during the first 3 months of pregnancy.
- if you are breast-feeding an infant. Benzodiazepines may pass into the breast milk and cause drowsiness, unusually slow heartbeat, shortness of breath, or troubled breathing in infants of mothers taking this medicine.
- if you have any of the following medical problems: asthma, bronchitis, emphysema, or other chronic lung disease; epilepsy or history of convulsions; hyperactivity (in children); kidney or lifer disease; mental depression or illness; myasthania gravis, porphyria.

Treatment

This medication is used to relieve or prevent the symptoms of your medical problem. Benzodiazepines are mainly used as antianxiety agents, anticonvulsants, or sedatives. Take them as directed. Do not take more of them and do not take them more often than recommended on the label, unless otherwise directed by your doctor. Benzodiazepine tranquilizing drugs can be abused if taken for long periods of time and it is possible to develop withdrawal symptoms if you discontinue the therapy abruptly.

Side effects

Along with the needed effects, a medicine may cause some unwanted effects. Minor side effects are: bitter taste in the mouth, dizziness, drowsiness, depression, constipation, dry mouth, excessive salivation, fatigue, flushing, headache, heartburn, loss of appetite, nausea, nervousness, sweating or vomiting. As your body adjusts to the medicine, these side effects should disappear.
- Tell your doctor about any side effects that are persistent or particularly bothersome. It is especially important to tell your doctor about:
  Blurred or double vision
  Chest pain
  Difficulty in urinating
  Fainting or falling
  Fever or hallucinations
  Joint pain
  Mouth sores
  Nightmares
  Palpitations
  Severe depression
  Shortness of breath
  Slurred speech
  Uncoordinated movements
  Unusual tiredness
  Yellowing of the skin

Interactions

This medicine may interact with several other drugs. Be sure to tell your doctor about any medications you are currently taking. This medicine will add to the effects of alcohol, and CNS depressants.

Storage

Store at room temperature in tightly closed, light-resistant-resistant containers. Keep out of the reach of children since overdose may be especially dangerous in children.

SERENTIL

Properties
This medicine contains as active ingredient mesoridazine, a phenothiazine derivative. Phenothiazines are a family of medicines used to treat nervous, mental, and emotional conditions. Some are used to control anxiety, restlessness, nausea and vomiting, and severe hiccups. This medicine is available only with your doctor's prescription.

Before using this medicine
Before you use this medicine check with your doctor, or pharmacist:
- if you ever had any unusual or allergic reaction to phenothiazine medicines.
- if you are on a low-salt, low-sugar, or any other special diet, or if you are allergic to any substance, such as sulfites or other preservatives or dyes.
- if you are pregnant or intend to become pregnant while using this medicine. Although phenothiazines have not been shown to cause birth defects, some side effects such as jaundice and muscle tremors have occurred in a few newborns whose mothers received phenothiazines during pregnancy.
- if you are breast-feeding an infant. Although this medicine has not been shown to cause problems in humans but the chance does exist since some phenothiazines are known to pass into the breast milk.
- if you have any of the following medical problems:
Alcoholism
Blood disease
Difficult urination
Enlarged prostate
Glaucoma
Heart or blood vessel disease
Liver or lung disease
Parkinson's disease
Stomach ulcers

Treatment
This medication is prescribed to treat the symptoms of certain types of mental illness or emotional problems. In order to avoid stomach irritation, you can take the tablet or capsule forms of this medication with a meal or with a glass of water or milk (unless your doctor or pharmacist directs you to do otherwise).

Side effects
Along with the needed effects, a medicine may cause some unwanted effects. Minor side effects are: blurred vision, constipation, decreased sweating, diarrhea, dizziness, drooling, drowsiness, dry mouth, fatigue, jitteriness, menstrual irregularities, nasal congestion, restlessness, tremors, vomiting, or weight gain.
- Tell your doctor about any side effects that are persistent or particularly bothersome. It is especially important to tell your doctor about:
Breast enlargement
Chest pain or convulsions
Darkened skin
Difficulty in swallowing
Fainting or fever
Involuntary movements
Palpitations or sleep disorders
Rash or sore throat
Uncoordinated movements
Unusual bleeding or bruising
Visual disturbances
Yellowing of the eyes or skin

Interactions
This medicine may interact with several other drugs such as barbiturates, sleeping pills, narcotics, other tranquilizers, or any other medication that may produce a sedative effect. Avoid alcohol.

Storage
Store this medication as directed on the label. Keep out of the reach of children.

SIBELIUM

Properties
This medicine contains flunarizine as active ingredient. It is a so-called calcium channel blocker, working by blocking the passage of calcium into heart and smooth muscle. Since calcium is an essential factor in muscle contraction, any medicine that affects calcium in this way will interfere with the contraction of these muscles.

The medicine works by:
♦ reducing the work that the heart must perform;
♦ reducing the normal arterial blood pressure;
♦ increasing oxygen to the heart muscle.

The medicine is prescribed for the treatment of attacks of angina pectoris, irregular heartbeat, and high blood pressure. In many cases it can be used for the treatment and prevention of migraine.

Before using this medicine
Before you use this medicine check with your doctor, or pharmacist:
– if you ever had any unusual or allergic reaction to this medicine or any calcium channel blocker;
– if you are pregnant or intend to become pregnant while using this medicine;
– if you have low blood pressure;
– if you have kidney or lifer disease;
– if you are breast-feeding an infant;
– if you easily get a rash or intensity sunburn in areas exposed to sun or ultraviolet light.

Treatment
This medication is used for treatment of heart conditions (for instance, angina pectoris) and high blood pressure. Tablets, capsules or extended-release tablets should be taken with liquid. The usual dose amounts to 30 to 100 milligrams a day.

For safe and effective use of medicine:
♦ Follow your doctor's instructions if this medicine was prescribed.
♦ Follow the manufacturer's package directions if you are treating yourself.

Side effects
Along with the needed effects, a medicine may cause some unwanted effects. Possible side effects include:
Tiredness
Changes in heartbeat
Wheezing
Cough
Shortness of breath
Dizziness
Fainting
Numbness in hands and feet
Tingling in hands and feet
Difficult urination
Constipation

Overdose
The following symptoms may be a sign of overdose:
Unusually fast heartbeat
Unusually slow heartbeat
Loss of consciousness
Cardiac arrest
■ Call a doctor or hospital emergency room for instructions. If necessary start first aid immediately.

Interactions
The effect of this medicine may cause a blood pressure drop if taken together with antihypertensives. Cimetidine may increase the effect of the calcium blocker.

The simultaneous use of diuretics and calcium channel blockers may cause dangerous blood pressure drop.
■ Be sure to tell your doctor about any medications you are currently taking.

Storage
Capsules, tablets, etc. should be stored at room temperature; store away from heat and direct light. Keep out of reach of children, since this medicine may be dangerous in children.

SINEQUAN

Properties

This medicine contains doxepin as active ingredient. It belongs to the group of medicines known as tricyclic antidepressants or 'mood elevators.' It is used to relieve mental depression and depression that sometimes occurs with anxiety. The medication gradually relieves, but doesn't cure, symptoms of depression. The medication may also be used for the treatment of narcolepsy, bulimia, painic attacks, cocaine withdrawal, attention deficit disorder.

Before using this medicine

Before you use this medicine check with your doctor, or pharmacist:
- if you ever had any unusual or allergic reaction to any tricyclic antidepressant, maprotiline or trazodone.
- if you are on a low-salt, low-sugar, or any other special diet, or if you are allergic to any substance, such as sulfites or other preservatives or dyes.
- if you are pregnant or intend to become pregnant while using this medicine. There have been reports of newborns suffering from heart, breathing, and urinary problems when their mothers had taken tricyclic antidepressants before delivery.
- if you are breast-feeding an infant. Some tricyclic antidepressants pass into the breast milk.

Treatment

Take this medicine only as directed by your doctor, to benefit your condition as much as possible. Do not take more of it, do not take it more often, and do not take it for a longer period of time than your doctor ordered.

To lessen stomach upset, take this medicine with food, even for a daily bedtime dose, unless your doctor has told you to take it on an empty stomach. If you forget your once-a-day bedtime dose, don't take it more than 3 hours late. If more than 3 hours, wait for next scheduled dose;.

Sometimes this medicine must be taken for several weeks before you begin to feel better.

Side effects

Along with the needed effects, a medicine may cause some unwanted effects. Side effects that usually do not require medical attention: difficult or frequent urination; decreased sex drive; muscle aches; abnormal dreams; nasal congestion; weakness and faintness when arising from bed or chair; back pain.
- Other side effects that should be reported to your doctor immediately are:
  Hallucinations
  Shakiness
  Dizziness or fainting
  Blurred vision, eye pain
  Irregular heartbeat or slow pulse
  Inflamed tongue
  Abdominal pain
  Jaundice
  Hair loss, rash
  Fever, chills
  Joint pain
  Palpitations

Interactions

This medicine may interact with several other drugs such as anticoagulants, anticholinergics, cold remedies, oral contraceptives, seizure medicines, sleeping medicines, thyroid medicines, etc.
- Be sure to tell your doctor about any medications you are currently taking.

Storage

Tablets, capsules, etc. should be stored at room temperature in tightly closed, light-resistant containers as directed by your pharmacist. Keep out of reach of children since overdose is especially dangerous in young children. Do not store in the bathroom medicine cabinet because the heat or moisture may cause the medicine to break down. Keep the liquid form of the medicine from freezing.

SK-AMITRIPTYLINE

Properties
This medicine contains amitriptyline as active ingredient. It belongs to the group of medicines known as tricyclic antidepressants or 'mood elevators.' It is used to relieve mental depression and depression that sometimes occurs with anxiety. The medication gradually relieves, but doesn't cure, symptoms of depression. The medication may also be used for the treatment of narcolepsy, bulimia, painic attacks, cocaine withdrawal, attention deficit disorder.

Before using this medicine
Before you use this medicine check with your doctor, or pharmacist:
- if you ever had any unusual or allergic reaction to any tricyclic antidepressant, maprotiline or trazodone.
- if you are on a low-salt, low-sugar, or any other special diet, or if you are allergic to any substance, such as sulfites or other preservatives or dyes.
- if you are pregnant or intend to become pregnant while using this medicine. There have been reports of newborns suffering from heart, breathing, and urinary problems when their mothers had taken tricyclic antidepressants before delivery.
- if you are breast-feeding an infant. Some tricyclic antidepressants pass into the breast milk.

Treatment
Take this medicine only as directed by your doctor, to benefit your condition as much as possible. Do not take more of it, do not take it more often, and do not take it for a longer period of time than your doctor ordered.

To lessen stomach upset, take this medicine with food, even for a daily bedtime dose, unless your doctor has told you to take it on an empty stomach. If you forget your once-a-day bedtime dose, don't take it more than 3 hours late. If more than 3 hours, wait for next scheduled dose;.

Sometimes this medicine must be taken for several weeks before you begin to feel better.

Side effects
Along with the needed effects, a medicine may cause some unwanted effects. Side effects that usually do not require medical attention: difficult or frequent urination; decreased sex drive; muscle aches; abnormal dreams; nasal congestion; weakness and faintness when arising from bed or chair; back pain.
- Other side effects that should be reported to your doctor immediately are:
  Hallucinations
  Shakiness
  Dizziness or fainting
  Blurred vision, eye pain
  Irregular heartbeat or slow pulse
  Inflamed tongue
  Abdominal pain
  Jaundice
  Hair loss, rash
  Fever, chills
  Joint pain
  Palpitations

Interactions
This medicine may interact with several other drugs such as anticoagulants, anticholinergics, cold remedies, oral contraceptives, seizure medicines, sleeping medicines, thyroid medicines, etc.
- Be sure to tell your doctor about any medications you are currently taking.

Storage
Tablets, capsules, etc. should be stored at room temperature in tightly closed, light-resistant containers as directed by your pharmacist. Keep out of reach of children since overdose is especially dangerous in young children. Do not store in the bathroom medicine cabinet because the heat or moisture may cause the medicine to break down. Keep the liquid form of the medicine from freezing.

SK-ERYTHROMYCIN

Properties
This medicine contains erythromycin as active ingredient. This antibiotic is prescribed to treat infections caused by bacteria. They will not work for colds, flu, or other virus infections. Erythromycins are available only with your doctor's prescription.

Before using this medicine
Before you use this medicine check with your doctor, or pharmacist:
- if you ever had any unusual or allergic reaction to any of the erythromycins.
- if you are on a low-salt, low-sugar, or any other special diet, or if you are allergic to any substance, such as sulfites or other preservatives or dyes.
- if you are pregnant or intend to become pregnant while using this medicine. Although erythromycins have not been shown to cause birth defects or other problems in humans, the chance always exists.
- if you are breast-feeding an infant. Most erythromycins pass into the breast milk. Although erythromycins have not been shown to cause problems in humans, the chance always exists.
- if you have lifer disease.

Treatment
This medication belongs to the general family of medicines called antibiotics. It is used to treat a wide variety of bacterial infections. It is also used to treat infections in persons who are allergic to penicillin. Erythromycins are also used to prevent "strep" infections in patients with a history of rheumatic heart disease. They may also be used in Legionnaires' disease and for other problems as determined by your doctor.
- Keep taking this medicine for the full time of treatment even if you begin to feel better after a few days; do not miss any doses. This is especially important if you have a "strep" infection since serious heart problems could develop later if your infection is not cleared up completely.
- If you do miss a dose of this medicine, take it as soon as possible. This will help to keep a constant amount of medicine in the blood. However, if it is almost time for your next dose, skip the missed dose and go back to your regular dosing schedule.
- This medication has been prescribed for your current infection only. Another infection later on, or one that someone else has, may require a different medicine. You should not give your medicine to other people or use it for other infections, unless your doctor specifically directs you to do so.

Side effects
Along with the needed effects, a medicine may cause some unwanted effects. Side effects that usually do not require medical attention: abdominal cramps, black tongue, cough, diarrhea, fatigue, irritation of the mouth, loss of appetite, nausea, or vomiting. These side effects should disappear as your body adjusts to the medication.
- Other side effects that should be reported to your doctor immediately are:
Fever
Hearing loss
Hives or rash
Rectal or vaginal itching
Yellowing of the eyes or skin

Interactions
This medicine may interact with several other drugs such as anticoagulants, theophylline preparations, carbamazepine, etc.
- Be sure to tell your doctor about any medications you are currently taking.

Storage
Tablets, capsules, etc. should be stored at room temperature in tightly closed, light-resistant containers as directed by your pharmacist.

SK-HYDROCHLOROTHIAZIDE

Properties
This medicine contains as active ingredient hydrochlorothiazide, a thiazide-like diuretic. Thiazide or thiazide-like diuretics are prescribed to treat high blood pressure (hypertension). They are also used to reduce fluid accumulation in the body caused by conditions such as heart failure, cirrhosis, kidney disease, and the long-term use of some medications. Thiazide diuretics may also be used for other conditions as determined by your doctor.

Before using this medicine
Before you use this medicine check with your doctor, or pharmacist:
- if you ever had any unusual or allergic reaction to sulfonamides (sulfa drugs) or any of the thiazide diuretics.
- if you are on a low-salt, low-sugar, or any other special diet, or if you are allergic to any substance, such as sulfites or other preservatives or dyes.
- if you are pregnant or intend to become pregnant while using this medicine. When this medicine is used during pregnancy, it may cause side effects including jaundice, blood problems, and low potassium in the newborn.
- if you are breast-feeding an infant. Although this medicine has not been shown to cause problems in humans, the chance always exists since thiazide diuretics pass into breast milk.
- if you have any of the following medical problems:
Diabetes
Gout
Kidney disease
Liver disease
Lupus erythematosus
Pancreas disease

Treatment
This medication is used to treat high blood pressure (hypertension) and also to help reduce the amount of water in the body by increasing the flow of urine. This medicine will not cure your high blood pressure but it does help control it. You must continue to take it - even if you feel well - if you expect to keep your blood pressure down. You may have to take high blood pressure medicine for the rest of your life.

Thiazide diuretics may cause an unusual feeling of tiredness when you begin to take them. You may also notice an increase in urine or in frequency of urination. To keep this from affecting sleep:
- if you are to take a single dose a day, take it in the morning after breakfast;
- if you are to take more than one dose, take the last one not later than 6 p.m.

Side effects
Along with the needed effects, a medicine may cause some unwanted effects. Side effects that usually do not require medical attention: decreased sexual ability; dizziness or lightheadedness when standing up; increased sensitivity of skin to sunlight; loss of appetite; upset stomach.
- Side effects that should be reported to your doctor: black, tarry stools; blood in urine or stools; cough or hoarseness; fever or chills; joint pain; lower back or side pains; painful or difficult urination; pinpoint red spots on skin; skin rash or hives; stomach pain (severe) with nausea; unusual bleeding or bruising; yellow eyes or skin. This medicine may cause a loss of potassium from your body. Signs of too much potassium loss are: dryness of mouth; increased thirst; mood changes; muscle cramps or pain; nausea or vomiting; unusual tiredness or weakness; weak or irregular heartbeat.

Interactions
This medicine may interact with several other drugs.
- Be sure to tell your doctor about any medications you are currently taking.

Storage
Store at room temperature in a tightly closed container.

SK-PENICILLIN G

Properties
This medicine contains penicillin G as active ingredient. Penicillins are prescribed to treat infections caused by bacteria. They will not work for colds, flu, or other virus infections. There are several different kinds of penicillins. Each is used to treat different kinds of infections.

Before using this medicine
Before you use this medicine check with your doctor, or pharmacist:
- if you ever had any unusual or allergic reaction to any of the penicillins, cefalosporins, griseofulvin, or penicillamine. Serious reactions may occur in patients who are allergic to penicillins.
- if you are on a low-salt, low-sugar, or any other special diet, or if you are allergic to any substance, such as sulfites or other preservatives or dyes.
- if you are pregnant or intend to become pregnant while using this medicine. Although penicillins have not been shown to cause problems in humans, the chance always exists.
- if you are breast-feeding an infant. Most penicillins (except amdinocillin) pass into the breast milk. Even though only small amounts may pass, allergic reaction, diarrhea, fungal infection, and skin rash may occur in the infant.
- if you have any of the following medical problems:
  Allergy
  Asthma
  Bleeding problems
  Eczema
  Hay fever, hives
  Kidney disease
  Liver disease
  Mononucleosis
  Stomach or intestinal disease

Treatment
This medication is used to treat an infection caused by bacteria. Most penicillins are best taken with a full glass (8 ounces) of water on an empty stomach, some are best taken with a snack or meal. Follow your doctor's or pharmacist's directions on how to take your medicine.
- ◆ Keep taking this medicine for the full time of treatment even if you begin to feel better after a few days; do not miss any doses. This is especially important if you have a "strep" infection since serious heart problems could develop later if your infection is not cleared up completely.
- ◆ If you do miss a dose of this medicine, take it as soon as possible. However, if it is almost time for your next dose, skip the missed dose and go back to your regular dosing schedule.

Side effects
Along with the needed effects, a medicine may cause some unwanted effects. Side effects that usually do not require medical attention: diarrhea; nausea or vomiting; sore mouth or tongue.
- ◆ Stop taking this medicine and get emergency help immediately if you notice: difficulty in breathing; light-headedness; skin rash, hives, itching; wheezing.

Other side effects that should be reported to your doctor immediately are: abdominal bloating; blood in urine; convulsions (seizures); decreased amount of urine; diarrhea (watery and severe) which may also be bloody; fever; joint pain; sore throat and fever; stomach or abdominal cramps and pain; unusual bleeding or bruising.

Interactions
This medicine may interact with several other drugs such as anticoagulants, diarrhea medicines, heparin, ibuprofen, oral contraceptives, potassium-containing medicines, etc.
- ■ Be sure to tell your doctor about any medications you are currently taking.

Storage
Tablets, capsules, etc. should be stored as directed by your pharmacist or according to instructions on the label.

SK-PENICILLIN VK

Properties

This medicine contains penicillin V as active ingredient. Penicillins are prescribed to treat infections caused by bacteria. They will not work for colds, flu, or other virus infections. There are several different kinds of penicillins. Each is used to treat different kinds of infections.

Before using this medicine

Before you use this medicine check with your doctor, or pharmacist:

- if you ever had any unusual or allergic reaction to any of the penicillins, cefalosporins, griseofulvin, or penicillamine. Serious reactions may occur in patients who are allergic to penicillins.
- if you are on a low-salt, low-sugar, or any other special diet, or if you are allergic to any substance, such as sulfites or other preservatives or dyes.
- if you are pregnant or intend to become pregnant while using this medicine. Although penicillins have not been shown to cause problems in humans, the chance always exists.
- if you are breast-feeding an infant. Most penicillins (except amdinocillin) pass into the breast milk. Even though only small amounts may pass, allergic reaction, diarrhea, fungal infection, and skin rash may occur in the infant.
- if you have any of the following medical problems:
  Allergy
  Asthma
  Bleeding problems
  Eczema
  Hay fever, hives
  Kidney disease
  Liver disease
  Mononucleosis
  Stomach or intestinal disease

Treatment

This medication is used to treat an infection caused by bacteria. Most penicillins are best taken with a full glass (8 ounces) of water on an empty stomach, some are best taken with a snack or meal. Follow your doctor's or pharmacist's directions on how to take your medicine.

- Keep taking this medicine for the full time of treatment even if you begin to feel better after a few days; do not miss any doses. This is especially important if you have a "strep" infection since serious heart problems could develop later if your infection is not cleared up completely.
- If you do miss a dose of this medicine, take it as soon as possible. However, if it is almost time for your next dose, skip the missed dose and go back to your regular dosing schedule.

Side effects

Along with the needed effects, a medicine may cause some unwanted effects. Side effects that usually do not require medical attention: diarrhea; nausea or vomiting; sore mouth or tongue.

- Stop taking this medicine and get emergency help immediately if you notice: difficulty in breathing; lightheadedness; skin rash, hives, itching; wheezing.

Other side effects that should be reported to your doctor immediately are: abdominal bloating; blood in urine; convulsions (seizures); decreased amount of urine; diarrhea (watery and severe) which may also be bloody; fever; joint pain; sore throat and fever; stomach or abdominal cramps and pain; unusual bleeding or bruising.

Interactions

This medicine may interact with several other drugs such as anticoagulants, diarrhea medicines, heparin, ibuprofen, oral contraceptives, potassium-containing medicines, etc.

- Be sure to tell your doctor about any medications you are currently taking.

Storage

Tablets, capsules, etc. should be stored as directed by your pharmacist or according to instructions on the label.

SK-PHENOBARBITAL

Properties

This medicine contains as active ingredient the barbiturate phenobarbital. Barbiturates belong to the group of medicines called central nervous system depressants (medicines that slow down the nervous system).

Barbiturates may partially block nerve impulses at nerve-cell connections. They may be used to treat insomnia (sleeplessness) by helping patients fall asleep. Also, they may be used to relieve anxiety or tension. Some of the barbiturates are used as anticonvulsants to help control convulsions in certain disorders or diseases, such as epilepsy. If too much of the drug is used, it may become habit-forming (causing mental or physical dependence).

Before using this medicine

Before you use this medicine check with your doctor, or pharmacist:
- if you ever had any unusual or allergic reaction to this medicine or one of its components.
- if you are on a low-salt, low-sugar, or any other special diet, or if you are allergic to preservatives or dyes.
- if you are pregnant or intend to become pregnant while using this medicine, since barbiturates have been shown to increase the chance of birth defects in humans. Taking barbiturates regularly during the last 3 months of pregnancy may cause the baby to become dependent on the medicine. This may lead to withdrawal side effects in the baby after birth.
- if you have any of the following medical problems:
Anemia (severe)
Diabetes mellitus (sugar disease)
Hyperactivity (in children)
Kidney or lifer disease
Mental depression
Overactive thyroid

Treatment

This medication is used to treat the symptoms of your medical condition. Barbiturates act in the central nervous system; some of their side effects are also caused by actions in the central nervous system. Use this medicine as directed by your doctor. Do not use more of it, do not use it more often, and do not use it for a longer period of time than your doctor ordered.
- If you are taking this medication on a regular schedule and you miss a dose, take the missed dose as soon as possible, unless it is almost time for your next dose. In that case do not take the missed dose at all.
- If a barbiturate is used for a long time, it may become habit-forming. Physical dependence may lead to withdrawal side effects when you stop taking this medicine.

Side effects

Along with the needed effects, a medicine may cause some unwanted effects. These side effects may go away during treatment as your body adjusts to the medicine. Such minor side effects are: depression, confusion, diarrhea, nausea, vomiting, joint or muscle pain, slurred speech, hallucinations, headache, decreased sex drive.
- Check with your doctor immediately if any of the following side effects occur:
Rash or hives
Face, lip or eyelid swelling
Sore throat, fever
Agitation
Slow heartbeat
Difficult breathing or chest pain

Interactions

This medicine may interact with several other drugs such as medicines acting on the central nervous system (e.g., antihistamines; beta-adrenergic blockers; MAO inhibitors; mind-altering drugs; nabilone; antidepressants; clozapine; anticonvulsants).

Storage

The medicine should be stored at room temperature in a tightly closed, light-resistant container. Keep out of reach of children since overdose is very dangerous in children.

SK-POTASSIUM CHLORIDE

Properties

This medicine contains potassium chloride as active ingredient; it is used to treat or prevent potassium deficiency, especially potassium deficiency that is caused by the use of diuretics (water pills).

Potassium is needed to maintain good health. Potassium supplements may be needed by patients who do not have enough potassium in their regular diet and by those who have lost too much potassium because of illness or treatment with certain medicines.

Since too much potassium may also cause health problems, most potassium supplements are available only with your doctor's prescription.

Before using this medicine

Before you use this medicine check with your doctor, or pharmacist:

- if you ever had any unusual or allergic reaction to potassium preparations;
- if you are on a low-salt, low-sugar, or any other special diet, or if you are allergic to any substance, such as sulfites or other preservatives or dyes.
- if you are pregnant or intend to become pregnant while using this medicine. Although potassium supplements have not been shown to cause problems in humans, the chance always exists.
- if you are breast-feeding an infant. Although this medicine has not been shown to cause problems in humans, the chance always exists since small amounts of potassium pass into the breast milk.
- if you have any of the following medical problems:
Addison's disease
Heart disease
Diarrhea
Kidney disease
Stomach ulcer

Treatment

This medication is used to relieve or prevent the symptoms of your medical problem. Take them as directed. Do not take more of them and do not take them more often than recommended on the label, unless otherwise directed by your doctor. To do so may increase the chance of side effects.

In order to avoid stomach irritation, you should take potassium supplements with food or immediately after a meal. If you miss a dose of this medication, take the missed dose as soon as possible, unless it is within two hours of the next scheduled dose;.

Side effects

The following minor side effects may occur:

Diarrhea
Nausea
Stomach Pains
Vomiting.

These side effects should disappear as your body adjusts to the medication. Tell your doctor about any side effects that are persistent or particularly bothersome. It is especially important to tell your doctor about anxiety; bloody or black, tarry stools; confusion; difficulty in breathing; numbness or tingling in the arms, legs, or feet; palpitations; severe abdominal pain; or unusual weakness.

Interactions

This medicine interacts with several other drugs such as adrenocorticosteroids, antimuscarinics, calcium-containing medicines; heart medicines such as digitalis or digoxin; laxatives; other potassium-containing medicines.

- Be sure to tell your doctor about any medications you are currently taking.

Storage

Tablets, elixir, etc. should be stored at room temperature in tightly closed containers. Store away from heat and direct light. Keep out of reach of children, since overdose may be very dangerous in children. Do not keep outdated medicine or medicine no longer needed. Flush the contents of the container down the toilet, unless otherwise directed.

SK-PRAMINE

Properties
This medicine contains imipramine as active ingredient. It belongs to the group of medicines known as tricyclic antidepressants or 'mood elevators.' It is used to relieve mental depression and depression that sometimes occurs with anxiety. The medication gradually relieves, but doesn't cure, symptoms of depression. The medication may also be used for the treatment of narcolepsy, bulimia, painic attacks, cocaine withdrawal, attention deficit disorder.

Before using this medicine
Before you use this medicine check with your doctor, or pharmacist:
- if you ever had any unusual or allergic reaction to any tricyclic antidepressant, maprotiline or trazodone.
- if you are on a low-salt, low-sugar, or any other special diet, or if you are allergic to any substance, such as sulfites or other preservatives or dyes.
- if you are pregnant or intend to become pregnant while using this medicine. There have been reports of newborns suffering from heart, breathing, and urinary problems when their mothers had taken tricyclic antidepressants before delivery.
- if you are breast-feeding an infant. Some tricyclic antidepressants pass into the breast milk.

Treatment
Take this medicine only as directed by your doctor, to benefit your condition as much as possible. Do not take more of it, do not take it more often, and do not take it for a longer period of time than your doctor ordered.
To lessen stomach upset, take this medicine with food, even for a daily bedtime dose, unless your doctor has told you to take it on an empty stomach. If you forget your once-a-day bedtime dose, don't take it more than 3 hours late. If more than 3 hours, wait for next scheduled dose;.
Sometimes this medicine must be taken for several weeks before you begin to feel better.

Side effects
Along with the needed effects, a medicine may cause some unwanted effects. Side effects that usually do not require medical attention: difficult or frequent urination; decreased sex drive; muscle aches; abnormal dreams; nasal congestion; weakness and faintness when arising from bed or chair; back pain.
- Other side effects that should be reported to your doctor immediately are:
Hallucinations
Shakiness
Dizziness or fainting
Blurred vision, eye pain
Irregular heartbeat or slow pulse
Inflamed tongue
Abdominal pain
Jaundice
Hair loss, rash
Fever, chills
Joint pain
Palpitations

Interactions
This medicine may interact with several other drugs such as anticoagulants, anticholinergics, cold remedies, oral contraceptives, seizure medicines, sleeping medicines, thyroid medicines, etc.
- Be sure to tell your doctor about any medications you are currently taking.

Storage
Tablets, capsules, etc. should be stored at room temperature in tightly closed, light-resistant containers as directed by your pharmacist. Keep out of reach of children since overdose is especially dangerous in young children. Do not store in the bathroom medicine cabinet because the heat or moisture may cause the medicine to break down. Keep the liquid form of the medicine from freezing.

SK-SOXAZOLE

Properties
This medicine contains sulfisoxazole, a sulfonamide, as active ingredient. Sulfonamides are prescribed to treat infections caused by bacteria. They will not work for colds, flu, or other virus infections.

Before using this medicine
Before you use this medicine check with your doctor:
- if you ever had any unusual or allergic reaction to any of the compounds of the medicine.
- if you are on a low-salt, low-sugar, or any other special diet, or if you are allergic to any substance, such as sulfites or other preservatives or dyes.
- if you are pregnant or intend to become pregnant while using this medicine. Although sulfonamides have not been shown to cause defects in humans, the chance may exists.
- if you are breast-feeding an infant. Most sulfonamides pass into the breast milk in small amounts and may cause unwanted effects in infants with some specific conditions.
- if you have any of the following medical problems:
Kidney disease
Liver disease
Porphyria
Deficiency of enzymes such as G6PD

Treatment
This medication is used to treat an infection caused by bacteria. Most sulfonamides are best taken with a full glass (8 ounces) of water on an empty stomach, either one hour before or two hours after a meal. Follow your doctor's or pharmacist's directions on how to take your medicine.
- Keep taking this medicine for the full time of treatment even if you begin to feel better after a few days; do not miss any doses.
- If you do miss a dose of this medicine, take the missed dose immediately.
- This medication works best when the level of medicine in your bloodstream (and urine) is kept constant. It is best, therefore, to take the doses at evenly spaced intervals day and night. if you take two doses a day, the doses should be spaced 12 hours apart.

Side effects
Along with the needed effects, a medicine may cause some unwanted effects. Side effects that usually do not require medical attention: abdominal pain, diarrhea, dizziness, headache, loss of appetite, nausea, sore mouth, or vomiting. These side effects should disappear as your body adjusts to the medication.
Sulfonamides can increase sensitivity to sunlight. It is, therefore, important to avoid prolonged exposure to sunlight and sunlamps.

Tell your doctor about any side effects that are persistent or particularly bothersome. It is especially important to tell your doctor about:
Bloody urine
Difficult urination
Difficulty in breathing
Difficulty in swallowing
Fever or hallucinations
Itching, rash, or pale skin
Joint pain, lower back pain
Ringing in the ears
Sore throat
Swollen or inflamed tongue
Tingling in hands or feet
Unusual bleeding
Yellowing of the eyes or skin

Interactions
This medicine may interact with several other drugs such as anticoagulants, oral antidiabetic agents, aspirin, some antibiotics, or anticancer drugs.
- Be sure to tell your doctor about any medications you are currently taking.

Storage
Tablets, capsules, suspension, etc. should be stored at room temperature as directed by your pharmacist or according to instructions on the label.

SLO-BID GYROCAPS

Properties

This medicine contains theophylline as active ingredient; it is used to treat or prevent breathing problems (wheezing and shortness of breath) caused by asthma, bronchitis, or emphysema. This medication belongs to a group known as xanthine-derivative bronchodilators. They work by opening up the bronchial tubes or air passages of the lungs and increasing the flow of air through them. These medicines are available only with your doctor's prescription.

Before using this medicine

Before you use this medicine check with your doctor, or pharmacist:
- if you ever had any unusual or allergic reaction to xanthine-derivative bronchodilators.
- if you are on a low-salt, low-sugar, or any other special diet, or if you are allergic to any substance, such as sulfites or other preservatives or dyes.
- if you are pregnant or intend to become pregnant while using this medicine.
- if you are breast-feeding an infant. Theophylline passes into the breast milk and may cause irritability, fretfulness, or trouble in sleeping in infants of mothers taking this medicine.
- if you have any of the following medical problems:
  Diarrhea
  Enlarged prostate
  Fibrocystic breast disease
  Heart disease
  Stomach ulcer

Treatment

This medication is used to relieve or prevent the symptoms of your medical problem. Take them as directed. Do not take more of them and do not take them more often than recommended on the label, unless otherwise directed by your doctor. To do so may increase the chance of side effects. The medicine should be taken on an empty stomach 30 to 60 minutes before a meal or two hours after a meal. Try not to miss any doses of this medication. If you do miss a dose, take the missed dose as soon as possible, unless it is almost time for the next dose. Do not double the next dose. It works best when taken with a glass of water.

Side effects

The following minor side effects may occur:
  Dizziness Or Flushing
  Headache
  Diarrhea
  Heartburn
  Increased Urination
  Insomnia
  Nervousness Or Irritability
  Loss Of Appetite
  Nausea Or Stomach Upset
  Stomach Pain.

These side effects should disappear as your body adjusts to the medication. Tell your doctor about any side effects that are persistent or particularly bothersome. It is especially important to tell your doctor about black, tarry stools; confusion; convulsions; difficulty in breathing; fainting; muscle twitching; palpitations; rash; severe abdominal pain; or unusual weakness.

Interactions

This medicine interacts with several other drugs such as diuretics, reserpine, beta blockers, phenytoin, lithium, phenobarbital, birth control pills, and other medications.
- Be sure to tell your doctor about any medications you are currently taking.

Storage

Tablets, capsules, liquid and suspension should be stored at room temperature in tightly closed containers. Store away from heat and direct light. Keep out of reach of children, since overdose may be very dangerous in children. Discard any outdated medication.

SLO-PHYLLIN

Properties
This medicine contains theophylline as active ingredient; it is used to treat or prevent breathing problems (wheezing and shortness of breath) caused by asthma, bronchitis, or emphysema. This medication belongs to a group known as xanthine-derivative bronchodilators. They work by opening up the bronchial tubes or air passages of the lungs and increasing the flow of air through them. These medicines are available only with your doctor's prescription.

Before using this medicine
Before you use this medicine check with your doctor, or pharmacist:
- if you ever had any unusual or allergic reaction to xanthine-derivative bronchodilators.
- if you are on a low-salt, low-sugar, or any other special diet, or if you are allergic to any substance, such as sulfites or other preservatives or dyes.
- if you are pregnant or intend to become pregnant while using this medicine.
- if you are breast-feeding an infant. Theophylline passes into the breast milk and may cause irritability, fretfulness, or trouble in sleeping in infants of mothers taking this medicine.
- if you have any of the following medical problems:
Diarrhea
Enlarged prostate
Fibrocystic breast disease
Heart disease
Stomach ulcer

Treatment
This medication is used to relieve or prevent the symptoms of your medical problem. Take them as directed. Do not take more of them and do not take them more often than recommended on the label, unless otherwise directed by your doctor. To do so may increase the chance of side effects. The medicine should be taken on an empty stomach 30 to 60 minutes before a meal or two hours after a meal. Try not to miss any doses of this medication. If you do miss a dose, take the missed dose as soon as possible, unless it is almost time for the next dose. Do not double the next dose. It works best when taken with a glass of water.

Side effects
The following minor side effects may occur:
Dizziness Or Flushing
Headache
Diarrhea
Heartburn
Increased Urination
Insomnia
Nervousness Or Irritability
Loss Of Appetite
Nausea Or Stomach Upset
Stomach Pain.
These side effects should disappear as your body adjusts to the medication. Tell your doctor about any side effects that are persistent or particularly bothersome. It is especially important to tell your doctor about black, tarry stools; confusion; convulsions; difficulty in breathing; fainting; muscle twitching; palpitations; rash; severe abdominal pain; or unusual weakness.

Interactions
This medicine interacts with several other drugs such as diuretics, reserpine, beta blockers, phenytoin, lithium, phenobarbital, birth control pills, and other medications.
- Be sure to tell your doctor about any medications you are currently taking.

Storage
Tablets, capsules, liquid and suspension should be stored at room temperature in tightly closed containers. Store away from heat and direct light. Keep out of reach of children, since overdose may be very dangerous in children. Discard any outdated medication.

SLOW-K

Properties

This medicine contains potassium chloride as active ingredient; it is used to treat or prevent potassium deficiency, especially potassium deficiency that is caused by the use of diuretics (water pills).

Potassium is needed to maintain good health. Potassium supplements may be needed by patients who do not have enough potassium in their regular diet and by those who have lost too much potassium because of illness or treatment with certain medicines.

Since too much potassium may also cause health problems, most potassium supplements are available only with your doctor's prescription.

Before using this medicine

Before you use this medicine check with your doctor, or pharmacist:

- if you ever had any unusual or allergic reaction to potassium preparations;
- if you are on a low-salt, low-sugar, or any other special diet, or if you are allergic to any substance, such as sulfites or other preservatives or dyes.
- if you are pregnant or intend to become pregnant while using this medicine. Although potassium supplements have not been shown to cause problems in humans, the chance always exists.
- if you are breast-feeding an infant. Although this medicine has not been shown to cause problems in humans, the chance always exists since small amounts of potassium pass into the breast milk.
- if you have any of the following medical problems:
Addison's disease
Heart disease
Diarrhea
Kidney disease
Stomach ulcer

Treatment

This medication is used to relieve or prevent the symptoms of your medical problem. Take them as directed. Do not take more of them and do not take them more often than recommended on the label, unless otherwise directed by your doctor. To do so may increase the chance of side effects.

In order to avoid stomach irritation, you should take potassium supplements with food or immediately after a meal. If you miss a dose of this medication, take the missed dose as soon as possible, unless it is within two hours of the next scheduled dose;.

Side effects

The following minor side effects may occur:

Diarrhea
Nausea
Stomach Pains
Vomiting.

These side effects should disappear as your body adjusts to the medication. Tell your doctor about any side effects that are persistent or particularly bothersome. It is especially important to tell your doctor about anxiety; bloody or black, tarry stools; confusion; difficulty in breathing; numbness or tingling in the arms, legs, or feet; palpitations; severe abdominal pain; or unusual weakness.

Interactions

This medicine interacts with several other drugs such as adrenocorticosteroids, antimuscarinics, calcium-containing medicines; heart medicines such as digitalis or digoxin; laxatives; other potassium-containing medicines.

- Be sure to tell your doctor about any medications you are currently taking.

Storage

Tablets, elixir, etc. should be stored at room temperature in tightly closed containers. Store away from heat and direct light. Keep out of reach of children, since overdose may be very dangerous in children. Do not keep outdated medicine or medicine no longer needed. Flush the contents of the container down the toilet, unless otherwise directed.

SLOPHYLLIN GYROCAPS

Properties
This medicine contains theophylline as active ingredient; it is used to treat or prevent breathing problems (wheezing and shortness of breath) caused by asthma, bronchitis, or emphysema. This medication belongs to a group known as xanthine-derivative bronchodilators. They work by opening up the bronchial tubes or air passages of the lungs and increasing the flow of air through them. These medicines are available only with your doctor's prescription.

Before using this medicine
Before you use this medicine check with your doctor, or pharmacist:
- if you ever had any unusual or allergic reaction to xanthine-derivative bronchodilators.
- if you are on a low-salt, low-sugar, or any other special diet, or if you are allergic to any substance, such as sulfites or other preservatives or dyes.
- if you are pregnant or intend to become pregnant while using this medicine.
- if you are breast-feeding an infant. Theophylline passes into the breast milk and may cause irritability, fretfulness, or trouble in sleeping in infants of mothers taking this medicine.
- if you have any of the following medical problems:
  Diarrhea
  Enlarged prostate
  Fibrocystic breast disease
  Heart disease
  Stomach ulcer

Treatment
This medication is used to relieve or prevent the symptoms of your medical problem. Take them as directed. Do not take more of them and do not take them more often than recommended on the label, unless otherwise directed by your doctor. To do so may increase the chance of side effects. The medicine should be taken on an empty stomach 30 to 60 minutes before a meal or two hours after a meal. Try not to miss any doses of this medication. If you do miss a dose, take the missed dose as soon as possible, unless it is almost time for the next dose. Do not double the next dose. It works best when taken with a glass of water.

Side effects
The following minor side effects may occur:
  Dizziness Or Flushing
  Headache
  Diarrhea
  Heartburn
  Increased Urination
  Insomnia
  Nervousness Or Irritability
  Loss Of Appetite
  Nausea Or Stomach Upset
  Stomach Pain.
These side effects should disappear as your body adjusts to the medication. Tell your doctor about any side effects that are persistent or particularly bothersome. It is especially important to tell your doctor about black, tarry stools; confusion; convulsions; difficulty in breathing; fainting; muscle twitching; palpitations; rash; severe abdominal pain; or unusual weakness.

Interactions
This medicine interacts with several other drugs such as diuretics, reserpine, beta blockers, phenytoin, lithium, phenobarbital, birth control pills, and other medications.
- Be sure to tell your doctor about any medications you are currently taking.

Storage
Tablets, capsules, liquid and suspension should be stored at room temperature in tightly closed containers. Store away from heat and direct light. Keep out of reach of children, since overdose may be very dangerous in children. Discard any outdated medication.

SLYN-LL

Properties

This medicine contains phendimetrazine as active ingredient; it is prescribed for appetite suppression.

Appetite suppressants are used in the short-term (a few weeks) treatment of obesity. In a few weeks (6 to 12), these medicines in combination with dieting, exercise, and changes in eating habits can help patients lose weight. However, since their appetite reducing effect is only temporary, they are useful only for the first weeks of dieting until new eating habits are established.

Before using this medicine

Before you use this medicine check with your doctor, or pharmacist:
- if you ever had any unusual or allergic reaction to any of the compounds of this medicine.
- if you are on a low-salt, low-sugar, or any other special diet, or if you are allergic to any substance, such as sulfites or other preservatives or dyes.
- if you are pregnant, intend to become pregnant or breast-feeding an infant while using this medicine.
- if you have any of the following medical problems:
  Diabetes mellitus (sugar diabetes)
  Epilepsy
  Glaucoma
  Heart or blood vessel disease
  High blood pressure
  Mental illness (severe)

Treatment

This medication is used to relieve or prevent the symptoms of your medical problem. Take them as directed. Do not take more of them and do not take them more often than recommended on the label. If too much of the drug is taken, it may become habit-forming.

The medicine produces central nervous system stimulation, and it should not be taken by people with heart disease or high blood pressure.

If you think this medicine is not working as well after you have taken it for a few weeks, do not increase the dose. Instead, check with your doctor.

Side effects

The following minor side effects may occur: irritability, nervousness, restlessness, trouble in sleeping.

These side effects should disappear as your body adjusts to the medication. Tell your doctor about any side effects that are persistent or particularly bothersome. It is especially important to tell your doctor about:
  Mental depression
  Nausea or vomiting
  Stomach cramps or pain
  Trembling
  Unusual tiredness or weakness
- Discontinue use of the drug; call your doctor right away. Adverse reactions and side effects may be more frequent and severe in people over age 60 than in younger persons.

Interactions

This medicine interacts with several other drugs such as antihypertensives, other appetite suppressants, caffeine, central nervous system depressants, central nervous system stimulants, furazolidone, guanethidine, hydralazine, MAO inhibitors, methyldopa, molindone, phenothiazines, rauwolfia alkaloids, sodium bicarbonate. Interaction with alcoholic beverages may produce drowsiness, sleepiness, and/or inability to concentrate.
- Be sure to tell your doctor about any medications you are currently taking.

Storage

This medicine should be stored at room temperature in tightly closed containers. Store away from heat and direct light. Keep out of reach of children, since overdose may be very dangerous in children.

Do not store this medicine in the bathroom medicine cabinet because the heat and moisture cause the medicine to break down. Do not keep outdated medicine or medicine no longer needed. Flush the contents of the container down the toilet.

SMZ-TMP

Properties
This medicine contains sulfamethoxa-zole, a sulfonamide, and trimethoprim as active ingredients. Sulfonamides are prescribed to treat infections caused by bacteria. They will not work for colds, flu, or other virus infections.

Before using this medicine
Before you use this medicine check with your doctor:
- if you ever had any unusual or aller-gic reaction to any of the compounds of the medicine.
- if you are on a low-salt, low-sugar, or any other special diet, or if you are allergic to any substance, such as sul-fites or other preservatives or dyes.
- if you are pregnant or intend to be-come pregnant while using this medicine. Although sulfonamides have not been shown to cause defects in humans, the chance may exists.
- if you are breast-feeding an infant. Most sulfonamides pass into the breast milk in small amounts and may cause unwanted effects in in-fants with some specific conditions.
- if you have any of the following medical problems:
Kidney disease
Liver disease
Porphyria
Deficiency of enzymes such as G6PD

Treatment
This medication is used to treat an in-fection caused by bacteria. Most sul-fonamides are best taken with a full glass (8 ounces) of water on an empty stomach, either one hour before or two hours after a meal. Follow your doctor's or pharmacist's directions on how to take your medicine.
- Keep taking this medicine for the full time of treatment even if you begin to feel better after a few days; do not miss any doses.
- If you do miss a dose of this medi-cine, take the missed dose immedia-tely.
- This medication works best when the level of medicine in your blood-stream (and urine) is kept constant. It is best, therefore, to take the doses at evenly spaced intervals day and night. if you take two doses a day, the doses should be spaced 12 hours apart.

Side effects
Along with the needed effects, a medi-cine may cause some unwanted effects. Side effects that usually do not require medical attention: abdominal pain, diar-rhea, dizziness, headache, loss of appe-tite, nausea, sore mouth, or vomiting. These side effects should disappear as your body adjusts to the medication.
Sulfonamides can increase sensitivity to sunlight. It is, therefore, important to avoid prolonged exposure to sunlight and sunlamps.
Tell your doctor about any side ef-fects that are persistent or particularly bothersome. It is especially important to tell your doctor about:
Bloody urine
Difficult urination
Difficulty in breathing
Difficulty in swallowing
Fever or hallucinations
Itching, rash, or pale skin
Joint pain, lower back pain
Ringing in the ears
Sore throat
Swollen or inflamed tongue
Tingling in hands or feet
Unusual bleeding
Yellowing of the eyes or skin

Interactions
This medicine may interact with several other drugs such as anticoagulants, oral antidiabetic agents, aspirin, some antibi-otics, or anticancer drugs.
- Be sure to tell your doctor about any medications you are currently taking.

Storage
Tablets, capsules, suspension, etc. should be stored at room temperature as directed by your pharmacist or ac-cording to instructions on the label.

SOLFOTON

Properties
This medicine contains as active ingredient the barbiturate phenobarbital. Barbiturates belong to the group of medicines called central nervous system depressants (medicines that slow down the nervous system).

Barbiturates may partially block nerve impulses at nerve-cell connections. They may be used to treat insomnia (sleeplessness) by helping patients fall asleep. Also, they may be used to relieve anxiety or tension. Some of the barbiturates are used as anticonvulsants to help control convulsions in certain disorders or diseases, such as epilepsy. If too much of the drug is used, it may become habit-forming (causing mental or physical dependence).

Before using this medicine
Before you use this medicine check with your doctor, or pharmacist:
– if you ever had any unusual or allergic reaction to this medicine or one of its components.
– if you are on a low-salt, low-sugar, or any other special diet, or if you are allergic to preservatives or dyes.
– if you are pregnant or intend to become pregnant while using this medicine, since barbiturates have been shown to increase the chance of birth defects in humans. Taking barbiturates regularly during the last 3 months of pregnancy may cause the baby to become dependent on the medicine. This may lead to withdrawal side effects in the baby after birth.
– if you have any of the following medical problems:
Anemia (severe)
Diabetes mellitus (sugar disease)
Hyperactivity (in children)
Kidney or lifer disease
Mental depression
Overactive thyroid

Treatment
This medication is used to treat the symptoms of your medical condition. Barbiturates act in the central nervous system; some of their side effects are also caused by actions in the central nervous system. Use this medicine as directed by your doctor. Do not use more of it, do not use it more often, and do not use it for a longer period of time than your doctor ordered.
- If you are taking this medication on a regular schedule and you miss a dose, take the missed dose as soon as possible, unless it is almost time for your next dose. In that case do not take the missed dose at all.
- If a barbiturate is used for a long time, it may become habit-forming. Physical dependence may lead to withdrawal side effects when you stop taking this medicine.

Side effects
Along with the needed effects, a medicine may cause some unwanted effects. These side effects may go away during treatment as your body adjusts to the medicine. Such minor side effects are: depression, confusion, diarrhea, nausea, vomiting, joint or muscle pain, slurred speech, hallucinations, headache, decreased sex drive.
- Check with your doctor immediately if any of the following side effects occur:
Rash or hives
Face, lip or eyelid swelling
Sore throat, fever
Agitation
Slow heartbeat
Difficult breathing or chest pain

Interactions
This medicine may interact with several other drugs such as medicines acting on the central nervous system (e.g., antihistamines; beta-adrenergic blockers; MAO inhibitors; mind-altering drugs; nabilone; antidepressants; clozapine; anticonvulsants).

Storage
The medicine should be stored at room temperature in a tightly closed, light-resistant container. Keep out of reach of children since overdose is very dangerous in children.

SOMOPHYLLIN-12

Properties
This medicine contains theophylline as active ingredient; it is used to treat or prevent breathing problems (wheezing and shortness of breath) caused by asthma, bronchitis, or emphysema. This medication belongs to a group known as xanthine-derivative bronchodilators. They work by opening up the bronchial tubes or air passages of the lungs and increasing the flow of air through them. These medicines are available only with your doctor's prescription.

Before using this medicine
Before you use this medicine check with your doctor, or pharmacist:
- if you ever had any unusual or allergic reaction to xanthine-derivative bronchodilators.
- if you are on a low-salt, low-sugar, or any other special diet, or if you are allergic to any substance, such as sulfites or other preservatives or dyes.
- if you are pregnant or intend to become pregnant while using this medicine.
- if you are breast-feeding an infant. Theophylline passes into the breast milk and may cause irritability, fretfulness, or trouble in sleeping in infants of mothers taking this medicine.
- if you have any of the following medical problems:
Diarrhea
Enlarged prostate
Fibrocystic breast disease
Heart disease
Stomach ulcer

Treatment
This medication is used to relieve or prevent the symptoms of your medical problem. Take them as directed. Do not take more of them and do not take them more often than recommended on the label, unless otherwise directed by your doctor. To do so may increase the chance of side effects. The medicine should be taken on an empty stomach 30 to 60 minutes before a meal or two hours after a meal. Try not to miss any doses of this medication. If you do miss a dose, take the missed dose as soon as possible, unless it is almost time for the next dose. Do not double the next dose. It works best when taken with a glass of water.

Side effects
The following minor side effects may occur:
  Dizziness Or Flushing
  Headache
  Diarrhea
  Heartburn
  Increased Urination
  Insomnia
  Nervousness Or Irritability
  Loss Of Appetite
  Nausea Or Stomach Upset
  Stomach Pain.
These Interaction with alcoholic beverages may producedrowsiness, sleepiness, and/or inability to concentrate.
side effects should disappear as your body adjusts to the medication. Tell your doctor about any side effects that are persistent or particularly bothersome. It is especially important to tell your doctor about black, tarry stools; confusion; convulsions; difficulty in breathing; fainting; muscle twitching; palpitations; rash; severe abdominal pain; or unusual weakness.

Interactions
This medicine interacts with several other drugs such as diuretics, reserpine, beta blockers, phenytoin, lithium, phenobarbital, birth control pills, and other medications.
- Be sure to tell your doctor about any medications you are currently taking.

Storage
Tablets, capsules, liquid and suspension should be stored at room temperature in tightly closed containers. Store away from heat and direct light. Keep out of reach of children, since overdose may be very dangerous in children. Discard any outdated medication.

SOMOPHYLLIN-CRT

Properties
This medicine contains theophylline as active ingredient; it is used to treat or prevent breathing problems (wheezing and shortness of breath) caused by asthma, bronchitis, or emphysema. This medication belongs to a group known as xanthine-derivative bronchodilators. They work by opening up the bronchial tubes or air passages of the lungs and increasing the flow of air through them. These medicines are available only with your doctor's prescription.

Before using this medicine
Before you use this medicine check with your doctor, or pharmacist:
- if you ever had any unusual or allergic reaction to xanthine-derivative bronchodilators.
- if you are on a low-salt, low-sugar, or any other special diet, or if you are allergic to any substance, such as sulfites or other preservatives or dyes.
- if you are pregnant or intend to become pregnant while using this medicine.
- if you are breast-feeding an infant. Theophylline passes into the breast milk and may cause irritability, fretfulness, or trouble in sleeping in infants of mothers taking this medicine.
- if you have any of the following medical problems:
Diarrhea
Enlarged prostate
Fibrocystic breast disease
Heart disease
Stomach ulcer

Treatment
This medication is used to relieve or prevent the symptoms of your medical problem. Take them as directed. Do not take more of them and do not take them more often than recommended on the label, unless otherwise directed by your doctor. To do so may increase the chance of side effects. The medicine should be taken on an empty stomach 30 to 60 minutes before a meal or two hours after a meal. Try not to miss any doses of this medication. If you do miss a dose, take the missed dose as soon as possible, unless it is almost time for the next dose. Do not double the next dose. It works best when taken with a glass of water.

Side effects
The following minor side effects may occur:
Dizziness Or Flushing
Headache
Diarrhea
Heartburn
Increased Urination
Insomnia
Nervousness Or Irritability
Loss Of Appetite
Nausea Or Stomach Upset
Stomach Pain.
These side effects should disappear as your body adjusts to the medication. Tell your doctor about any side effects that are persistent or particularly bothersome. It is especially important to tell your doctor about black, tarry stools; confusion; convulsions; difficulty in breathing; fainting; muscle twitching; palpitations; rash; severe abdominal pain; or unusual weakness.

Interactions
This medicine interacts with several other drugs such as diuretics, reserpine, beta blockers, phenytoin, lithium, phenobarbital, birth control pills, and other medications.
- Be sure to tell your doctor about any medications you are currently taking.

Storage
Tablets, capsules, liquid and suspension should be stored at room temperature in tightly closed containers. Store away from heat and direct light. Keep out of reach of children, since overdose may be very dangerous in children. Discard any outdated medication.

SORATE

Properties
This medicine contains isosorbide dinitrate as active ingredient. Nitrates improve the supply of blood and oxygen to the heart.

Before using this medicine
Before you use this medicine check with your doctor, or pharmacist:
- if you ever had any unusual or allergic reaction to nitrates or nitrites.
- if you are on a low-salt, low-sugar, or any other special diet, or if you are allergic to any substance, such as sulfites or other preservatives or dyes.
- if you are pregnant or intend to become pregnant while using this medicine. Although nitrates have not been shown to cause problems in humans, the chance always exists.
- if you are breast-feeding an infant.
- if you have recently had a heart attack or stroke.
- if you have any of the following medical problems:
  Anemia
  Glaucoma
  Intestinal problems
  Overactive thyroid
- if you are now taking any of the following medicines or types of medicines:
  Antihypertensives
  Asthma or hay fever medicine
  Cold medicine
  Decongestant
  Medicine for appetite control
  Narcotic
  Pain medicine
  Sinus congestion medicine

Treatment
This medication is used to treat and prevent angina (chest pain). Nitroglycerin is a vasodilator, which relaxes the muscles of the blood vessels, causing an increase in the oxygen supply to the heart. The oral tablets, capsules, ointment and patches do not act quickly; they are used to prevent chest pain. The sublingual tablets and oral spray act quickly and can be used to relieve chest pain after it has started.

- Take this medicine exactly as directed by your doctor or pharmacist. It will work only if taken correctly.
- If you are taking this medicine regularly and you miss a dose, take it as soon as possible. However, if your next scheduled dose; is within 2 hours (or within 6 hours for extended-release capsules or tablets), skip the missed dose and go back to your regular dosing schedule.
- If you have been taking this medicine regularly for several weeks or more, do not suddenly stop using it. Stopping suddenly may bring on attacks of angina.

Side effects
There are a number of side effects that usually do not require medical attention. These possible side effects may go away during treatment; however, if they continue or are bothersome, check with your doctor, nurse, or pharmacist. More common are: dizziness, lightheadedness, or fainting when standing up; fast pulse; flushing of face and neck; headache; nausea or vomiting.

Side effects that should be reported to your doctor are: blurred vision; dry mouth; severe or prolonged headache; skin rash.

Interactions
This medicine may interact with several other drugs such as tricyclic antidepressants and cough medicines. Before starting to take or apply nitroglycerin, be sure to tell your doctor about any medications you are currently taking.

Storage
Tablets, capsules, and oral spray should be stored as in a tightly capped bottle in a cool, dry place. Ointment and patches should be stored at room temperature in their original containers. Keep out of reach of children. Do not keep outdated medicine or medicine no longer needed.

SORBITRATE

Properties
This medicine contains isosorbide dinitrate as active ingredient. Nitrates improve the supply of blood and oxygen to the heart.

Before using this medicine
Before you use this medicine check with your doctor, or pharmacist:
- if you ever had any unusual or allergic reaction to nitrates or nitrites.
- if you are on a low-salt, low-sugar, or any other special diet, or if you are allergic to any substance, such as sulfites or other preservatives or dyes.
- if you are pregnant or intend to become pregnant while using this medicine. Although nitrates have not been shown to cause problems in humans, the chance always exists.
- if you are breast-feeding an infant.
- if you have recently had a heart attack or stroke.
- if you have any of the following medical problems:
  Anemia
  Glaucoma
  Intestinal problems
  Overactive thyroid
- if you are now taking any of the following medicines or types of medicines:
  Antihypertensives
  Asthma or hay fever medicine
  Cold medicine
  Decongestant
  Medicine for appetite control
  Narcotic
  Pain medicine
  Sinus congestion medicine

Treatment
This medication is used to treat and prevent angina (chest pain). Nitroglycerin is a vasodilator, which relaxes the muscles of the blood vessels, causing an increase in the oxygen supply to the heart. The oral tablets, capsules, ointment and patches do not act quickly; they are used to prevent chest pain. The sublingual tablets and oral spray act quickly and can be used to relieve chest pain after it has started.

- Take this medicine exactly as directed by your doctor or pharmacist. It will work only if taken correctly.
- If you are taking this medicine regularly and you miss a dose, take it as soon as possible. However, if your next scheduled dose; is within 2 hours (or within 6 hours for extended-release capsules or tablets), skip the missed dose and go back to your regular dosing schedule.
- If you have been taking this medicine regularly for several weeks or more, do not suddenly stop using it. Stopping suddenly may bring on attacks of angina.

Side effects
There are a number of side effects that usually do not require medical attention. These possible side effects may go away during treatment; however, if they continue or are bothersome, check with your doctor, nurse, or pharmacist. More common are: dizziness, lightheadedness, or fainting when standing up; fast pulse; flushing of face and neck; headache; nausea or vomiting.

Side effects that should be reported to your doctor are: blurred vision; dry mouth; severe or prolonged headache; skin rash.

Interactions
This medicine may interact with several other drugs such as tricyclic antidepressants and cough medicines. Before starting to take or apply nitroglycerin, be sure to tell your doctor about any medications you are currently taking.

Storage
Tablets, capsules, and oral spray should be stored as in a tightly capped bottle in a cool, dry place. Ointment and patches should be stored at room temperature in their original containers. Keep out of reach of children. Do not keep outdated medicine or medicine no longer needed.

SPARINE

Properties
This medicine contains as active ingredient promazine, a phenothiazine derivative. Phenothiazines are a family of medicines used to treat nervous, mental, and emotional conditions. Some are used to control anxiety, restlessness, nausea and vomiting, and severe hiccups. This medicine is available only with your doctor's prescription.

Before using this medicine
Before you use this medicine check with your doctor, or pharmacist:
- if you ever had any unusual or allergic reaction to phenothiazine medicines.
- if you are on a low-salt, low-sugar, or any other special diet, or if you are allergic to any substance, such as sulfites or other preservatives or dyes.
- if you are pregnant or intend to become pregnant while using this medicine. Although phenothiazines have not been shown to cause birth defects, some side effects such as jaundice and muscle tremors have occurred in a few newborns whose mothers received phenothiazines during pregnancy.
- if you are breast-feeding an infant. Although this medicine has not been shown to cause problems in humans but the chance does exist since some phenothiazines are known to pass into the breast milk.
- if you have any of the following medical problems:
Alcoholism
Blood disease
Difficult urination
Enlarged prostate
Glaucoma
Heart or blood vessel disease
Liver or lung disease
Parkinson's disease
Stomach ulcers

Treatment
This medication is prescribed to treat the symptoms of certain types of mental illness or emotional problems. In order to avoid stomach irritation, you can take the tablet or capsule forms of this medication with a meal or with a glass of water or milk (unless your doctor or pharmacist directs you to do otherwise).

Side effects
Along with the needed effects, a medicine may cause some unwanted effects.
Minor side effects are: blurred vision, constipation, decreased sweating, diarrhea, dizziness, drooling, drowsiness, dry mouth, fatigue, jitteriness, menstrual irregularities, nasal congestion, restlessness, tremors, vomiting, or weight gain.
- Tell your doctor about any side effects that are persistent or particularly bothersome. It is especially important to tell your doctor about:
Breast enlargement
Chest pain or convulsions
Darkened skin
Difficulty in swallowing
Fainting or fever
Involuntary movements
Palpitations or sleep disorders
Rash or sore throat
Uncoordinated movements
Unusual bleeding or bruising
Visual disturbances
Yellowing of the eyes or skin

Interactions
This medicine may interact with several other drugs such as barbiturates, sleeping pills, narcotics, other tranquilizers, or any other medication that may produce a sedative effect. Avoid alcohol.

Storage
Store this medication as directed on the label. Keep out of the reach of children.

SPRX-1/3

Properties

This medicine contains phendimetrazine as active ingredient; it is prescribed for appetite suppression.

Appetite suppressants are used in the short-term (a few weeks) treatment of obesity. In a few weeks (6 to 12), these medicines in combination with dieting, exercise, and changes in eating habits can help patients lose weight. However, since their appetite reducing effect is only temporary, they are useful only for the first weeks of dieting until new eating habits are established.

Before using this medicine

Before you use this medicine check with your doctor, or pharmacist:
- if you ever had any unusual or allergic reaction to any of the compounds of this medicine.
- if you are on a low-salt, low-sugar, or any other special diet, or if you are allergic to any substance, such as sulfites or other preservatives or dyes.
- if you are pregnant, intend to become pregnant or breast-feeding an infant while using this medicine.
- if you have any of the following medical problems:
Diabetes mellitus (sugar diabetes)
Epilepsy
Glaucoma
Heart or blood vessel disease
High blood pressure
Mental illness (severe)

Treatment

This medication is used to relieve or prevent the symptoms of your medical problem. Take them as directed. Do not take more of them and do not take them more often than recommended on the label. If too much of the drug is taken, it may become habit-forming.

The medicine produces central nervous system stimulation, and it should not be taken by people with heart disease or high blood pressure.

If you think this medicine is not working as well after you have taken it for a few weeks, do not increase the dose. Instead, check with your doctor.

Side effects

The following minor side effects may occur: irritability, nervousness, restlessness, trouble in sleeping.

These side effects should disappear as your body adjusts to the medication. Tell your doctor about any side effects that are persistent or particularly bothersome. It is especially important to tell your doctor about:
Mental depression
Nausea or vomiting
Stomach cramps or pain
Trembling
Unusual tiredness or weakness
- Discontinue use of the drug; call your doctor right away. Adverse reactions and side effects may be more frequent and severe in people over age 60 than in younger persons.

Interactions

This medicine interacts with several other drugs such as antihypertensives, other appetite suppressants, caffeine, central nervous system depressants, central nervous system stimulants, furazolidone, guanethidine, hydralazine, MAO inhibitors, methyldopa, molindone, phenothiazines, rauwolfia alkaloids, sodium bicarbonate. Interaction with alcoholic beverages may produce drowsiness, sleepiness, and/or inability to concentrate.
- Be sure to tell your doctor about any medications you are currently taking.

Storage

This medicine should be stored at room temperature in tightly closed containers. Store away from heat and direct light. Keep out of reach of children, since overdose may be very dangerous in children.

Do not store this medicine in the bathroom medicine cabinet because the heat and moisture cause the medicine to break down. Do not keep outdated medicine or medicine no longer needed. Flush the contents of the container down the toilet.

STADOL

Properties
This medicine contains as active ingredient butorphanol. It is a narcotic analgesic that acts directly on the central nervous system (brain and spinal cord). It is used to relieve pain or to suppress coughing.

Before using this medicine
Before you use this medicine check with your doctor, or pharmacist:
- if you ever had any unusual or allergic reaction to this medicine or one of its components.
- if you are on a low-salt, low-sugar, or any other special diet, or if you are allergic to any substance, such as sulfites or other preservatives or dyes.
- if you are pregnant or intend to become pregnant while using this medicine. Studies on birth defects have not been done in humans. Too much use of narcotics during pregnancy may cause the baby to become dependent on the medicine.
- if you are breast-feeding an infant. Although this medicine has not been shown to cause problems in humans, it passes into the breast milk in small amounts.
- if you have any of the following medical problems:
  Brain disease or head injury
  Colitis
  Convulsions
  Emphysema, asthma, or chronic lung disease
  Enlarged prostate
  Gallbladder disease or gallstones
  Heart disease
  Kidney or lifer disease
  Underactive thyroid

Treatment
This medication is used to relieve pain or to suppress coughing. Narcotic analgesics act in the central nervous system; some of their side effects are also caused by actions in the central nervous system.
- If you are taking this medication on a regular schedule and you miss a dose, take the missed dose as soon as possible, unless it is almost time for your next dose. In that case do not take the missed dose at all.
- If a narcotic analgesic is used for a long time, it may become habit-forming (causing mental or physical dependence). Physical dependence may lead to withdrawal side effects when you stop taking this medicine.

Unless otherwise directed by your doctor or pharmacist take this as directed. Do not take more of them and do not take them more often than recommended on the label. Children up to 12 years of age should not take this medicine more than 3 times a day or for more than 5 days in a row.

Side effects
Along with the needed effects, a medicine may cause some unwanted effects. These side effects may go away during treatment as your body adjusts to the medicine. Such minor side effects are: constipation, dizziness, drowsiness, dry mouth, false sense of well-being, flushing, light-headedness, loss or appetite, nausea, painful or difficult urination, or sweating.
- Check with your doctor immediately if any of the following side effects occur:
  Anxiety or breathing difficulties
  Excitation or restlessness
  Fatigue, palpitations
  Rash, sore throat and fever
  Tremors or weakness

Interactions
This medicine may interact with several other drugs such as medicines acting on the central nervous system (e.g., antidepressants, tranquilizers), cimetidine, nitrates, quinidine, etc.
- Be sure to tell your doctor about any medications you are currently taking.

Storage
Tablets, elixir, suppository etc. should be stored at room temperature in a tightly closed, light-resistant container.

STATEX

Properties
This medicine contains as active ingredient morphine.

It is a narcotic analgesic that acts directly on the central nervous system (brain and spinal cord). It is used to relieve pain or to suppress coughing.

Before using this medicine
Before you use this medicine check with your doctor, or pharmacist:
- if you ever had any unusual or allergic reaction to this medicine or one of its components.
- if you are on a low-salt, low-sugar, or any other special diet, or if you are allergic to any substance, such as sulfites or other preservatives or dyes.
- if you are pregnant or intend to become pregnant while using this medicine. Studies on birth defects have not been done in humans. Too much use of narcotics during pregnancy may cause the baby to become dependent on the medicine.
- if you are breast-feeding an infant. Although this medicine has not been shown to cause problems in humans, it passes into the breast milk in small amounts.
- if you have any of the following medical problems:
Brain disease or head injury
Colitis
Convulsions
Emphysema, asthma, or chronic lung disease
Enlarged prostate
Gallbladder disease or gallstones
Heart disease
Kidney or lifer disease
Underactive thyroid

Treatment
This medication is used to relieve pain or to suppress coughing. Narcotic analgesics act in the central nervous system; some of their side effects are also caused by actions in the central nervous system.
- If you are taking this medication on a regular schedule and you miss a dose, take the missed dose as soon as possible, unless it is almost time for your next dose. In that case do not take the missed dose at all.
- If a narcotic analgesic is used for a long time, it may become habit-forming (causing mental or physical dependence). Physical dependence may lead to withdrawal side effects when you stop taking this medicine.
Unless otherwise directed by your doctor or pharmacist take this as directed. Do not take more of them and do not take them more often than recommended on the label. Children up to 12 years of age should not take this medicine more than 3 times a day or for more than 5 days in a row.

Side effects
Along with the needed effects, a medicine may cause some unwanted effects. These side effects may go away during treatment as your body adjusts to the medicine. Such minor side effects are: constipation, dizziness, drowsiness, dry mouth, false sense of well-being, flushing, light-headedness, loss or appetite, nausea, painful or difficult urination, or sweating.
- Check with your doctor immediately if any of the following side effects occur:
Anxiety or breathing difficulties
Excitation or restlessness
Fatigue, palpitations
Rash, sore throat and fever
Tremors or weakness

Interactions
This medicine may interact with several other drugs such as medicines acting on the central nervous system (e.g., antidepressants, tranquilizers), cimetidine, nitrates, quinidine, etc.
- Be sure to tell your doctor about any medications you are currently taking.

Storage
Tablets, elixir, suppository etc. should be stored at room temperature in a tightly closed, light-resistant container.

STATOBEX

Properties
This medicine contains phendimetrazine as active ingredient; it is prescribed for appetite suppression.
Appetite suppressants are used in the short-term (a few weeks) treatment of obesity. In a few weeks (6 to 12), these medicines in combination with dieting, exercise, and changes in eating habits can help patients lose weight. However, since their appetite reducing effect is only temporary, they are useful only for the first weeks of dieting until new eating habits are established.

Before using this medicine
Before you use this medicine check with your doctor, or pharmacist:
- if you ever had any unusual or allergic reaction to any of the compounds of this medicine.
- if you are on a low-salt, low-sugar, or any other special diet, or if you are allergic to any substance, such as sulfites or other preservatives or dyes.
- if you are pregnant, intend to become pregnant or breast-feeding an infant while using this medicine.
- if you have any of the following medical problems:
  Diabetes mellitus (sugar diabetes)
  Epilepsy
  Glaucoma
  Heart or blood vessel disease
  High blood pressure
  Mental illness (severe)

Treatment
This medication is used to relieve or prevent the symptoms of your medical problem. Take them as directed. Do not take more of them and do not take them more often than recommended on the label. If too much of the drug is taken, it may become habit-forming.
The medicine produces central nervous system stimulation, and it should not be taken by people with heart disease or high blood pressure.
If you think this medicine is not working as well after you have taken it for a few weeks, do not increase the dose. Instead, check with your doctor.

Side effects
The following minor side effects may occur: irritability, nervousness, restlessness, trouble in sleeping.
These side effects should disappear as your body adjusts to the medication. Tell your doctor about any side effects that are persistent or particularly bothersome. It is especially important to tell your doctor about:
  Mental depression
  Nausea or vomiting
  Stomach cramps or pain
  Trembling
  Unusual tiredness or weakness
- Discontinue use of the drug; call your doctor right away. Adverse reactions and side effects may be more frequent and severe in people over age 60 than in younger persons.

Interactions
This medicine interacts with several other drugs such as antihypertensives, other appetite suppressants, caffeine, central nervous system depressants, central nervous system stimulants, furazolidone, guanethidine, hydralazine, MAO inhibitors, methyldopa, molindone, phenothiazines, rauwolfia alkaloids, sodium bicarbonate. Interaction with alcoholic beverages may produce drowsiness, sleepiness, and/or inability to concentrate.
- Be sure to tell your doctor about any medications you are currently taking.

Storage
This medicine should be stored at room temperature in tightly closed containers. Store away from heat and direct light. Keep out of reach of children, since overdose may be very dangerous in children.
Do not store this medicine in the bathroom medicine cabinet because the heat and moisture cause the medicine to break down. Do not keep outdated medicine or medicine no longer needed. Flush the contents of the container down the toilet.

STILPHOSTROL

Properties
This medicine contains diethylstilboestrol as active ingredient. The medicine is prescribed for treatment of estrogen deficiency; it restores normal estrogen levels in tissues. There is no evidence that this drug is effective for nervous symptoms or depression occurring during menopause. They should not be used to treat this condition; they should be used only to replace the estrogen that is naturally absent after menopause.

Before using this medicine
Before you use this medicine check with your doctor, or pharmacist:
- if you ever had any unusual or allergic reaction to estrogens;
- if you are pregnant or intend to become pregnant within three months;
- if you are breast-feeding an infant;
- if you have any of the following medical problems:
  Diabetes
  Breast cancer
  Fibrocystic breast disease
  Fibroid uterine tumors
  Endometriosis
  Migraine headaches
  Epilepsy
  Porphyria
  High blood pressure
  Asthma
  Congestive heart failure
  Kidney disease
  Gallstones

Treatment
This medication is used to treat estrogen deficiency, specific symptoms of menopause, estrogen-deficiency osteoporosis, atrophic vaginitis, prostate cancer.
For safe and effective use of this medicine:
- Follow your doctor's instructions if this medicine was prescribed.
- Follow the manufacturer's package directions if you are treating yourself.
- Estrogens have been reported to increase the risk of endometrial carcinoma.

Side effects
Along with the needed effects, a medicine may cause some unwanted effects. Possible side effects include:
  Stomach cramps
  Profuse bleeding
  Appetite loss
  Nausea and vomiting
  Swollen breasts
  Change in menstruation
  Rash, skin blisters
  Depression
  Dizziness

Overdose
The following symptoms may indicate an overdose:
  Nausea and vomiting
  Fluid retention
  Breast enlargement
  Abnormal vaginal bleeding
- Call a doctor or hospital emergency room for instructions.

Interactions
This medicine may interact with several other drugs such as adrenocorticosteroids, antidepressants, oral antidiabetics, insulin, phenobarbital, primidone.
- Be sure to tell your doctor about any medications you are currently taking.

Storage
Capsules, tablets, vaginal cream, transdermal patches, etc. should be stored at room temperature; store away from heat and direct light. Keep out of reach of children, since this medicine may be dangerous in children.

SULAR

Properties
This medicine contains nisoldipine as active ingredient. It is a so-called calcium channel blocker, working by blocking the passage of calcium into heart and smooth muscle. Since calcium is an essential factor in muscle contraction, any medicine that affects calcium in this way will interfere with the contraction of these muscles.

The medicine works by:
◆ reducing the work that the heart must perform;
◆ reducing the normal arterial blood pressure;
◆ increasing oxygen to the heart muscle.

The medicine is prescribed for the treatment of attacks of angina pectoris, irregular heartbeat, and high blood pressure. In many cases it can be used for the treatment and prevention of migraine.

Before using this medicine
Before you use this medicine check with your doctor, or pharmacist:
– if you ever had any unusual or allergic reaction to this medicine or any calcium channel blocker;
– if you are pregnant or intend to become pregnant while using this medicine;
– if you have low blood pressure;
– if you have kidney or lifer disease;
– if you are breast-feeding an infant;
– if you easily get a rash or intensity sunburn in areas exposed to sun or ultraviolet light.

Treatment
This medication is used for treatment of heart conditions (for instance, angina pectoris) and high blood pressure. Tablets, capsules or extended-release tablets should be taken with liquid. The usual dose amounts to 30 to 100 milligrams a day.

For safe and effective use of medicine:
◆ Follow your doctor's instructions if this medicine was prescribed.
◆ Follow the manufacturer's package directions if you are treating yourself.

Side effects
Along with the needed effects, a medicine may cause some unwanted effects. Possible side effects include:
Tiredness
Changes in heartbeat
Wheezing
Cough
Shortness of breath
Dizziness
Fainting
Numbness in hands and feet
Tingling in hands and feet
Difficult urination
Constipation

Overdose
The following symptoms may be a sign of overdose:
Unusually fast heartbeat
Unusually slow heartbeat
Loss of consciousness
Cardiac arrest
■ Call a doctor or hospital emergency room for instructions. If necessary start first aid immediately.

Interactions
The effect of this medicine may cause a blood pressure drop if taken together with antihypertensives. Cimetidine may increase the effect of the calcium blocker.

The simultaneous use of diuretics and calcium channel blockers may cause dangerous blood pressure drop.
■ Be sure to tell your doctor about any medications you are currently taking.

Storage
Capsules, tablets, etc. should be stored at room temperature; store away from heat and direct light. Keep out of reach of children, since this medicine may be dangerous in children.

SULFACYTINE

Properties
This medicine contains sulfacytine, a sulfonamide, as active ingredient. Sulfonamides are prescribed to treat infections caused by bacteria. They will not work for colds, flu, or other virus infections.

Before using this medicine
Before you use this medicine check with your doctor:
- if you ever had any unusual or allergic reaction to any of the compounds of the medicine.
- if you are on a low-salt, low-sugar, or any other special diet, or if you are allergic to any substance, such as sulfites or other preservatives or dyes.
- if you are pregnant or intend to become pregnant while using this medicine. Although sulfonamides have not been shown to cause defects in humans, the chance may exists.
- if you are breast-feeding an infant. Most sulfonamides pass into the breast milk in small amounts and may cause unwanted effects in infants with some specific conditions.
- if you have any of the following medical problems:
  Kidney disease
  Liver disease
  Porphyria
  Deficiency of enzymes such as G6PD

Treatment
This medication is used to treat an infection caused by bacteria. Most sulfonamides are best taken with a full glass (8 ounces) of water on an empty stomach, either one hour before or two hours after a meal. Follow your doctor's or pharmacist's directions on how to take your medicine.
- Keep taking this medicine for the full time of treatment even if you begin to feel better after a few days; do not miss any doses.
- If you do miss a dose of this medicine, take the missed dose immediately.
- This medication works best when the level of medicine in your bloodstream (and urine) is kept constant. It is best, therefore, to take the doses at evenly spaced intervals day and night. if you take two doses a day, the doses should be spaced 12 hours apart.

Side effects
Along with the needed effects, a medicine may cause some unwanted effects. Side effects that usually do not require medical attention: abdominal pain, diarrhea, dizziness, headache, loss of appetite, nausea, sore mouth, or vomiting. These side effects should disappear as your body adjusts to the medication.

Sulfonamides can increase sensitivity to sunlight. It is, therefore, important to avoid prolonged exposure to sunlight and sunlamps.

Tell your doctor about any side effects that are persistent or particularly bothersome. It is especially important to tell your doctor about:
  Bloody urine
  Difficult or painful urination
  Difficulty in breathing
  Difficulty in swallowing
  Fever or hallucinations
  Itching, rash, or pale skin
  Joint pain, lower back pain
  Ringing in the ears
  Sore throat
  Swollen or inflamed tongue
  Tingling in hands or feet
  Unusual bleeding, bruising
  Yellowing of the eyes or skin

Interactions
This medicine may interact with several other drugs such as anticoagulants, oral antidiabetic agents, aspirin, some antibiotics, or anticancer drugs.
- Be sure to tell your doctor about any medications you are currently taking.

Storage
Tablets, capsules, suspension, etc. should be stored at room temperature as directed by your pharmacist or according to instructions on the label.

SULFADIAZINE

Properties
This medicine contains sulfadiazine, a sulfonamide, as active ingredient. Sulfonamides are prescribed to treat infections caused by bacteria. They will not work for colds, flu, or other virus infections.

Before using this medicine
Before you use this medicine check with your doctor:
- if you ever had any unusual or allergic reaction to any of the compounds of the medicine.
- if you are on a low-salt, low-sugar, or any other special diet, or if you are allergic to any substance, such as sulfites or other preservatives or dyes.
- if you are pregnant or intend to become pregnant while using this medicine. Although sulfonamides have not been shown to cause defects in humans, the chance may exists.
- if you are breast-feeding an infant. Most sulfonamides pass into the breast milk in small amounts and may cause unwanted effects in infants with some specific conditions.
- if you have any of the following medical problems:
Kidney disease
Liver disease
Porphyria
Deficiency of enzymes such as G6PD

Treatment
This medication is used to treat an infection caused by bacteria. Most sulfonamides are best taken with a full glass (8 ounces) of water on an empty stomach, either one hour before or two hours after a meal. Follow your doctor's or pharmacist's directions on how to take your medicine.
- Keep taking this medicine for the full time of treatment even if you begin to feel better after a few days; do not miss any doses.
- If you do miss a dose of this medicine, take the missed dose immediately.
- This medication works best when the level of medicine in your bloodstream (and urine) is kept constant. It is best, therefore, to take the doses at evenly spaced intervals day and night. if you take two doses a day, the doses should be spaced 12 hours apart.

Side effects
Along with the needed effects, a medicine may cause some unwanted effects. Side effects that usually do not require medical attention: abdominal pain, diarrhea, dizziness, headache, loss of appetite, nausea, sore mouth, or vomiting. These side effects should disappear as your body adjusts to the medication.
Sulfonamides can increase sensitivity to sunlight. It is, therefore, important to avoid prolonged exposure to sunlight and sunlamps.
Tell your doctor about any side effects that are persistent or particularly bothersome. It is especially important to tell your doctor about:
Bloody urine
Difficult urination
Difficulty in breathing
Difficulty in swallowing
Fever or hallucinations
Itching, rash, or pale skin
Joint pain, lower back pain
Ringing in the ears
Sore throat
Swollen or inflamed tongue
Tingling in hands or feet
Unusual bleeding
Yellowing of the eyes or skin

Interactions
This medicine may interact with several other drugs such as anticoagulants, oral antidiabetic agents, aspirin, some antibiotics, or anticancer drugs.
- Be sure to tell your doctor about any medications you are currently taking.

Storage
Tablets, capsules, suspension, etc. should be stored at room temperature as directed by your pharmacist or according to instructions on the label.

SULFAFURAZOLE

Properties

This medicine contains sulfixazole, a sulfonamide, as active ingredient. Sulfonamides are prescribed to treat infections caused by bacteria. They will not work for colds, flu, or other virus infections.

Before using this medicine

Before you use this medicine check with your doctor:
- if you ever had any unusual or allergic reaction to any of the compounds of the medicine.
- if you are on a low-salt, low-sugar, or any other special diet, or if you are allergic to any substance, such as sulfites or other preservatives or dyes.
- if you are pregnant or intend to become pregnant while using this medicine. Although sulfonamides have not been shown to cause defects in humans, the chance may exists.
- if you are breast-feeding an infant. Most sulfonamides pass into the breast milk in small amounts and may cause unwanted effects in infants with some specific conditions.
- if you have any of the following medical problems:
Kidney disease
Liver disease
Porphyria
Deficiency of enzymes such as G6PD

Treatment

This medication is used to treat an infection caused by bacteria. Most sulfonamides are best taken with a full glass (8 ounces) of water on an empty stomach, either one hour before or two hours after a meal. Follow your doctor's or pharmacist's directions on how to take your medicine.
- Keep taking this medicine for the full time of treatment even if you begin to feel better after a few days; do not miss any doses.
- If you do miss a dose of this medicine, take the missed dose immediately.
- This medication works best when the level of medicine in your bloodstream (and urine) is kept constant. It is best, therefore, to take the doses at evenly spaced intervals day and night. if you take two doses a day, the doses should be spaced 12 hours apart.

Side effects

Along with the needed effects, a medicine may cause some unwanted effects. Side effects that usually do not require medical attention: abdominal pain, diarrhea, dizziness, headache, loss of appetite, nausea, sore mouth, or vomiting. These side effects should disappear as your body adjusts to the medication.
Sulfonamides can increase sensitivity to sunlight. It is, therefore, important to avoid prolonged exposure to sunlight and sunlamps.

Tell your doctor about any side effects that are persistent or particularly bothersome. It is especially important to tell your doctor about:
Bloody urine
Difficult urination
Difficulty in breathing
Difficulty in swallowing
Fever or hallucinations
Itching, rash, or pale skin
Joint pain, lower back pain
Ringing in the ears
Sore throat
Swollen or inflamed tongue
Tingling in hands or feet
Unusual bleeding
Yellowing of the eyes or skin

Interactions

This medicine may interact with several other drugs such as anticoagulants, oral antidiabetic agents, aspirin, some antibiotics, or anticancer drugs.
- Be sure to tell your doctor about any medications you are currently taking.

Storage

Tablets, capsules, suspension, etc. should be stored at room temperature as directed by your pharmacist or according to instructions on the label.

SULFAMETHIAZOLE

Properties

This medicine contains sulfamethiazole, a sulfonamide, as active ingredient. Sulfonamides are prescribed to treat infections caused by bacteria. They will not work for colds, flu, or other virus infections.

Before using this medicine

Before you use this medicine check with your doctor:

– if you ever had any unusual or allergic reaction to any of the compounds of the medicine.
– if you are on a low-salt, low-sugar, or any other special diet, or if you are allergic to any substance, such as sulfites or other preservatives or dyes.
– if you are pregnant or intend to become pregnant while using this medicine. Although sulfonamides have not been shown to cause defects in humans, the chance may exists.
– if you are breast-feeding an infant. Most sulfonamides pass into the breast milk in small amounts and may cause unwanted effects in infants with some specific conditions.
– if you have any of the following medical problems:
Kidney disease
Liver disease
Porphyria
Deficiency of enzymes such as G6PD

Treatment

This medication is used to treat an infection caused by bacteria. Most sulfonamides are best taken with a full glass (8 ounces) of water on an empty stomach, either one hour before or two hours after a meal. Follow your doctor's or pharmacist's directions on how to take your medicine.

■ Keep taking this medicine for the full time of treatment even if you begin to feel better after a few days; do not miss any doses.
■ If you do miss a dose of this medicine, take the missed dose immediately.
■ This medication works best when the level of medicine in your bloodstream (and urine) is kept constant. It is best, therefore, to take the doses at evenly spaced intervals day and night. if you take two doses a day, the doses should be spaced 12 hours apart.

Side effects

Along with the needed effects, a medicine may cause some unwanted effects. Side effects that usually do not require medical attention: abdominal pain, diarrhea, dizziness, headache, loss of appetite, nausea, sore mouth, or vomiting. These side effects should disappear as your body adjusts to the medication.

Sulfonamides can increase sensitivity to sunlight. It is, therefore, important to avoid prolonged exposure to sunlight and sunlamps.

Tell your doctor about any side effects that are persistent or particularly bothersome. It is especially important to tell your doctor about:
Bloody urine
Difficult urination
Difficulty in breathing
Difficulty in swallowing
Fever or hallucinations
Itching, rash, or pale skin
Joint pain, lower back pain
Ringing in the ears
Sore throat
Swollen or inflamed tongue
Tingling in hands or feet
Unusual bleeding
Yellowing of the eyes or skin

Interactions

This medicine may interact with several other drugs such as anticoagulants, oral antidiabetic agents, aspirin, some antibiotics, or anticancer drugs.
■ Be sure to tell your doctor about any medications you are currently taking.

Storage

Tablets, capsules, suspension, etc. should be stored at room temperature as directed by your pharmacist or according to instructions on the label.

SULFAMETHOXAZOLE

Properties
This medicine contains sulfamethoxazole, a sulfonamide, as active ingredient. Sulfonamides are prescribed to treat infections caused by bacteria. They will not work for colds, flu, or other virus infections.

Before using this medicine
Before you use this medicine check with your doctor:
- if you ever had any unusual or allergic reaction to any of the compounds of the medicine.
- if you are on a low-salt, low-sugar, or any other special diet, or if you are allergic to any substance, such as sulfites or other preservatives or dyes.
- if you are pregnant or intend to become pregnant while using this medicine. Although sulfonamides have not been shown to cause defects in humans, the chance may exists.
- if you are breast-feeding an infant. Most sulfonamides pass into the breast milk in small amounts and may cause unwanted effects in infants with some specific conditions.
- if you have any of the following medical problems:
Kidney disease
Liver disease
Porphyria
Deficiency of enzymes such as G6PD

Treatment
This medication is used to treat an infection caused by bacteria. Most sulfonamides are best taken with a full glass (8 ounces) of water on an empty stomach, either one hour before or two hours after a meal. Follow your doctor's or pharmacist's directions on how to take your medicine.
- Keep taking this medicine for the full time of treatment even if you begin to feel better after a few days; do not miss any doses.
- If you do miss a dose of this medicine, take the missed dose immediately.
- This medication works best when the level of medicine in your bloodstream (and urine) is kept constant. It is best, therefore, to take the doses at evenly spaced intervals day and night. if you take two doses a day, the doses should be spaced 12 hours apart.

Side effects
Along with the needed effects, a medicine may cause some unwanted effects. Side effects that usually do not require medical attention: abdominal pain, diarrhea, dizziness, headache, loss of appetite, nausea, sore mouth, or vomiting. These side effects should disappear as your body adjusts to the medication.

Sulfonamides can increase sensitivity to sunlight. It is, therefore, important to avoid prolonged exposure to sunlight and sunlamps.

Tell your doctor about any side effects that are persistent or particularly bothersome. It is especially important to tell your doctor about:
Bloody urine
Difficult urination
Difficulty in breathing
Difficulty in swallowing
Fever or hallucinations
Itching, rash, or pale skin
Joint pain, lower back pain
Ringing in the ears
Sore throat
Swollen or inflamed tongue
Tingling in hands or feet
Unusual bleeding, bruising
Yellowing of the eyes or skin

Interactions
This medicine may interact with several other drugs such as anticoagulants, oral antidiabetic agents, aspirin, some antibiotics, or anticancer drugs.
- Be sure to tell your doctor about any medications you are currently taking.

Storage
Tablets, capsules, suspension, etc. should be stored at room temperature as directed by your pharmacist or according to instructions on the label.

SULFASIN

Properties
This medicine contains sulfisoxasole, a sulfonamide, as active ingredient. Sulfonamides are prescribed to treat infections caused by bacteria. They will not work for colds, flu, or other virus infections.

Before using this medicine
Before you use this medicine check with your doctor:
- if you ever had any unusual or allergic reaction to any of the compounds of the medicine.
- if you are on a low-salt, low-sugar, or any other special diet, or if you are allergic to any substance, such as sulfites or other preservatives or dyes.
- if you are pregnant or intend to become pregnant while using this medicine. Although sulfonamides have not been shown to cause defects in humans, the chance may exists.
- if you are breast-feeding an infant. Most sulfonamides pass into the breast milk in small amounts and may cause unwanted effects in infants with some specific conditions.
- if you have any of the following medical problems:
  Kidney disease
  Liver disease
  Porphyria
  Deficiency of enzymes such as G6PD

Treatment
This medication is used to treat an infection caused by bacteria. Most sulfonamides are best taken with a full glass (8 ounces) of water on an empty stomach, either one hour before or two hours after a meal. Follow your doctor's or pharmacist's directions on how to take your medicine.
- Keep taking this medicine for the full time of treatment even if you begin to feel better after a few days; do not miss any doses.
- If you do miss a dose of this medicine, take the missed dose immediately.
- This medication works best when the level of medicine in your bloodstream (and urine) is kept constant. It is best, therefore, to take the doses at evenly spaced intervals day and night. if you take two doses a day, the doses should be spaced 12 hours apart.

Side effects
Along with the needed effects, a medicine may cause some unwanted effects. Side effects that usually do not require medical attention: abdominal pain, diarrhea, dizziness, headache, loss of appetite, nausea, sore mouth, or vomiting. These side effects should disappear as your body adjusts to the medication.
Sulfonamides can increase sensitivity to sunlight. It is, therefore, important to avoid prolonged exposure to sunlight and sunlamps.

Tell your doctor about any side effects that are persistent or particularly bothersome. It is especially important to tell your doctor about:
  Bloody urine
  Difficult urination
  Difficulty in breathing
  Difficulty in swallowing
  Fever or hallucinations
  Itching, rash, or pale skin
  Joint pain, lower back pain
  Ringing in the ears
  Sore throat
  Swollen or inflamed tongue
  Tingling in hands or feet
  Unusual bleeding
  Yellowing of the eyes or skin

Interactions
This medicine may interact with several other drugs such as anticoagulants, oral antidiabetic agents, aspirin, some antibiotics, or anticancer drugs.
- Be sure to tell your doctor about any medications you are currently taking.

Storage
Tablets, capsules, suspension, etc. should be stored at room temperature as directed by your pharmacist or according to instructions on the label.

SULFISOXASOLE

Properties
This medicine contains sulfisoxasole, a sulfonamide, as active ingredient. Sulfonamides are prescribed to treat infections caused by bacteria. They will not work for colds, flu, or other virus infections.

Before using this medicine
Before you use this medicine check with your doctor:
- if you ever had any unusual or allergic reaction to any of the compounds of the medicine.
- if you are on a low-salt, low-sugar, or any other special diet, or if you are allergic to any substance, such as sulfites or other preservatives or dyes.
- if you are pregnant or intend to become pregnant while using this medicine. Although sulfonamides have not been shown to cause defects in humans, the chance may exists.
- if you are breast-feeding an infant. Most sulfonamides pass into the breast milk in small amounts and may cause unwanted effects in infants with some specific conditions.
- if you have any of the following medical problems:
Kidney disease
Liver disease
Porphyria
Deficiency of enzymes such as G6PD

Treatment
This medication is used to treat an infection caused by bacteria. Most sulfonamides are best taken with a full glass (8 ounces) of water on an empty stomach, either one hour before or two hours after a meal. Follow your doctor's or pharmacist's directions on how to take your medicine.
- Keep taking this medicine for the full time of treatment even if you begin to feel better after a few days; do not miss any doses.
- If you do miss a dose of this medicine, take the missed dose immediately.
- This medication works best when the level of medicine in your bloodstream (and urine) is kept constant. It is best, therefore, to take the doses at evenly spaced intervals day and night. if you take two doses a day, the doses should be spaced 12 hours apart.

Side effects
Along with the needed effects, a medicine may cause some unwanted effects. Side effects that usually do not require medical attention: abdominal pain, diarrhea, dizziness, headache, loss of appetite, nausea, sore mouth, or vomiting. These side effects should disappear as your body adjusts to the medication.
Sulfonamides can increase sensitivity to sunlight. It is, therefore, important to avoid prolonged exposure to sunlight and sunlamps.

Tell your doctor about any side effects that are persistent or particularly bothersome. It is especially important to tell your doctor about:
Bloody urine
Difficult urination
Difficulty in breathing
Difficulty in swallowing
Fever or hallucinations
Itching, rash, or pale skin
Joint pain, lower back pain
Ringing in the ears
Sore throat
Swollen or inflamed tongue
Tingling in hands or feet
Unusual bleeding
Yellowing of the eyes or skin

Interactions
This medicine may interact with several other drugs such as anticoagulants, oral antidiabetic agents, aspirin, some antibiotics, or anticancer drugs.
- Be sure to tell your doctor about any medications you are currently taking.

Storage
Tablets, capsules, suspension, etc. should be stored at room temperature as directed by your pharmacist or according to instructions on the label.

SUPRAX

Properties

This medicine contains cephalosporin as active ingredient. Cephalosporins belong to the general family of medicines called antibiotics, used in the treatment of infections caused by bacteria. They work by killing bacteria or preventing their growth. Cephalosporins will not work for colds, flu, or other viral infections.

Before using this medicine

Before you use this medicine check with your doctor:

- if you ever had any unusual or allergic reaction to any of the cephalosporins, penicillins, penicillin-like medicines, or penicillamine.
- if you are on a low-salt, low-sugar, or any other special diet, or if you are allergic to any substance, such as sulfites or other preservatives or dyes.
- if you are pregnant or intend to become pregnant while using this medicine. Although cephalosporins have not been shown to cause birth defects or other problems in humans, the chance always exists.
- if you are breast-feeding an infant. Most cephalosporins pass into the breast milk, usually in small amounts.
- if you have any of the following medical problems:
  Bleeding problem
  Kidney or lifer disease

Treatment

This medication belongs to the general family of medicines called antibiotics. It is used to treat a wide variety of bacterial infections. It is also used to treat infections in persons who are allergic to penicillin.

- Keep taking this medicine for the full time of treatment even if you begin to feel better after a few days; do not miss any doses.
- If you do miss a dose of this medicine, take it as soon as possible. This will help to keep a constant amount of medicine in the blood. However, if it is almost time for your next dose, skip the missed dose and go back to your regular dosing schedule.
- This medication has been prescribed for your current infection only. Another infection later on, or one that someone else has, may require a different medicine. You should not give your medicine to other people or use it for other infections, unless your doctor specifically directs you to do so.
- Take the medicine at the same times each day, 1 hour before or 2 hours after eating.

Side effects

Along with the needed effects, a medicine may cause some unwanted effects. Side effects that usually do not require medical attention: rectal itching, oral or vaginal white spots, mild diarrhea. These side effects should disappear as your body adjusts to the medication.

- Other side effects that should be reported to your doctor immediately are:
  Hives, rash
  Intense itching
  Faintness soon after a dose
  Difficulty in breathing
  Nausea and vomiting
  Severe diarrhea
  Unusual weakness or tiredness
  Bleeding or bruising

Interactions

This medicine may interact with several other drugs such as anticoagulants, theophylline preparations, probenecid, tetracyclines, etc.

- Be sure to tell your doctor about any medications you are currently taking.

Storage

Tablets, capsules, etc. should be stored at room temperature. Store the liquid form in the refrigerator. Keep out of the reach of children. Do not keep outdated medicine or medicine no longer needed.

SUSTAIRE

Properties
This medicine contains theophylline as active ingredient; it is used to treat or prevent breathing problems (wheezing and shortness of breath) caused by asthma, bronchitis, or emphysema. This medication belongs to a group known as xanthine-derivative bronchodilators. They work by opening up the bronchial tubes or air passages of the lungs and increasing the flow of air through them. These medicines are available only with your doctor's prescription.

Before using this medicine
Before you use this medicine check with your doctor, or pharmacist:
- if you ever had any unusual or allergic reaction to xanthine-derivative bronchodilators.
- if you are on a low-salt, low-sugar, or any other special diet, or if you are allergic to any substance, such as sulfites or other preservatives or dyes.
- if you are pregnant or intend to become pregnant while using this medicine.
- if you are breast-feeding an infant. Theophylline passes into the breast milk and may cause irritability, fretfulness, or trouble in sleeping in infants of mothers taking this medicine.
- if you have any of the following medical problems:
Diarrhea
Enlarged prostate
Fibrocystic breast disease
Heart disease
Stomach ulcer

Treatment
This medication is used to relieve or prevent the symptoms of your medical problem. Take them as directed. Do not take more of them and do not take them more often than recommended on the label, unless otherwise directed by your doctor. To do so may increase the chance of side effects. The medicine should be taken on an empty stomach 30 to 60 minutes before a meal or two hours after a meal. Try not to miss any doses of this medication. If you do miss a dose, take the missed dose as soon as possible, unless it is almost time for the next dose. Do not double the next dose. It works best when taken with a glass of water.

Side effects
The following minor side effects may occur:
Dizziness Or Flushing
Headache
Diarrhea
Heartburn
Increased Urination
Insomnia
Nervousness Or Irritability
Loss Of Appetite
Nausea Or Stomach Upset
Stomach Pain.
These side effects should disappear as your body adjusts to the medication. Tell your doctor about any side effects that are persistent or particularly bothersome. It is especially important to tell your doctor about black, tarry stools; confusion; convulsions; difficulty in breathing; fainting; muscle twitching; palpitations; rash; severe abdominal pain; or unusual weakness.

Interactions
This medicine interacts with several other drugs such as diuretics, reserpine, beta blockers, phenytoin, lithium, phenobarbital, birth control pills, and other medications.
- Be sure to tell your doctor about any medications you are currently taking.

Storage
Tablets, capsules, liquid and suspension should be stored at room temperature in tightly closed containers. Store away from heat and direct light. Keep out of reach of children, since overdose may be very dangerous in children. Discard any outdated medication.

SYMPHASIC

Properties

This medicine contains norethindrone and ethinyl estradiol as active ingredients. It is an oral contraceptive prescribed to prevent pregnancy and/or to regulate menstrual periods.

The drug works by altering the mucus at the cervix entrance to prevent the entry of sperm. It also alters the uterus lining to resist implantation of the fertilized egg. Oral contraceptives create the same chemical atmosphere in blood that exists during pregnancy.

Before using this medicine

Before you use this medicine check with your doctor, or pharmacist:
- if you ever had any unusual or allergic reaction to estrogens or progestogen;
- if you are pregnant or want to become pregnant within three months;
- if you are breast-feeding an infant;
- if you have any of the following medical problems:
  Diabetes
  Ailments of the breast
  Disorders of the uterus
  Migraine or epilepsy
  High blood pressure
  Asthma or heart conditions
  Kidney disease
  Gallstones

Treatment

This medication is used to prevent pregnancy or to regulate menstrual periods.

Adverse reactions

Along with the needed effects, a medicine may cause some unwanted effects or adverse reactions.
- *An increased risk of the following adverse reactions has been associated with the use of oral contraceptives:*
  Thrombophlebitis
  Venous thrombosis
  Arterial thromboembolism
  Pulmonary (lung) embolism
  Myocardial infarction
  Cerebral hemorrhage
  Cerebral thrombosis
  Hypertension
  Gallbladder disease
  Hepatic (liver) hepatomas
  Benign lifer tumors
- *The following adverse reactions have been reported in patients receiving oral contraceptives and are believed to be drug-related:*
  Nausea and vomiting
  Abdominal cramps
  Breakthrough bleeding
  Spotting
  Change in menstrual flow
  Amenorrhea
  Temporary infertility
  Edema
  Breast changes
  Weight changes
  Cholestatic jaundice
  Migraine
  Rash (allergic)
  Mental depression
  Vaginal candidiasis

Interactions

This medicine may interact with several other drugs such as antibiotics, anticoagulants, anticonvulsants, antidepressants, oral antidiabetics, antihistamines, barbiturates, oral hypoglycemics, insulin, meperidine.
- Be sure to tell your doctor about any medications you are currently taking.

Storage

Tablets should be stored at room temperature; store away from heat and direct light. Keep out of reach of children, since this medicine may be dangerous in children.

SYN-DILTIAZEM

Properties
This medicine contains diltiazem as active ingredient. It is a so-called calcium channel blocker, working by blocking the passage of calcium into heart and smooth muscle. Since calcium is an essential factor in muscle contraction, any medicine that affects calcium in this way will interfere with the contraction of these muscles.

The medicine works by:
♦ reducing the work that the heart must perform;
♦ reducing the normal arterial blood pressure;
♦ increasing oxygen to the heart muscle.

The medicine is prescribed for the treatment of attacks of angina pectoris, irregular heartbeat, and high blood pressure. In many cases it can be used for the treatment and prevention of migraine.

Before using this medicine
Before you use this medicine check with your doctor, or pharmacist:
- if you ever had any unusual or allergic reaction to this medicine or any calcium channel blocker;
- if you are pregnant or intend to become pregnant while using this medicine;
- if you have low blood pressure;
- if you have kidney or lifer disease;
- if you are breast-feeding an infant;
- if you easily get a rash or intensity sunburn in areas exposed to sun or ultraviolet light.

Treatment
This medication is used for treatment of heart conditions (for instance, angina pectoris) and high blood pressure. Tablets, capsules or extended-release tablets should be taken with liquid. The usual dose amounts to 30 to 100 milligrams a day.

For safe and effective use of medicine:
♦ Follow your doctor's instructions if this medicine was prescribed.
♦ Follow the manufacturer's package directions if you are treating yourself.

Side effects
Along with the needed effects, a medicine may cause some unwanted effects. Possible side effects include:
Tiredness
Changes in heartbeat
Wheezing
Cough
Shortness of breath
Dizziness
Fainting
Numbness in hands and feet
Tingling in hands and feet
Difficult urination
Constipation

Overdose
The following symptoms may be a sign of overdose:
Unusually fast heartbeat
Unusually slow heartbeat
Loss of consciousness
Cardiac arrest
■ Call a doctor or hospital emergency room for instructions. If necessary start first aid immediately.

Interactions
The effect of this medicine may cause a blood pressure drop if taken together with antihypertensives. Cimetidine may increase the effect of the calcium blocker.

The simultaneous use of diuretics and calcium channel blockers may cause dangerous blood pressure drop.
■ Be sure to tell your doctor about any medications you are currently taking.

Storage
Capsules, tablets, etc. should be stored at room temperature; store away from heat and direct light. Keep out of reach of children, since this medicine may be dangerous in children.

TACE

Properties
This medicine contains estrogen as active ingredient. The medicine is prescribed for treatment of estrogen deficiency; it restores normal estrogen levels in tissues. There is no evidence that this drug is effective for nervous symptoms or depression occurring during menopause. They should not be used to treat this condition; they should be used only to replace the estrogen that is naturally absent after menopause.

Before using this medicine
Before you use this medicine check with your doctor, or pharmacist:
- if you ever had any unusual or allergic reaction to estrogens;
- if you are pregnant or intend to become pregnant within three months;
- if you are breast-feeding an infant;
- if you have any of the following medical problems:
  Diabetes
  Breast cancer
  Fibrocystic breast disease
  Fibroid uterine tumors
  Endometriosis
  Migraine headaches
  Epilepsy
  Porphyria
  High blood pressure
  Asthma
  Congestive heart failure
  Kidney disease
  Gallstones

Treatment
This medication is used to treat estrogen deficiency, specific symptoms of menopause, estrogen-deficiency osteoporosis, atrophic vaginitis, prostate cancer.

For safe and effective use of this medicine:
- Follow your doctor's instructions if this medicine was prescribed.
- Follow the manufacturer's package directions if you are treating yourself.
- Estrogens have been reported to increase the risk of endometrial carcinoma.

Side effects
Along with the needed effects, a medicine may cause some unwanted effects. Possible side effects include:
  Stomach cramps
  Profuse bleeding
  Appetite loss
  Nausea and vomiting
  Swollen breasts
  Change in menstruation
  Rash, skin blisters
  Depression
  Dizziness

Overdose
The following symptoms may indicate an overdose:
  Nausea and vomiting
  Fluid retention
  Breast enlargement
  Abnormal vaginal bleeding
- Call a doctor or hospital emergency room for instructions.

Interactions
This medicine may interact with several other drugs such as adrenocorticosteroids, antidepressants, oral antidiabetics, insulin, phenobarbital, primidone.
- Be sure to tell your doctor about any medications you are currently taking.

Storage
Capsules, tablets, vaginal cream, transdermal patches, etc. should be stored at room temperature; store away from heat and direct light. Keep out of reach of children, since this medicine may be dangerous in children.

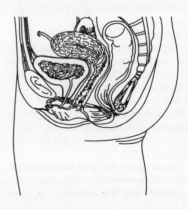

TALBUTAL

Properties
This medicine contains as active ingredient the barbiturate talbutal. Barbiturates belong to the group of medicines called central nervous system depressants (medicines that slow down the nervous system).

Barbiturates may partially block nerve impulses at nerve-cell connections. They may be used to treat insomnia (sleeplessness) by helping patients fall asleep. Also, they may be used to relieve anxiety or tension. Some of the barbiturates are used as anticonvulsants to help control convulsions in certain disorders or diseases, such as epilepsy. If too much of the drug is used, it may become habit-forming (causing mental or physical dependence).

Before using this medicine
Before you use this medicine check with your doctor, or pharmacist:
- if you ever had any unusual or allergic reaction to this medicine or one of its components.
- if you are on a low-salt, low-sugar, or any other special diet, or if you are allergic to preservatives or dyes.
- if you are pregnant or intend to become pregnant while using this medicine, since barbiturates have been shown to increase the chance of birth defects in humans. Taking barbiturates regularly during the last 3 months of pregnancy may cause the baby to become dependent on the medicine. This may lead to withdrawal side effects in the baby after birth.
- if you have any of the following medical problems:
  Anemia (severe)
  Diabetes mellitus (sugar disease)
  Hyperactivity (in children)
  Kidney or lifer disease
  Mental depression
  Overactive thyroid

Treatment
This medication is used to treat the symptoms of your medical condition. Barbiturates act in the central nervous system; some of their side effects are also caused by actions in the central nervous system. Use this medicine as directed by your doctor. Do not use more of it, do not use it more often, and do not use it for a longer period of time than your doctor ordered.
- If you are taking this medication on a regular schedule and you miss a dose, take the missed dose as soon as possible, unless it is almost time for your next dose. In that case do not take the missed dose at all.
- If a barbiturate is used for a long time, it may become habit-forming. Physical dependence may lead to withdrawal side effects when you stop taking this medicine.

Side effects
Along with the needed effects, a medicine may cause some unwanted effects. These side effects may go away during treatment as your body adjusts to the medicine. Such minor side effects are: depression, confusion, diarrhea, nausea, vomiting, joint or muscle pain, slurred speech, hallucinations, headache, decreased sex drive.
- Check with your doctor immediately if any of the following side effects occur:
  Rash or hives
  Face, lip or eyelid swelling
  Sore throat, fever
  Agitation
  Slow heartbeat
  Difficult breathing or chest pain

Interactions
This medicine may interact with several other drugs such as medicines acting on the central nervous system (e.g., antihistamines; beta-adrenergic blockers; MAO inhibitors; mind-altering drugs; nabilone; antidepressants; clozapine; anticonvulsants).

Storage
The medicine should be stored at room temperature in a tightly closed, light-resistant container. Keep out of reach of children since overdose is very dangerous in children.

TEMAZEPAM

Properties
This medicine contains as active ingredient temazepam, a benzodiazepine preparation. Benzodiazepines belong to the group of psychoactive medicines that influence the activity of the brain. Some are used to relieve nervousness or tension. It is effective for this purpose for short periods. Others are used for sleeplessness or to relax muscles or relieve muscle spasm. The benzodiazepines may also be used for other conditions as determined by your doctor.

Before using this medicine
Before you use this medicine check with your doctor:
- if you ever had any unusual or allergic reaction to benzodiazepines.
- if you are on a low-salt, low-sugar, or any other special diet, or if you are allergic to any substance, such as sulfites or other preservatives or dyes.
- if you are pregnant or intend to become pregnant while using this medicine. Some benzodiazepines have been reported to increase the chance of birth defects when used during the first 3 months of pregnancy.
- if you are breast-feeding an infant. Benzodiazepines may pass into the breast milk and cause drowsiness, unusually slow heartbeat, shortness of breath, or troubled breathing in infants of mothers taking this medicine.
- if you have any of the following medical problems: asthma, bronchitis, emphysema, or other chronic lung disease; epilepsy or history of convulsions; hyperactivity (in children); kidney or lifer disease; mental depression or illness; myasthania gravis, porphyria.

Treatment
This medication is used to relieve or prevent the symptoms of your medical problem. Benzodiazepines are mainly used as antianxiety agents, anticonvulsants, or sedatives. Take them as directed. Do not take more of them and do not take them more often than recommended on the label, unless otherwise directed by your doctor. Benzodiazepine tranquilizing drugs can be abused if taken for long periods of time and it is possible to develop withdrawal symptoms if you discontinue the therapy abruptly.

Side effects
Along with the needed effects, a medicine may cause some unwanted effects. Minor side effects are: bitter taste in the mouth, dizziness, drowsiness, depression, constipation, dry mouth, excessive salivation, fatigue, flushing, headache, heartburn, loss of appetite, nausea, nervousness, sweating or vomiting. As your body adjusts to the medicine, these side effects should disappear.
- Tell your doctor about any side effects that are persistent or particularly bothersome. It is especially important to tell your doctor about:
Blurred or double vision
Chest pain
Difficulty in urinating
Fainting or falling
Fever or hallucinations
Joint pain
Mouth sores
Nightmares
Palpitations
Severe depression
Shortness of breath
Slurred speech
Uncoordinated movements
Unusual tiredness
Yellowing of the skin

Interactions
This medicine may interact with several other drugs. This medicine will add to the effects of alcohol, and CNS depressants.
- Be sure to tell your doctor about any medications you are currently taking.

Storage
Store at room temperature in tightly closed, light-resistant-resistant containers. Keep out of the reach of children since overdose may be especially dangerous in children.

TENUATE

Properties

This medicine contains diethylpropion as active ingredient; it is prescribed for appetite suppression.

Appetite suppressants are used in the short-term (a few weeks) treatment of obesity. In a few weeks (6 to 12), these medicines in combination with dieting, exercise, and changes in eating habits can help patients lose weight. However, since their appetite reducing effect is only temporary, they are useful only for the first weeks of dieting until new eating habits are established.

Before using this medicine

Before you use this medicine check with your doctor, or pharmacist:

- if you ever had any unusual or allergic reaction to any of the compounds of this medicine.
- if you are on a low-salt, low-sugar, or any other special diet, or if you are allergic to any substance, such as sulfites or other preservatives or dyes.
- if you are pregnant, intend to become pregnant or breast-feeding an infant while using this medicine.
- if you have any of the following medical problems:
  Diabetes mellitus
  Epilepsy
  Glaucoma
  Heart disease
  High blood pressure
  Mental illness (severe)

Treatment

This medication is used to relieve or prevent the symptoms of your medical problem.

Take them as directed. Do not take more of them and do not take them more often than recommended on the label. If too much of the drug is taken, it may become habit-forming.

- The medicine produces central nervous system stimulation, and it should not be taken by people with heart disease or high blood pressure.
- If you think this medicine is not working as well after you have taken it for a few weeks, do not increase the dose. Instead, check with your doctor.

Side effects

The following minor side effects may occur: irritability, nervousness, restlessness, trouble in sleeping.

These side effects should disappear as your body adjusts to the medication. Tell your doctor about any side effects that are persistent or particularly bothersome. It is especially important to tell your doctor about:
  Mental depression
  Nausea or vomiting
  Stomach cramps or pain
  Trembling
  Unusual tiredness

- Discontinue use of the drug; call your doctor right away. Adverse reactions and side effects may be more frequent and severe in people over age 60 than in younger persons.

Interactions

This medicine interacts with several other drugs such as antihypertensives, other appetite suppressants, caffeine, central nervous system depressants, central nervous system stimulants, furazolidone, guanethidine, hydralazine, MAO inhibitors, methyldopa, molindone, phenothiazines, rauwolfia alkaloids, sodium bicarbonate.

- Be sure to tell your doctor about any medications you are currently taking. Interaction with alcoholic beverages may produce drowsiness, sleepiness, and/or inability to concentrate.

Storage

This medicine should be stored at room temperature in tightly closed containers. Store away from heat and direct light. Keep out of reach of children, since overdose may be very dangerous in children.

Do not store this medicine in the bathroom medicine cabinet because the heat and moisture cause the medicine to break down. Do not keep outdated medicine or medicine no longer needed. Flush the contents of the container down the toilet.

TEPANIL

Properties
This medicine contains diethylpropion as active ingredient; it is prescribed for appetite suppression.

Appetite suppressants are used in the short-term (a few weeks) treatment of obesity. In a few weeks (6 to 12), these medicines in combination with dieting, exercise, and changes in eating habits can help patients lose weight. However, since their appetite reducing effect is only temporary, they are useful only for the first weeks of dieting until new eating habits are established.

Before using this medicine
Before you use this medicine check with your doctor, or pharmacist:
- if you ever had any unusual or allergic reaction to any of the compounds of this medicine.
- if you are on a low-salt, low-sugar, or any other special diet, or if you are allergic to any substance, such as sulfites or other preservatives or dyes.
- if you are pregnant, intend to become pregnant or breast-feeding an infant while using this medicine.
- if you have any of the following medical problems:
  Diabetes mellitus
  Epilepsy
  Glaucoma
  Heart disease
  High blood pressure
  Mental illness (severe)

Treatment
This medication is used to relieve or prevent the symptoms of your medical problem. Take them as directed.

Do not take more of them and do not take them more often than recommended on the label. If too much of the drug is taken, it may become habit-forming.
- The medicine produces central nervous system stimulation, and it should not be taken by people with heart disease or high blood pressure.
- If you think this medicine is not working as well after you have taken it for a few weeks, do not increase the dose. Instead, check with your doctor.

Side effects
The following minor side effects may occur: irritability, nervousness, restlessness, trouble in sleeping.

These side effects should disappear as your body adjusts to the medication. Tell your doctor about any side effects that are persistent or particularly bothersome. It is especially important to tell your doctor about:
  Mental depression
  Nausea or vomiting
  Stomach cramps or pain
  Trembling
  Unusual tiredness
- Discontinue use of the drug; call your doctor right away. Adverse reactions and side effects may be more frequent and severe in people over age 60 than in younger persons.

Interactions
This medicine interacts with several other drugs such as antihypertensives, other appetite suppressants, caffeine, central nervous system depressants, central nervous system stimulants, furazolidone, guanethidine, hydralazine, MAO inhibitors, methyldopa, molindone, phenothiazines, rauwolfia alkaloids, sodium bicarbonate.
- Be sure to tell your doctor about any medications you are currently taking.
Interaction with alcoholic beverages may produce drowsiness, sleepiness, and/or inability to concentrate.

Storage
This medicine should be stored at room temperature in tightly closed containers. Store away from heat and direct light. Keep out of reach of children, since overdose may be very dangerous in children.

Do not store this medicine in the bathroom medicine cabinet because the heat and moisture cause the medicine to break down. Do not keep outdated medicine or medicine no longer needed. Flush the contents of the container down the toilet.

TERAMINE

Properties
This medicine contains phentermine as active ingredient; it is prescribed for appetite suppression.

Appetite suppressants are used in the short-term (a few weeks) treatment of obesity. In a few weeks (6 to 12), these medicines in combination with dieting, exercise, and changes in eating habits can help patients lose weight. However, since their appetite reducing effect is only temporary, they are useful only for the first weeks of dieting until new eating habits are established.

Before using this medicine
Before you use this medicine check with your doctor, or pharmacist:
- if you ever had any unusual or allergic reaction to any of the compounds of this medicine.
- if you are on a low-salt, low-sugar, or any other special diet, or if you are allergic to any substance, such as sulfites or other preservatives or dyes.
- if you are pregnant, intend to become pregnant or breast-feeding an infant while using this medicine.
- if you have any of the following medical problems:
  Diabetes mellitus
  Epilepsy
  Glaucoma
  Heart disease
  High blood pressure
  Mental illness (severe)

Treatment
This medication is used to relieve or prevent the symptoms of your medical problem.

Take them as directed. Do not take more of them and do not take them more often than recommended on the label. If too much of the drug is taken, it may become habit-forming.
- The medicine produces central nervous system stimulation, and it should not be taken by people with heart disease or high blood pressure.
- If you think this medicine is not working as well after you have taken it for a few weeks, do not increase the dose. Instead, check with your doctor.

Side effects
The following minor side effects may occur: irritability, nervousness, restlessness, trouble in sleeping.

These side effects should disappear as your body adjusts to the medication. Tell your doctor about any side effects that are persistent or particularly bothersome. It is especially important to tell your doctor about:
  Mental depression
  Nausea or vomiting
  Stomach cramps or pain
  Trembling
  Unusual tiredness
- Discontinue use of the drug; call your doctor right away. Adverse reactions and side effects may be more frequent and severe in people over age 60 than in younger persons.

Interactions
This medicine interacts with several other drugs such as antihypertensives, other appetite suppressants, caffeine, central nervous system depressants, central nervous system stimulants, furazolidone, guanethidine, hydralazine, MAO inhibitors, methyldopa, molindone, phenothiazines, rauwolfia alkaloids, sodium bicarbonate.
- Be sure to tell your doctor about any medications you are currently taking.
Interaction with alcoholic beverages may produce drowsiness, sleepiness, and/or inability to concentrate.

Storage
This medicine should be stored at room temperature in tightly closed containers. Store away from heat and direct light. Keep out of reach of children, since overdose may be very dangerous in children.

Do not store this medicine in the bathroom medicine cabinet because the heat and moisture cause the medicine to break down. Do not keep outdated medicine or medicine no longer needed. Flush the contents of the container down the toilet.

THEO-24

Properties
This medicine contains theophylline as active ingredient; it is used to treat or prevent breathing problems (wheezing and shortness of breath) caused by asthma, bronchitis, or emphysema. This medication belongs to a group known as xanthine-derivative bronchodilators. They work by opening up the bronchial tubes or air passages of the lungs and increasing the flow of air through them. These medicines are available only with your doctor's prescription.

Before using this medicine
Before you use this medicine check with your doctor, or pharmacist:
- if you ever had any unusual or allergic reaction to xanthine-derivative bronchodilators.
- if you are on a low-salt, low-sugar, or any other special diet, or if you are allergic to any substance, such as sulfites or other preservatives or dyes.
- if you are pregnant or intend to become pregnant while using this medicine.
- if you are breast-feeding an infant. Theophylline passes into the breast milk and may cause irritability, fretfulness, or trouble in sleeping in infants of mothers taking this medicine.
- if you have any of the following medical problems:
Diarrhea
Enlarged prostate
Fibrocystic breast disease
Heart disease
Stomach ulcer

Treatment
This medication is used to relieve or prevent the symptoms of your medical problem. Take them as directed. Do not take more of them and do not take them more often than recommended on the label, unless otherwise directed by your doctor. To do so may increase the chance of side effects. The medicine should be taken on an empty stomach 30 to 60 minutes before a meal or two hours after a meal. Try not to miss any doses of this medication. If you do miss a dose, take the missed dose as soon as possible, unless it is almost time for the next dose. Do not double the next dose. It works best when taken with a glass of water.

Side effects
The following minor side effects may occur:
Dizziness Or Flushing
Headache
Diarrhea
Heartburn
Increased Urination
Insomnia
Nervousness Or Irritability
Loss Of Appetite
Nausea Or Stomach Upset
Stomach Pain.
These side effects should disappear as your body adjusts to the medication. Tell your doctor about any side effects that are persistent or particularly bothersome. It is especially important to tell your doctor about black, tarry stools; confusion; convulsions; difficulty in breathing; fainting; muscle twitching; palpitations; rash; severe abdominal pain; or unusual weakness.

Interactions
This medicine interacts with several other drugs such as diuretics, reserpine, beta blockers, phenytoin, lithium, phenobarbital, birth control pills, and other medications.
- Be sure to tell your doctor about any medications you are currently taking.

Storage
Tablets, capsules, liquid and suspension should be stored at room temperature in tightly closed containers. Store away from heat and direct light. Keep out of reach of children, since overdose may be very dangerous in children. Discard any outdated medication.

THEOBID DURACAPS

Properties

This medicine contains theophylline as active ingredient; it is used to treat or prevent breathing problems (wheezing and shortness of breath) caused by asthma, bronchitis, or emphysema. This medication belongs to a group known as xanthine-derivative bronchodilators. They work by opening up the bronchial tubes or air passages of the lungs and increasing the flow of air through them. These medicines are available only with your doctor's prescription.

Before using this medicine

Before you use this medicine check with your doctor, or pharmacist:

- if you ever had any unusual or allergic reaction to xanthine-derivative bronchodilators.
- if you are on a low-salt, low-sugar, or any other special diet, or if you are allergic to any substance, such as sulfites or other preservatives or dyes.
- if you are pregnant or intend to become pregnant while using this medicine.
- if you are breast-feeding an infant. Theophylline passes into the breast milk and may cause irritability, fretfulness, or trouble in sleeping in infants of mothers taking this medicine.
- if you have any of the following medical problems:
Diarrhea
Enlarged prostate
Fibrocystic breast disease
Heart disease
Stomach ulcer

Treatment

This medication is used to relieve or prevent the symptoms of your medical problem. Take them as directed. Do not take more of them and do not take them more often than recommended on the label, unless otherwise directed by your doctor. To do so may increase the chance of side effects. The medicine should be taken on an empty stomach 30 to 60 minutes before a meal or two hours after a meal. Try not to miss any doses of this medication. If you do miss a dose, take the missed dose as soon as possible, unless it is almost time for the next dose. Do not double the next dose. It works best when taken with a glass of water.

Side effects

The following minor side effects may occur:

Dizziness Or Flushing
Headache
Diarrhea
Heartburn
Increased Urination
Insomnia
Nervousness Or Irritability
Loss Of Appetite
Nausea Or Stomach Upset
Stomach Pain.

These side effects should disappear as your body adjusts to the medication. Tell your doctor about any side effects that are persistent or particularly bothersome. It is especially important to tell your doctor about black, tarry stools; confusion; convulsions; difficulty in breathing; fainting; muscle twitching; palpitations; rash; severe abdominal pain; or unusual weakness.

Interactions

This medicine interacts with several other drugs such as diuretics, reserpine, beta blockers, phenytoin, lithium, phenobarbital, birth control pills, and other medications.

- Be sure to tell your doctor about any medications you are currently taking.

Storage

Tablets, capsules, liquid and suspension should be stored at room temperature in tightly closed containers. Store away from heat and direct light. Keep out of reach of children, since overdose may be very dangerous in children. Discard any outdated medication.

THIAZIDE

Properties
This medicine contains as active ingredient trichlormethiazide, a thiazide-like diuretic. Thiazide or thiazide-like diuretics are prescribed to treat high blood pressure (hypertension). They are also used to reduce fluid accumulation in the body caused by conditions such as heart failure, cirrhosis, kidney disease, and the long-term use of some medications. Thiazide diuretics may also be used for other conditions as determined by your doctor.

Before using this medicine
Before you use this medicine check with your doctor, or pharmacist:
- if you ever had any unusual or allergic reaction to sulfonamides (sulfa drugs) or any of the thiazide diuretics.
- if you are on a low-salt, low-sugar, or any other special diet, or if you are allergic to any substance, such as sulfites or other preservatives or dyes.
- if you are pregnant or intend to become pregnant while using this medicine. When this medicine is used during pregnancy, it may cause side effects including jaundice, blood problems, and low potassium in the newborn.
- if you are breast-feeding an infant. Although this medicine has not been shown to cause problems in humans, the chance always exists since thiazide diuretics pass into breast milk.
- if you have any of the following medical problems:
Diabetes
Gout
Kidney disease
Liver disease
Lupus erythematosus
Pancreas disease

Treatment
This medication is used to treat high blood pressure (hypertension) and also to help reduce the amount of water in the body by increasing the flow of urine. This medicine will not cure your high blood pressure but it does help control it. You must continue to take it - even if you feel well - if you expect to keep your blood pressure down. You may have to take high blood pressure medicine for the rest of your life.

Thiazide diuretics may cause an unusual feeling of tiredness when you begin to take them. You may also notice an increase in urine or in frequency of urination. To keep this from affecting sleep:
- if you are to take a single dose a day, take it in the morning after breakfast;
- if you are to take more than one dose, take the last one not later than 6 p.m.

Side effects
Along with the needed effects, a medicine may cause some unwanted effects. Side effects that usually do not require medical attention: decreased sexual ability; dizziness or lightheadedness when standing up; increased sensitivity of skin to sunlight; loss of appetite; upset stomach.
- Side effects that should be reported to your doctor: black, tarry stools; blood in urine or stools; cough or hoarseness; fever or chills; joint pain; lower back or side pains; painful or difficult urination; pinpoint red spots on skin; skin rash or hives; stomach pain (severe) with nausea; unusual bleeding or bruising; yellow eyes or skin. This medicine may cause a loss of potassium from your body. Signs of too much potassium loss are: dryness of mouth; increased thirst; mood changes; muscle cramps or pain; nausea or vomiting; unusual tiredness or weakness; weak or irregular heartbeat.

Interactions
This medicine may interact with several other drugs.
- Be sure to tell your doctor about any medications you are currently taking.

Storage
Store at room temperature in a tightly closed container.

THIORIDAZINE

Properties

This medicine contains as active ingredient thioridazine, a phenothiazine derivative. Phenothiazines are a family of medicines used to treat nervous, mental, and emotional conditions. Some are used to control anxiety, restlessness, nausea and vomiting, and severe hiccups. This medicine is available only with your doctor's prescription.

Before using this medicine

Before you use this medicine check with your doctor, or pharmacist:
- if you ever had any unusual or allergic reaction to phenothiazine medicines.
- if you are on a low-salt, low-sugar, or any other special diet, or if you are allergic to any substance, such as sulfites or other preservatives or dyes.
- if you are pregnant or intend to become pregnant while using this medicine. Although phenothiazines have not been shown to cause birth defects, some side effects such as jaundice and muscle tremors have occurred in a few newborns whose mothers received phenothiazines during pregnancy.
- if you are breast-feeding an infant. Although this medicine has not been shown to cause problems in humans but the chance does exist since some phenothiazines are known to pass into the breast milk.
- if you have any of the following medical problems:
  Alcoholism
  Blood disease
  Difficult urination
  Enlarged prostate
  Glaucoma
  Heart or blood vessel disease
  Liver or lung disease
  Parkinson's disease
  Stomach ulcers

Treatment

This medication is prescribed to treat the symptoms of certain types of mental illness or emotional problems. In order to avoid stomach irritation, you can take the tablet or capsule forms of this medication with a meal or with a glass of water or milk (unless your doctor or pharmacist directs you to do otherwise).

Side effects

Along with the needed effects, a medicine may cause some unwanted effects.
Minor side effects are: blurred vision, constipation, decreased sweating, diarrhea, dizziness, drooling, drowsiness, dry mouth, fatigue, jitteriness, menstrual irregularities, nasal congestion, restlessness, tremors, vomiting, or weight gain.
- Tell your doctor about any side effects that are persistent or particularly bothersome. It is especially important to tell your doctor about:
  Breast enlargement
  Chest pain or convulsions
  Darkened skin
  Difficulty in swallowing
  Fainting or fever
  Involuntary movements
  Palpitations or sleep disorders
  Rash or sore throat
  Uncoordinated movements
  Unusual bleeding or bruising
  Visual disturbances
  Yellowing of the eyes or skin

Interactions

This medicine may interact with several other drugs such as barbiturates, sleeping pills, narcotics, other tranquilizers, or any other medication that may produce a sedative effect. Avoid alcohol.

Storage

Store this medication as directed on the label. Keep out of the reach of children.

THIOSULFIDE

Properties
This medicine contains sulfamethiazole, a sulfonamide, as active ingredient. Sulfonamides are prescribed to treat infections caused by bacteria. They will not work for colds, flu, or other virus infections.

Before using this medicine
Before you use this medicine check with your doctor:
- if you ever had any unusual or allergic reaction to any of the compounds of the medicine.
- if you are on a low-salt, low-sugar, or any other special diet, or if you are allergic to any substance, such as sulfites or other preservatives or dyes.
- if you are pregnant or intend to become pregnant while using this medicine. Although sulfonamides have not been shown to cause defects in humans, the chance may exists.
- if you are breast-feeding an infant. Most sulfonamides pass into the breast milk in small amounts and may cause unwanted effects in infants with some specific conditions.
- if you have any of the following medical problems:
  Kidney disease
  Liver disease
  Porphyria
  Deficiency of enzymes such as G6PD

Treatment
This medication is used to treat an infection caused by bacteria. Most sulfonamides are best taken with a full glass (8 ounces) of water on an empty stomach, either one hour before or two hours after a meal. Follow your doctor's or pharmacist's directions on how to take your medicine.
- Keep taking this medicine for the full time of treatment even if you begin to feel better after a few days; do not miss any doses.
- If you do miss a dose of this medicine, take the missed dose immediately.
- This medication works best when the level of medicine in your bloodstream (and urine) is kept constant. It is best, therefore, to take the doses at evenly spaced intervals day and night. if you take two doses a day, the doses should be spaced 12 hours apart.

Side effects
Along with the needed effects, a medicine may cause some unwanted effects. Side effects that usually do not require medical attention: abdominal pain, diarrhea, dizziness, headache, loss of appetite, nausea, sore mouth, or vomiting. These side effects should disappear as your body adjusts to the medication.
Sulfonamides can increase sensitivity to sunlight. It is, therefore, important to avoid prolonged exposure to sunlight and sunlamps.

Tell your doctor about any side effects that are persistent or particularly bothersome. It is especially important to tell your doctor about:
Bloody urine
Difficult urination
Difficulty in breathing
Difficulty in swallowing
Fever or hallucinations
Itching, rash, or pale skin
Joint pain, lower back pain
Ringing in the ears
Sore throat
Swollen or inflamed tongue
Tingling in hands or feet
Unusual bleeding
Yellowing of the eyes or skin

Interactions
This medicine may interact with several other drugs such as anticoagulants, oral antidiabetic agents, aspirin, some antibiotics, or anticancer drugs.
- Be sure to tell your doctor about any medications you are currently taking.

Storage
Tablets, capsules, suspension, etc. should be stored at room temperature as directed by your pharmacist or according to instructions on the label.

THIOSULFIDE FORTE

Properties
This medicine contains sulfamethiazole, a sulfonamide, as active ingredient. Sulfonamides are prescribed to treat infections caused by bacteria. They will not work for colds, flu, or other virus infections.

Before using this medicine
Before you use this medicine check with your doctor:
- if you ever had any unusual or allergic reaction to any of the compounds of the medicine.
- if you are on a low-salt, low-sugar, or any other special diet, or if you are allergic to any substance, such as sulfites or other preservatives or dyes.
- if you are pregnant or intend to become pregnant while using this medicine. Although sulfonamides have not been shown to cause defects in humans, the chance may exists.
- if you are breast-feeding an infant. Most sulfonamides pass into the breast milk in small amounts and may cause unwanted effects in infants with some specific conditions.
- if you have any of the following medical problems:
Kidney disease
Liver disease
Porphyria
Deficiency of enzymes such as G6PD

Treatment
This medication is used to treat an infection caused by bacteria. Most sulfonamides are best taken with a full glass (8 ounces) of water on an empty stomach, either one hour before or two hours after a meal. Follow your doctor's or pharmacist's directions on how to take your medicine.
- Keep taking this medicine for the full time of treatment even if you begin to feel better after a few days; do not miss any doses.
- If you do miss a dose of this medicine, take the missed dose immediately.
- This medication works best when the level of medicine in your bloodstream (and urine) is kept constant. It is best, therefore, to take the doses at evenly spaced intervals day and night. if you take two doses a day, the doses should be spaced 12 hours apart.

Side effects
Along with the needed effects, a medicine may cause some unwanted effects. Side effects that usually do not require medical attention: abdominal pain, diarrhea, dizziness, headache, loss of appetite, nausea, sore mouth, or vomiting. These side effects should disappear as your body adjusts to the medication.
Sulfonamides can increase sensitivity to sunlight. It is, therefore, important to avoid prolonged exposure to sunlight and sunlamps.

Tell your doctor about any side effects that are persistent or particularly bothersome. It is especially important to tell your doctor about:
Bloody urine
Difficult urination
Difficulty in breathing
Difficulty in swallowing
Fever or hallucinations
Itching, rash, or pale skin
Joint pain, lower back pain
Ringing in the ears
Sore throat
Swollen or inflamed tongue
Tingling in hands or feet
Unusual bleeding
Yellowing of the eyes or skin

Interactions
This medicine may interact with several other drugs such as anticoagulants, oral antidiabetic agents, aspirin, some antibiotics, or anticancer drugs.
- Be sure to tell your doctor about any medications you are currently taking.

Storage
Tablets, capsules, suspension, etc. should be stored at room temperature as directed by your pharmacist or according to instructions on the label.

THIURETIC

Properties
This medicine contains as active ingredient hydrochlorothiazide, a thiazide-like diuretic. Thiazide or thiazide-like diuretics are prescribed to treat high blood pressure (hypertension). They are also used to reduce fluid accumulation in the body caused by conditions such as heart failure, cirrhosis, kidney disease, and the long-term use of some medications. Thiazide diuretics may also be used for other conditions as determined by your doctor.

Before using this medicine
Before you use this medicine check with your doctor, or pharmacist:
- if you ever had any unusual or allergic reaction to sulfonamides (sulfa drugs) or any of the thiazide diuretics.
- if you are on a low-salt, low-sugar, or any other special diet, or if you are allergic to any substance, such as sulfites or other preservatives or dyes.
- if you are pregnant or intend to become pregnant while using this medicine. When this medicine is used during pregnancy, it may cause side effects including jaundice, blood problems, and low potassium in the newborn.
- if you are breast-feeding an infant. Although this medicine has not been shown to cause problems in humans, the chance always exists since thiazide diuretics pass into breast milk.
- if you have any of the following medical problems:
  Diabetes
  Gout
  Kidney disease
  Liver disease
  Lupus erythematosus
  Pancreas disease

Treatment
This medication is used to treat high blood pressure (hypertension) and also to help reduce the amount of water in the body by increasing the flow of urine. This medicine will not cure your high blood pressure but it does help control it. You must continue to take it - even if you feel well - if you expect to keep your blood pressure down. You may have to take high blood pressure medicine for the rest of your life.

Thiazide diuretics may cause an unusual feeling of tiredness when you begin to take them. You may also notice an increase in urine or in frequency of urination. To keep this from affecting sleep:
- if you are to take a single dose a day, take it in the morning after breakfast;
- if you are to take more than one dose, take the last one not later than 6 p.m.

Side effects
Along with the needed effects, a medicine may cause some unwanted effects. Side effects that usually do not require medical attention: decreased sexual ability; dizziness or lightheadedness when standing up; increased sensitivity of skin to sunlight; loss of appetite; upset stomach.
- Side effects that should be reported to your doctor: black, tarry stools; blood in urine or stools; cough or hoarseness; fever or chills; joint pain; lower back or side pains; painful or difficult urination; pinpoint red spots on skin; skin rash or hives; stomach pain (severe) with nausea; unusual bleeding or bruising; yellow eyes or skin. This medicine may cause a loss of potassium from your body. Signs of too much potassium loss are: dryness of mouth; increased thirst; mood changes; muscle cramps or pain; nausea or vomiting; unusual tiredness or weakness; weak or irregular heartbeat.

Interactions
This medicine may interact with several other drugs.
- Be sure to tell your doctor about any medications you are currently taking.

Storage
Store at room temperature in a tightly closed container.

THOR-PROM

Properties

This medicine contains as active ingredient chlorpromazine, a phenothiazine derivative. Phenothiazines are a family of medicines used to treat nervous, mental, and emotional conditions. Some are used to control anxiety, restlessness, nausea and vomiting, and severe hiccups. This medicine is available only with your doctor's prescription.

Before using this medicine

Before you use this medicine check with your doctor, or pharmacist:

- if you ever had any unusual or allergic reaction to phenothiazine medicines.
- if you are on a low-salt, low-sugar, or any other special diet, or if you are allergic to any substance, such as sulfites or other preservatives or dyes.
- if you are pregnant or intend to become pregnant while using this medicine. Although phenothiazines have not been shown to cause birth defects, some side effects such as jaundice and muscle tremors have occurred in a few newborns whose mothers received phenothiazines during pregnancy.
- if you are breast-feeding an infant. Although this medicine has not been shown to cause problems in humans but the chance does exist since some phenothiazines are known to pass into the breast milk.
- if you have any of the following medical problems:
  Alcoholism
  Blood disease
  Difficult urination
  Enlarged prostate
  Glaucoma
  Heart or blood vessel disease
  Liver or lung disease
  Parkinson's disease
  Stomach ulcers

Treatment

This medication is prescribed to treat the symptoms of certain types of mental illness or emotional problems. In order to avoid stomach irritation, you can take the tablet or capsule forms of this medication with a meal or with a glass of water or milk (unless your doctor or pharmacist directs you to do otherwise).

Side effects

Along with the needed effects, a medicine may cause some unwanted effects. Minor side effects are: blurred vision, constipation, decreased sweating, diarrhea, dizziness, drooling, drowsiness, dry mouth, fatigue, jitteriness, menstrual irregularities, nasal congestion, restlessness, tremors, vomiting, or weight gain.

- Tell your doctor about any side effects that are persistent or particularly bothersome. It is especially important to tell your doctor about:
  Breast enlargement
  Chest pain or convulsions
  Darkened skin
  Difficulty in swallowing
  Fainting or fever
  Involuntary movements
  Palpitations or sleep disorders
  Rash or sore throat
  Uncoordinated movements
  Unusual bleeding or bruising
  Visual disturbances
  Yellowing of the eyes or skin

Interactions

This medicine may interact with several other drugs such as barbiturates, sleeping pills, narcotics, other tranquilizers, or any other medication that may produce a sedative effect. Avoid alcohol.

Storage

Store this medication as directed on the label. Keep out of the reach of children.

THORAZINE

Properties
This medicine contains as active ingredient chlorpromazine, a phenothiazine derivative. Phenothiazines are a family of medicines used to treat nervous, mental, and emotional conditions. Some are used to control anxiety, restlessness, nausea and vomiting, and severe hiccups. This medicine is available only with your doctor's prescription.

Before using this medicine
Before you use this medicine check with your doctor, or pharmacist:
- if you ever had any unusual or allergic reaction to phenothiazine medicines.
- if you are on a low-salt, low-sugar, or any other special diet, or if you are allergic to any substance, such as sulfites or other preservatives or dyes.
- if you are pregnant or intend to become pregnant while using this medicine. Although phenothiazines have not been shown to cause birth defects, some side effects such as jaundice and muscle tremors have occurred in a few newborns whose mothers received phenothiazines during pregnancy.
- if you are breast-feeding an infant. Although this medicine has not been shown to cause problems in humans but the chance does exist since some phenothiazines are known to pass into the breast milk.
- if you have any of the following medical problems:
Alcoholism
Blood disease
Difficult urination
Enlarged prostate
Glaucoma
Heart or blood vessel disease
Liver or lung disease
Parkinson's disease
Stomach ulcers

Treatment
This medication is prescribed to treat the symptoms of certain types of mental illness or emotional problems. In order to avoid stomach irritation, you can take the tablet or capsule forms of this medication with a meal or with a glass of water or milk (unless your doctor or pharmacist directs you to do otherwise).

Side effects
Along with the needed effects, a medicine may cause some unwanted effects.
Minor side effects are: blurred vision, constipation, decreased sweating, diarrhea, dizziness, drooling, drowsiness, dry mouth, fatigue, jitteriness, menstrual irregularities, nasal congestion, restlessness, tremors, vomiting, or weight gain.
- Tell your doctor about any side effects that are persistent or particularly bothersome. It is especially important to tell your doctor about:
Breast enlargement
Chest pain or convulsions
Darkened skin
Difficulty in swallowing
Fainting or fever
Involuntary movements
Palpitations or sleep disorders
Rash or sore throat
Uncoordinated movements
Unusual bleeding or bruising
Visual disturbances
Yellowing of the eyes or skin

Interactions
This medicine may interact with several other drugs such as barbiturates, sleeping pills, narcotics, other tranquilizers, or any other medication that may produce a sedative effect. Avoid alcohol.

Storage
Store this medication as directed on the label. Keep out of the reach of children.

TICAR

Properties
This medicine contains ticarcillin (penicillin) as active ingredient. Penicillins are prescribed to treat infections caused by bacteria. They will not work for colds, flu, or other virus infections. There are several different kinds of penicillins. Each is used to treat different kinds of infections.

Before using this medicine
Before you use this medicine check with your doctor, or pharmacist:
- if you ever had any unusual or allergic reaction to any of the penicillins, cefalosporins, griseofulvin, or penicillamine. Serious reactions may occur in patients who are allergic to penicillins.
- if you are on a low-salt, low-sugar, or any other special diet, or if you are allergic to any substance, such as sulfites or other preservatives or dyes.
- if you are pregnant or intend to become pregnant while using this medicine. Although penicillins have not been shown to cause problems in humans, the chance always exists.
- if you are breast-feeding an infant. Most penicillins (except amdinocillin) pass into the breast milk. Even though only small amounts may pass, allergic reaction, diarrhea, fungal infection, and skin rash may occur in the infant.
- if you have any of the following medical problems:
  Allergy
  Asthma
  Bleeding problems
  Eczema
  Hay fever, hives
  Kidney disease
  Liver disease
  Mononucleosis
  Stomach or intestinal disease

Treatment
This medication is used to treat an infection caused by bacteria. Most penicillins are best taken with a full glass (8 ounces) of water on an empty stomach, some are best taken with a snack or meal. Follow your doctor's or pharmacist's directions on how to take your medicine.
- ◆ Keep taking this medicine for the full time of treatment even if you begin to feel better after a few days; do not miss any doses. This is especially important if you have a "strep" infection since serious heart problems could develop later if your infection is not cleared up completely.
- ◆ If you do miss a dose of this medicine, take it as soon as possible. However, if it is almost time for your next dose, skip the missed dose and go back to your regular dosing schedule.

Side effects
Along with the needed effects, a medicine may cause some unwanted effects. Side effects that usually do not require medical attention: diarrhea; nausea or vomiting; sore mouth or tongue.
- ◆ Stop taking this medicine and get emergency help immediately if you notice: difficulty in breathing; light-headedness; skin rash, hives, itching; wheezing.

  Other side effects that should be reported to your doctor immediately are: abdominal bloating; blood in urine; convulsions (seizures); decreased amount of urine; diarrhea (watery and severe) which may also be bloody; fever; joint pain; sore throat and fever; stomach or abdominal cramps and pain; unusual bleeding or bruising.

Interactions
This medicine may interact with several other drugs such as anticoagulants, diarrhea medicines, heparin, ibuprofen, oral contraceptives, potassium-containing medicines, etc.
- ■ Be sure to tell your doctor about any medications you are currently taking.

Storage
Tablets, capsules, etc. should be stored as directed by your pharmacist or according to instructions on the label.

TICARCILLIN

Properties

This medicine contains ticarcillin (penicillin) as active ingredient. Penicillins are prescribed to treat infections caused by bacteria. They will not work for colds, flu, or other virus infections. There are several different kinds of penicillins. Each is used to treat different kinds of infections.

Before using this medicine

Before you use this medicine check with your doctor, or pharmacist:

- if you ever had any unusual or allergic reaction to any of the penicillins, cefalosporins, griseofulvin, or penicillamine. Serious reactions may occur in patients who are allergic to penicillins.
- if you are on a low-salt, low-sugar, or any other special diet, or if you are allergic to any substance, such as sulfites or other preservatives or dyes.
- if you are pregnant or intend to become pregnant while using this medicine. Although penicillins have not been shown to cause problems in humans, the chance always exists.
- if you are breast-feeding an infant. Most penicillins (except amdinocillin) pass into the breast milk. Even though only small amounts may pass, allergic reaction, diarrhea, fungal infection, and skin rash may occur in the infant.
- if you have any of the following medical problems:
  Allergy
  Asthma
  Bleeding problems
  Eczema
  Hay fever, hives
  Kidney disease
  Liver disease
  Mononucleosis
  Stomach or intestinal disease

Treatment

This medication is used to treat an infection caused by bacteria. Most penicillins are best taken with a full glass (8 ounces) of water on an empty stomach, some are best taken with a snack or meal. Follow your doctor's or pharmacist's directions on how to take your medicine.

- ◆ Keep taking this medicine for the full time of treatment even if you begin to feel better after a few days; do not miss any doses. This is especially important if you have a "strep" infection since serious heart problems could develop later if your infection is not cleared up completely.
- ◆ If you do miss a dose of this medicine, take it as soon as possible. However, if it is almost time for your next dose, skip the missed dose and go back to your regular dosing schedule.

Side effects

Along with the needed effects, a medicine may cause some unwanted effects. Side effects that usually do not require medical attention: diarrhea; nausea or vomiting; sore mouth or tongue.

- ◆ Stop taking this medicine and get emergency help immediately if you notice: difficulty in breathing; lightheadedness; skin rash, hives, itching; wheezing.

Other side effects that should be reported to your doctor immediately are: abdominal bloating; blood in urine; convulsions (seizures); decreased amount of urine; diarrhea (watery and severe) which may also be bloody; fever; joint pain; sore throat and fever; stomach or abdominal cramps and pain; unusual bleeding or bruising.

Interactions

This medicine may interact with several other drugs such as anticoagulants, diarrhea medicines, heparin, ibuprofen, oral contraceptives, potassium-containing medicines, etc.

- ▪ Be sure to tell your doctor about any medications you are currently taking.

Storage

Tablets, capsules, etc. should be stored as directed by your pharmacist or according to instructions on the label.

TIMENTIN

Properties
This medicine contains ticarcillin (penicillin) and clavulanate as active ingredients. Penicillins are prescribed to treat infections caused by bacteria. They will not work for colds, flu, or other virus infections. There are several different kinds of penicillins. Each is used to treat different kinds of infections.

Before using this medicine
Before you use this medicine check with your doctor, or pharmacist:
- if you ever had any unusual or allergic reaction to any of the penicillins, cefalosporins, griseofulvin, or penicillamine. Serious reactions may occur in patients who are allergic to penicillins.
- if you are on a low-salt, low-sugar, or any other special diet, or if you are allergic to any substance, such as sulfites or other preservatives or dyes.
- if you are pregnant or intend to become pregnant while using this medicine. Although penicillins have not been shown to cause problems in humans, the chance always exists.
- if you are breast-feeding an infant. Most penicillins (except amdinocillin) pass into the breast milk. Even though only small amounts may pass, allergic reaction, diarrhea, fungal infection, and skin rash may occur in the infant.
- if you have any of the following medical problems:
Allergy
Asthma
Bleeding problems
Eczema
Hay fever, hives
Kidney disease
Liver disease
Mononucleosis
Stomach or intestinal disease

Treatment
This medication is used to treat an infection caused by bacteria. Most penicillins are best taken with a full glass (8 ounces) of water on an empty stomach, some are best taken with a snack or meal. Follow your doctor's or pharmacist's directions on how to take your medicine.
- Keep taking this medicine for the full time of treatment even if you begin to feel better after a few days; do not miss any doses. This is especially important if you have a "strep" infection since serious heart problems could develop later if your infection is not cleared up completely.
- If you do miss a dose of this medicine, take it as soon as possible. However, if it is almost time for your next dose, skip the missed dose and go back to your regular dosing schedule.

Side effects
Along with the needed effects, a medicine may cause some unwanted effects. Side effects that usually do not require medical attention: diarrhea; nausea or vomiting; sore mouth or tongue.
- Stop taking this medicine and get emergency help immediately if you notice: difficulty in breathing; lightheadedness; skin rash, hives, itching; wheezing.

Other side effects that should be reported to your doctor immediately are: abdominal bloating; blood in urine; convulsions (seizures); decreased amount of urine; diarrhea (watery and severe) which may also be bloody; fever; joint pain; sore throat and fever; stomach or abdominal cramps and pain; unusual bleeding or bruising.

Interactions
This medicine may interact with several other drugs such as anticoagulants, diarrhea medicines, heparin, ibuprofen, oral contraceptives, potassium-containing medicines, etc.
- Be sure to tell your doctor about any medications you are currently taking.

Storage
Tablets, capsules, etc. should be stored as directed by your pharmacist or according to instructions on the label.

TINDAL

Properties

This medicine contains as active ingredient acetophenazine, a phenothiazine derivative. Phenothiazines are a family of medicines used to treat nervous, mental, and emotional conditions. Some are used to control anxiety, restlessness, nausea and vomiting, and severe hiccups. This medicine is available only with your doctor's prescription.

Before using this medicine

Before you use this medicine check with your doctor, or pharmacist:
- if you ever had any unusual or allergic reaction to phenothiazine medicines.
- if you are on a low-salt, low-sugar, or any other special diet, or if you are allergic to any substance, such as sulfites or other preservatives or dyes.
- if you are pregnant or intend to become pregnant while using this medicine. Although phenothiazines have not been shown to cause birth defects, some side effects such as jaundice and muscle tremors have occurred in a few newborns whose mothers received phenothiazines during pregnancy.
- if you are breast-feeding an infant. Although this medicine has not been shown to cause problems in humans but the chance does exist since some phenothiazines are known to pass into the breast milk.
- if you have any of the following medical problems:
  Alcoholism
  Blood disease
  Difficult urination
  Enlarged prostate
  Glaucoma
  Heart or blood vessel disease
  Liver or lung disease
  Parkinson's disease
  Stomach ulcers

Treatment

This medication is prescribed to treat the symptoms of certain types of mental illness or emotional problems. In order to avoid stomach irritation, you can take the tablet or capsule forms of this medication with a meal or with a glass of water or milk (unless your doctor or pharmacist directs you to do otherwise).

Side effects

Along with the needed effects, a medicine may cause some unwanted effects. Minor side effects are: blurred vision, constipation, decreased sweating, diarrhea, dizziness, drooling, drowsiness, dry mouth, fatigue, jitteriness, menstrual irregularities, nasal congestion, restlessness, tremors, vomiting, or weight gain.
- Tell your doctor about any side effects that are persistent or particularly bothersome. It is especially important to tell your doctor about:
  Breast enlargement
  Chest pain or convulsions
  Darkened skin
  Difficulty in swallowing
  Fainting or fever
  Involuntary movements .
  Palpitations or sleep disorders
  Rash or sore throat
  Uncoordinated movements
  Unusual bleeding or bruising
  Visual disturbances
  Yellowing of the eyes

Interactions

This medicine may interact with several other drugs such as barbiturates, sleeping pills, narcotics, other tranquilizers, or any other medication that may produce a sedative effect. Avoid alcohol.

Storage

Store this medication as directed on the label. Keep out of the reach of children.

TIPRAMINE

Properties
This medicine contains imipramine as active ingredient. It belongs to the group of medicines known as tricyclic antidepressants or 'mood elevators.' It is used to relieve mental depression and depression that sometimes occurs with anxiety. The medication gradually relieves, but doesn't cure, symptoms of depression. The medication may also be used for the treatment of narcolepsy, bulimia, painic attacks, cocaine withdrawal, attention deficit disorder.

Before using this medicine
Before you use this medicine check with your doctor, or pharmacist:
- if you ever had any unusual or allergic reaction to any tricyclic antidepressant, maprotiline or trazodone.
- if you are on a low-salt, low-sugar, or any other special diet, or if you are allergic to any substance, such as sulfites or other preservatives or dyes.
- if you are pregnant or intend to become pregnant while using this medicine. There have been reports of newborns suffering from heart, breathing, and urinary problems when their mothers had taken tricyclic antidepressants before delivery.
- if you are breast-feeding an infant. Some tricyclic antidepressants pass into the breast milk.

Treatment
Take this medicine only as directed by your doctor, to benefit your condition as much as possible. Do not take more of it, do not take it more often, and do not take it for a longer period of time than your doctor ordered.

To lessen stomach upset, take this medicine with food, even for a daily bedtime dose, unless your doctor has told you to take it on an empty stomach. If you forget your once-a-day bedtime dose, don't take it more than 3 hours late. If more than 3 hours, wait for next scheduled dose;.

Sometimes this medicine must be taken for several weeks before you begin to feel better.

Side effects
Along with the needed effects, a medicine may cause some unwanted effects. Side effects that usually do not require medical attention: difficult or frequent urination; decreased sex drive; muscle aches; abnormal dreams; nasal congestion; weakness and faintness when arising from bed or chair; back pain.
- Other side effects that should be reported to your doctor immediately are:
  Hallucinations
  Shakiness
  Dizziness or fainting
  Blurred vision, eye pain
  Irregular heartbeat or slow pulse
  Inflamed tongue
  Abdominal pain
  Jaundice
  Hair loss, rash
  Fever, chills
  Joint pain
  Palpitations

Interactions
This medicine may interact with several other drugs such as anticoagulants, anticholinergics, cold remedies, oral contraceptives, seizure medicines, sleeping medicines, thyroid medicines, etc.
- Be sure to tell your doctor about any medications you are currently taking.

Storage
Tablets, capsules, etc. should be stored at room temperature in tightly closed, light-resistant containers as directed by your pharmacist. Keep out of reach of children since overdose is especially dangerous in young children. Do not store in the bathroom medicine cabinet because the heat or moisture may cause the medicine to break down. Keep the liquid form of the medicine from freezing.

TOFRANIL

Properties
This medicine contains imipramine as active ingredient. It belongs to the group of medicines known as tricyclic antidepressants or 'mood elevators.' It is used to relieve mental depression and depression that sometimes occurs with anxiety. The medication gradually relieves, but doesn't cure, symptoms of depression. The medication may also be used for the treatment of narcolepsy, bulimia, painic attacks, cocaine withdrawal, attention deficit disorder.

Before using this medicine
Before you use this medicine check with your doctor, or pharmacist:
- if you ever had any unusual or allergic reaction to any tricyclic antidepressant, maprotiline or trazodone.
- if you are on a low-salt, low-sugar, or any other special diet, or if you are allergic to any substance, such as sulfites or other preservatives or dyes.
- if you are pregnant or intend to become pregnant while using this medicine. There have been reports of newborns suffering from heart, breathing, and urinary problems when their mothers had taken tricyclic antidepressants before delivery.
- if you are breast-feeding an infant. Some tricyclic antidepressants pass into the breast milk.

Treatment
Take this medicine only as directed by your doctor, to benefit your condition as much as possible. Do not take more of it, do not take it more often, and do not take it for a longer period of time than your doctor ordered.

To lessen stomach upset, take this medicine with food, even for a daily bedtime dose, unless your doctor has told you to take it on an empty stomach. If you forget your once-a-day bedtime dose, don't take it more than 3 hours late. If more than 3 hours, wait for next scheduled dose;.

Sometimes this medicine must be taken for several weeks before you begin to feel better.

Side effects
Along with the needed effects, a medicine may cause some unwanted effects. Side effects that usually do not require medical attention: difficult or frequent urination; decreased sex drive; muscle aches; abnormal dreams; nasal congestion; weakness and faintness when arising from bed or chair; back pain.
- Other side effects that should be reported to your doctor immediately are:
  Hallucinations
  Shakiness
  Dizziness or fainting
  Blurred vision, eye pain
  Irregular heartbeat or slow pulse
  Inflamed tongue
  Abdominal pain
  Jaundice
  Hair loss, rash
  Fever, chills
  Joint pain
  Palpitations

Interactions
This medicine may interact with several other drugs such as anticoagulants, anticholinergics, cold remedies, oral contraceptives, seizure medicines, sleeping medicines, thyroid medicines, etc.
- Be sure to tell your doctor about any medications you are currently taking.

Storage
Tablets, capsules, etc. should be stored at room temperature in tightly closed, light-resistant containers as directed by your pharmacist. Keep out of reach of children since overdose is especially dangerous in young children. Do not store in the bathroom medicine cabinet because the heat or moisture may cause the medicine to break down. Keep the liquid form of the medicine from freezing.

TORA

Properties
This medicine contains phentermine as active ingredient; it is prescribed for appetite suppression.

Appetite suppressants are used in the short-term (a few weeks) treatment of obesity. In a few weeks (6 to 12), these medicines in combination with dieting, exercise, and changes in eating habits can help patients lose weight. However, since their appetite reducing effect is only temporary, they are useful only for the first weeks of dieting until new eating habits are established.

Before using this medicine
Before you use this medicine check with your doctor, or pharmacist:
- if you ever had any unusual or allergic reaction to any of the compounds of this medicine.
- if you are on a low-salt, low-sugar, or any other special diet, or if you are allergic to any substance, such as sulfites or other preservatives or dyes.
- if you are pregnant, intend to become pregnant or breast-feeding an infant while using this medicine.
- if you have any of the following medical problems:
  Diabetes mellitus
  Epilepsy
  Glaucoma
  Heart disease
  High blood pressure
  Mental illness (severe)

Treatment
This medication is used to relieve or prevent the symptoms of your medical problem. Take them as directed.

Do not take more of them and do not take them more often than recommended on the label. If too much of the drug is taken, it may become habit-forming.
- The medicine produces central nervous system stimulation, and it should not be taken by people with heart disease or high blood pressure.
- If you think this medicine is not working as well after you have taken it for a few weeks, do not increase the dose. Instead, check with your doctor.

Side effects
The following minor side effects may occur: irritability, nervousness, restlessness, trouble in sleeping.

These side effects should disappear as your body adjusts to the medication. Tell your doctor about any side effects that are persistent or particularly bothersome. It is especially important to tell your doctor about:
  Mental depression
  Nausea or vomiting
  Stomach cramps or pain
  Trembling
  Unusual tiredness
- Discontinue use of the drug; call your doctor right away. Adverse reactions and side effects may be more frequent and severe in people over age 60 than in younger persons.

Interactions
This medicine interacts with several other drugs such as antihypertensives, other appetite suppressants, caffeine, central nervous system depressants, central nervous system stimulants, furazolidone, guanethidine, hydralazine, MAO inhibitors, methyldopa, molindone, phenothiazines, rauwolfia alkaloids, sodium bicarbonate. Interaction with alcoholic beverages may produce drowsiness, sleepiness, and/or inability to concentrate.
- Be sure to tell your doctor about any medications you are currently taking.

Storage
This medicine should be stored at room temperature in tightly closed containers. Store away from heat and direct light. Keep out of reach of children, since overdose may be very dangerous in children. Do not store this medicine in the bathroom medicine cabinet because the heat and moisture cause the medicine to break down. Do not keep outdated medicine or medicine no longer needed. Flush the contents of the container down the toilet.

TRI-CYCLEN

Properties
This medicine contains norgestimate
and ethinyl estradiol as active ingredients. It is an oral contraceptive prescribed to prevent pregnancy and/or to
regulate menstrual periods.

The drug works by altering the mucus at the cervix entrance to prevent the
entry of sperm. It also alters the uterus
lining to resist implantation of the fertilized egg. Oral contraceptives create the
same chemical atmosphere in blood that
exists during pregnancy.

Before using this medicine
Before you use this medicine check
with your doctor, or pharmacist:
- if you ever had any unusual or allergic reaction to estrogens or progestogen;
- if you are pregnant or want to become pregnant within three months;
- if you are breast-feeding an infant;
- if you have any of the following
  medical problems:
  Diabetes
  Ailments of the breast
  Disorders of the uterus
  Migraine or epilepsy
  High blood pressure
  Asthma or heart conditions
  Kidney disease
  Gallstones

Treatment
This medication is used to prevent pregnancy or to regulate menstrual periods.

Adverse reactions
Along with the needed effects, a medi-
cine may cause some unwanted effects
or adverse reactions.
- *An increased risk of the following
  adverse reactions has been associa-
  ted with the use of oral contracep-
  tives:*
  Thrombophlebitis
  Venous thrombosis
  Arterial thromboembolism
  Pulmonary (lung) embolism
  Myocardial infarction
  Cerebral hemorrhage
  Cerebral thrombosis

Hypertension
Gallbladder disease
Hepatic (liver) hepatomas
Benign lifer tumors
- *The following adverse reactions have
  been reported in patients receiving
  oral contraceptives and are believed
  to be drug-related:*
  Nausea and vomiting
  Abdominal cramps
  Breakthrough bleeding
  Spotting
  Change in menstrual flow
  Amenorrhea
  Temporary infertility
  Edema
  Breast changes
  Weight changes
  Cholestatic jaundice
  Migraine
  Rash (allergic)
  Mental depression
  Vaginal candidiasis

Interactions
This medicine may interact with several
other drugs such as antibiotics, anticoagulants, anticonvulsants, antidepressants, oral antidiabetics, antihistamines,
barbiturates, oral hypoglycemics, insulin, meperidine.
- Be sure to tell your doctor about any
  medications you are currently taking.

Storage
Tablets should be stored at room temperature; store away from heat and direct light. Keep out of reach of children,
since this medicine may be dangerous
in children.

TRI-K

Properties

This medicine contains trikates as active ingredient; it is used to treat or prevent potassium deficiency, especially potassium deficiency that is caused by the use of diuretics (water pills).

Potassium is needed to maintain good health. Potassium supplements may be needed by patients who do not have enough potassium in their regular diet and by those who have lost too much potassium because of illness or treatment with certain medicines.

Since too much potassium may also cause health problems, most potassium supplements are available only with your doctor's prescription.

Before using this medicine

Before you use this medicine check with your doctor, or pharmacist:
- if you ever had any unusual or allergic reaction to potassium preparations;
- if you are on a low-salt, low-sugar, or any other special diet, or if you are allergic to any substance, such as sulfites or other preservatives or dyes.
- if you are pregnant or intend to become pregnant while using this medicine. Although potassium supplements have not been shown to cause problems in humans, the chance always exists.
- if you are breast-feeding an infant. Although this medicine has not been shown to cause problems in humans, the chance always exists since small amounts of potassium pass into the breast milk.
- if you have any of the following medical problems:
Addison's disease
Heart disease
Diarrhea
Kidney disease
Stomach ulcer

Treatment

This medication is used to relieve or prevent the symptoms of your medical problem. Take them as directed. Do not take more of them and do not take them more often than recommended on the label, unless otherwise directed by your doctor. To do so may increase the chance of side effects.

In order to avoid stomach irritation, you should take potassium supplements with food or immediately after a meal. If you miss a dose of this medication, take the missed dose as soon as possible, unless it is within two hours of the next scheduled dose;.

Side effects

The following minor side effects may occur:
Diarrhea
Nausea
Stomach Pains
Vomiting.

These side effects should disappear as your body adjusts to the medication. Tell your doctor about any side effects that are persistent or particularly bothersome. It is especially important to tell your doctor about anxiety; bloody or black, tarry stools; confusion; difficulty in breathing; numbness or tingling in the arms, legs, or feet; palpitations; severe abdominal pain; or unusual weakness.

Interactions

This medicine interacts with several other drugs such as adrenocorticosteroids, antimuscarinics, calcium-containing medicines; heart medicines such as digitalis or digoxin; laxatives; other potassium-containing medicines.
- Be sure to tell your doctor about any medications you are currently taking.

Storage

Tablets, elixir, etc. should be stored at room temperature in tightly closed containers. Store away from heat and direct light. Keep out of reach of children, since overdose may be very dangerous in children. Do not keep outdated medicine or medicine no longer needed. Flush the contents of the container down the toilet, unless otherwise directed.

TRIAZOLAM

Properties

This medicine contains as active ingredient triazolam, a benzodiazepine preparation. Benzodiazepines belong to the group of psychoactive medicines that influence the activity of the brain. Some are used to relieve nervousness or tension. It is effective for this purpose for short periods. Others are used for sleeplessness or to relax muscles or relieve muscle spasm. The benzodiazepines may also be used for other conditions as determined by your doctor.

Before using this medicine

Before you use this medicine check with your doctor:
- if you ever had any unusual or allergic reaction to benzodiazepines.
- if you are on a low-salt, low-sugar, or any other special diet, or if you are allergic to any substance, such as sulfites or other preservatives or dyes.
- if you are pregnant or intend to become pregnant while using this medicine. Some benzodiazepines have been reported to increase the chance of birth defects when used during the first 3 months of pregnancy.
- if you are breast-feeding an infant. Benzodiazepines may pass into the breast milk and cause drowsiness, unusually slow heartbeat, shortness of breath, or troubled breathing in infants of mothers taking this medicine.
- if you have any of the following medical problems: asthma, bronchitis, emphysema, or other chronic lung disease; epilepsy or history of convulsions; hyperactivity (in children); kidney or lifer disease; mental depression or illness; myasthania gravis, porphyria.

Treatment

This medication is used to relieve or prevent the symptoms of your medical problem. Benzodiazepines are mainly used as antianxiety agents, anticonvulsants, or sedatives. Take them as directed. Do not take more of them and do not take them more often than recommended on the label, unless otherwise directed by your doctor. Benzodiazepine tranquilizing drugs can be abused if taken for long periods of time and it is possible to develop withdrawal symptoms if you discontinue the therapy abruptly.

Side effects

Along with the needed effects, a medicine may cause some unwanted effects. Minor side effects are: bitter taste in the mouth, dizziness, drowsiness, depression, constipation, dry mouth, excessive salivation, fatigue, flushing, headache, heartburn, loss of appetite, nausea, nervousness, sweating or vomiting. As your body adjusts to the medicine, these side effects should disappear.

- Tell your doctor about any side effects that are persistent or particularly bothersome. It is especially important to tell your doctor about:
  Blurred or double vision
  Chest pain
  Difficulty in urinating
  Fainting or falling
  Fever or hallucinations
  Joint pain
  Mouth sores
  Nightmares
  Palpitations
  Severe depression
  Shortness of breath
  Slurred speech
  Uncoordinated movements
  Unusual tiredness
  Yellowing of the skin

Interactions

This medicine may interact with several other drugs. Be sure to tell your doctor about any medications you are currently taking. This medicine will add to the effects of alcohol, and CNS depressants.

Storage

Store at room temperature in tightly closed, light-resistant-resistant containers. Keep out of the reach of children since overdose may be especially dangerous in children.

TRICHLOREX

Properties

This medicine contains as active ingredient trichlormethiazide, a thiazide-like diuretic. Thiazide or thiazide-like diuretics are prescribed to treat high blood pressure (hypertension). They are also used to reduce fluid accumulation in the body caused by conditions such as heart failure, cirrhosis, kidney disease, and the long-term use of some medications. Thiazide diuretics may also be used for other conditions as determined by your doctor.

Before using this medicine

Before you use this medicine check with your doctor, or pharmacist:

- if you ever had any unusual or allergic reaction to sulfonamides (sulfa drugs) or any of the thiazide diuretics.
- if you are on a low-salt, low-sugar, or any other special diet, or if you are allergic to any substance, such as sulfites or other preservatives or dyes.
- if you are pregnant or intend to become pregnant while using this medicine. When this medicine is used during pregnancy, it may cause side effects including jaundice, blood problems, and low potassium in the newborn.
- if you are breast-feeding an infant. Although this medicine has not been shown to cause problems in humans, the chance always exists since thiazide diuretics pass into breast milk.
- if you have any of the following medical problems:
  Diabetes
  Gout
  Kidney disease
  Liver disease
  Lupus erythematosus
  Pancreas disease

Treatment

This medication is used to treat high blood pressure (hypertension) and also to help reduce the amount of water in the body by increasing the flow of urine. This medicine will not cure your high blood pressure but it does help control it. You must continue to take it - even if you feel well - if you expect to keep your blood pressure down. You may have to take high blood pressure medicine for the rest of your life.

Thiazide diuretics may cause an unusual feeling of tiredness when you begin to take them. You may also notice an increase in urine or in frequency of urination. To keep this from affecting sleep:

- if you are to take a single dose a day, take it in the morning after breakfast;
- if you are to take more than one dose, take the last one not later than 6 p.m.

Side effects

Along with the needed effects, a medicine may cause some unwanted effects. Side effects that usually do not require medical attention: decreased sexual ability; dizziness or lightheadedness when standing up; increased sensitivity of skin to sunlight; loss of appetite; upset stomach.

- Side effects that should be reported to your doctor: black, tarry stools; blood in urine or stools; cough or hoarseness; fever or chills; joint pain; lower back or side pains; painful or difficult urination; pinpoint red spots on skin; skin rash or hives; stomach pain (severe) with nausea; unusual bleeding or bruising; yellow eyes or skin. This medicine may cause a loss of potassium from your body. Signs of too much potassium loss are: dryness of mouth; increased thirst; mood changes; muscle cramps or pain; nausea or vomiting; unusual tiredness or weakness; weak or irregular heartbeat.

Interactions

This medicine may interact with several other drugs.

- Be sure to tell your doctor about any medications you are currently taking.

Storage

Store at room temperature in a tightly closed container.

TRICLORMETHIAZIDE

Properties
This medicine contains as active ingredient triclormethiazide, a thiazide-like diuretic. Thiazide or thiazide-like diuretics are prescribed to treat high blood pressure (hypertension). They are also used to reduce fluid accumulation in the body caused by conditions such as heart failure, cirrhosis, kidney disease, and the long-term use of some medications. Thiazide diuretics may also be used for other conditions as determined by your doctor.

Before using this medicine
Before you use this medicine check with your doctor, or pharmacist:
- if you ever had any unusual or allergic reaction to sulfonamides (sulfa drugs) or any of the thiazide diuretics.
- if you are on a low-salt, low-sugar, or any other special diet, or if you are allergic to any substance, such as sulfites or other preservatives or dyes.
- if you are pregnant or intend to become pregnant while using this medicine. When this medicine is used during pregnancy, it may cause side effects including jaundice, blood problems, and low potassium in the newborn.
- if you are breast-feeding an infant. Although this medicine has not been shown to cause problems in humans, the chance always exists since thiazide diuretics pass into breast milk.
- if you have any of the following medical problems:
Diabetes
Gout
Kidney disease
Liver disease
Lupus erythematosus
Pancreas disease

Treatment
This medication is used to treat high blood pressure (hypertension) and also to help reduce the amount of water in the body by increasing the flow of urine. This medicine will not cure your high blood pressure but it does help

control it. You must continue to take it - even if you feel well - if you expect to keep your blood pressure down. You may have to take high blood pressure medicine for the rest of your life.

Thiazide diuretics may cause an unusual feeling of tiredness when you begin to take them. You may also notice an increase in urine or in frequency of urination. To keep this from affecting sleep:
- if you are to take a single dose a day, take it in the morning after breakfast;
- if you are to take more than one dose, take the last one not later than 6 p.m.

Side effects
Along with the needed effects, a medicine may cause some unwanted effects. Side effects that usually do not require medical attention: decreased sexual ability; dizziness or lightheadedness when standing up; increased sensitivity of skin to sunlight; loss of appetite; upset stomach.
- Side effects that should be reported to your doctor: black, tarry stools; blood in urine or stools; cough or hoarseness; fever or chills; joint pain; lower back or side pains; painful or difficult urination; pinpoint red spots on skin; skin rash or hives; stomach pain (severe) with nausea; unusual bleeding or bruising; yellow eyes or skin. This medicine may cause a loss of potassium from your body. Signs of too much potassium loss are: dryness of mouth; increased thirst; mood changes; muscle cramps or pain; nausea or vomiting; unusual tiredness or weakness; weak or irregular heartbeat.

Interactions
This medicine may interact with several other drugs.
- Be sure to tell your doctor about any medications you are currently taking.

Storage
Store at room temperature in a tightly closed container.

TRIDESILON

Properties

This medicine contains desonide, a corticosteroid, as active ingredient. Corticosteroids are used to help relieve redness, swelling, itching, inflammation, and discomfort of many skin problems. They exert this effect by interfering with natural body mechanisms that produce the rash, itching, or inflammation. They do not cure the underlying cause of the skin problem. This medication is applied to the skin.

Before using this medicine

Before you use this medicine check with your doctor, or pharmacist:
- if you ever had any unusual or allergic reaction to corticosteroids.
- if you are allergic to any substance, such as sulfites or other preservatives or dyes.
- if you are pregnant or intend to become pregnant while using this medicine. Studies have shown that corticosteroids applied to the skin in large amounts or over long periods of time can be the cause of birth defects.
- if you are breast-feeding an infant. Some corticosteroids pass into breast milk and may interfere with the infant's growth.

Treatment

Do not use this medicine more often or for a longer time than ordered. To do so may increase absorption through the skin and the chance of side effects. In addition, too much use, especially on areas with thinner skin (for example, face, armpits, groin), may result in thinning of the skin and stretch marks.

Before applying this medication, wash your hands. than, unless your doctor or pharmacist gives you different instructions, gently wash the area where the medication is to be applied. With a clean towel pat the area dry. Apply a small amount of the medication to the affected area in a thin layer. Do not bandage the area unless your doctor tells you to do so.

If you miss a dose of this medication, apply the dose as soon as possible, unless it is almost time for the next application.

- ◆ Do not use this medicine for other skin problems without first checking with your doctor. You should not use a topical corticosteroid if you have a virus disease (such as herpes), fungal infection of the skin (such as athlete's foot), or tuberculosis of the skin.

Side effects

There are a number of side effects that usually do not require medical attention. Minor side effects are:
Acne
Burning sensations
Itching
Rash
Skin dryness

These possible side effects may go away during treatment; however, if they continue or are bothersome, check with your doctor, nurse, or pharmacist. Tell your doctor about any side effects that are persistent or particularly bothersome, such as:
Blistering
Increased hair growth
Irritation of the affected area
Loss of skin
Secondary infection in the area being treated
Thinning of the skin with easy bruising

Interactions

None known as long as it is used according to the directions given to you by your doctor or pharmacist.

Storage

Cream, ointment, lotion, gel, spray, and aerosol should be stored at room temperature in tightly closed containers. This medication should never be frozen.

TRIFLUPERAZINE

Properties
This medicine contains as active ingredient trifluperazine, a phenothiazine derivative. Phenothiazines are a family of medicines used to treat nervous, mental, and emotional conditions. Some are used to control anxiety, restlessness, nausea and vomiting, and severe hiccups. This medicine is available only with your doctor's prescription.

Before using this medicine
Before you use this medicine check with your doctor, or pharmacist:
- if you ever had any unusual or allergic reaction to phenothiazine medicines.
- if you are on a low-salt, low-sugar, or any other special diet, or if you are allergic to any substance, such as sulfites or other preservatives or dyes.
- if you are pregnant or intend to become pregnant while using this medicine. Although phenothiazines have not been shown to cause birth defects, some side effects such as jaundice and muscle tremors have occurred in a few newborns whose mothers received phenothiazines during pregnancy.
- if you are breast-feeding an infant. Although this medicine has not been shown to cause problems in humans but the chance does exist since some phenothiazines are known to pass into the breast milk.
- if you have any of the following medical problems:
  Alcoholism
  Blood disease
  Difficult urination
  Enlarged prostate
  Glaucoma
  Heart or blood vessel disease
  Liver or lung disease
  Parkinson's disease
  Stomach ulcers

Treatment
This medication is prescribed to treat the symptoms of certain types of mental illness or emotional problems. In order to avoid stomach irritation, you can take the tablet or capsule forms of this medication with a meal or with a glass of water or milk (unless your doctor or pharmacist directs you to do otherwise).

Side effects
Along with the needed effects, a medicine may cause some unwanted effects. Minor side effects are: blurred vision, constipation, decreased sweating, diarrhea, dizziness, drooling, drowsiness, dry mouth, fatigue, jitteriness, menstrual irregularities, nasal congestion, restlessness, tremors, vomiting, or weight gain.
- Tell your doctor about any side effects that are persistent or particularly bothersome. It is especially important to tell your doctor about:
  Breast enlargement
  Chest pain or convulsions
  Darkened skin
  Difficulty in swallowing
  Fainting or fever
  Involuntary movements
  Palpitations or sleep disorders
  Rash or sore throat
  Uncoordinated movements
  Unusual bleeding or bruising
  Visual disturbances
  Yellowing of the eyes or skin

Interactions
This medicine may interact with several other drugs such as barbiturates, sleeping pills, narcotics, other tranquilizers, or any other medication that may produce a sedative effect. Avoid alcohol.

Storage
Store this medication as directed on the label. Keep out of the reach of children.

TRIKATES

Properties

This medicine contains trikates chloride as active ingredient; it is used to treat or prevent potassium deficiency, especially potassium deficiency that is caused by the use of diuretics (water pills).

Potassium is needed to maintain good health. Potassium supplements may be needed by patients who do not have enough potassium in their regular diet and by those who have lost too much potassium because of illness or treatment with certain medicines.

Since too much potassium may also cause health problems, most potassium supplements are available only with your doctor's prescription.

Before using this medicine

Before you use this medicine check with your doctor, or pharmacist:

- if you ever had any unusual or allergic reaction to potassium preparations;
- if you are on a low-salt, low-sugar, or any other special diet, or if you are allergic to any substance, such as sulfites or other preservatives or dyes.
- if you are pregnant or intend to become pregnant while using this medicine. Although potassium supplements have not been shown to cause problems in humans, the chance always exists.
- if you are breast-feeding an infant. Although this medicine has not been shown to cause problems in humans, the chance always exists since small amounts of potassium pass into the breast milk.
- if you have any of the following medical problems:
  Addison's disease
  Heart disease
  Diarrhea
  Kidney disease
  Stomach ulcer

Treatment

This medication is used to relieve or prevent the symptoms of your medical problem. Take them as directed. Do not take more of them and do not take them more often than recommended on the label, unless otherwise directed by your doctor. To do so may increase the chance of side effects.

In order to avoid stomach irritation, you should take potassium supplements with food or immediately after a meal. If you miss a dose of this medication, take the missed dose as soon as possible, unless it is within two hours of the next scheduled dose;.

Side effects

The following minor side effects may occur:
  Diarrhea
  Nausea
  Stomach Pains
  Vomiting.

These side effects should disappear as your body adjusts to the medication. Tell your doctor about any side effects that are persistent or particularly bothersome. It is especially important to tell your doctor about anxiety; bloody or black, tarry stools; confusion; difficulty in breathing; numbness or tingling in the arms, legs, or feet; palpitations; severe abdominal pain; or unusual weakness.

Interactions

This medicine interacts with several other drugs such as adrenocorticosteroids, antimuscarinics, calcium-containing medicines; heart medicines such as digitalis or digoxin; laxatives; other potassium-containing medicines.
- Be sure to tell your doctor about any medications you are currently taking.

Storage

Tablets, elixir, etc. should be stored at room temperature in tightly closed containers. Store away from heat and direct light. Keep out of reach of children, since overdose may be very dangerous in children. Do not keep outdated medicine or medicine no longer needed. Flush the contents of the container down the toilet, unless otherwise directed.

TRILAFON

Properties
This medicine contains as active ingredient perphenazine, a phenothiazine derivative. Phenothiazines are a family of medicines used to treat nervous, mental, and emotional conditions. Some are used to control anxiety, restlessness, nausea and vomiting, and severe hiccups. This medicine is available only with your doctor's prescription.

Before using this medicine
Before you use this medicine check with your doctor, or pharmacist:
- if you ever had any unusual or allergic reaction to phenothiazine medicines.
- if you are on a low-salt, low-sugar, or any other special diet, or if you are allergic to any substance, such as sulfites or other preservatives or dyes.
- if you are pregnant or intend to become pregnant while using this medicine. Although phenothiazines have not been shown to cause birth defects, some side effects such as jaundice and muscle tremors have occurred in a few newborns whose mothers received phenothiazines during pregnancy.
- if you are breast-feeding an infant. Although this medicine has not been shown to cause problems in humans but the chance does exist since some phenothiazines are known to pass into the breast milk.
- if you have any of the following medical problems:
Alcoholism
Blood disease
Difficult urination
Enlarged prostate
Glaucoma
Heart or blood vessel disease
Liver or lung disease
Parkinson's disease
Stomach ulcers

Treatment
This medication is prescribed to treat the symptoms of certain types of mental illness or emotional problems. In order to avoid stomach irritation, you can take the tablet or capsule forms of this medication with a meal or with a glass of water or milk (unless your doctor or pharmacist directs you to do otherwise).

Side effects
Along with the needed effects, a medicine may cause some unwanted effects. Minor side effects are: blurred vision, constipation, decreased sweating, diarrhea, dizziness, drooling, drowsiness, dry mouth, fatigue, jitteriness, menstrual irregularities, nasal congestion, restlessness, tremors, vomiting, or weight gain.
- Tell your doctor about any side effects that are persistent or particularly bothersome. It is especially important to tell your doctor about:
Breast enlargement
Chest pain or convulsions
Darkened skin
Difficulty in swallowing
Fainting or fever
Involuntary movements
Palpitations or sleep disorders
Rash or sore throat
Uncoordinated movements
Unusual bleeding or bruising
Visual disturbances
Yellowing of the eyes or skin

Interactions
This medicine may interact with several other drugs such as barbiturates, sleeping pills, narcotics, other tranquilizers, or any other medication that may produce a sedative effect. Avoid alcohol.

Storage
Store this medication as directed on the label. Keep out of the reach of children.

TRIMCAPS

Properties

This medicine contains phendimetrazine as active ingredient; it is prescribed for appetite suppression.

Appetite suppressants are used in the short-term (a few weeks) treatment of obesity. In a few weeks (6 to 12), these medicines in combination with dieting, exercise, and changes in eating habits can help patients lose weight. However, since their appetite reducing effect is only temporary, they are useful only for the first weeks of dieting until new eating habits are established.

Before using this medicine

Before you use this medicine check with your doctor, or pharmacist:
- if you ever had any unusual or allergic reaction to any of the compounds of this medicine.
- if you are on a low-salt, low-sugar, or any other special diet, or if you are allergic to any substance, such as sulfites or other preservatives or dyes.
- if you are pregnant, intend to become pregnant or breast-feeding an infant while using this medicine.
- if you have any of the following medical problems:
  Diabetes mellitus (sugar diabetes)
  Epilepsy
  Glaucoma
  Heart or blood vessel disease
  High blood pressure
  Mental illness (severe)

Treatment

This medication is used to relieve or prevent the symptoms of your medical problem. Take them as directed. Do not take more of them and do not take them more often than recommended on the label. If too much of the drug is taken, it may become habit-forming.
The medicine produces central nervous system stimulation, and it should not be taken by people with heart disease or high blood pressure.
If you think this medicine is not working as well after you have taken it for a few weeks, do not increase the dose. Instead, check with your doctor.

Side effects

The following minor side effects may occur: irritability, nervousness, restlessness, trouble in sleeping.

These side effects should disappear as your body adjusts to the medication. Tell your doctor about any side effects that are persistent or particularly bothersome. It is especially important to tell your doctor about:
  Mental depression
  Nausea or vomiting
  Stomach cramps or pain
  Trembling
  Unusual tiredness or weakness
- Discontinue use of the drug; call your doctor right away. Adverse reactions and side effects may be more frequent and severe in people over age 60 than in younger persons.

Interactions

This medicine interacts with several other drugs such as antihypertensives, other appetite suppressants, caffeine, central nervous system depressants, central nervous system stimulants, furazolidone, guanethidine, hydralazine, MAO inhibitors, methyldopa, molindone, phenothiazines, rauwolfia alkaloids, sodium bicarbonate.
- Be sure to tell your doctor about any medications you are currently taking.
Interaction with alcoholic beverages may produce drowsiness, sleepiness, and/or inability to concentrate.

Storage

This medicine should be stored at room temperature in tightly closed containers. Store away from heat and direct light. Keep out of reach of children, since overdose may be very dangerous in children.

Do not store this medicine in the bathroom medicine cabinet because the heat and moisture cause the medicine to break down. Do not keep outdated medicine or medicine no longer needed. Flush the contents of the container down the toilet.

TRIMSTAT

Properties
This medicine contains phendimetrazine as active ingredient; it is prescribed for appetite suppression.

Appetite suppressants are used in the short-term (a few weeks) treatment of obesity. In a few weeks (6 to 12), these medicines in combination with dieting, exercise, and changes in eating habits can help patients lose weight. However, since their appetite reducing effect is only temporary, they are useful only for the first weeks of dieting until new eating habits are established.

Before using this medicine
Before you use this medicine check with your doctor, or pharmacist:
- if you ever had any unusual or allergic reaction to any of the compounds of this medicine.
- if you are on a low-salt, low-sugar, or any other special diet, or if you are allergic to any substance, such as sulfites or other preservatives or dyes.
- if you are pregnant, intend to become pregnant or breast-feeding an infant while using this medicine.
- if you have any of the following medical problems:
  Diabetes mellitus (sugar diabetes)
  Epilepsy
  Glaucoma
  Heart or blood vessel disease
  High blood pressure
  Mental illness (severe)

Treatment
This medication is used to relieve or prevent the symptoms of your medical problem. Take them as directed. Do not take more of them and do not take them more often than recommended on the label. If too much of the drug is taken, it may become habit-forming.

The medicine produces central nervous system stimulation, and it should not be taken by people with heart disease or high blood pressure.

If you think this medicine is not working as well after you have taken it for a few weeks, do not increase the dose. Instead, check with your doctor.

Side effects
The following minor side effects may occur: irritability, nervousness, restlessness, trouble in sleeping.

These side effects should disappear as your body adjusts to the medication. Tell your doctor about any side effects that are persistent or particularly bothersome. It is especially important to tell your doctor about:
  Mental depression
  Nausea or vomiting
  Stomach cramps or pain
  Trembling
  Unusual tiredness or weakness
- Discontinue use of the drug; call your doctor right away. Adverse reactions and side effects may be more frequent and severe in people over age 60 than in younger persons.

Interactions
This medicine interacts with several other drugs such as antihypertensives, other appetite suppressants, caffeine, central nervous system depressants, central nervous system stimulants, furazolidone, guanethidine, hydralazine, MAO inhibitors, methyldopa, molindone, phenothiazines, rauwolfia alkaloids, sodium bicarbonate. Interaction with alcoholic beverages may produce drowsiness, sleepiness, and/or inability to concentrate.
- Be sure to tell your doctor about any medications you are currently taking.

Storage
This medicine should be stored at room temperature in tightly closed containers. Store away from heat and direct light. Keep out of reach of children, since overdose may be very dangerous in children.

Do not store this medicine in the bathroom medicine cabinet because the heat and moisture cause the medicine to break down. Do not keep outdated medicine or medicine no longer needed. Flush the contents of the container down the toilet.

TRIMTABS

Properties

This medicine contains phendimetrazine as active ingredient; it is prescribed for appetite suppression.

Appetite suppressants are used in the short-term (a few weeks) treatment of obesity. In a few weeks (6 to 12), these medicines in combination with dieting, exercise, and changes in eating habits can help patients lose weight. However, since their appetite reducing effect is only temporary, they are useful only for the first weeks of dieting until new eating habits are established.

Before using this medicine

Before you use this medicine check with your doctor, or pharmacist:
- if you ever had any unusual or allergic reaction to any of the compounds of this medicine.
- if you are on a low-salt, low-sugar, or any other special diet, or if you are allergic to any substance, such as sulfites or other preservatives or dyes.
- if you are pregnant, intend to become pregnant or breast-feeding an infant while using this medicine.
- if you have any of the following medical problems:
  Diabetes mellitus (sugar diabetes)
  Epilepsy
  Glaucoma
  Heart or blood vessel disease
  High blood pressure
  Mental illness (severe)

Treatment

This medication is used to relieve or prevent the symptoms of your medical problem. Take them as directed. Do not take more of them and do not take them more often than recommended on the label. If too much of the drug is taken, it may become habit-forming.

The medicine produces central nervous system stimulation, and it should not be taken by people with heart disease or high blood pressure.

If you think this medicine is not working as well after you have taken it for a few weeks, do not increase the dose. Instead, check with your doctor.

Side effects

The following minor side effects may occur: irritability, nervousness, restlessness, trouble in sleeping.

These side effects should disappear as your body adjusts to the medication. Tell your doctor about any side effects that are persistent or particularly bothersome. It is especially important to tell your doctor about:
  Mental depression
  Nausea or vomiting
  Stomach cramps or pain
  Trembling
  Unusual tiredness or weakness
- Discontinue use of the drug; call your doctor right away. Adverse reactions and side effects may be more frequent and severe in people over age 60 than in younger persons.

Interactions

This medicine interacts with several other drugs such as antihypertensives, other appetite suppressants, caffeine, central nervous system depressants, central nervous system stimulants, furazolidone, guanethidine, hydralazine, MAO inhibitors, methyldopa, molindone, phenothiazines, rauwolfia alkaloids, sodium bicarbonate. Interaction with alcoholic beverages may produce drowsiness, sleepiness, and/or inability to concentrate.
- Be sure to tell your doctor about any medications you are currently taking.

Storage

This medicine should be stored at room temperature in tightly closed containers. Store away from heat and direct light. Keep out of reach of children, since overdose may be very dangerous in children.

Do not store this medicine in the bathroom medicine cabinet because the heat and moisture cause the medicine to break down. Do not keep outdated medicine or medicine no longer needed. Flush the contents of the container down the toilet.

TUINAL

Properties

This medicine contains as active ingredient the barbiturate secobarbital. Barbiturates belong to the group of medicines called central nervous system depressants (medicines that slow down the nervous system).

Barbiturates may partially block nerve impulses at nerve-cell connections. They may be used to treat insomnia (sleeplessness) by helping patients fall asleep. Also, they may be used to relieve anxiety or tension. Some of the barbiturates are used as anticonvulsants to help control convulsions in certain disorders or diseases, such as epilepsy. If too much of the drug is used, it may become habit-forming (causing mental or physical dependence).

Before using this medicine

Before you use this medicine check with your doctor, or pharmacist:

- if you ever had any unusual or allergic reaction to this medicine or one of its components.
- if you are on a low-salt, low-sugar, or any other special diet, or if you are allergic to preservatives or dyes.
- if you are pregnant or intend to become pregnant while using this medicine, since barbiturates have been shown to increase the chance of birth defects in humans. Taking barbiturates regularly during the last 3 months of pregnancy may cause the baby to become dependent on the medicine. This may lead to withdrawal side effects in the baby after birth.
- if you have any of the following medical problems:
  Anemia (severe)
  Diabetes mellitus (sugar disease)
  Hyperactivity (in children)
  Kidney or lifer disease
  Mental depression
  Overactive thyroid

Treatment

This medication is used to treat the symptoms of your medical condition. Barbiturates act in the central nervous system; some of their side effects are also caused by actions in the central nervous system. Use this medicine as directed by your doctor. Do not use more of it, do not use it more often, and do not use it for a longer period of time than your doctor ordered.

- If you are taking this medication on a regular schedule and you miss a dose, take the missed dose as soon as possible, unless it is almost time for your next dose. In that case do not take the missed dose at all.
- If a barbiturate is used for a long time, it may become habit-forming. Physical dependence may lead to withdrawal side effects when you stop taking this medicine.

Side effects

Along with the needed effects, a medicine may cause some unwanted effects. These side effects may go away during treatment as your body adjusts to the medicine. Such minor side effects are: depression, confusion, diarrhea, nausea, vomiting, joint or muscle pain, slurred speech, hallucinations, headache, decreased sex drive.

- Check with your doctor immediately if any of the following side effects occur:
  Rash or hives
  Face, lip or eyelid swelling
  Sore throat, fever
  Agitation
  Slow heartbeat
  Difficult breathing or chest pain

Interactions

This medicine may interact with several other drugs such as medicines acting on the central nervous system (e.g., antihistamines; beta-adrenergic blockers; MAO inhibitors; mind-altering drugs; nabilone; antidepressants; clozapine; anticonvulsants).

Storage

The medicine should be stored at room temperature in a tightly closed, light-resistant container. Keep out of reach of children since overdose is very dangerous in children.

TWIN-K

Properties

This medicine contains potassium gluconate and potassium citrate chloride as active ingredient; it is used to treat or prevent potassium deficiency, especially potassium deficiency that is caused by the use of diuretics (water pills).

Potassium is needed to maintain good health. Potassium supplements may be needed by patients who do not have enough potassium in their regular diet and by those who have lost too much potassium because of illness or treatment with certain medicines.

Since too much potassium may also cause health problems, most potassium supplements are available only with your doctor's prescription.

Before using this medicine

Before you use this medicine check with your doctor, or pharmacist:

- if you ever had any unusual or allergic reaction to potassium preparations;
- if you are on a low-salt, low-sugar, or any other special diet, or if you are allergic to any substance, such as sulfites or other preservatives or dyes.
- if you are pregnant or intend to become pregnant while using this medicine. Although potassium supplements have not been shown to cause problems in humans, the chance always exists.
- if you are breast-feeding an infant. Although this medicine has not been shown to cause problems in humans, the chance always exists since small amounts of potassium pass into the breast milk.
- if you have any of the following medical problems:
  Addison's disease
  Heart disease
  Diarrhea
  Kidney disease
  Stomach ulcer

Treatment

This medication is used to relieve or prevent the symptoms of your medical problem. Take them as directed. Do not take more of them and do not take them more often than recommended on the label, unless otherwise directed by your doctor. To do so may increase the chance of side effects.

In order to avoid stomach irritation, you should take potassium supplements with food or immediately after a meal. If you miss a dose of this medication, take the missed dose as soon as possible, unless it is within two hours of the next scheduled dose;.

Side effects

The following minor side effects may occur:
  Diarrhea
  Nausea
  Stomach Pains
  Vomiting.

These side effects should disappear as your body adjusts to the medication. Tell your doctor about any side effects that are persistent or particularly bothersome. It is especially important to tell your doctor about anxiety; bloody or black, tarry stools; confusion; difficulty in breathing; numbness or tingling in the arms, legs, or feet; palpitations; severe abdominal pain; or unusual weakness.

Interactions

This medicine interacts with several other drugs such as adrenocorticosteroids, antimuscarinics, calcium-containing medicines; heart medicines such as digitalis or digoxin; laxatives; other potassium-containing medicines.

- Be sure to tell your doctor about any medications you are currently taking.

Storage

Tablets, elixir, etc. should be stored at room temperature in tightly closed containers. Store away from heat and direct light. Keep out of reach of children, since overdose may be very dangerous in children. Do not keep outdated medicine or medicine no longer needed. Flush the contents of the container down the toilet, unless otherwise directed.

TWIN-K-Cl

Properties
This medicine contains potassium gluconate, potassium citrate, and ammonium chloride as active ingredients; it is used to treat or prevent potassium deficiency, especially potassium deficiency that is caused by the use of diuretics (water pills).Potassium is needed to maintain good health. Potassium supplements may be needed by patients who do not have enough potassium in their regular diet and by those who have lost too much potassium because of illness or treatment with certain medicines.

Since too much potassium may also cause health problems, most potassium supplements are available only with your doctor's prescription.

Before using this medicine
Before you use this medicine check with your doctor, or pharmacist:
- if you ever had any unusual or allergic reaction to potassium preparations;
- if you are on a low-salt, low-sugar, or any other special diet, or if you are allergic to any substance, such as sulfites or other preservatives or dyes.
- if you are pregnant or intend to become pregnant while using this medicine. Although potassium supplements have not been shown to cause problems in humans, the chance always exists.
- if you are breast-feeding an infant. Although this medicine has not been shown to cause problems in humans, the chance always exists since small amounts of potassium pass into the breast milk.
- if you have any of the following medical problems:
Addison's disease
Heart disease
Diarrhea
Kidney disease
Stomach ulcer

Treatment
This medication is used to relieve or prevent the symptoms of your medical problem. Take them as directed. Do not take more of them and do not take them more often than recommended on the label, unless otherwise directed by your doctor. To do so may increase the chance of side effects.

In order to avoid stomach irritation, you should take potassium supplements with food or immediately after a meal. If you miss a dose of this medication, take the missed dose as soon as possible, unless it is within two hours of the next scheduled dose;.

Side effects
The following minor side effects may occur:
Diarrhea
Nausea
Stomach Pains
Vomiting.

These side effects should disappear as your body adjusts to the medication. Tell your doctor about any side effects that are persistent or particularly bothersome. It is especially important to tell your doctor about anxiety; bloody or black, tarry stools; confusion; difficulty in breathing; numbness or tingling in the arms, legs, or feet; palpitations; severe abdominal pain; or unusual weakness.

Interactions
This medicine interacts with several other drugs such as adrenocorticosteroids, antimuscarinics, calcium-containing medicines; heart medicines such as digitalis or digoxin; laxatives; other potassium-containing medicines.
- Be sure to tell your doctor about any medications you are currently taking.

Storage
Tablets, elixir, etc. should be stored at room temperature in tightly closed containers. Store away from heat and direct light. Keep out of reach of children, since overdose may be very dangerous in children. Do not keep outdated medicine or medicine no longer needed. Flush the contents of the container down the toilet, unless otherwise directed.

ULTRACEF

Properties
This medicine contains cephalosporin as active ingredient. Cephalosporins belong to the general family of medicines called antibiotics, used in the treatment of infections caused by bacteria. They work by killing bacteria or preventing their growth. Cephalosporins will not work for colds, flu, or other viral infections.

Before using this medicine
Before you use this medicine check with your doctor:
- if you ever had any unusual or allergic reaction to any of the cephalosporins, penicillins, penicillin-like medicines, or penicillamine.
- if you are on a low-salt, low-sugar, or any other special diet, or if you are allergic to any substance, such as sulfites or other preservatives or dyes.
- if you are pregnant or intend to become pregnant while using this medicine. Although cephalosporins have not been shown to cause birth defects or other problems in humans, the chance always exists.
- if you are breast-feeding an infant. Most cephalosporins pass into the breast milk, usually in small amounts.
- if you have any of the following medical problems:
Bleeding problem
Kidney or lifer disease

Treatment
This medication belongs to the general family of medicines called antibiotics. It is used to treat a wide variety of bacterial infections. It is also used to treat infections in persons who are allergic to penicillin.
- Keep taking this medicine for the full time of treatment even if you begin to feel better after a few days; do not miss any doses.
- If you do miss a dose of this medicine, take it as soon as possible. This will help to keep a constant amount of medicine in the blood. However, if it is almost time for your next dose, skip the missed dose and go back to your regular dosing schedule.
- This medication has been prescribed for your current infection only. Another infection later on, or one that someone else has, may require a different medicine. You should not give your medicine to other people or use it for other infections, unless your doctor specifically directs you to do so.
- Take the medicine at the same times each day, 1 hour before or 2 hours after eating.

Side effects
Along with the needed effects, a medicine may cause some unwanted effects. Side effects that usually do not require medical attention: rectal itching, oral or vaginal white spots, mild diarrhea. These side effects should disappear as your body adjusts to the medication.
- Other side effects that should be reported to your doctor immediately are:
Hives, rash
Intense itching
Faintness soon after a dose
Difficulty in breathing
Nausea and vomiting
Severe diarrhea
Unusual weakness or tiredness
Bleeding or bruising

Interactions
This medicine may interact with several other drugs such as anticoagulants, theophylline preparations, probenecid, tetracyclines, etc.
- Be sure to tell your doctor about any medications you are currently taking.

Storage
Tablets, capsules, etc. should be stored at room temperature. Store the liquid form in the refrigerator. Keep out of the reach of children. Do not keep outdated medicine or medicine no longer needed.

UNIFAST UNICELLES

Properties
This medicine contains phentermine as active ingredient; it is prescribed for appetite suppression.

Appetite suppressants are used in the short-term (a few weeks) treatment of obesity. In a few weeks (6 to 12), these medicines in combination with dieting, exercise, and changes in eating habits can help patients lose weight. However, since their appetite reducing effect is only temporary, they are useful only for the first weeks of dieting until new eating habits are established.

Before using this medicine
Before you use this medicine check with your doctor, or pharmacist:
- if you ever had any unusual or allergic reaction to any of the compounds of this medicine.
- if you are on a low-salt, low-sugar, or any other special diet, or if you are allergic to any substance, such as sulfites or other preservatives or dyes.
- if you are pregnant, intend to become pregnant or breast-feeding an infant while using this medicine.
- if you have any of the following medical problems:
  Diabetes mellitus
  Epilepsy
  Glaucoma
  Heart disease
  High blood pressure
  Mental illness (severe)

Treatment
This medication is used to relieve or prevent the symptoms of your medical problem.

Take them as directed. Do not take more of them and do not take them more often than recommended on the label. If too much of the drug is taken, it may become habit-forming.
- The medicine produces central nervous system stimulation, and it should not be taken by people with heart disease or high blood pressure.
- If you think this medicine is not working as well after you have taken it for a few weeks, do not increase the dose. Instead, check with your doctor.

Side effects
The following minor side effects may occur: irritability, nervousness, restlessness, trouble in sleeping.

These side effects should disappear as your body adjusts to the medication. Tell your doctor about any side effects that are persistent or particularly bothersome. It is especially important to tell your doctor about:
  Mental depression
  Nausea or vomiting
  Stomach cramps or pain
  Trembling
  Unusual tiredness
- Discontinue use of the drug; call your doctor right away. Adverse reactions and side effects may be more frequent and severe in people over age 60 than in younger persons.

Interactions
This medicine interacts with several other drugs such as antihypertensives, other appetite suppressants, caffeine, central nervous system depressants, central nervous system stimulants, furazolidone, guanethidine, hydralazine, MAO inhibitors, methyldopa, molindone, phenothiazines, rauwolfia alkaloids, sodium bicarbonate. Interaction with alcoholic beverages may produce drowsiness, sleepiness, and/or inability to concentrate.
- Be sure to tell your doctor about any medications you are currently taking.

Storage
This medicine should be stored at room temperature in tightly closed containers. Store away from heat and direct light. Keep out of reach of children, since overdose may be very dangerous in children.

Do not store this medicine in the bathroom medicine cabinet because the heat and moisture cause the medicine to break down. Do not keep outdated medicine or medicine no longer needed. Flush the contents of the container down the toilet.

UROBAK

Properties

This medicine contains sulfamethoxazole, a sulfonamide, as active ingredient. Sulfonamides are prescribed to treat infections caused by bacteria. They will not work for colds, flu, or other virus infections.

Before using this medicine

Before you use this medicine check with your doctor:

- if you ever had any unusual or allergic reaction to any of the compounds of the medicine.
- if you are on a low-salt, low-sugar, or any other special diet, or if you are allergic to any substance, such as sulfites or other preservatives or dyes.
- if you are pregnant or intend to become pregnant while using this medicine. Although sulfonamides have not been shown to cause defects in humans, the chance may exists.
- if you are breast-feeding an infant. Most sulfonamides pass into the breast milk in small amounts and may cause unwanted effects in infants with some specific conditions.
- if you have any of the following medical problems:
Kidney disease
Liver disease
Porphyria
Deficiency of enzymes such as G6PD

Treatment

This medication is used to treat an infection caused by bacteria. Most sulfonamides are best taken with a full glass (8 ounces) of water on an empty stomach, either one hour before or two hours after a meal. Follow your doctor's or pharmacist's directions on how to take your medicine.

- Keep taking this medicine for the full time of treatment even if you begin to feel better after a few days; do not miss any doses.
- If you do miss a dose of this medicine, take the missed dose immediately.
- This medication works best when the level of medicine in your bloodstream (and urine) is kept constant. It is best, therefore, to take the doses at evenly spaced intervals day and night. if you take two doses a day, the doses should be spaced 12 hours apart.

Side effects

Along with the needed effects, a medicine may cause some unwanted effects. Side effects that usually do not require medical attention: abdominal pain, diarrhea, dizziness, headache, loss of appetite, nausea, sore mouth, or vomiting. These side effects should disappear as your body adjusts to the medication.

Sulfonamides can increase sensitivity to sunlight. It is, therefore, important to avoid prolonged exposure to sunlight and sunlamps.

Tell your doctor about any side effects that are persistent or particularly bothersome. It is especially important to tell your doctor about:
Bloody urine
Difficult urination
Difficulty in breathing
Difficulty in swallowing
Fever or hallucinations
Itching, rash, or pale skin
Joint pain, lower back pain
Ringing in the ears
Sore throat
Swollen or inflamed tongue
Tingling in hands or feet
Unusual bleeding
Yellowing of the eyes or skin

Interactions

This medicine may interact with several other drugs such as anticoagulants, oral antidiabetic agents, aspirin, some antibiotics, or anticancer drugs.

- Be sure to tell your doctor about any medications you are currently taking.

Storage

Tablets, capsules, suspension, etc. should be stored at room temperature as directed by your pharmacist or according to instructions on the label.

UTICILLIN VK

Properties

This medicine contains penicillin V as active ingredient. Penicillins are prescribed to treat infections caused by bacteria. They will not work for colds, flu, or other virus infections. There are several different kinds of penicillins. Each is used to treat different kinds of infections.

Before using this medicine

Before you use this medicine check with your doctor, or pharmacist:

- if you ever had any unusual or allergic reaction to any of the penicillins, cefalosporins, griseofulvin, or penicillamine. Serious reactions may occur in patients who are allergic to penicillins.
- if you are on a low-salt, low-sugar, or any other special diet, or if you are allergic to any substance, such as sulfites or other preservatives or dyes.
- if you are pregnant or intend to become pregnant while using this medicine. Although penicillins have not been shown to cause problems in humans, the chance always exists.
- if you are breast-feeding an infant. Most penicillins (except amdinocillin) pass into the breast milk. Even though only small amounts may pass, allergic reaction, diarrhea, fungal infection, and skin rash may occur in the infant.
- if you have any of the following medical problems:
  Allergy
  Asthma
  Bleeding problems
  Eczema
  Hay fever, hives
  Kidney disease
  Liver disease
  Mononucleosis
  Stomach or intestinal disease

Treatment

This medication is used to treat an infection caused by bacteria. Most penicillins are best taken with a full glass (8 ounces) of water on an empty stomach, some are best taken with a snack or meal. Follow your doctor's or pharmacist's directions on how to take your medicine.

- ◆ Keep taking this medicine for the full time of treatment even if you begin to feel better after a few days; do not miss any doses. This is especially important if you have a "strep" infection since serious heart problems could develop later if your infection is not cleared up completely.
- ◆ If you do miss a dose of this medicine, take it as soon as possible. However, if it is almost time for your next dose, skip the missed dose and go back to your regular dosing schedule.

Side effects

Along with the needed effects, a medicine may cause some unwanted effects. Side effects that usually do not require medical attention: diarrhea; nausea or vomiting; sore mouth or tongue.

- ◆ Stop taking this medicine and get emergency help immediately if you notice: difficulty in breathing; lightheadedness; skin rash, hives, itching; wheezing.

Other side effects that should be reported to your doctor immediately are: abdominal bloating; blood in urine; convulsions (seizures); decreased amount of urine; diarrhea (watery and severe) which may also be bloody; fever; joint pain; sore throat and fever; stomach or abdominal cramps and pain; unusual bleeding or bruising.

Interactions

This medicine may interact with several other drugs such as anticoagulants, diarrhea medicines, heparin, ibuprofen, oral contraceptives, potassium-containing medicines, etc.

- ■ Be sure to tell your doctor about any medications you are currently taking.

Storage

Tablets, capsules, etc. should be stored as directed by your pharmacist or according to instructions on the label.

UTICORT

Properties
This medicine contains betamethasone, a corticosteroid, as active ingredient. Corticosteroids are used to help relieve redness, swelling, itching, inflammation, and discomfort of many skin problems. They exert this effect by interfering with natural body mechanisms that produce the rash, itching, or inflammation. They do not cure the underlying cause of the skin problem. This medication is applied to the skin.

Before using this medicine
Before you use this medicine check with your doctor, or pharmacist:
- if you ever had any unusual or allergic reaction to corticosteroids.
- if you are allergic to any substance, such as sulfites or other preservatives or dyes.
- if you are pregnant or intend to become pregnant while using this medicine. Studies have shown that corticosteroids applied to the skin in large amounts or over long periods of time can be the cause of birth defects.
- if you are breast-feeding an infant. Some corticosteroids pass into breast milk and may interfere with the infant's growth.

Treatment
Do not use this medicine more often or for a longer time than ordered. To do so may increase absorption through the skin and the chance of side effects. In addition, too much use, especially on areas with thinner skin (for example, face, armpits, groin), may result in thinning of the skin and stretch marks.

Before applying this medication, wash your hands. than, unless your doctor or pharmacist gives you different instructions, gently wash the area where the medication is to be applied. With a clean towel pat the area dry. Apply a small amount of the medication to the affected area in a thin layer. Do not bandage the area unless your doctor tells you to do so.

If you miss a dose of this medication, apply the dose as soon as possible, unless it is almost time for the next application.

- ◆ Do not use this medicine for other skin problems without first checking with your doctor. You should not use a topical corticosteroid if you have a virus disease (such as herpes), fungal infection of the skin (such as athlete's foot), or tuberculosis of the skin.

Side effects
There are a number of side effects that usually do not require medical attention. Minor side effects are:
Acne
Burning sensations
Itching
Rash
Skin dryness
These possible side effects may go away during treatment; however, if they continue or are bothersome, check with your doctor, nurse, or pharmacist. Tell your doctor about any side effects that are persistent or particularly bothersome, such as:
Blistering
Increased hair growth
Irritation of the affected area
Loss of skin
Secondary infection in the area being treated
Thinning of the skin with easy bruising

Interactions
None known as long as it is used according to the directions given to you by your doctor or pharmacist.

Storage
Cream, ointment, lotion, gel, spray, and aerosol should be stored at room temperature in tightly closed containers. This medication should never be frozen.

VALERGEN

Properties
This medicine contains estrogen as active ingredient. The medicine is prescribed for treatment of estrogen deficiency; it restores normal estrogen levels in tissues. There is no evidence that this drug is effective for nervous symptoms or depression occurring during menopause. They should not be used to treat this condition; they should be used only to replace the estrogen that is naturally absent after menopause.

Before using this medicine
Before you use this medicine check with your doctor, or pharmacist:
- if you ever had any unusual or allergic reaction to estrogens;
- if you are pregnant or intend to become pregnant within three months;
- if you are breast-feeding an infant;
- if you have any of the following medical problems:
  Diabetes
  Breast cancer
  Fibrocystic breast disease
  Fibroid uterine tumors
  Endometriosis
  Migraine headaches
  Epilepsy
  Porphyria
  High blood pressure
  Asthma
  Congestive heart failure
  Kidney disease
  Gallstones

Treatment
This medication is used to treat estrogen deficiency, specific symptoms of menopause, estrogen-deficiency osteoporosis, atrophic vaginitis, prostate cancer.
For safe and effective use of this medicine:
- Follow your doctor's instructions if this medicine was prescribed.
- Follow the manufacturer's package directions if you are treating yourself.
- Estrogens have been reported to increase the risk of endometrial carcinoma.

Side effects
Along with the needed effects, a medicine may cause some unwanted effects. Possible side effects include:
  Stomach cramps
  Profuse bleeding
  Appetite loss
  Nausea and vomiting
  Swollen breasts
  Change in menstruation
  Rash, skin blisters
  Depression
  Dizziness

Overdose
The following symptoms may indicate an overdose:
  Nausea and vomiting
  Fluid retention
  Breast enlargement
  Abnormal vaginal bleeding
- Call a doctor or hospital emergency room for instructions.

Interactions
This medicine may interact with several other drugs such as adrenocorticosteroids, antidepressants, oral antidiabetics, insulin, phenobarbital, primidone.
- Be sure to tell your doctor about any medications you are currently taking.

Storage
Capsules, tablets, vaginal cream, transdermal patches, etc. should be stored at room temperature; store away from heat and direct light. Keep out of reach of children, since this medicine may be dangerous in children.

VALISONE

Properties
This medicine contains betamethasone, a corticosteroid, as active ingredient. Corticosteroids are used to help relieve redness, swelling, itching, inflammation, and discomfort of many skin problems. They exert this effect by interfering with natural body mechanisms that produce the rash, itching, or inflammation. They do not cure the underlying cause of the skin problem. This medication is applied to the skin.

Before using this medicine
Before you use this medicine check with your doctor, or pharmacist:
- if you ever had any unusual or allergic reaction to corticosteroids.
- if you are allergic to any substance, such as sulfites or other preservatives or dyes.
- if you are pregnant or intend to become pregnant while using this medicine. Studies have shown that corticosteroids applied to the skin in large amounts or over long periods of time can be the cause of birth defects.
- if you are breast-feeding an infant. Some corticosteroids pass into breast milk and may interfere with the infant's growth.

Treatment
Do not use this medicine more often or for a longer time than ordered. To do so may increase absorption through the skin and the chance of side effects. In addition, too much use, especially on areas with thinner skin (for example, face, armpits, groin), may result in thinning of the skin and stretch marks.

Before applying this medication, wash your hands. than, unless your doctor or pharmacist gives you different instructions, gently wash the area where the medication is to be applied. With a clean towel pat the area dry. Apply a small amount of the medication to the affected area in a thin layer. Do not bandage the area unless your doctor tells you to do so.

If you miss a dose of this medication, apply the dose as soon as possible, unless it is almost time for the next application.

- ◆ Do not use this medicine for other skin problems without first checking with your doctor. You should not use a topical corticosteroid if you have a virus disease (such as herpes), fungal infection of the skin (such as athlete's foot), or tuberculosis of the skin.

Side effects
There are a number of side effects that usually do not require medical attention. Minor side effects are:
   Acne
   Burning sensations
   Itching
   Rash
   Skin dryness
These possible side effects may go away during treatment; however, if they continue or are bothersome, check with your doctor, nurse, or pharmacist. Tell your doctor about any side effects that are persistent or particularly bothersome, such as:
   Blistering
   Increased hair growth
   Irritation of the affected area
   Loss of skin
   Secondary infection in the area being treated
   Thinning of the skin with easy bruising

Interactions
None known as long as it is used according to the directions given to you by your doctor or pharmacist.

Storage
Cream, ointment, lotion, gel, spray, and aerosol should be stored at room temperature in tightly closed containers. This medication should never be frozen.

VALIUM

Properties

This medicine contains as active ingredient diazepam, a benzodiazepine preparation. Benzodiazepines belong to the group of psychoactive medicines that influence the activity of the brain. Some are used to relieve nervousness or tension. It is effective for this purpose for short periods. Others are used for sleeplessness or to relax muscles or relieve muscle spasm. The benzodiazepines may also be used for other conditions as determined by your doctor.

Before using this medicine

Before you use this medicine check with your doctor:

- if you ever had any unusual or allergic reaction to benzodiazepines.
- if you are on a low-salt, low-sugar, or any other special diet, or if you are allergic to any substance, such as sulfites or other preservatives or dyes.
- if you are pregnant or intend to become pregnant while using this medicine. Some benzodiazepines have been reported to increase the chance of birth defects when used during the first 3 months of pregnancy.
- if you are breast-feeding an infant. Benzodiazepines may pass into the breast milk and cause drowsiness, unusually slow heartbeat, shortness of breath, or troubled breathing in infants of mothers taking this medicine.
- if you have any of the following medical problems: asthma, bronchitis, emphysema, or other chronic lung disease; epilepsy or history of convulsions; hyperactivity (in children); kidney or lifer disease; mental depression or illness; myasthania gravis, porphyria.

Treatment

This medication is used to relieve or prevent the symptoms of your medical problem. Benzodiazepines are mainly used as antianxiety agents, anticonvulsants, or sedatives. Take them as directed. Do not take more of them and do not take them more often than recommended on the label, unless otherwise directed by your doctor. Benzodiazepine tranquilizing drugs can be abused if taken for long periods of time and it is possible to develop withdrawal symptoms if you discontinue the therapy abruptly.

Side effects

Along with the needed effects, a medicine may cause some unwanted effects. Minor side effects are: bitter taste in the mouth, dizziness, drowsiness, depression, constipation, dry mouth, excessive salivation, fatigue, flushing, headache, heartburn, loss of appetite, nausea, nervousness, sweating or vomiting. As your body adjusts to the medicine, these side effects should disappear.

- Tell your doctor about any side effects that are persistent or particularly bothersome. It is especially important to tell your doctor about:
  Blurred or double vision
  Chest pain
  Difficulty in urinating
  Fainting or falling
  Fever or hallucinations
  Joint pain
  Mouth sores
  Nightmares
  Palpitations
  Severe depression
  Shortness of breath
  Slurred speech
  Uncoordinated movements
  Unusual tiredness
  Yellowing of the skin

Interactions

This medicine may interact with several other drugs. This medicine will add to the effects of alcohol, and CNS depressants.

- Be sure to tell your doctor about any medications you are currently taking.

Storage

Store at room temperature in tightly closed, light-resistant-resistant containers. Keep out of the reach of children since overdose may be especially dangerous in children.

VALNAC

Properties
This medicine contains betamethasone, a corticosteroid, as active ingredient. Corticosteroids are used to help relieve redness, swelling, itching, inflammation, and discomfort of many skin problems. They exert this effect by interfering with natural body mechanisms that produce the rash, itching, or inflammation. They do not cure the underlying cause of the skin problem. This medication is applied to the skin.

Before using this medicine
Before you use this medicine check with your doctor, or pharmacist:
- if you ever had any unusual or allergic reaction to corticosteroids.
- if you are allergic to any substance, such as sulfites or other preservatives or dyes.
- if you are pregnant or intend to become pregnant while using this medicine. Studies have shown that corticosteroids applied to the skin in large amounts or over long periods of time can be the cause of birth defects.
- if you are breast-feeding an infant. Some corticosteroids pass into breast milk and may interfere with the infant's growth.

Treatment
Do not use this medicine more often or for a longer time than ordered. To do so may increase absorption through the skin and the chance of side effects. In addition, too much use, especially on areas with thinner skin (for example, face, armpits, groin), may result in thinning of the skin and stretch marks.

Before applying this medication, wash your hands. than, unless your doctor or pharmacist gives you different instructions, gently wash the area where the medication is to be applied. With a clean towel pat the area dry. Apply a small amount of the medication to the affected area in a thin layer. Do not bandage the area unless your doctor tells you to do so.

If you miss a dose of this medication, apply the dose as soon as possible, unless it is almost time for the next application.
- ◆ Do not use this medicine for other skin problems without first checking with your doctor. You should not use a topical corticosteroid if you have a virus disease (such as herpes), fungal infection of the skin (such as athlete's foot), or tuberculosis of the skin.

Side effects
There are a number of side effects that usually do not require medical attention. Minor side effects are:
Acne
Burning sensations
Itching
Rash
Skin dryness

These possible side effects may go away during treatment; however, if they continue or are bothersome, check with your doctor, nurse, or pharmacist. Tell your doctor about any side effects that are persistent or particularly bothersome, such as:
Blistering
Increased hair growth
Irritation of the affected area
Loss of skin
Secondary infection in the area being treated
Thinning of the skin with easy bruising

Interactions
None known as long as it is used according to the directions given to you by your doctor or pharmacist.

Storage
Cream, ointment, lotion, gel, spray, and aerosol should be stored at room temperature in tightly closed containers. This medication should never be frozen.

VALRELEASE

Properties
This medicine contains as active ingredient diazepam, a benzodiazepine preparation. Benzodiazepines belong to the group of psychoactive medicines that influence the activity of the brain. Some are used to relieve nervousness or tension. It is effective for this purpose for short periods. Others are used for sleeplessness or to relax muscles or relieve muscle spasm. The benzodiazepines may also be used for other conditions as determined by your doctor.

Before using this medicine
Before you use this medicine check with your doctor:
- if you ever had any unusual or allergic reaction to benzodiazepines.
- if you are on a low-salt, low-sugar, or any other special diet, or if you are allergic to any substance, such as sulfites or other preservatives or dyes.
- if you are pregnant or intend to become pregnant while using this medicine. Some benzodiazepines have been reported to increase the chance of birth defects when used during the first 3 months of pregnancy.
- if you are breast-feeding an infant. Benzodiazepines may pass into the breast milk and cause drowsiness, unusually slow heartbeat, shortness of breath, or troubled breathing in infants of mothers taking this medicine.
- if you have any of the following medical problems: asthma, bronchitis, emphysema, or other chronic lung disease; epilepsy or history of convulsions; hyperactivity (in children); kidney or lifer disease; mental depression or illness; myasthania gravis, porphyria.

Treatment
This medication is used to relieve or prevent the symptoms of your medical problem. Benzodiazepines are mainly used as antianxiety agents, anticonvulsants, or sedatives. Take them as directed. Do not take more of them and do not take them more often than recommended on the label, unless otherwise directed by your doctor. Benzodiazepine tranquilizing drugs can be abused if taken for long periods of time and it is possible to develop withdrawal symptoms if you discontinue the therapy abruptly.

Side effects
Along with the needed effects, a medicine may cause some unwanted effects. Minor side effects are: bitter taste in the mouth, dizziness, drowsiness, depression, constipation, dry mouth, excessive salivation, fatigue, flushing, headache, heartburn, loss of appetite, nausea, nervousness, sweating or vomiting. As your body adjusts to the medicine, these side effects should disappear.
- Tell your doctor about any side effects that are persistent or particularly bothersome. It is especially important to tell your doctor about:
  Blurred or double vision
  Chest pain
  Difficulty in urinating
  Fainting or falling
  Fever or hallucinations
  Joint pain
  Mouth sores
  Nightmares
  Palpitations
  Severe depression
  Shortness of breath
  Slurred speech
  Uncoordinated movements
  Unusual tiredness
  Yellowing of the skin

Interactions
This medicine may interact with several other drugs. This medicine will add to the effects of alcohol, and CNS depressants.
- Be sure to tell your doctor about any medications you are currently taking.

Storage
Store at room temperature in tightly closed, light-resistant-resistant containers. Keep out of the reach of children since overdose may be especially dangerous in children.

VANTIN

Properties

This medicine contains cephalosporin as active ingredient. Cephalosporins belong to the general family of medicines called antibiotics, used in the treatment of infections caused by bacteria. They work by killing bacteria or preventing their growth. Cephalosporins will not work for colds, flu, or other viral infections.

Before using this medicine

Before you use this medicine check with your doctor:

– if you ever had any unusual or allergic reaction to any of the cephalosporins, penicillins, penicillin-like medicines, or penicillamine.
– if you are on a low-salt, low-sugar, or any other special diet, or if you are allergic to any substance, such as sulfites or other preservatives or dyes.
– if you are pregnant or intend to become pregnant while using this medicine. Although cephalosporins have not been shown to cause birth defects or other problems in humans, the chance always exists.
– if you are breast-feeding an infant. Most cephalosporins pass into the breast milk, usually in small amounts.
– if you have any of the following medical problems:
Bleeding problem
Kidney or lifer disease

Treatment

This medication belongs to the general family of medicines called antibiotics. It is used to treat a wide variety of bacterial infections. It is also used to treat infections in persons who are allergic to penicillin.

■ Keep taking this medicine for the full time of treatment even if you begin to feel better after a few days; do not miss any doses.
■ If you do miss a dose of this medicine, take it as soon as possible. This will help to keep a constant amount of medicine in the blood. However, if it is almost time for your next dose, skip the missed dose and go back to your regular dosing schedule.
■ This medication has been prescribed for your current infection only. Another infection later on, or one that someone else has, may require a different medicine. You should not give your medicine to other people or use it for other infections, unless your doctor specifically directs you to do so.
■ Take the medicine at the same times each day, 1 hour before or 2 hours after eating.

Side effects

Along with the needed effects, a medicine may cause some unwanted effects. Side effects that usually do not require medical attention: rectal itching, oral or vaginal white spots, mild diarrhea. These side effects should disappear as your body adjusts to the medication.

■ Other side effects that should be reported to your doctor immediately are:
Hives, rash
Intense itching
Faintness soon after a dose
Difficulty in breathing
Nausea and vomiting
Severe diarrhea
Unusual weakness or tiredness
Bleeding or bruising

Interactions

This medicine may interact with several other drugs such as anticoagulants, theophylline preparations, probenecid, tetracyclines, etc.

■ Be sure to tell your doctor about any medications you are currently taking.

Storage

Tablets, capsules, etc. should be stored at room temperature. Store the liquid form in the refrigerator. Keep out of the reach of children. Do not keep outdated medicine or medicine no longer needed.

VASCOR

Properties

This medicine contains bepridil as active ingredient. It is a so-called calcium channel blocker, working by blocking the passage of calcium into heart and smooth muscle. Since calcium is an essential factor in muscle contraction, any medicine that affects calcium in this way will interfere with the contraction of these muscles.

The medicine works by:
♦ reducing the work that the heart must perform;
♦ reducing the normal arterial blood pressure;
♦ increasing oxygen to the heart muscle.

The medicine is prescribed for the treatment of attacks of angina pectoris, irregular heartbeat, and high blood pressure. In many cases it can be used for the treatment and prevention of migraine.

Before using this medicine

Before you use this medicine check with your doctor, or pharmacist:
- if you ever had any unusual or allergic reaction to this medicine or any calcium channel blocker;
- if you are pregnant or intend to become pregnant while using this medicine;
- if you have low blood pressure;
- if you have kidney or lifer disease;
- if you are breast-feeding an infant;
- if you easily get a rash or intensity sunburn in areas exposed to sun or ultraviolet light.

Treatment

This medication is used for treatment of heart conditions (for instance, angina pectoris) and high blood pressure. Tablets, capsules or extended-release tablets should be taken with liquid. The usual dose amounts to 30 to 100 milligrams a day.

For safe and effective use of medicine:
♦ Follow your doctor's instructions if this medicine was prescribed.
♦ Follow the manufacturer's package directions if you are treating yourself.

Side effects

Along with the needed effects, a medicine may cause some unwanted effects. Possible side effects include:
Tiredness
Changes in heartbeat
Wheezing
Cough
Shortness of breath
Dizziness
Fainting
Numbness in hands and feet
Tingling in hands and feet
Difficult urination
Constipation

Overdose

The following symptoms may be a sign of overdose:
Unusually fast heartbeat
Unusually slow heartbeat
Loss of consciousness
Cardiac arrest
■ Call a doctor or hospital emergency room for instructions. If necessary start first aid immediately.

Interactions

The effect of this medicine may cause a blood pressure drop if taken together with antihypertensives. Cimetidine may increase the effect of the calcium blocker.

The simultaneous use of diuretics and calcium channel blockers may cause dangerous blood pressure drop.
■ Be sure to tell your doctor about any medications you are currently taking.

Storage

Capsules, tablets, etc. should be stored at room temperature; store away from heat and direct light. Keep out of reach of children, since this medicine may be dangerous in children.

VAZEPAM

Properties
This medicine contains as active ingredient diazepam, a benzodiazepine preparation. Benzodiazepines belong to the group of psychoactive medicines that influence the activity of the brain. Some are used to relieve nervousness or tension. It is effective for this purpose for short periods. Others are used for sleeplessness or to relax muscles or relieve muscle spasm. The benzodiazepines may also be used for other conditions as determined by your doctor.

Before using this medicine
Before you use this medicine check with your doctor:
- if you ever had any unusual or allergic reaction to benzodiazepines.
- if you are on a low-salt, low-sugar, or any other special diet, or if you are allergic to any substance, such as sulfites or other preservatives or dyes.
- if you are pregnant or intend to become pregnant while using this medicine. Some benzodiazepines have been reported to increase the chance of birth defects when used during the first 3 months of pregnancy.
- if you are breast-feeding an infant. Benzodiazepines may pass into the breast milk and cause drowsiness, unusually slow heartbeat, shortness of breath, or troubled breathing in infants of mothers taking this medicine.
- if you have any of the following medical problems: asthma, bronchitis, emphysema, or other chronic lung disease; epilepsy or history of convulsions; hyperactivity (in children); kidney or lifer disease; mental depression or illness; myasthania gravis, porphyria.

Treatment
This medication is used to relieve or prevent the symptoms of your medical problem. Benzodiazepines are mainly used as antianxiety agents, anticonvulsants, or sedatives. Take them as directed. Do not take more of them and do not take them more often than recommended on the label, unless otherwise directed by your doctor. Benzodiazepine tranquilizing drugs can be abused if taken for long periods of time and it is possible to develop withdrawal symptoms if you discontinue the therapy abruptly.

Side effects
Along with the needed effects, a medicine may cause some unwanted effects. Minor side effects are: bitter taste in the mouth, dizziness, drowsiness, depression, constipation, dry mouth, excessive salivation, fatigue, flushing, headache, heartburn, loss of appetite, nausea, nervousness, sweating or vomiting. As your body adjusts to the medicine, these side effects should disappear.
- Tell your doctor about any side effects that are persistent or particularly bothersome. It is especially important to tell your doctor about:
  Blurred or double vision
  Chest pain
  Difficulty in urinating
  Fainting or falling
  Fever or hallucinations
  Joint pain
  Mouth sores
  Nightmares
  Palpitations
  Severe depression
  Shortness of breath
  Slurred speech
  Uncoordinated movements
  Unusual tiredness
  Yellowing of the skin

Interactions
This medicine may interact with several other drugs. This medicine will add to the effects of alcohol, and CNS depressants.
- Be sure to tell your doctor about any medications you are currently taking.

Storage
Store at room temperature in tightly closed, light-resistant-resistant containers. Keep out of the reach of children since overdose may be especially dangerous in children.

V-CILLIN K

Properties
This medicine contains penicillin V as active ingredient. Penicillins are prescribed to treat infections caused by bacteria. They will not work for colds, flu, or other virus infections. There are several different kinds of penicillins. Each is used to treat different kinds of infections.

Before using this medicine
Before you use this medicine check with your doctor, or pharmacist:
- if you ever had any unusual or allergic reaction to any of the penicillins, cefalosporins, griseofulvin, or penicillamine. Serious reactions may occur in patients who are allergic to penicillins.
- if you are on a low-salt, low-sugar, or any other special diet, or if you are allergic to any substance, such as sulfites or other preservatives or dyes.
- if you are pregnant or intend to become pregnant while using this medicine. Although penicillins have not been shown to cause problems in humans, the chance always exists.
- if you are breast-feeding an infant. Most penicillins (except amdinocillin) pass into the breast milk. Even though only small amounts may pass, allergic reaction, diarrhea, fungal infection, and skin rash may occur in the infant.
- if you have any of the following medical problems:
Allergy
Asthma
Bleeding problems
Eczema
Hay fever, hives
Kidney disease
Liver disease
Mononucleosis
Stomach or intestinal disease

Treatment
This medication is used to treat an infection caused by bacteria. Most penicillins are best taken with a full glass (8 ounces) of water on an empty stomach, some are best taken with a snack or meal. Follow your doctor's or pharmacist's directions on how to take your medicine.
- ◆ Keep taking this medicine for the full time of treatment even if you begin to feel better after a few days; do not miss any doses. This is especially important if you have a "strep" infection since serious heart problems could develop later if your infection is not cleared up completely.
- ◆ If you do miss a dose of this medicine, take it as soon as possible. However, if it is almost time for your next dose, skip the missed dose and go back to your regular dosing schedule.

Side effects
Along with the needed effects, a medicine may cause some unwanted effects. Side effects that usually do not require medical attention: diarrhea; nausea or vomiting; sore mouth or tongue.
- ◆ Stop taking this medicine and get emergency help immediately if you notice: difficulty in breathing; light-headedness; skin rash, hives, itching; wheezing.

Other side effects that should be reported to your doctor immediately are: abdominal bloating; blood in urine; convulsions (seizures); decreased amount of urine; diarrhea (watery and severe) which may also be bloody; fever; joint pain; sore throat and fever; stomach or abdominal cramps and pain; unusual bleeding or bruising.

Interactions
This medicine may interact with several other drugs such as anticoagulants, diarrhea medicines, heparin, ibuprofen, oral contraceptives, potassium-containing medicines, etc.
- ■ Be sure to tell your doctor about any medications you are currently taking.

Storage
Tablets, capsules, etc. should be stored as directed by your pharmacist or according to instructions on the label.

VEETIDS

Properties
This medicine contains penicillin V as active ingredient. Penicillins are prescribed to treat infections caused by bacteria. They will not work for colds, flu, or other virus infections. There are several different kinds of penicillins. Each is used to treat different kinds of infections.

Before using this medicine
Before you use this medicine check with your doctor, or pharmacist:
- if you ever had any unusual or allergic reaction to any of the penicillins, cefalosporins, griseofulvin, or penicillamine. Serious reactions may occur in patients who are allergic to penicillins.
- if you are on a low-salt, low-sugar, or any other special diet, or if you are allergic to any substance, such as sulfites or other preservatives or dyes.
- if you are pregnant or intend to become pregnant while using this medicine. Although penicillins have not been shown to cause problems in humans, the chance always exists.
- if you are breast-feeding an infant. Most penicillins (except amdinocillin) pass into the breast milk. Even though only small amounts may pass, allergic reaction, diarrhea, fungal infection, and skin rash may occur in the infant.
- if you have any of the following medical problems:
Allergy
Asthma
Bleeding problems
Eczema
Hay fever, hives
Kidney disease
Liver disease
Mononucleosis
Stomach or intestinal disease

Treatment
This medication is used to treat an infection caused by bacteria. Most penicillins are best taken with a full glass (8 ounces) of water on an empty stomach, some are best taken with a snack or meal. Follow your doctor's or pharmacist's directions on how to take your medicine.
- ◆ Keep taking this medicine for the full time of treatment even if you begin to feel better after a few days; do not miss any doses. This is especially important if you have a "strep" infection since serious heart problems could develop later if your infection is not cleared up completely.
- ◆ If you do miss a dose of this medicine, take it as soon as possible. However, if it is almost time for your next dose, skip the missed dose and go back to your regular dosing schedule.

Side effects
Along with the needed effects, a medicine may cause some unwanted effects. Side effects that usually do not require medical attention: diarrhea; nausea or vomiting; sore mouth or tongue.
- ◆ Stop taking this medicine and get emergency help immediately if you notice: difficulty in breathing; lightheadedness; skin rash, hives, itching; wheezing.
Other side effects that should be reported to your doctor immediately are: abdominal bloating; blood in urine; convulsions (seizures); decreased amount of urine; diarrhea (watery and severe) which may also be bloody; fever; joint pain; sore throat and fever; stomach or abdominal cramps and pain; unusual bleeding or bruising.

Interactions
This medicine may interact with several other drugs such as anticoagulants, diarrhea medicines, heparin, ibuprofen, oral contraceptives, potassium-containing medicines, etc.
- ■ Be sure to tell your doctor about any medications you are currently taking.

Storage
Tablets, capsules, etc. should be stored as directed by your pharmacist or according to instructions on the label.

VERAPAMIL

Properties
This medicine contains verapamil as active ingredient. It is a so-called calcium channel blocker, working by blocking the passage of calcium into heart and smooth muscle. Since calcium is an essential factor in muscle contraction, any medicine that affects calcium in this way will interfere with the contraction of these muscles.

The medicine works by:
♦ reducing the work that the heart must perform;
♦ reducing the normal arterial blood pressure;
♦ increasing oxygen to the heart muscle.

The medicine is prescribed for the treatment of attacks of angina pectoris, irregular heartbeat, and high blood pressure. In many cases it can be used for the treatment and prevention of migraine.

Before using this medicine
Before you use this medicine check with your doctor, or pharmacist:
– if you ever had any unusual or allergic reaction to this medicine or any calcium channel blocker;
– if you are pregnant or intend to become pregnant while using this medicine;
– if you have low blood pressure;
– if you have kidney or lifer disease;
– if you are breast-feeding an infant;
– if you easily get a rash or intensity sunburn in areas exposed to sun or ultraviolet light.

Treatment
This medication is used for treatment of heart conditions (for instance, angina pectoris) and high blood pressure. Tablets, capsules or extended-release tablets should be taken with liquid. The usual dose amounts to 30 to 100 milligrams a day.

For safe and effective use of medicine:
♦ Follow your doctor's instructions if this medicine was prescribed.
♦ Follow the manufacturer's package directions if you are treating yourself.

Side effects
Along with the needed effects, a medicine may cause some unwanted effects. Possible side effects include:
    Tiredness
    Changes in heartbeat
    Wheezing
    Cough
    Shortness of breath
    Dizziness
    Fainting
    Numbness in hands and feet
    Tingling in hands and feet
    Difficult urination
    Constipation

Overdose
The following symptoms may be a sign of overdose:
    Unusually fast heartbeat
    Unusually slow heartbeat
    Loss of consciousness
    Cardiac arrest
■ Call a doctor or hospital emergency room for instructions. If necessary start first aid immediately.

Interactions
The effect of this medicine may cause a blood pressure drop if taken together with antihypertensives. Cimetidine may increase the effect of the calcium blocker.

The simultaneous use of diuretics and calcium channel blockers may cause dangerous blood pressure drop.
■ Be sure to tell your doctor about any medications you are currently taking.

Storage
Capsules, tablets, etc. should be stored at room temperature; store away from heat and direct light. Keep out of reach of children, since this medicine may be dangerous in children.

VERELAN

Properties

This medicine contains verapamil as active ingredient. It is a so-called calcium channel blocker, working by blocking the passage of calcium into heart and smooth muscle. Since calcium is an essential factor in muscle contraction, any medicine that affects calcium in this way will interfere with the contraction of these muscles.

The medicine works by:
◆ reducing the work that the heart must perform;
◆ reducing the normal arterial blood pressure;
◆ increasing oxygen to the heart muscle.

The medicine is prescribed for the treatment of attacks of angina pectoris, irregular heartbeat, and high blood pressure. In many cases it can be used for the treatment and prevention of migraine.

Before using this medicine

Before you use this medicine check with your doctor, or pharmacist:
– if you ever had any unusual or allergic reaction to this medicine or any calcium channel blocker;
– if you are pregnant or intend to become pregnant while using this medicine;
– if you have low blood pressure;
– if you have kidney or lifer disease;
– if you are breast-feeding an infant;
– if you easily get a rash or intensity sunburn in areas exposed to sun or ultraviolet light.

Treatment

This medication is used for treatment of heart conditions (for instance, angina pectoris) and high blood pressure. Tablets, capsules or extended-release tablets should be taken with liquid. The usual dose amounts to 30 to 100 milligrams a day.

For safe and effective use of medicine:
◆ Follow your doctor's instructions if this medicine was prescribed.
◆ Follow the manufacturer's package directions if you are treating yourself.

Side effects

Along with the needed effects, a medicine may cause some unwanted effects. Possible side effects include:
Tiredness
Changes in heartbeat
Wheezing
Cough
Shortness of breath
Dizziness
Fainting
Numbness in hands and feet
Tingling in hands and feet
Difficult urination
Constipation

Overdose

The following symptoms may be a sign of overdose:
Unusually fast heartbeat
Unusually slow heartbeat
Loss of consciousness
Cardiac arrest
■ Call a doctor or hospital emergency room for instructions. If necessary start first aid immediately.

Interactions

The effect of this medicine may cause a blood pressure drop if taken together with antihypertensives. Cimetidine may increase the effect of the calcium blocker.

The simultaneous use of diuretics and calcium channel blockers may cause dangerous blood pressure drop.
■ Be sure to tell your doctor about any medications you are currently taking.

Storage

Capsules, tablets, etc. should be stored at room temperature; store away from heat and direct light. Keep out of reach of children, since this medicine may be dangerous in children.

VIAGRA

Properties
This medicine contains sildenafil citrate as active ingredient. It is indicated for the treatment of erectile dysfunction. The studies that established benefit demonstrated improvements in success rates for sexual intercourse compared with placebo.

Erectile dysfunction is the consistent inability to achieve and/or maintain an erection sufficient for satisfactory sexual activity. That means not just an occasional problem, but one that has been occurring repeatedly for a period of time.

Before using this medicine
A thorough medical history and physical examination should be undertaken to diagnose erectile dysfunction, determine potential underlying causes, and identify appropriate treatment.

Agents for the treatment of erectile dysfunction should be used with caution in patients with anatomical deformation of the penis (such as angulation, cavernosal fibrosis or Peyronie's disease), or in patients who have conditions which may predispose them to priapism (such as sickle cell anemia, multiple myeloma, or leukemia).

Treatment
This medication is used for treatment of erectile dysfunction. For safe and effective use of medicine:
- Follow your doctor's instructions if this medicine was prescribed.
- Follow the manufacturer's package directions if you are treating yourself.

The use of this medicine offers no protection against sexually transmitted diseases. Counseling of patients about the protective measures necessary to guard against sexually transmitted diseases, including HIV, may be considered.

Adverse reactions
Viagra was administered to over 3700 patients (aged 19-87) during clinical trials worldwide. Over 500 patients were treated for longer than one year. In placebo-controlled clinical studies, the discontinuation rate due to adverse events for Viagra (2.5 percent) was not significantly different from placebo (2.3 percent). The adverse events were generally transient and mild to moderate in nature.

Side effects
Along with the needed effects, a medicine may cause some unwanted effects. Possible side effects include:
- Headache
- Flushing
- Dyspepsia
- Nasal congestion
- Urinary tract infection
- Abnormal vision
- Diarrhea
- Dizziness
- Rash

Overdose
In studies with healthy volunteers of single doses up to 800 mg adverse events were similar to those seen at lower doses but incidence rates were increased.

In cases of overdose, standard supportive measures should be adopted as required.
- Call a doctor or hospital emergency room for instructions. If necessary start first aid immediately.

Interactions
- Be sure to tell your doctor about any medications you are currently taking.

Storage
Tablets should be stored at room temperature; store away from heat and direct light. Keep out of reach of children, since this medicine may be dangerous in children.

VIVELLE

Properties
This medicine contains estrogen as active ingredient. The medicine is prescribed for treatment of estrogen deficiency; it restores normal estrogen levels in tissues. There is no evidence that this drug is effective for nervous symptoms or depression occurring during menopause. They should not be used to treat this condition; they should be used only to replace the estrogen that is naturally absent after menopause.

Before using this medicine
Before you use this medicine check with your doctor, or pharmacist:
- if you ever had any unusual or allergic reaction to estrogens;
- if you are pregnant or intend to become pregnant within three months;
- if you are breast-feeding an infant;
- if you have any of the following medical problems:
    Diabetes
    Breast cancer
    Fibrocystic breast disease
    Fibroid uterine tumors
    Endometriosis
    Migraine headaches
    Epilepsy
    Porphyria
    High blood pressure
    Asthma
    Congestive heart failure
    Kidney disease
    Gallstones

Treatment
This medication is used to treat estrogen deficiency, specific symptoms of menopause, estrogen-deficiency osteoporosis, atrophic vaginitis, prostate cancer.
For safe and effective use of this medicine:
- Follow your doctor's instructions if this medicine was prescribed.
- Follow the manufacturer's package directions if you are treating yourself.
- Estrogens have been reported to increase the risk of endometrial carcinoma.

Side effects
Along with the needed effects, a medicine may cause some unwanted effects. Possible side effects include:
    Stomach cramps
    Profuse bleeding
    Appetite loss
    Nausea and vomiting
    Swollen breasts
    Change in menstruation
    Rash, skin blisters
    Depression
    Dizziness

Overdose
The following symptoms may indicate an overdose:
    Nausea and vomiting
    Fluid retention
    Breast enlargement
    Abnormal vaginal bleeding
- Call a doctor or hospital emergency room for instructions.

Interactions
This medicine may interact with several other drugs such as adrenocorticosteroids, antidepressants, oral antidiabetics, insulin, phenobarbital, primidone.
- Be sure to tell your doctor about any medications you are currently taking.

Storage
Capsules, tablets, vaginal cream, transdermal patches, etc. should be stored at room temperature; store away from heat and direct light. Keep out of reach of children, since this medicine may be dangerous in children.

VIVOL

Properties
This medicine contains as active ingredient diazepam, a benzodiazepine preparation. Benzodiazepines belong to the group of psychoactive medicines that influence the activity of the brain. Some are used to relieve nervousness or tension. It is effective for this purpose for short periods. Others are used for sleeplessness or to relax muscles or relieve muscle spasm. The benzodiazepines may also be used for other conditions as determined by your doctor.

Before using this medicine
Before you use this medicine check with your doctor:
- if you ever had any unusual or allergic reaction to benzodiazepines.
- if you are on a low-salt, low-sugar, or any other special diet, or if you are allergic to any substance, such as sulfites or other preservatives or dyes.
- if you are pregnant or intend to become pregnant while using this medicine. Some benzodiazepines have been reported to increase the chance of birth defects when used during the first 3 months of pregnancy.
- if you are breast-feeding an infant. Benzodiazepines may pass into the breast milk and cause drowsiness, unusually slow heartbeat, shortness of breath, or troubled breathing in infants of mothers taking this medicine.
- if you have any of the following medical problems: asthma, bronchitis, emphysema, or other chronic lung disease; epilepsy or history of convulsions; hyperactivity (in children); kidney or lifer disease; mental depression or illness; myasthania gravis, porphyria.

Treatment
This medication is used to relieve or prevent the symptoms of your medical problem. Benzodiazepines are mainly used as antianxiety agents, anticonvulsants, or sedatives. Take them as directed. Do not take more of them and do not take them more often than recommended on the label, unless otherwise directed by your doctor. Benzodiazepine tranquilizing drugs can be abused if taken for long periods of time and it is possible to develop withdrawal symptoms if you discontinue the therapy abruptly.

Side effects
Along with the needed effects, a medicine may cause some unwanted effects. Minor side effects are: bitter taste in the mouth, dizziness, drowsiness, depression, constipation, dry mouth, excessive salivation, fatigue, flushing, headache, heartburn, loss of appetite, nausea, nervousness, sweating or vomiting. As your body adjusts to the medicine, these side effects should disappear.
- Tell your doctor about any side effects that are persistent or particularly bothersome. It is especially important to tell your doctor about:
Blurred or double vision
Chest pain
Difficulty in urinating
Fainting or falling
Fever or hallucinations
Joint pain
Mouth sores
Nightmares
Palpitations
Severe depression
Shortness of breath
Slurred speech
Uncoordinated movements
Unusual tiredness
Yellowing of the skin

Interactions
This medicine may interact with several other drugs. This medicine will add to the effects of alcohol, and CNS depressants.
- Be sure to tell your doctor about any medications you are currently taking.

Storage
Store at room temperature in tightly closed, light-resistant-resistant containers. Keep out of the reach of children since overdose may be especially dangerous in children.

VK

Properties

This medicine contains penicillin V as active ingredient. Penicillins are prescribed to treat infections caused by bacteria. They will not work for colds, flu, or other virus infections. There are several different kinds of penicillins. Each is used to treat different kinds of infections.

Before using this medicine

Before you use this medicine check with your doctor, or pharmacist:

- if you ever had any unusual or allergic reaction to any of the penicillins, cefalosporins, griseofulvin, or penicillamine. Serious reactions may occur in patients who are allergic to penicillins.
- if you are on a low-salt, low-sugar, or any other special diet, or if you are allergic to any substance, such as sulfites or other preservatives or dyes.
- if you are pregnant or intend to become pregnant while using this medicine. Although penicillins have not been shown to cause problems in humans, the chance always exists.
- if you are breast-feeding an infant. Most penicillins (except amdinocillin) pass into the breast milk. Even though only small amounts may pass, allergic reaction, diarrhea, fungal infection, and skin rash may occur in the infant.
- if you have any of the following medical problems:
Allergy
Asthma
Bleeding problems
Eczema
Hay fever, hives
Kidney disease
Liver disease
Mononucleosis
Stomach or intestinal disease

Treatment

This medication is used to treat an infection caused by bacteria. Most penicillins are best taken with a full glass (8 ounces) of water on an empty stomach, some are best taken with a snack or meal. Follow your doctor's or pharmacist's directions on how to take your medicine.

- Keep taking this medicine for the full time of treatment even if you begin to feel better after a few days; do not miss any doses. This is especially important if you have a "strep" infection since serious heart problems could develop later if your infection is not cleared up completely.
- If you do miss a dose of this medicine, take it as soon as possible. However, if it is almost time for your next dose, skip the missed dose and go back to your regular dosing schedule.

Side effects

Along with the needed effects, a medicine may cause some unwanted effects. Side effects that usually do not require medical attention: diarrhea; nausea or vomiting; sore mouth or tongue.

- Stop taking this medicine and get emergency help immediately if you notice: difficulty in breathing; lightheadedness; skin rash, hives, itching; wheezing.

Other side effects that should be reported to your doctor immediately are: abdominal bloating; blood in urine; convulsions (seizures); decreased amount of urine; diarrhea (watery and severe) which may also be bloody; fever; joint pain; sore throat and fever; stomach or abdominal cramps and pain; unusual bleeding or bruising.

Interactions

This medicine may interact with several other drugs such as anticoagulants, diarrhea medicines, heparin, ibuprofen, oral contraceptives, potassium-containing medicines, etc.

- Be sure to tell your doctor about any medications you are currently taking.

Storage

Tablets, capsules, etc. should be stored as directed by your pharmacist or according to instructions on the label.

WEHGEN

Properties
This medicine contains estrone as active ingredient. The medicine is prescribed for treatment of estrogen deficiency; it restores normal estrogen levels in tissues. There is no evidence that this drug is effective for nervous symptoms or depression occurring during menopause. They should not be used to treat this condition; they should be used only to replace the estrogen that is naturally absent after menopause.

Before using this medicine
Before you use this medicine check with your doctor, or pharmacist:
- if you ever had any unusual or allergic reaction to estrogens;
- if you are pregnant or intend to become pregnant within three months;
- if you are breast-feeding an infant;
- if you have any of the following medical problems:
  Diabetes
  Breast cancer
  Fibrocystic breast disease
  Fibroid uterine tumors
  Endometriosis
  Migraine headaches
  Epilepsy
  Porphyria
  High blood pressure
  Asthma
  Congestive heart failure
  Kidney disease
  Gallstones

Treatment
This medication is used to treat estrogen deficiency, specific symptoms of menopause, estrogen-deficiency osteoporosis, atrophic vaginitis, prostate cancer.
For safe and effective use of this medicine:
- ◆ Follow your doctor's instructions if this medicine was prescribed.
- ◆ Follow the manufacturer's package directions if you are treating yourself.
- ◆ Estrogens have been reported to increase the risk of endometrial carcinoma.

Side effects
Along with the needed effects, a medicine may cause some unwanted effects. Possible side effects include:
  Stomach cramps
  Profuse bleeding
  Appetite loss
  Nausea and vomiting
  Swollen breasts
  Change in menstruation
  Rash, skin blisters
  Depression
  Dizziness

Overdose
The following symptoms may indicate an overdose:
  Nausea and vomiting
  Fluid retention
  Breast enlargement
  Abnormal vaginal bleeding
- ■ Call a doctor or hospital emergency room for instructions.

Interactions
This medicine may interact with several other drugs such as adrenocorticosteroids, antidepressants, oral antidiabetics, insulin, phenobarbital, primidone.
- ■ Be sure to tell your doctor about any medications you are currently taking.

Storage
Capsules, tablets, vaginal cream, transdermal patches, etc. should be stored at room temperature; store away from heat and direct light. Keep out of reach of children, since this medicine may be dangerous in children.

WEHLESS

Properties

This medicine contains phendimetrazine as active ingredient; it is prescribed for appetite suppression.

Appetite suppressants are used in the short-term (a few weeks) treatment of obesity. In a few weeks (6 to 12), these medicines in combination with dieting, exercise, and changes in eating habits can help patients lose weight. However, since their appetite reducing effect is only temporary, they are useful only for the first weeks of dieting until new eating habits are established.

Before using this medicine

Before you use this medicine check with your doctor, or pharmacist:

- if you ever had any unusual or allergic reaction to any of the compounds of this medicine.
- if you are on a low-salt, low-sugar, or any other special diet, or if you are allergic to any substance, such as sulfites or other preservatives or dyes.
- if you are pregnant, intend to become pregnant or breast-feeding an infant while using this medicine.
- if you have any of the following medical problems:
  Diabetes mellitus (sugar diabetes)
  Epilepsy
  Glaucoma
  Heart or blood vessel disease
  High blood pressure
  Mental illness (severe)

Treatment

This medication is used to relieve or prevent the symptoms of your medical problem. Take them as directed. Do not take more of them and do not take them more often than recommended on the label. If too much of the drug is taken, it may become habit-forming.

The medicine produces central nervous system stimulation, and it should not be taken by people with heart disease or high blood pressure.

If you think this medicine is not working as well after you have taken it for a few weeks, do not increase the dose. Instead, check with your doctor.

Side effects

The following minor side effects may occur: irritability, nervousness, restlessness, trouble in sleeping.

These side effects should disappear as your body adjusts to the medication. Tell your doctor about any side effects that are persistent or particularly bothersome. It is especially important to tell your doctor about:

Mental depression
Nausea or vomiting
Stomach cramps or pain
Trembling
Unusual tiredness or weakness

- Discontinue use of the drug; call your doctor right away. Adverse reactions and side effects may be more frequent and severe in people over age 60 than in younger persons.

Interactions

This medicine interacts with several other drugs such as antihypertensives, other appetite suppressants, caffeine, central nervous system depressants, central nervous system stimulants, furazolidone, guanethidine, hydralazine, MAO inhibitors, methyldopa, molindone, phenothiazines, rauwolfia alkaloids, sodium bicarbonate. Interaction with alcoholic beverages may produce drowsiness, sleepiness, and/or inability to concentrate.

- Be sure to tell your doctor about any medications you are currently taking.

Storage

This medicine should be stored at room temperature in tightly closed containers. Store away from heat and direct light. Keep out of reach of children, since overdose may be very dangerous in children.

Do not store this medicine in the bathroom medicine cabinet because the heat and moisture cause the medicine to break down. Do not keep outdated medicine or medicine no longer needed. Flush the contents of the container down the toilet.

WEIGHTROL

Properties

This medicine contains phendimetrazine as active ingredient; it is prescribed for appetite suppression.

Appetite suppressants are used in the short-term (a few weeks) treatment of obesity. In a few weeks (6 to 12), these medicines in combination with dieting, exercise, and changes in eating habits can help patients lose weight. However, since their appetite reducing effect is only temporary, they are useful only for the first weeks of dieting until new eating habits are established.

Before using this medicine

Before you use this medicine check with your doctor, or pharmacist:
- if you ever had any unusual or allergic reaction to any of the compounds of this medicine.
- if you are on a low-salt, low-sugar, or any other special diet, or if you are allergic to any substance, such as sulfites or other preservatives or dyes.
- if you are pregnant, intend to become pregnant or breast-feeding an infant while using this medicine.
- if you have any of the following medical problems:
  Diabetes mellitus (sugar diabetes)
  Epilepsy
  Glaucoma
  Heart or blood vessel disease
  High blood pressure
  Mental illness (severe)

Treatment

This medication is used to relieve or prevent the symptoms of your medical problem. Take them as directed. Do not take more of them and do not take them more often than recommended on the label. If too much of the drug is taken, it may become habit-forming.

The medicine produces central nervous system stimulation, and it should not be taken by people with heart disease or high blood pressure.

If you think this medicine is not working as well after you have taken it for a few weeks, do not increase the dose. Instead, check with your doctor.

Side effects

The following minor side effects may occur: irritability, nervousness, restlessness, trouble in sleeping.

These side effects should disappear as your body adjusts to the medication. Tell your doctor about any side effects that are persistent or particularly bothersome. It is especially important to tell your doctor about:
  Mental depression
  Nausea or vomiting
  Stomach cramps or pain
  Trembling
  Unusual tiredness or weakness
- Discontinue use of the drug; call your doctor right away. Adverse reactions and side effects may be more frequent and severe in people over age 60 than in younger persons.

Interactions

This medicine interacts with several other drugs such as antihypertensives, other appetite suppressants, caffeine, central nervous system depressants, central nervous system stimulants, furazolidone, guanethidine, hydralazine, MAO inhibitors, methyldopa, molindone, phenothiazines, rauwolfia alkaloids, sodium bicarbonate. Interaction with alcoholic beverages may produce drowsiness, sleepiness, and/or inability to concentrate
- Be sure to tell your doctor about any medications you are currently taking.

Storage

This medicine should be stored at room temperature in tightly closed containers. Store away from heat and direct light. Keep out of reach of children, since overdose may be very dangerous in children.

Do not store this medicine in the bathroom medicine cabinet because the heat and moisture cause the medicine to break down. Do not keep outdated medicine or medicine no longer needed. Flush the contents of the container down the toilet.

WYAMYCIN E

Properties

This medicine contains erythromycin as active ingredient. This antibiotic is prescribed to treat infections caused by bacteria. They will not work for colds, flu, or other virus infections. Erythromycins are available only with your doctor's prescription.

Before using this medicine

Before you use this medicine check with your doctor, or pharmacist:

- if you ever had any unusual or allergic reaction to any of the erythromycins.
- if you are on a low-salt, low-sugar, or any other special diet, or if you are allergic to any substance, such as sulfites or other preservatives or dyes.
- if you are pregnant or intend to become pregnant while using this medicine. Although erythromycins have not been shown to cause birth defects or other problems in humans, the chance always exists.
- if you are breast-feeding an infant. Most erythromycins pass into the breast milk. Although erythromycins have not been shown to cause problems in humans, the chance always exists.
- if you have lifer disease.

Treatment

This medication belongs to the general family of medicines called antibiotics. It is used to treat a wide variety of bacterial infections. It is also used to treat infections in persons who are allergic to penicillin. Erythromycins are also used to prevent "strep" infections in patients with a history of rheumatic heart disease. They may also be used in Legionnaires' disease and for other problems as determined by your doctor.

- Keep taking this medicine for the full time of treatment even if you begin to feel better after a few days; do not miss any doses. This is especially important if you have a "strep" infection since serious heart problems could develop later if your infection is not cleared up completely.

- If you do miss a dose of this medicine, take it as soon as possible. This will help to keep a constant amount of medicine in the blood. However, if it is almost time for your next dose, skip the missed dose and go back to your regular dosing schedule.
- This medication has been prescribed for your current infection only. Another infection later on, or one that someone else has, may require a different medicine. You should not give your medicine to other people or use it for other infections, unless your doctor specifically directs you to do so.

Side effects

Along with the needed effects, a medicine may cause some unwanted effects. Side effects that usually do not require medical attention: abdominal cramps, black tongue, cough, diarrhea, fatigue, irritation of the mouth, loss of appetite, nausea, or vomiting. These side effects should disappear as your body adjusts to the medication.

- Other side effects that should be reported to your doctor immediately are:
  Fever
  Hearing loss
  Hives or rash
  Rectal or vaginal itching
  Yellowing of the eyes or skin

Interactions

This medicine may interact with several other drugs such as anticoagulants, theophylline preparations, carbamazepine, etc.

- Be sure to tell your doctor about any medications you are currently taking.

Storage

Tablets, capsules, etc. should be stored at room temperature in tightly closed, light-resistant containers as directed by your pharmacist.

WYAMYCIN S

Properties
This medicine contains erythromycin as active ingredient. This antibiotic is prescribed to treat infections caused by bacteria. They will not work for colds, flu, or other virus infections. Erythromycins are available only with your doctor's prescription.

Before using this medicine
Before you use this medicine check with your doctor, or pharmacist:
- if you ever had any unusual or allergic reaction to any of the erythromycins.
- if you are on a low-salt, low-sugar, or any other special diet, or if you are allergic to any substance, such as sulfites or other preservatives or dyes.
- if you are pregnant or intend to become pregnant while using this medicine. Although erythromycins have not been shown to cause birth defects or other problems in humans, the chance always exists.
- if you are breast-feeding an infant. Most erythromycins pass into the breast milk. Although erythromycins have not been shown to cause problems in humans, the chance always exists.
- if you have lifer disease.

Treatment
This medication belongs to the general family of medicines called antibiotics. It is used to treat a wide variety of bacterial infections. It is also used to treat infections in persons who are allergic to penicillin. Erythromycins are also used to prevent "strep" infections in patients with a history of rheumatic heart disease. They may also be used in Legionnaires' disease and for other problems as determined by your doctor.
- Keep taking this medicine for the full time of treatment even if you begin to feel better after a few days; do not miss any doses. This is especially important if you have a "strep" infection since serious heart problems could develop later if your infection is not cleared up completely.
- If you do miss a dose of this medicine, take it as soon as possible. This will help to keep a constant amount of medicine in the blood. However, if it is almost time for your next dose, skip the missed dose and go back to your regular dosing schedule.
- This medication has been prescribed for your current infection only. Another infection later on, or one that someone else has, may require a different medicine. You should not give your medicine to other people or use it for other infections, unless your doctor specifically directs you to do so.

Side effects
Along with the needed effects, a medicine may cause some unwanted effects. Side effects that usually do not require medical attention: abdominal cramps, black tongue, cough, diarrhea, fatigue, irritation of the mouth, loss of appetite, nausea, or vomiting. These side effects should disappear as your body adjusts to the medication.
- Other side effects that should be reported to your doctor immediately are:
  Fever
  Hearing loss
  Hives or rash
  Rectal or vaginal itching
  Yellowing of the eyes or skin

Interactions
This medicine may interact with several other drugs such as anticoagulants, theophylline preparations, carbamazepine, etc.
- Be sure to tell your doctor about any medications you are currently taking.

Storage
Tablets, capsules, etc. should be stored at room temperature in tightly closed, light-resistant containers as directed by your pharmacist.

WYCILLIN

Properties
This medicine contains penicillin G as active ingredient. Penicillins are prescribed to treat infections caused by bacteria. They will not work for colds, flu, or other virus infections. There are several different kinds of penicillins. Each is used to treat different kinds of infections.

Before using this medicine
Before you use this medicine check with your doctor, or pharmacist:
- if you ever had any unusual or allergic reaction to any of the penicillins, cefalosporins, griseofulvin, or penicillamine. Serious reactions may occur in patients who are allergic to penicillins.
- if you are on a low-salt, low-sugar, or any other special diet, or if you are allergic to any substance, such as sulfites or other preservatives or dyes.
- if you are pregnant or intend to become pregnant while using this medicine. Although penicillins have not been shown to cause problems in humans, the chance always exists.
- if you are breast-feeding an infant. Most penicillins (except amdinocillin) pass into the breast milk. Even though only small amounts may pass, allergic reaction, diarrhea, fungal infection, and skin rash may occur in the infant.
- if you have any of the following medical problems:
  Allergy
  Asthma
  Bleeding problems
  Eczema
  Hay fever, hives
  Kidney disease
  Liver disease
  Mononucleosis
  Stomach or intestinal disease

Treatment
This medication is used to treat an infection caused by bacteria. Most penicillins are best taken with a full glass (8 ounces) of water on an empty stomach, some are best taken with a snack or meal. Follow your doctor's or pharmacist's directions on how to take your medicine.
- ◆ Keep taking this medicine for the full time of treatment even if you begin to feel better after a few days; do not miss any doses. This is especially important if you have a "strep" infection since serious heart problems could develop later if your infection is not cleared up completely.
- ◆ If you do miss a dose of this medicine, take it as soon as possible. However, if it is almost time for your next dose, skip the missed dose and go back to your regular dosing schedule.

Side effects
Along with the needed effects, a medicine may cause some unwanted effects. Side effects that usually do not require medical attention: diarrhea; nausea or vomiting; sore mouth or tongue.
- ◆ Stop taking this medicine and get emergency help immediately if you notice: difficulty in breathing; lightheadedness; skin rash, hives, itching; wheezing.

Other side effects that should be reported to your doctor immediately are: abdominal bloating; blood in urine; convulsions (seizures); decreased amount of urine; diarrhea (watery and severe) which may also be bloody; fever; joint pain; sore throat and fever; stomach or abdominal cramps and pain; unusual bleeding or bruising.

Interactions
This medicine may interact with several other drugs such as anticoagulants, diarrhea medicines, heparin, ibuprofen, oral contraceptives, potassium-containing medicines, etc.
- ■ Be sure to tell your doctor about any medications you are currently taking.

Storage
Tablets, capsules, etc. should be stored as directed by your pharmacist or according to instructions on the label.

X-TROZINE

Properties
This medicine contains phendi-metrazine as active ingredient; it is prescribed for appetite suppression.

Appetite suppressants are used in the short-term (a few weeks) treatment of obesity. In a few weeks (6 to 12), these medicines in combination with dieting, exercise, and changes in eating habits can help patients lose weight. However, since their appetite reducing effect is only temporary, they are useful only for the first weeks of dieting until new eating habits are established.

Before using this medicine
Before you use this medicine check with your doctor, or pharmacist:
- if you ever had any unusual or allergic reaction to any of the compounds of this medicine.
- if you are on a low-salt, low-sugar, or any other special diet, or if you are allergic to any substance, such as sulfites or other preservatives or dyes.
- if you are pregnant, intend to become pregnant or breast-feeding an infant while using this medicine.
- if you have any of the following medical problems:
Diabetes mellitus (sugar diabetes)
Epilepsy
Glaucoma
Heart or blood vessel disease
High blood pressure
Mental illness (severe)

Treatment
This medication is used to relieve or prevent the symptoms of your medical problem. Take them as directed. Do not take more of them and do not take them more often than recommended on the label. If too much of the drug is taken, it may become habit-forming.

The medicine produces central nervous system stimulation, and it should not be taken by people with heart disease or high blood pressure.

If you think this medicine is not working as well after you have taken it for a few weeks, do not increase the dose. Instead, check with your doctor.

Side effects
The following minor side effects may occur: irritability, nervousness, restlessness, trouble in sleeping.

These side effects should disappear as your body adjusts to the medication. Tell your doctor about any side effects that are persistent or particularly bothersome. It is especially important to tell your doctor about:
Mental depression
Nausea or vomiting
Stomach cramps or pain
Trembling
Unusual tiredness or weakness
- Discontinue use of the drug; call your doctor right away. Adverse reactions and side effects may be more frequent and severe in people over age 60 than in younger persons.

Interactions
This medicine interacts with several other drugs such as antihypertensives, other appetite suppressants, caffeine, central nervous system depressants, central nervous system stimulants, furazolidone, guanethidine, hydralazine, MAO inhibitors, methyldopa, molindone, phenothiazines, rauwolfia alkaloids, sodium bicarbonate. Interaction with alcoholic beverages may produce drowsiness, sleepiness, and/or inability to concentrate.
- Be sure to tell your doctor about any medications you are currently taking.

Storage
This medicine should be stored at room temperature in tightly closed containers. Store away from heat and direct light. Keep out of reach of children, since overdose may be very dangerous in children.

Do not store this medicine in the bathroom medicine cabinet because the heat and moisture cause the medicine to break down. Do not keep outdated medicine or medicine no longer needed. Flush the contents of the container down the toilet.

ZAPEX

Properties

This medicine contains as active ingredient oxazepam, a benzodiazepine preparation. Benzodiazepines belong to the group of psychoactive medicines that influence the activity of the brain. Some are used to relieve nervousness or tension. It is effective for this purpose for short periods. Others are used for sleeplessness or to relax muscles or relieve muscle spasm. The benzodiazepines may also be used for other conditions as determined by your doctor.

Before using this medicine

Before you use this medicine check with your doctor:
- if you ever had any unusual or allergic reaction to benzodiazepines.
- if you are on a low-salt, low-sugar, or any other special diet, or if you are allergic to any substance, such as sulfites or other preservatives or dyes.
- if you are pregnant or intend to become pregnant while using this medicine. Some benzodiazepines have been reported to increase the chance of birth defects when used during the first 3 months of pregnancy.
- if you are breast-feeding an infant. Benzodiazepines may pass into the breast milk and cause drowsiness, unusually slow heartbeat, shortness of breath, or troubled breathing in infants of mothers taking this medicine.
- if you have any of the following medical problems: asthma, bronchitis, emphysema, or other chronic lung disease; epilepsy or history of convulsions; hyperactivity (in children); kidney or lifer disease; mental depression or illness; myasthania gravis, porphyria.

Treatment

This medication is used to relieve or prevent the symptoms of your medical problem. Benzodiazepines are mainly used as antianxiety agents, anticonvulsants, or sedatives. Take them as directed. Do not take more of them and do not take them more often than recommended on the label, unless otherwise directed by your doctor. Benzodiazepine tranquilizing drugs can be abused if taken for long periods of time and it is possible to develop withdrawal symptoms if you discontinue the therapy abruptly.

Side effects

Along with the needed effects, a medicine may cause some unwanted effects. Minor side effects are: bitter taste in the mouth, dizziness, drowsiness, depression, constipation, dry mouth, excessive salivation, fatigue, flushing, headache, heartburn, loss of appetite, nausea, nervousness, sweating or vomiting. As your body adjusts to the medicine, these side effects should disappear.

- Tell your doctor about any side effects that are persistent or particularly bothersome. It is especially important to tell your doctor about:
Blurred or double vision
Chest pain
Difficulty in urinating
Fainting or falling
Fever or hallucinations
Joint pain
Mouth sores
Nightmares
Palpitations
Severe depression
Shortness of breath
Slurred speech
Uncoordinated movements
Unusual tiredness
Yellowing of the skin

Interactions

This medicine may interact with several other drugs. This medicine will add to the effects of alcohol, and CNS depressants.

- Be sure to tell your doctor about any medications you are currently taking.

Storage

Store at room temperature in tightly closed, light-resistant-resistant containers. Keep out of the reach of children since overdose may be especially dangerous in children.

ZAROXOLON

Properties
This medicine contains as active ingredient metolazone, a thiazide-like diuretic. Thiazide or thiazide-like diuretics are prescribed to treat high blood pressure (hypertension). They are also used to reduce fluid accumulation in the body caused by conditions such as heart failure, cirrhosis, kidney disease, and the long-term use of some medications. Thiazide diuretics may also be used for other conditions as determined by your doctor.

Before using this medicine
Before you use this medicine check with your doctor, or pharmacist:
- if you ever had any unusual or allergic reaction to sulfonamides (sulfa drugs) or any of the thiazide diuretics.
- if you are on a low-salt, low-sugar, or any other special diet, or if you are allergic to any substance, such as sulfites or other preservatives or dyes.
- if you are pregnant or intend to become pregnant while using this medicine. When this medicine is used during pregnancy, it may cause side effects including jaundice, blood problems, and low potassium in the newborn.
- if you are breast-feeding an infant. Although this medicine has not been shown to cause problems in humans, the chance always exists since thiazide diuretics pass into breast milk.
- if you have any of the following medical problems:
Diabetes
Gout
Kidney disease
Liver disease
Lupus erythematosus
Pancreas disease

Treatment
This medication is used to treat high blood pressure (hypertension) and also to help reduce the amount of water in the body by increasing the flow of urine. This medicine will not cure your high blood pressure but it does help control it. You must continue to take it - even if you feel well - if you expect to keep your blood pressure down. You may have to take high blood pressure medicine for the rest of your life.

Thiazide diuretics may cause an unusual feeling of tiredness when you begin to take them. You may also notice an increase in urine or in frequency of urination. To keep this from affecting sleep:
- if you are to take a single dose a day, take it in the morning after breakfast;
- if you are to take more than one dose, take the last one not later than 6 p.m.

Side effects
Along with the needed effects, a medicine may cause some unwanted effects. Side effects that usually do not require medical attention: decreased sexual ability; dizziness or lightheadedness when standing up; increased sensitivity of skin to sunlight; loss of appetite; upset stomach.
- Side effects that should be reported to your doctor: black, tarry stools; blood in urine or stools; cough or hoarseness; fever or chills; joint pain; lower back or side pains; painful or difficult urination; pinpoint red spots on skin; skin rash or hives; stomach pain (severe) with nausea; unusual bleeding or bruising; yellow eyes or skin. This medicine may cause a loss of potassium from your body. Signs of too much potassium loss are: dryness of mouth; increased thirst; mood changes; muscle cramps or pain; nausea or vomiting; unusual tiredness or weakness; weak or irregular heartbeat.

Interactions
This medicine may interact with several other drugs.
- Be sure to tell your doctor about any medications you are currently taking.

Storage
Store at room temperature in a tightly closed container.

ZETRAN

Properties
This medicine contains as active ingredient diazepam, a benzodiazepine preparation. Benzodiazepines belong to the group of psychoactive medicines that influence the activity of the brain. Some are used to relieve nervousness or tension. It is effective for this purpose for short periods. Others are used for sleeplessness or to relax muscles or relieve muscle spasm. The benzodiazepines may also be used for other conditions as determined by your doctor.

Before using this medicine
Before you use this medicine check with your doctor:
- if you ever had any unusual or allergic reaction to benzodiazepines.
- if you are on a low-salt, low-sugar, or any other special diet, or if you are allergic to any substance, such as sulfites or other preservatives or dyes.
- if you are pregnant or intend to become pregnant while using this medicine. Some benzodiazepines have been reported to increase the chance of birth defects when used during the first 3 months of pregnancy.
- if you are breast-feeding an infant. Benzodiazepines may pass into the breast milk and cause drowsiness, unusually slow heartbeat, shortness of breath, or troubled breathing in infants of mothers taking this medicine.
- if you have any of the following medical problems: asthma, bronchitis, emphysema, or other chronic lung disease; epilepsy or history of convulsions; hyperactivity (in children); kidney or lifer disease; mental depression or illness; myasthania gravis, porphyria.

Treatment
This medication is used to relieve or prevent the symptoms of your medical problem. Benzodiazepines are mainly used as antianxiety agents, anticonvulsants, or sedatives. Take them as directed. Do not take more of them and do not take them more often than recommended on the label, unless otherwise directed by your doctor. Benzodiazepine tranquilizing drugs can be abused if taken for long periods of time and it is possible to develop withdrawal symptoms if you discontinue the therapy abruptly.

Side effects
Along with the needed effects, a medicine may cause some unwanted effects. Minor side effects are: bitter taste in the mouth, dizziness, drowsiness, depression, constipation, dry mouth, excessive salivation, fatigue, flushing, headache, heartburn, loss of appetite, nausea, nervousness, sweating or vomiting. As your body adjusts to the medicine, these side effects should disappear.
- Tell your doctor about any side effects that are persistent or particularly bothersome. It is especially important to tell your doctor about:
  Blurred or double vision
  Chest pain
  Difficulty in urinating
  Fainting or falling
  Fever or hallucinations
  Joint pain
  Mouth sores
  Nightmares
  Palpitations
  Severe depression
  Shortness of breath
  Slurred speech
  Uncoordinated movements
  Unusual tiredness
  Yellowing of the skin

Interactions
This medicine may interact with several other drugs. This medicine will add to the effects of alcohol, and CNS depressants.
- Be sure to tell your doctor about any medications you are currently taking.

Storage
Store at room temperature in tightly closed, light-resistant-resistant containers. Keep out of the reach of children since overdose may be especially dangerous in children.

ZOCOR

Properties

This medicine contains simvastatin as active ingredient. It is a medicine that lowers blood cholesterol levels caused by low-density lipoproteins (LDL). Cholesterol plays an important role in the genesis of atherosclerosis, and thus in heart conditions such as angina pectoris and myocardial infarction. It may be used in combination with a low-fat diet to slow the progression of atherosclerosis in patients with coronary heart diseases and high cholesterol levels.

The effect of this medicine is caused by the inhibition of a particular enzyme in the lifer.

Before using this medicine

Before you use this medicine check with your doctor, or pharmacist:
- if you ever had any unusual or allergic reaction to this medicine or any HMG-CoA reductase inhibitors;
- if you are pregnant or intend to become pregnant while using this medicine;
- if you are breast-feeding an infant;
- if you take immunosuppressive medicines;
- if you have low blood pressure;
- if you have disorders of abnormalities of hormones of endocrine glands;
- if you have active lifer disease;
- if you have an active infection or are suffering from chronic infections of the gastrointestinal system;
- if you have a seizure disorder or epilepsy.

Treatment

This medication is prescribed for lowering blood cholesterol levels caused by low-density lipoprotein (LDL) in persons who have not improved by exercising, dieting or using other methods. It is also used in combination with a low-fat diet to slow the progression of atherosclerosis.

If you forget to take a dose of this medicine, take it as soon as you remember up to two hours late. If more than two hours late, wait for the next scheduled dose;. People over 60 years of age are likely to have more adverse effects and are more sensitive to the medicine.

Tablets or capsules should be taken with liquid. If you have problems taking the whole tablets, you may crumble them and take with liquid or food.

For safe and effective use of medicine:
- ◆ Follow your doctor's instructions if this medicine was prescribed.
- ◆ Follow the manufacturer's package directions if you are treating yourself.

Side effects

Along with the needed effects, a medicine may cause some unwanted effects. Possible side effects include:
Muscle ache
Blurred vision
Fever
Nausea
Constipation
Tiredness
Weakness
Dizziness
Impotence
Headache
Skin rash
Dizziness
Insomnia

Interactions

It may increase the effect of digoxin. With the simultaneous use of gemfibrozil there is an increased risk of heart and kidney problems and muscle inflammation.
- ■ Be sure to tell your doctor about any medications you are currently taking.

Storage

Capsules and tablets should be stored at room temperature; store away from heat and direct light. Keep out of reach of children, since the medicine acts by inhibiting an enzyme in the lifer. Therefore this drug is not recommended for infants and children.

ZOLOFT

Properties
This medicine contains sertraline as active ingredient. It is an antidepressant drug that has a specific effect on certain areas of the brain. The medicine is known to affect serotonin, one of the chemicals in the brain called neurotransmitters or chemical messengers, that play a role in the steering of psychoactive behavior. It is prescribed for the treatment of depressive disorders.

Before using this medicine
Before you use this medicine check with your doctor, or pharmacist:
- if you ever had any unusual or allergic reaction to this medicine or any psychoactive drug;
- if you are allergic to any medicines, foods or other substances;
- if you are pregnant or intend to become pregnant while using this medicine (animal studies have shown toxic effects to developing fetuses);
- if you are breast-feeding an infant.

Treatment
This medication is used for treatment of certain types of mental depression and obsessive-compulsive disorders.

Tablets should be swallowed with liquid. If you forget to take a dose of this medicine, take it as soon as you remember up to two hours late. If more than two hours, wait for the next scheduled dose;. In patients over 60 years of age, adverse reactions may be more frequent and severe than in younger persons.

For safe and effective use of medicine:
♦ Follow your doctor's instructions if this medicine was prescribed.
♦ Follow the manufacturer's package directions if you are treating yourself.

Side effects
Along with the needed effects, a medicine may cause some unwanted effects. Possible side effects include:
Rash, itchy skin
Headache
Nervousness
Increased sweating
Nausea
Insomnia
Anxiety
Joint pain
Nightmares
Sensory changes
Decreased sex drive
Dry mouth
Changes in heartbeat
Flushing
Painful menstruation
Tremors

Overdose
The following symptoms may be a sign of overdose:
Seizures
Agitation
Violent vomiting
■ Call a doctor or hospital emergency room for instructions. If necessary, give first aid immediately.

Interactions
The effect of this medicine may be increased by other antidepressants. Lithium, may increase the occurrence of side effects. Anticoagulants may cause an increase in anticoagulation. Alcohol will sometimes augment the depression.
■ Be sure to tell your doctor about any medications you are currently taking.

Storage
The tablets should be stored at room temperature; store away from heat and direct light. Keep out of reach of children, since this medicine may be dangerous to children.

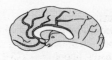
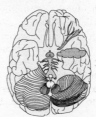

IV   Directory

Guide to Directory

Names of medicines appearing in bold type are described in this book.

In regular type two names of medicines are mentioned; the description of the first one is similar to the second one; look under the second name for a full description.

A

ACCURBRON
ACETAPHENAZINE
ACLOMETASONE
DIPROPRIONATE
ACLOVATE
Acticort   Betamethasone
ADALAT
ADIPEX-P
ADIPIN
ADIPOST
ADPHEN
AEROLATE
Ala-cort   Benisone
ALPHATREX
Alprazolam   Diazepam
ALURATE
ALZAPAM
Amcil   Novopen
Amdinocillin   Penicillin
Aminophyllin   Aerolate
AMITRIL
AMITRIPTYLINE
AMLODIPINE
AMOBARBITAL
Amoline   Accurbron
AMOXAPINE
Amoxil   Penicillin
Ampicillin   Novopen
Ampicin   Permapen
Ampilean   Penicillin
AMYTAL
ANABOLIN
ANADROL
ANAFRANIL
ANAPOLON 50
ANAVAR
ANCEF
ANDRO 100
ANDRO-CYP 100
ANDROID
ANDROLONE
ANDRONAQ-50
ANDRONATE
ANDROPOSITORY 100
ANDRYL 200
ANG-0-SPAN
Anhydron   Thiazide
ANOREX
Anspor   Cefanex
ANTACEF
AON-Cl
APO-AMITRIPTYLINE
APO-CEPHALEX

APO-FLURAZEPAM
APO-IMIPRAMINE
APO-NIFED
APO-OXAZEPAM
Apo-oxtriphylline   Accurbron
Apo-Pen VK   Penicillin
APO-SULFATRIM
APROBARBITAL
AQUAPHYLLIN
Aquatac   Thiazide
AQUATENSEN
AQUEST
Aristocort   Betamethasone
ASENDIN
ASMALIX
Asminil   Aerolate
ATIVAN
AUGMENTIN
AVENTYL
Azlin   Wycillin
Azlocillin   Peniclllin

B

Bacampicillin   Novopen
BACARATE
Bactocill   Penicillin
BACTRIM
BARBITA
BAYON
Baypen   Penicillin
BEBEN
BEEPEN-VK
BENISONE
BENZPHETAMINE
Benzthiazide   Thiazide
BEPADIN
BEPRIDIL
BETA-VAL
BETACORT SCALP LOTION
BETADERM
BETAMETHASONE
BETAPEN-VK
BETATREX
BETNOLATE
BIAXIN
Bicillin   Penicillin
BI-K
BONTRIL PDM
BREVICON
BRONKODYL
BRONKODYL S-R
BUTABARBITAL
BUTACE

BUTALAN
BUTALBITAL
BUTATRAN
BUTICAPS
BUTISOL
BUTORPHANOL

C

C.E.S.
C-LEXIN
CALAN
Calecort   Betaderm
Carbenicillin   Penicillin
CARDENE
CARDILATE
CARDIZEM
CECLOR
CEFACLOR
Cefadroxil   Cefanex
Cefadyl   Apo-Cephadex
Cefamandole   Cefotan
CEFANEX
Cefazolin   Cefixime
CEFIXIME
CEFIZOX
CEFOBID
CEFOBINE
Cefonizid   Cefotan
Ceforanide   Ultracef
Ceforazine   Keftab
Ceforperazone   Cefanex
CEFOTAN
Cefotaxime   Suprax
CEFOTETAN
Cefoxitin   Cefanex
CEFROZIL
Ceftazidime   Ceclor
CEFTIN
Ceftizoxime   Nu-cephalex
Ceftriaxone   Cefixime
Cefuroxine   Suprax
CEFZIL
CELESTODERM
CENA-K
CENTRAX
Cephalexin   Cefanex
Cephalotin   Ceclor
Ceporex   Keftab
Cetacort   Betaderm
Choledyl   Asmalix
Chlordiazepoxide Diazepam
Chlorothiazide   Thiazide
CHLOROTRIANISENE

CHLORPROMAZINE
Chlorthalidone   Hydrodiuril
CIMETIDINE
CLAFORAN
CLARITIN
CLIMARA
CLINAGEN LA 40
Clinicort   Betamethasone
CLOBETASOL PROPIONATE
CLOCORTOLONE
CLODERM
CLOMIPRAMINE
Clonopin   Diazepam
CLORAZINE
Cloxacillin   Penicillin
Cloxapen   Novopen
Cloxilean   Megacillin
Coactin   Novopen
CO-TRIMOXAZOLE
CODEINE
Compazine   Chlorpromazine
CONGEST
CONSTANT-T
CORONEX
Corophyllin   Duraphyl
Cortaid   Celestoderm
Cortate   Beben
Cortef   Alphatrex
Corticreme   Dermabet
Cortoderm   Beben
Cortril   Betamethasone
COTRIM
Cremocort   Celestoderm
Crystapen   Megacillin
Cyclacillin   Penicillin
Cyclapen   Novopen
CYCLEN
CYCLOCORT
Cyclothiazide   Thiazide

D

DAPEX-37.5
DAY-BARB
DECA-DURABOLIN
Decaderm   Betaderm
Decaspray   Celestoderm
Delacort   Betamethasone
DELADIOL-40
DELATEST
DELATESTRYL
DELESTROGEN
DEMER-IDINE
DEMEROL

DEMOVATE
DEMULEN
DEP ANDRO
DEPGYNOGEN
DEPO ESTRADIOL
DEPO-TESTOSTERONE
DEPOGEN
DEPOTEST
DERMABET

Dermacort	Betamethasone
Dermtex	Dermabet

DES
DESIPRAMINE
DESOGEN
DESONIDE
DESOWEN

Dexamethasone	Betamethasone

DI-AP-TROL

Diachlor	Thiazide
Diaqua	Duretic

DIAZEPAM INTENSOL

Dicloxacillin	Penicillin

DICODID
DIDREX
DIETHYLPROPION
DIETHYLSTILBESTROL
DIHYDROMORPHINONE
DILACOR-XR
DILATRATE SR
DILAUDID

Dilin	Asmalix
Dilor	Lixolin

DILTIAZEM
DIOVAL 40
DIPROLENE
DIPROSONE

Diucardon	Thiazide

DIULO
DIURESE

Diurigen	Thiuretic
Diuril	Thiazide

DOLOPHINE
DOXEPIN

Droxine	Lixolin
Duotrate	Isordil

DURA-ESTRIN
DURABOLIN
DURACILLIN A.S.
DURAGEN
DURAMORPH RF
DURAPHYL
DURATEST
DURATHATE 200
DURETIC
DURICEF

Dycill	Penicillin
Dyflex	Aerolate
Dylline	Asmalix

DYNA CIRC

Dy-phyl-lin	Duraphyl

DYREXAN-OD

E

E-CYPLONATE
E.E.S.
E-MYCIN
E-MYCIN E
ECTOSONE
ELAVIL

Eldecort	Betamethasone

ELICOPHYLLIN
ELIXICON
ELIXOMIN
EM-K-10%
EMITRIP
ENDEP
ENDURON
ENOVIL
EPIMORPH
ERAMYCIN
ERY-TAB
ERYC
ERYPAR
ERYPED
ERYTHRITOL TETRANITRATE
ERYTHROCIN
ERYTHROMID
ERYTHROMYCIN
ESIDRIX
ESTINYL
ESTRACE
ESTRADERM
ESTRADIOL
ESTRO-A
ESTROGEN
ESTROJECT-L.A.
ESTRONE
ESTROPIPATE
ETHON
ETHRIL
ETHYLESTRENOL
ETHYNIL ESTRADIOL
EVERONE

F

FASTIN

FELODIPINE
FEMOGEX
Florone — Dermabet
Fluidil — Thiazide
FLUNARIZINE
Fluocet — Betamethasone
Fluoderm — Betaderm
Fluolar — Cetestoderm
Fluonid — Betatrex
FLUOXYMESTERONE
FLUPHENAZINE
FLURAZEPAM
Flurosyn — Beben
Flutex — Betamethasone
FOILLECORT — Betaderm
FORTAZ

G

GAMAZOLE
GANTANOL
GANTRISIN
GARDENAL
GEMONIL
GENCEPT
GENORA
Geocillin — Penicillin
Geopen — Megacillin
GLYCERYL TRINITRATE
Gynecort — Betamethasone
GYNOGEN L.A.

H

HALAZEPAM
HALCION
HALOTESTIN
HISTERONE
HONVOL
Hybolin — Anabolin
HYBOLIN DECANOATE
HYCODAN
Hyderm — Betamethasone
Hydrex — Thiazide
HYDRO-T
HYDRO-Z-50
Hydrochlor — Thiazide
HYDROCHLOROTHIAZIDE
Hydrocortisone — Betamethasone
HYDRODIURIL
HYDROMAL
Hydromox — Thiazide
HYDROZIDE-50

Hygroton — Thiazide
Hylidone — Hydrodiuril
HYREX-105

I

ILOSONE
ILOTYCIN
ILOTYCIN (Ophthalmic)
IMIPRAMINE
IMITREX
IMPRIL
Indapamide — Thiazide
IONAMIN
ISO-BID
ISOCHRON
ISONATE
ISONATE TR
ISOPTIN
ISOPTO CETAMIDE (Ophthalmic)
ISOPTO FENICOL (Ophthalmic)
ISORBIDE DINITRATE
ISORDIL
ISOTRATE
ISRADIPINE

J

JANIMINE
JENEST

K

K-DUR
K-G ELIXIR
K-LOR
K-LYTE/Cl
K-TAB/Cl
KAO-NOR
KAOCHLOR
KAON
KATO
KAY CIEL
KAYLIXIR
KEACHLOR-EFF
KEFLET
Keflex — Cefanex
Keflin Neutral — Cefanex
KEFTAB
KEFZOL
Kenac — Betamethasone
Kenalog — Celestoderm

KESTRONE-5
KLAVIKORDAL
KLOR-CON
KLORVESS
KLORVESS 10%
KLOTRIX
KOLYUM

L

LABID
Lacticare   Betaderm
Lamoxactam   Cefanex
Lanacort   Betamethasone
LANOPHYLLIN
LANSPORAZOLE
LARGACTIL
Latamoxef   Cefanex
Ledercillin-VK Penicillin
LEVLEN
LEVO-DROMORAN
LEVORA
LEVORPHANOL
Librium   Diazepam
LIPO-GANTRISIN
LIQUIFILM (Ophthalmic)
LIQUOPHYLLINE
Lixaminol   Labid
LIXOLIN
LO/OVRAL
Locoid   Betamethasone
LODRANE
LOESTRIN
LORAZEPAM
LOSEC
LOTREL
LOTUSATE
Lozol   Thiazide
Lufyllin   Aerolate
LUMINAL

M

M S CONTIN
M.O.S.
Malogen   Anadrol
Malogex   Durabolin
MANDOL
MANNEST
MARVELON
Maxibolin   Anabolin
MAXIVATE
MAZANOR

MAZINDOL
MEBARAL
Mecillinam   Penicillin
Medilium   Diazepam
MEFOXIN
MEGACILLIN
MELFIAT
MELLARIL
MENAVAL-20
MENEST
MEPERIDINE
MEPHOBARBITAL
MESORIDAZINE
METADERM
METAHYDRIN
Metandren   Anabolin
METHADONE
METHADOSE
METHARBITAL
Methicillin   Penicillin
METHOXANOL
METHYCLOTHIAZIDE
METOLAZONE
METRA
Mezlin   Permapen
Mezlocillin   Penicillin
Microcort   Betamethasone
MICRO EXTENCAPS K 10
MICRO-K
MICROSULFON
MICROX
MICTRIN
MILLAZINE
MIN-OVRAL
MINESTRIN
Mitran   Flurazepam
MODECATE
MODICON
MODITEN
MONOCID
MORPHINE
MORPHITEC
Moxam   Cefanex
Moxilean   Penicillin
Murcil   Diazepam
MYCITRACIN (Ophthalmic)

N

N.E.E.
N-G-C
NADOPEN-V
Nafcillinn   Penicillin
NALBUPHINE

Nallpen	Pfizerpen	Novolexin	Cefanex
Nancrobolic	Aanabolin	**NOVOPEN-G**	
Nandrolone	Durabolin	**NOVOPEN-VK**	
Naptrate	Cardilate	**NOVOPENTOBARB**	
NAQUA		Novopoxide	Diazepam
Naturetin	Thiazide	**NOVORIDAZINE**	
Neampicil	Penicillin	**NOVORYTHRO**	
NECON		**NOVOSECOBARB**	
NEFEDIPINE		**NOVOSOXAZOLE**	
NELOVA		Novothalidone	Thiazide
NELULEN		**NOVOTRIMEL**	
NEMBUTAL		Novotriphyl	Duraphyl
NEO-BARB		**NOVOTRIPTYN**	
Neo-Durabolic	Anabolin	Nu-Amoxi	Penicillin
NEO-ESTRONE		**NU-CEPHALEX**	
NEOCIDEN (Ophthalmic)		**NU-NIFED**	
NEOMYCIN (Ophthalmic)		Nu-Pen	Novopen
NEOSPORIN (Ophthalmic)		**NUBAIN**	
NEOTAL (Ophthalmic)		Nutracort	Betamethasone
NEOTRICIN (Ophthalmic)			
NICARDIPINE			
NIONG		**O**	
NISOLDIPINE			
NITRO-BID		**OBALAN**	
NITRO-BON		**OBE-NIX**	
NITROCAP		**OBEPHEN**	
Nitrodisc	Sorbitrate	**OBERMINE**	
Nitrodur	Isonate	**OBESTIN-30**	
NITROGLYCERINE		**OBEVAL**	
NITROGLYN		**OBY-TRIM**	
Nitrol	Niong	**OCU-CHLOR OPHTHALMIC**	
NITROLIN		**OINTMENT**	
NITRO-LONG		**OCU-MYCIN (Ophthalmic)**	
NITRONET		**OCU-SPOR-B (Ophthalmic)**	
NITRONG		**OCU-SULF-10 Ophthalmic)**	
NITROSPAN		**OCUFLOX (Ophthalmic)**	
NITROSPAT		**OCUTRICIN (Ophthalmic)**	
Nitrostat	Cardilate	**OFLOXACIN (Ophthalmic)**	
NITRO-TIME		**OGEN**	
NOBESINE-75		**OMEPRAZOLE**	
NORCEPT-E		Omnipen	Novopen
NORDETTE		Onset	Cardilate
NORETHIN		**OPHTHACET (Ophthalmic)**	
NORFLOXACIN (Ophthalmic)		Ora-Testryl	Anabolin
NORINYL 1		Orbenin	Penicillin
NORLESTRIN		**ORETIC**	
NORPRAMIN		Oreton	Durabolin
NORTRIPTYLINE		**ORMAZINE**	
NORVASC		**ORTHO**	
Novamoxin	Ticar	**ORTHO-CEPT**	
NOVOBETAMET		**ORTHO-CYCLEN**	
Novocloxin	Penicillin	**ORTHO-EST**	
NOVOFLUPAM		**ORTHO-NOVUM**	
Novoflurazine	Largactil	**ORTHO-TRI-CYCLEN**	
NOVOHYDRAZIDE		**OVCON**	

OVRAL
Oxacillin — Penicillin
Oxandrolone — Durabolin
Oxitriphyllin — Asmalix
OX-PAM
Oxalactam — Cefanex
OXAZEPAM
Oxymetholone — Anabolin
Oxystat — Lixolin

P

Palarol — Lodrane
PAMELOR
PANTOPON
PARMINE
Pathocil — Penicillin
PAVERAL
PAXIL
PAXIPAM
PBR/12
PCE DISPERTAB
PEDIAMYCIN
PEN VEE K
PENAPAR VK
Penbritin — Penicillin
Penecort — Betamethasone
PENICILLIN V
PENTAMYCETIN (Ophthalmic)
PENTIDS
PENTOBARBITAL
Pentol — Cardilate
Pentraspan — Isonate
Pentritol — Isordil
Pentylan — Coronex
Pen Vee — Novopen
PERMAPEN
PERMITIL
PERPHENAZINE
PERTOFRANE
PETHADOL
PETHIDINE
PFIZERPEN
PHENAZINE
PHENDIMETRAZINE
PHENOBARB
PHENOBARBITAL
PHENTAMINE
PHENTERMINE
PHENTROL
PHENZINE
Phyllocontin — Elixicon
PIPERACILLIN
PIPERAZINE

PIPRACIL
PLEGINE
PLENDIL
PMS AMITRIPTYLINE
PMS IMIPRAMINE
PMS THEOPHYLLINE
P.N. OPHTHALMIC (Ophthalmic)
Polyxcillin — Penicillin
Polymox — Novopen
POLYMYXIN B Ophthalmic)
Polythiazide — Thiazide
POTACHLOR
POTAGE
POTASALAN
POTASSINE
POTASSIUM ACETATE
POTASSIUM BICARBONATE
POTASSIUM CHLORIDE
POTASSIUM GLUCONATE
POTASSIUM TRIPLEX
PRAZEPAM
PRECEF
PRELU-2
PREMARIN
PREMPHASE
PREVACID
PRILOSEC
Principen — Penicillin
PROCARDIA
PROCHLORPERAZINE
PROKLAR
PROLIXIN
PROLIXIN DECANOATE
PROMAPAR
PROMAZ
PROMAZINE
Protophylline — Labid
PROTRIN
PROTRIPTYINE
PROZAC
PROZINE
PULMOPHYLLINE
PVF-K — Penicillin

Q

QUIBRON-T
QUINESTROL
Quinetazone — Thiazide

R

REGIBON

RENEDIL
Renese   Thiazide
RENOQUID
Reposans   Diazepam
Resicort   Betamethasone
RESPBID
RESTORIL
Rhulicort   Betamethasone
RISPERAL
Rival   Flurazepam
Rivotril   Diazepam
RMS UNISERTS
RO-CEF
ROBICILLIN VK
ROBIDONE
ROBIMYCIN
ROCEPHIN
ROUBAC
ROXANOL
RP-MYCIN

S

Saluron   Thiazide
SANOREX
SARISOL NO.2
SECOBARBITAL
SECONAL
SEDAPAP
Seffin   Cefanex
Sensacort   Betaderm
SEPTRA
SERAL
SERAX
Sereen   Diazepam
SERENTIL
SIBELIUM
SINEQUAN
SK-AMITRIPTYLINE
SK-Ampicillin   Penicillin
SK-ERYTHROMYCIN
SK-HYDROCHLOROTHIAZIDE
SK-PENICILLIN G
SK-PENICILLIN VK
SK-PHENOBARBITAL
SK-POTASSIUM CHLORIDE
SK-PRAMINE
SK-SOXAZOLE
SLO-BID GYROCAPS
SLO-PHYLLIN
SLOPHYLLIN GYROCAPS
SLOW-K
SLYN-LL
SMZ-TMP

Solazine   Acetaphenazine
SOLFOTON
Solium   Diazepam
SOMOPHYLLIN-12
SOMOPHYLLIN-CRT
Sonazine   Chlorpromazine
SORATE
SORBITRATE
SPARINE
Spectrobid   Permapen
SPRX-1/3
STADOL
Stanozolol   Durabolin
Staphcillin   Penicillin
STATEX
STATOBEX
Stelazine   Largactil
STILPHOSTROL
SULAR
SULFACYTINE
SULFADIAZINE
SULFAFURAZOLE
SULFAMETHIAZOLE
SULFAMETHOXAZOLE
SULFASIN
SULFISOXASOLE
Sumox   Wycillin
Supen   Penicillin
SUPRAX
Suprazine   Acetaphenazine
Sustachron   Cardilate
SUSTAIRE
SYMPHASIC
Synacort   Betamethasone
Synalar   Betaderm
SYN-DILTIAZEM
Synemol   Alphatrex
Synophylate   Aerolate

T

TACE
TALBUTAL
Tegopen   Penicillin
TEMAZEPAM
TENUATE
TEPANIL
TERAMINE
Terfluzine   Acetaphenazine
Testa-C   Durabolin
Testamone   Anadrol
Testaqua   Anavar
Testex   Delatest
Testoject   Anabolin

Testone	Durabolin	**TRIMSTAT**	
Testosterone	Anadrol	**TRIMTABS**	
Testred	Durabolin	Triphyllin	Eloximin
Testrin	Android	**TUINAL**	
Thalidone	Thiazide	**TWIN-K**	
THEO-24		**TWIN-K-Cl**	
THEOBID DURACAPS			
Theobron	Accurbron		
Theoclair	Labid	**U**	
Theoclear	Aerolate		
Theochron	Asmalix	**ULTRACEF**	
Theo-dur	Accurbron	Unicort	Betamethasone
Theo-lix	Duraphyl	**UNIFAST UNICELLES**	
Theolixir	Aerolate	Unipen	Penicillin
Theon	Labid	Uniphyl	Accurbron
Theophyl	Accurbron	Uridon	Thiazide
Theophylline	Lodrane	**UROBAK**	
Theospan	Aerolate	**UTICILLIN VK**	
Theostat	Accurbron	**UTICORT**	
Theo-time	Lixolin	Utimox	Penicillin
Theovent	Lodrane		
THIAZIDE			
THIORIDAZINE		**V**	
THIOSULFIDE			
THIOSULFIDE FORTE			
THIURETIC		**VALERGEN**	
THOR-PROM		**VALISONE**	
THORAZINE		**VALIUM**	
TICAR		**VALNAC**	
TICARCILLIN		**VALRELEASE**	
TIMENTIN		**VANTIN**	
TINDAL		**VASCOR**	
TIPRAMINE		**VAZEPAM**	
TOFRANIL		**V-CILLIN-K**	
Topicort	Betamethasone	**VEETIDS**	
TORA		Velosef	Cefanex
Totacillin	Penicillin	**VERAPAMIL**	
Tranxene	Diazepam	**VERELAN**	
Trates	Cardilate	Vesprin	Chlorpromazine
TRI-CYCLEN		**VIAGRA**	
TRI-K		Virilon	Anabolin
Triacet	Betamethasone	**VIVELLE**	
Triaderm	Betaderm	**VIVOL**	
Trialean	Cetestoderm	**VK**	
Triamalone	Betamethasone		
TRIAZOLAM		**W**	
TRICHLOREX			
TRICLORMETHIAZIDE		**WEHGEN**	
TRIDESILON		**WEHLESS**	
TRIFLUPERAZINE		**WEIGHTROL**	
Triflupromazine	Chlorpromazine	Westcort	Betamethasone
TRIKATES		Winstrol	Durabolin
TRILAFON		**WYAMYCIN E**	
TRIMCAPS		**WYAMYCIN S**	
Trimox	Penicillin	**WYCILLIN**	

Wymox   Penicillin

X

Xannax   Flurazepam
X-TROZINE

Z

ZAPEX
ZAROXOLON
ZETRAN
Zinacef   Cefanex
ZOCOR
ZOLOFT